Every Decker book is accompanied by a CD-ROM.

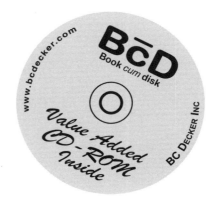

The disk appears in the front of each copy, in its own sealed jacket. Affixed to the front of the book will be a distinctive BcD sticker **"Book *cum* disk"**.

The disk contains the complete text and illustrations of the book, in fully searchable PDF files. The book and disk will be sold *only* as a package; neither will be available independently, and no prices will be available for the items individually.

BC Decker Inc is committed to providing high quality electronic publications that will compliment traditional information and learning methods.

We trust you will find the Book/CD Package invaluable and invite your comments and suggestions.

Brian C. Decker
CEO and Publisher

American Cancer Society
Atlas of Clinical Oncology

Published

Blumgart, Fong, Jarnagin	*Hepatobiliary Cancer (2001)*
Cameron	*Pancreatic Cancer (2001)*
Char	*Tumors of the Eye and Ocular Adnexa (2001)*
Eifel, Levenback	*Cancer of the Female Lower Genital Tract (2001)*
Prados	*Brain Cancer (2001)*
Shah	*Cancer of the Head and Neck (2001)*
Silverman	*Oral Cancer (1998)*
Sober, Haluska	*Skin Cancer (2001)*
Wiernik	*Adult Leukemias (2001)*
Willett	*Cancer of the Lower Gastrointestinal Tract (2001)*
Winchester, Winchester	*Breast Cancer (2000)*

Forthcoming

Carroll, Grossfeld, Reese	*Prostate Cancer (2002)*
Clark, Duh, Jahan, Perrier	*Endocrine Tumors (2002)*
Droller	*Urothelial Cancer (2002)*
Fuller, Seiden, Young	*Uterine and Endometrial Cancer (2003)*
Ginsberg	*Lung Cancer (2001)*
Grossbard	*Malignant Lymphomas (2001)*
Ozols	*Ovarian Cancer (2002)*
Pollock	*Soft Tissue Sarcomas (2001)*
Posner, Weichselbaum	*Cancer of the Upper Gastrointestinal Tract (2001)*
Raghavan	*Germ Cell Tumors (2002)*
Steele, Richie	*Kidney Tumors (2003)*
Volberding	*Viral and Immunological Malignancies (2003)*
Yasko	*Bone Tumors (2002)*

American Cancer Society
Atlas of Clinical Oncology

Editors

GLENN D. STEELE JR, MD
Geisinger Health System

THEODORE L. PHILLIPS, MD
University of California

BRUCE A. CHABNER, MD
Harvard Medical School

Managing Editor

TED S. GANSLER, MD, MBA
Director of Health Content, American Cancer Society

American Cancer Society
Atlas of Clinical Oncology

Brain Cancer

Michael Prados, MD

Charles B. Wilson Chair of Neurological Surgery
Professor
Department of Neurological Surgery
University of California San Francisco
San Francisco, California

2002
BC Decker Inc
Hamilton • London

BC Decker Inc
20 Hughson Street South
P.O. Box 620, LCD 1
Hamilton, Ontario L8N 3K7
Tel: 905-522-7017; 1-800-568-7281
Fax: 905-522-7839; 1-888-311-4987
E-mail: info@bcdecker.com
Website: www.bcdecker.com

© 2002 American Cancer Society

All rights reserved. No part of this publication may be reproduced, stored in a retrieval system, or transmitted, in any form or by any means, electronic, mechanical, photocopying, recording, or otherwise, without prior written permission from the publisher.

02 03 04 05 / UTP / 9 8 7 6 5 4 3 2 1

ISBN 1–55009–098–4
Printed in Canada

Sales and Distribution

United States
BC Decker Inc
P.O. Box 785
Lewiston, NY 14092-0785
Tel: 905-522-7017; 1-800-568-7281
Fax: 905-522-7839; 1-888-311-4987
E-mail: info@bcdecker.com
Website: www.bcdecker.com

Canada
BC Decker Inc
20 Hughson Street South
P.O. Box 620, LCD 1
Hamilton, Ontario L8N 3K7
Tel: 905-522-7017; 1-800-568-7281
Fax: 905-522-7839; 1-888-311-4987
E-mail: info@bcdecker.com
Website: www.bcdecker.com

Foreign Rights
John Scott & Company
International Publishers' Agency
P.O. Box 878
Kimberton, PA 19442
Tel: 610-827-1640
Fax: 610-827-1671
E-mail: jsco@voicenet.com

U.K., Europe, Scandinavia, Middle East
Harcourt Publishers Limited
Customer Service Department
Foots Cray High Street
Sidcup, Kent
DA14 5HP, UK
Tel: 44 (0) 208 308 5760
Fax: 44 (0) 181 308 5702
E-mail: cservice@harcourt_brace.com

Australia, New Zealand
Harcourt Australia Pty Limited
Customer Service Department
STM Division
Locked Bag 16
St. Peters, New South Wales, 2044
Australia
Tel: 61 02 9517-8999
Fax: 61 02 9517-2249
E-mail: stmp@harcourt.com.au
Website: www.harcourt.com.au

Japan
Igaku-Shoin Ltd.
Foreign Publications Department
3-24-17 Hongo
Bunkyo-ku, Tokyo, Japan 113-8719
Tel: 81 3 3817 5680
Fax: 81 3 3815 6776
E-mail: fd@igaku-shoin.co.jp

Singapore, Malaysia, Thailand, Philippines, Indonesia, Vietnam, Pacific Rim, Korea
Harcourt Asia Pte Limited
583 Orchard Road
#09/01, Forum
Singapore 238884
Tel: 65-737-3593
Fax: 65-753-2145

Notice: The authors and publisher have made every effort to ensure that the patient care recommended herein, including choice of drugs and drug dosages, is in accord with the accepted standard and practice at the time of publication. However, since research and regulation constantly change clinical standards, the reader is urged to check the product information sheet included in the package of each drug, which includes recommended doses, warnings, and contraindications. This is particularly important with new or infrequently used drugs.

Contributors

ADEKUNLE M. ADESINA, MD, PHD
Department of Pathology
University of Oklahoma Health Sciences Center
Oklahoma City, Oklahoma
Histopathology of Primary Tumors of the Central Nervous System

FRED G. BARKER II, MD
Department of Surgery and Neurosurgery
Harvard Medical School
Brain Tumor Center Neurological Service
Massachusetts General Hospital
Boston, Massachusetts
Surgery for Brain Tumors

GLENN BAUMAN, MD, FRCP(C)
University of Western Ontario
London Regional Cancer Centre
London, Ontario
External Beam Radiotherapy

MITCHEL S. BERGER, MD
Department of Neurological Surgery
University of California San Francisco
San Francisco, California
Interstitial Brachytherapy
Surgical Considerations in Childhood Brain Tumors

ANDREW W. BOLLEN, DVM, MD
Department of Pathology
University of California San Francisco
San Francisco, California
Molecular Genetics of Malignant Glioma
Meningiomas

MELISSA L. BONDY, PHD
Department of Epidemiology
University of Texas MD Anderson Cancer Center
Houston, Texas
Epidemiology of Primary Brain Tumors

ROGER A. BRUMBACK, MD
Department of Pathology
Creighton University School of Medicine
St. Joseph Hospital
Omaha, Nebraska
Histopathology of Primary Tumors of the Central Nervous System

ERIC BURTON, MD
Department of Neuro-Oncology
Brain Tumor Research Center
University of California San Francisco
San Francisco, California
Management of Primary Malignant Brain Tumors in Adults

GARY R. CAPUTO, MD
Department of Radiology
University of California San Francisco
San Francisco, California
Positron Emission Tomography Imaging of Brain Tumors

SUDHA CHALLA, MD
Department of Radiology
Downstate Medical Center
Brooklyn, New York
Positron Emission Tomography Imaging of Brain Tumors

MARC C. CHAMBERLAIN, MD
Departments of Neurology and Neurosurgery
University of Southern California/Norris
  Comprehensive Cancer Center
Los Angeles, California
Diagnosis and Treatment of Neoplastic Meningitis

SUSAN M. CHANG, MD
Department of Neurological Surgery
University of California San Francisco
San Francisco, California
Clinical Trials and Experimental Chemotherapy

PENGCHIN CHEN, PHD
Department of Epidemiology and Biostatistics
University of California San Francisco
San Francisco, California
Molecular Genetics of Malignant Glioma

CYNTHIA T. CHIN, MD
Department of Radiology
University of California San Francisco
San Francisco, California
*Magnetic Resonance Imaging of Central
  Nervous System Tumors*

WILLIAM P. DILLON, MD
Departments of Radiology, Neurology, and
  Neurological Surgery
University of California San Francisco
San Francisco, California
*Magnetic Resonance Imaging of Central
  Nervous System Tumors*

HOWARD A. FINE, MD
Neuro-Oncology Branch
National Cancer Institute
Bethesda, Maryland
*Systemic Chemotherapy of Central Nervous
  System Tumors*

JUAN FUEYO, MD
Department of Neuro-Oncology
University of Texas MD Anderson
  Cancer Center
Houston, Texas
Gene Therapy Approaches

CANDELARIA GOMEZ-MANZANO, MD
Department of Neuro-Oncology
University of Texas MD Anderson Cancer Center
Houston, Texas
Gene Therapy Approaches

RANDALL A. HAWKINS, MD, PHD
Department of Radiology
Nuclear Medicine Program
University of California San Francisco
San Francisco, California
*Positron Emission Tomography Imaging
  of Brain Tumors*

MARK A. ISRAEL, MD
Departments of Pediatrics and Neurological
  Surgery
University of California San Francisco
San Francisco, California
Molecular Genetics of Malignant Glioma

G. EVREN KELES, MD
Department of Neurological Surgery
University of California San Francisco
San Francisco, California
Interstitial Brachytherapy
*Surgical Considerations in Childhood
  Brain Tumors*

DAVID A. LARSON, PHD, MD
Department of Radiation Oncology
University of California San Francisco
San Francisco, California
External Beam Radiotherapy
Interstitial Brachytherapy
Radiosurgery for Brain Tumors
Meningiomas

RICHARD W. LEECH, MD
Department of Pathology
University of Oklahoma Health Sciences Center
Oklahoma City, Oklahoma
*Histopathology of Primary Tumors
  of the Central Nervous System*

FRANK S. LIEBERMAN, MD
Department of Neurology
University of Pittsburgh School of Medicine
Pittsburgh, Pennsylvania
Paraneoplastic Syndromes

AKIO MANTANI, MD, PHD
Department of Neurological Surgery
Brain Tumor Research Center
University of California San Francisco
San Francisco, California
Molecular Genetics of Malignant Glioma

MICHAEL W. MCDERMOTT, MD, FRCSC
Department of Neurological Surgery
University of California San Francisco
San Francisco, California
Radiosurgery for Brain Tumors
Meningiomas

YURIKO MINN, MS
Department of Neurology
Stanford University School of Medicine
Stanford, California
Epidemiology of Primary Brain Tumors

MARTIN KELLY NICHOLAS, MD, PHD
Department of Neurological Surgery
University of California San Francisco
San Francisco, California
Familial Brain Tumor Syndromes

EDWARD PAN, MD
Department of Neurological Surgery
University of California San Francisco
San Francisco, California
Familial Brain Tumor Syndromes

MICHAEL PRADOS, MD
Department of Neurological Surgery
University of California San Francisco
San Francisco, California
Management of Primary Malignant Brain Tumors in Adults
Evaluation and Management of Pediatric Brain Tumors
Meningiomas
Future Directions

ALFREDO QUINONES-HINOJOSA, MD
Department of Neurological Surgery
University of California San Francisco
San Francisco, California
Meningiomas

WILLIAM S. ROSENBERG, MD
Department of Neurological Surgery
University of California San Francisco
San Francisco, California
Spinal Tumors

CAROLYN RUSSO, MD
Department of Pediatrics
University of California San Francisco
San Francisco, California
Evaluation and Management of Pediatric Brain Tumors

EDWARD G. SHAW, MD
Department of Radiation Oncology
Wake Forest University School of Medicine
Winston-Salem, North Carolina
Management of Low-Grade Gliomas in Adults

PENNY K. SNEED, MD
Department of Radiation Oncology
University of California San Francisco
San Francisco, California
Interstitial Brachytherapy
Radiosurgery for Brain Tumors
Metastatic Brain Tumors

PETER SZTRAMSKI, RN
Department of Perioperative Nursing
Massachusetts General Hospital
Boston, Massachusetts
Surgery for Brain Tumors

PHILIP V. THEODOSOPOULOS, MD
Department of Neurological Surgery
University of California San Francisco
San Francisco, California
Spinal Tumors
Evaluation and Management of Pediatric Brain Tumors

JANE H. UYEHARA-LOCK, MD
Department of Pathology
University of California San Francisco
San Francisco, California
Familial Brain Tumor Syndromes

KATHERINE E. WARREN, MD
Neuro-Oncology Branch
National Cancer Institute
Bethesda, Maryland
Systemic Chemotherapy of Central Nervous System Tumors

MARGARET WRENSCH, PhD
Department of Epidemiology and Biostatistics
University of California San Francisco
San Francisco, California
Epidemiology of Primary Brain Tumors

W.K. ALFRED YUNG, MD
Department of Neuro-Oncology
University of Texas MD Anderson Cancer Center
Houston, Texas
Gene Therapy Approaches

RANDA ZAKHARY, MD, PhD
Department of Neurological Surgery
University of California San Francisco
San Francisco, California
Radiosurgery for Brain Tumors

Contents

Preface xi

1. **Epidemiology of Primary Brain Tumors** 1
   Yuriko Minn, MS, Margaret Wrensch, PhD, Melissa L. Bondy, PhD

2. **Histopathology of Primary Tumors of the Central Nervous System** 16
   Adekunle M. Adesina, MD, PhD, Richard W. Leech, MD, Roger A. Brumback, MD

3. **Familial Brain Tumor Syndromes** 48
   Edward Pan, MD, Jane H. Uyehara-Lock, MD, Martin Kelly Nicholas, MD, PhD

4. **Molecular Genetics of Malignant Glioma** 93
   Akio Mantani, MD, PhD, Pengchin Chen PhD, Andrew W. Bollen, DVM, MD, Mark A. Israel, MD

5. **Magnetic Resonance Imaging of Central Nervous System Tumors** 104
   Cynthia T. Chin, MD, William P. Dillon, MD

6. **Positron Emission Tomography Imaging of Brain Tumors** 129
   Sudha Challa, MD, Randall A. Hawkins, MD, PhD, Gary R. Caputo, MD

7. **External Beam Radiotherapy** 142
   Glenn Bauman, MD, FRCP(C), David A. Larson, PhD, MD

8. **Interstitial Brachytherapy** 157
   G. Evren Keles, MD, Penny K. Sneed, MD, David A. Larson, PhD, MD, Mitchel S. Berger, MD

9. **Radiosurgery for Brain Tumors** 167
   Michael W. McDermott, MD, FRCSC, Penny K. Sneed, MD, Randa Zakhary, MD, PhD, David A. Larson, PhD, MD

10. **Systemic Chemotherapy of Central Nervous System Tumors** 193
    Katherine E. Warren, MD, Howard A. Fine, MD

11. **Clinical Trials and Experimental Chemotherapy** 211
    Susan M. Chang, MD

| 12 | **Gene Therapy Approaches** | 219 |

Candelaria Gomez-Manzano, MD, Juan Fueyo, MD, W.K. Alfred Yung, MD

| 13 | **Surgery for Brain Tumors** | 238 |

Fred G. Barker II, MD, Peter Sztramski, RN

| 14 | **Management of Primary Malignant Brain Tumors in Adults** | 262 |

Eric Burton, MD, Michael Prados, MD

| 15 | **Management of Low-Grade Gliomas in Adults** | 279 |

Edward G. Shaw, MD

| 16 | **Surgical Considerations in Childhood Brain Tumors** | 303 |

G. Evren Keles, MD, Mitchel S. Berger, MD

| 17 | **Evaluation and Management of Pediatric Brain Tumors** | 321 |

Carolyn Russo, MD, Philip V. Theodosopoulos, MD, Michael Prados, MD

| 18 | **Meningiomas** | 333 |

Michael W. McDermott, MD, FRCSC, Alfredo Quinones-Hinojosa, MD,
Andrew W. Bollen, DVM, MD, David A. Larson, PhD, MD, Michael Prados, MD

| 19 | **Spinal Tumors** | 365 |

William S. Rosenberg, MD, Philip V. Theodosopoulos, MD

| 20 | **Metastatic Brain Tumors** | 375 |

Penny K. Sneed, MD

| 21 | **Diagnosis and Treatment of Neoplastic Meningitis** | 391 |

Marc C. Chamberlain, MD

| 22 | **Paraneoplastic Syndromes** | 406 |

Frank S. Lieberman, MD

| 23 | **Future Directions** | 422 |

Michael Prados, MD

Index ... 426

Preface

Central nervous system tumors constitute a heterogeneous group of diseases that vary from benign, slow-growing lesions to aggressive malignancies that can cause death within a matter of months if left untreated. Each of these tumors has unique clinical, radiographic, and biologic characteristics that dictate, in part, their management. In general, the glial neoplasms that are seen commonly in adults include low-grade tumors such as the infiltrating astrocytoma, oligodendroglioma, and mixed low-grade tumors. Intermediate-grade tumors include anaplastic astrocytoma and anaplastic oligodendroglioma, or mixed anaplastic tumors. The most malignant glial neoplasm is glioblastoma multiforme. A variety of other tumors can be seen as well, such as meningioma and ependymoma. Brain tumors of childhood include pilocytic astrocytoma, primitive neuroectodermal tumors such as medulloblastoma, ependymoma, and a variety of rare tumor types such as the germ cell tumors and atypical rhabdoid tumors of the central nervous system.

The location of brain tumors presents a challenge regarding surgical approaches for diagnosis and attempts to remove tumors. Some tumors are surgically "curable," obviating the need for any additional therapy. Others present with clinical and radiographic findings that are felt to be so characteristic of a specific disease that a biopsy or surgical resection may not be indicated, particularly if the tumor is located within areas of brain where the risk of the procedure outweighs the potential benefit of obtaining tissue. For the most part, however, the goal of the neurosurgical oncologist is to remove as much tumor as is safely possible. Fortunately, with the advent of computer-assisted surgical navigation tools and functional neuroimaging, this is more of a reality today than in the past.

Once the diagnosis is made, therapy is based on accurate histologic confirmation of disease. Therapy is specific to each tumor type and may include irradiation, chemotherapy, observation, or treatment with investigational approaches. For the adult patient with malignant glioma, surgery and irradiation constitute the standard of care. Some patient groups may benefit from adjuvant chemotherapy, but much more clinical research is needed in this area. For the lower-grade gliomas, treatment may include irradiation or chemotherapy and, in some cases, observation alone. As with the malignant gliomas, much more research is needed to identify specific prognostic and predictive factors that will aid in the management of these diverse tumors. Treatment of children with brain tumors may differ significantly from treatment approaches used in adults. For instance, young babies and infants cannot tolerate the risks or long-term complications associated with irradiation, and many of the clinical research efforts in this setting are based on the use of chemotherapy. As a consequence, we have learned a great deal about the activity of drugs for various tumors that present in childhood and, in some cases, have used this information to guide therapy for adults. For example, because of the observation that chemotherapy may produce responses in low-grade gliomas in children, we now have begun to explore this approach in adults with similar kinds of tumors. Some tumors in children are rarely found in adults and present specific challenges. Despite these differences, there is opportunity for biologic research in both adults and children that may aid in our understanding of the initiation of the malignant phenotype that results in a brain tumor and that ultimately will result in better therapy.

There remain a number of practical issues related to the treatment and management of these diseases. The ability of the surgeon to remove more or less tumor tissue will affect survival expectations and, consequently, decisions regarding surgical management. There are various ways to deliver irradiation, but the use of these techniques should be based on risk-benefit ratios that are supported by rigorous clinical research rather than by bias. We need to identify more specific molecular markers to better characterize the pathology of the various kinds of tumors seen in the central nervous system. Standard histopathology has been important in helping us group certain patients into various risk groups, and it has been instrumental in the understanding of prognosis. However, with further review of these pathologically based risk factors, we now understand that other factors must play a role in further segregating subsets of patients who may deviate from the "median" expectation. For instance, we know that the age of a patient may be more prognostic than the pathologic diagnosis based on the tissue sample. A 40-year-old patient with glioblastoma multiforme will likely live twice as long as a 70-year-old patient with the same diagnosis, receiving the identical therapy. The biologic factors that influence this fact are still poorly understood. We also know that various cytogenetic changes present in tumor cells are beginning to help us identify patient groups who may be more likely to respond to chemotherapy. Numerous such examples exist, emphasizing the need for more intensive research into these cellular and molecular aspects of brain cancers.

We also need more research in neuroimaging. The current standard for imaging brain cancer is the use of magnetic resonance, and, although MR imaging is superior to computed tomography, it still provides only an indirect measure of the actual tumor burden and location of disease. We cannot directly image tumor cells within the brain. Effects of treatment, particularly irradiation, can appear similar to tumor using current MR techniques; this presents a challenge to the clinician as it confounds the interpretation of results of specific therapy as to whether a patient has progressed or has some toxicity of treatment. Fortunately, a great deal of research is ongoing using metabolic and biologic imaging paradigms that appear to help in the identification of extent and location of tumor. However, much more research is needed in this area, particularly as therapeutic approaches change over time.

New therapy is needed. Unfortunately, the usual outcome of patients with malignant brain tumors is to have a short period of disease control before progression and death. Surgery, irradiation, and standard cytotoxic chemotherapy have not been successful in producing long-term control of many of the tumors seen in the brain. Patients with glioblastoma multiforme have a median survival expectation of only 10 to 12 months, despite many years of intensive clinical research. Patients with lower-grade tumors have fared better, but median survival for anaplastic astrocytoma is 3 to 4 years, and for low-grade gliomas, only 7 to 10 years. Some childhood tumors have equally dismal prognoses, particularly diffuse intrinsic brainstem tumors and atypical rhabdoid tumors. For patients with nonglial tumors, there is more hope, and some patients with localized primitive neuroectodermal tumors and germ cell tumors will have prolonged disease-free survival or even be cured. The long-term effects of therapy must be taken into consideration, both for the patient who has achieved a cure and for those who will have chronic disease for many years.

Fortunately, there is an ever-increasing rate of biologic research ongoing for all of the tumors that will be discussed in this monograph. We now have a greater understanding of many of the molecular events that are associated with the maintenance of the malignant phenotype. We know more now about cell-cycle regulation and control, tumor cell invasion, and angiogenesis. We also have identified specific molecular markers and the genetic regulation for many of these events. We are attempting to understand the early initiating events associated with neogenesis, to try to complete the "loop" of initiation, malignant transformation, growth, and maintenance of brain cancers. Perhaps we finally will be able to reverse the malignant phenotype or at least stop the process with specific therapies directed at these targets. The acquisition of human tumor tissue is critical for further research and understanding of the biology of these tumors. It is only through this avenue of laboratory investigation that we will achieve the ultimate goal of long-term control and cure.

Michael Prados, MD
September 2001

Dedication

I would like to dedicate this book to my friend, colleague, and mentor Dr. Charles B. Wilson. His pioneering work helped shape a vision, and his leadership gave me the opportunity to develop a career in neuro-oncology.

Epidemiology of Primary Brain Tumors

YURIKO MINN, MS
MARGARET WRENSCH, PhD
MELISSA L. BONDY, PhD

A total of about 35,000 new cases of primary malignant and benign brain tumors are estimated to be diagnosed in the United States in 2001.[1] Just considering cancers (primary malignant tumors) of the brain and central nervous system, the American Cancer Society estimated 17,200 new cases and 13,100 deaths in 2001.[2] Brain tumor epidemiology attempts to improve the understanding of the distribution and causes of this disease. It is hoped that unraveling the etiology of brain tumors will be instrumental in preventing this devastating cancer. Descriptive epidemiologic studies characterize brain tumor incidence or mortality with respect to some demographic characteristics (ie, age, gender, geographic region, histologic type), whereas analytic epidemiologic studies provide information on possible risk factors. Analytic studies of brain tumors have either compared the risk of brain tumors in people with and without certain characteristics (cohort studies) or compared the past histories of people with and without brain tumors (case-control studies). Because of the relative rarity of brain tumors, most analytic studies of brain tumors are case-control studies. We[3–5] and others[6–8] have recently reviewed the epidemiology of brain tumors, so this chapter summarizes, rather than replicates, these more exhaustive reviews.

For a variety of reasons, there is still little known about the causes of brain tumors and which risk factors may pertain to which histologic subtypes. However, there has been an increasing interest in brain tumors in recent years. Improved diagnostic tools and molecular classification of tumors may help in understanding who gets brain tumors and why. In addition, with the Human Genome Project deciphering our genetic makeup, the growing research fields of brain tumor genetics and molecular epidemiology may help to determine which genes might make an individual susceptible or resistant to brain tumors and which genes might lead to particular sensitivity to environmental agents. This knowledge might eventually help to prevent brain tumors.

DESCRIPTIVE EPIDEMIOLOGY

Primary brain tumors are relatively rare compared to lung, breast, prostate, and colorectal cancers. However, primary brain and spinal cord tumors are among the top 10 causes of deaths due to cancer,[2] with over 13,000 people dying from them each year.[1] Brain tumors are the second most common cancer to arise in children, and childhood brain tumors account for approximately 9 percent of all primary brain tumors.[9]

The overall annual incidence rate of primary brain tumors in the United States is 11 to 12 per 100,000 persons, and 6 to 7 per 100,000 for primary malignant brain tumors.[9] The incidence of childhood primary brain tumors is 3.8 per 100,000 person-years, based on United States data from 1990 to 1994.[9] Glioma and other neuroepithelial tumors make up approximately 51 percent of brain tumors by histologic type, then meningiomas, 25 percent; sellar region tumors, 9 percent; cranial and spinal nerve tumors, 7 percent; central nervous system (CNS) lymphoma, 4 percent; and other brain tumor types, 4 percent.[9]

Age and Gender

The average age of onset for all primary brain tumors is 53 years, whereas for both glioblastoma and meningioma specifically, the average age of onset is 62 years.[1] However, age distributions vary by site and histologic types (Figures 1–1 and 1–2). Although there is a peak in the incidence of glioblastoma and astrocytoma for the elderly at ages 65 to 74 years, the incidence of meningioma continues to increase with increasing age. Since cancers are generally thought of as diseases of older age, the increasing incidence of most types of brain tumors with age could be due to length of exposure required for malignant transformation, the necessity of many genetic alterations prior to clinical disease, or poorer immune surveillance. An intriguing feature of brain tumor epidemiology is the peak in incidence in young children (Figure 1–3), some, but not all, of which is attributable to medulloblastoma or other tumors of primitive neuroectodermal origin.

The most consistent epidemiologic finding in brain tumors is that neuroepithelial tumors are more common among men, whereas meningeal tumors are more common among women.[9,10] Incidence rates of glioma are approximately 40 percent greater among males than females; rates of meningioma are approximately 80 percent greater among females than males.[9] The biologic or social differences that account for these consistently observed gender differences in brain tumor rates are not understood, but any comprehensive theory of the causes of brain tumors must account for these basic observations.

Time Trends in Incidence and Mortality

Increased brain tumor incidence and mortality of up to 300 percent over the past three decades in developed countries has been primarily observed in the elderly,[4,11] although the reported incidence of primary malignant brain tumors among children also has increased by approximately 35 percent from 1973 to 1994 in the United States.[12] These increases (particularly in the elderly) have been explained by improved diagnostic procedures such as computed tomography (CT) scanning and magnetic resonance

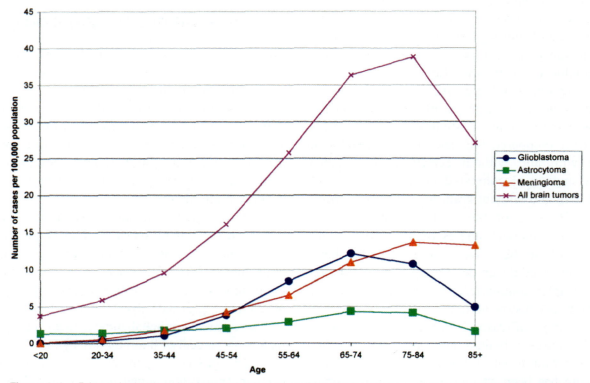

Figure 1–1. Primary brain tumor incidence rates by age at diagnosis for all and most common histologic types, 1990–1994. (Adapted from Central Brain Tumor Registry of the United States. 1997 annual report. Chicago (IL): CBTRUS; 1998.)

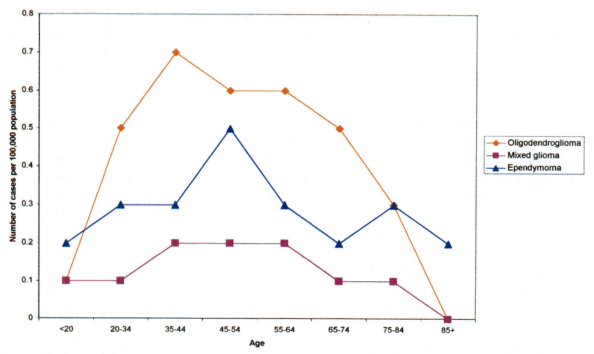

Figure 1–2. Primary brain tumor incidence rates by age at diagnosis of oligodendroglioma, mixed glioma, and ependymoma, 1990–1994. (Adapted from Central Brain Tumor Registry of the United States. 1997 annual report. Chicago (IL): CBTRUS; 1998.)

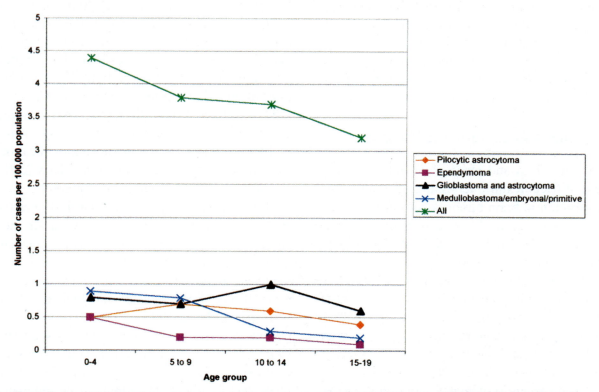

Figure 1–3. Childhood primary brain tumor incidence rates by age and histologic type, 1990–1994. (Adapted from Central Brain Tumor Registry of the United States. 1997 annual report. Chicago (IL): CBTRUS; 1998.)

imaging (MRI), greater availability of neurosurgeons, changing medical practices for the elderly, and increased life span. However, some researchers also suggest that increases in childhood brain tumor incidence might be due to changes in causal factors. Although environmental factors have been implicated in some analytic epidemiologic studies, few consistent factors have been identified. Because no strong risk factors have yet been identified for brain tumors, no attempts have been made to explain quantitatively the temporal trends on the basis of changes in environmental factors.

Comparing results across several descriptive studies is subject to many difficulties. Since incidence rates may vary among studies due to methodologic differences and definitions, there is a need for uniformity for brain tumor registration.[13] An accurate and unbiased registration method would help answer questions regarding the changing incidence of brain tumors. Cancer registries also should routinely track both benign and malignant forms of brain tumors. In addition to ascertainment biases due to health care availability and access, there are also difficulties due to the inherent complexity in brain tumor anatomic, pathologic, and clinical classification. Specifically, controversies about correct classification of some tumor histologies, especially mixed tumor types, may warrant increasing use of genetic markers in conjunction with neuropathologic diagnosis in the future.

Ethnic and Geographic Variation

Ascertainment bias and inconsistent reporting contribute to difficulties in interpreting geographic and ethnic variation in brain tumor occurrence. In countries or areas where health care is more accessible and developed, reported incidence rates of primary malignant brain tumors tend to be higher.[6,7] Ethnic distinctions and cultural or geographic differences in risk factors may also account for some of the variation in rates. For example, the rate of malignant brain tumors in Japan, an economically prosperous country, is less than half the rate of that in Northern Europe. As another example, in the United States, although Caucasians have higher rates of glioma than African Americans, rates of meningioma among African Americans and Caucasians are nearly equal; this would be difficult to attribute solely to differences in medical care access or diagnostic practices.[9] Even in countries that may have similar medical care, there is some variation in incidence rates; for example, these rates range from 5 to 6 per 100,000 in the United Kingdom and France but are about 10 per 100,000 in Sweden, Iceland, and Denmark.[14] However, the absolute variation in occurrence of brain tumors from high- to low-risk areas in the world is on the order of four- to fivefold as compared to the 20-fold differences observed for lung cancer or the 150-fold differences observed for melanoma.[6]

Survival Patterns

Improved survival is associated with histologic type and younger age within histologic type (Figure 1–4) for primary malignant brain tumors.[1] Patients with glioblastoma multiforme consistently show the worst survival rates for all age groups, and little progress in treatment has been noted for these tumors in the past 20 years. Some notable improvements have been reported for medulloblastoma, with 5-year survival rates increasing 20 percent from the 1970s to the 1980s, but survival rates have leveled off in recent years.[15] Five-year survival rate for all ages and all brain tumor types in the United States is 20 percent (95% CI: 0.18 to 0.22),[15] comparable to rates observed in Europe for men (16%) and women (23%).[14] Other prognostic factors that may predict overall survival or progression-free survival may include extent of resection and tumor location.[16,17] Current research is focusing on the identification of prognostic molecular and genetic markers.[18]

Two-year and 5-year relative survival rates (which are the observed probability of survival adjusted for age, sex, race, and calendar year) were 36.2 percent and 27.6 percent, respectively, for patients with primary malignant brain tumors in the United States SEER (Surveillance, Epidemiology, and End Results) areas between 1979 and 1993.[17] Relative survival in these patients decreased most rapidly in the first 2 years following diagnosis. However, there was some variation by tumor type. Five-year relative survival was less than 30 percent for glioblastoma multiforme and malignant glioma, not otherwise specified patients. The conditional probability of surviving an additional 3 years

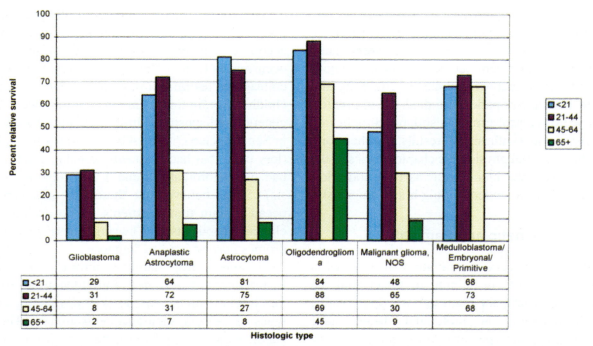

Figure 1–4. Two-year relative survival rates for primary malignant brain tumors by age groups, 1973–1994. (Adapted from Central Brain Tumor Registry of the United States. 1997 annual report. Chicago (IL): CBTRUS; 1998.)

after survival to 2 years for all brain and other CNS tumors was 76.2 percent (95% CI: 74.8% to 77.6%). In all histologies except glioblastoma, surviving to 5 years after survival to 2 years is greater than 60 percent.

Dismal improvement in survival for glioblastoma multiforme patients motivates the desire to determine significant factors associated with long-term survival. In a study conducted by Scott and colleagues,[19] 286 glioblastoma multiforme patients were identified. Of these, only five patients were long-term glioblastoma multiforme survivors, defined as surviving ≥ 3 years. Long-term survivors were significantly younger when compared to all glioblastoma multiforme patients. In addition, long-term survivors had a higher Karnofsky Performance Status (KPS) at diagnosis. Although not statistically significant, long-term glioblastoma multiforme patients tended to have fewer mitotic figures and a lower Ki-67 labeling index compared to controls. Interestingly, seven long-term survivors whose initial diagnosis was glioblastoma multiforme were excluded from this study because upon pathologic re-review, diagnosis was revised to malignant oligodendroglioma, malignant oligoastrocytoma, malignant astrocytoma, or medulloblastoma.

For all meningiomas combined (benign, atypical, and malignant), the overall 2-year and 5-year survival was 81 percent and 69 percent, respectively.[20] However, 5-year survival for malignant meningiomas was 54.6 percent. Age at diagnosis was a significant predictor of survival for patients with benign, atypical, and malignant meningiomas. In patients whose benign tumor had been completely resected, the 5-year tumor recurrence rate was 20.5 percent.

Grovas and colleagues[21] recently examined survival for childhood (birth to 14 years) brain tumors (astrocytomas, ependymomas, medulloblastomas, and unspecified brain/CNS tumors). Five-year survival for all brain tumors combined was 72 percent. In general, survival for children younger than 3 years of age was worse than that for older children.[22]

ANALYTIC STUDIES OF RISK FACTORS

Although the number of published epidemiologic studies of brain tumors has more than doubled since the 1980s, there is little consensus about the nature and magnitude associated with various risk factors. Identification of risk factors has been especially problematic due to the substantial heterogeneity of primary brain tumors; diagnostic inconsistencies due to differences in histologic diagnoses, definitions, and groupings; retrospective exposure assessments; and undefined pertinent latency periods. Methodologic differences between studies in eligibility and representativeness of patients studied, use of proxies, and choice of control groups also have complicated comparison and synthesis of results. Furthermore, certain biologic and physiologic characteristics of the brain itself (eg, the blood-brain barrier) add additional challenges to understanding brain tumor risk.

Genetic and Familial

As with other cancers, examination of genetics is playing a large role in helping us understand the pathogenesis of primary brain tumors. Specifically, recent cytogenetic and molecular studies have shown there are subtypes of tumors and tumor patterns within the larger homogeneous histologic categories such as glioblastoma (or astrocytoma).[23] Being able to accurately categorize brain tumors according to these alterations may help to form groups that are more homogeneous with respect to causes than are standard histologic groupings.

Cancers are believed to develop through accumulation of genetic alterations that allow the cells to grow out of control of normal regulatory mechanisms and/or escape destruction by the immune system. Inherited or acquired alterations in crucial cell-cycle–control genes such as p53, as well as chemical, physical, or biologic agents that damage DNA, are therefore considered candidate carcinogens. Genetic and familial factors implicated in brain tumors have been the subject of many studies and were recently reviewed by Bondy and colleagues.[5] Because of numerous studies and substantiating biologic plausibility, it is generally accepted that certain inherited genes may contribute to primary brain tumors.

The occurrence of brain tumors in individuals with hereditary syndromes, such as tuberous sclerosis, neurofibromatosis types 1 and 2, nevoid basal cell carcinoma syndrome, and syndromes involving adenomatous polyps, indicates genetic predisposition to brain tumors.[5] Genetic predisposition is defined as having a rare gene or chromosomal abnormality that greatly increases the chances of developing the tumor compared to the general population. However, genetic predisposition probably accounts for a very small percentage of brain tumor occurrences (5 to 10%).[24] For example, Narod and colleagues[24] estimated that only about 2 percent of childhood brain tumors in Great Britain were due to genetic predisposition. In a population-based study in San Francisco,[25] only 4 of 500 adults with glioma (less than 1%) had a known heritable syndrome (3 had neurofibromatosis and 1 had tuberous sclerosis). Some believe that these are underestimates because brain tumor patients do not routinely see clinical geneticists and because these genetic syndromes may be hard to diagnose.

In some cancer family syndromes (such as the Li-Fraumeni syndrome), individuals in affected families have an increased risk of developing certain types of cancers, including brain tumors. The now classic study linking Li-Fraumeni syndrome to alterations in the gene for p53 led to numerous studies of the importance of p53 in a wide variety of human cancers. With regard to brain tumors, germline p53 mutations have been found to be more frequent in patients with multifocal glioma, glioma and another primary malignancy, and a family history of cancer.[6]

In a population-based study of malignant glioma, Li and colleagues[26] reported that patients whose tumors had p53 mutations were more likely to have a first-degree relative affected with cancer (58% vs 42%), as well as a personal history of a previous cancer (17% vs 8%). Further research is underway to determine the frequency of p53 mutations and whether specific p53 mutations correlate with certain exposures. Studies of frequencies of alterations in other important cell-cycle regulators such as p16, RB, and MDM2 are also being conducted. Some work has been conducted to identify germline mutations in genes that are mutated, deleted, or amplified in sporadic gliomas. One such study found that there was no evidence of germline mutations of CDK4, p16, or p15.[27]

Although familial cancer aggregation often suggests a genetic etiology, common familial exposure to environmental agents may also contribute to the induction of brain tumors. Significant familial aggregation of brain tumors and of brain tumors with other cancers has been reported in some, but not other, studies, with relative risks of brain tumors ranging from nearly one to nine.[5,25,28] Some, but not all, studies of siblings have revealed a higher than expected frequency of sibs with brain tumors, which supports a genetic etiology; however, studies of twins have not.

In a family study of 250 childhood brain tumor patients, Bondy and colleagues showed by segregation analysis that the small amount of familial aggregation was due to multifactorial inheritance and could not be due to chance alone.[5] Segregation analyses of more than 600 adult glioma patients' families found a polygenic model best explained the pattern of occurrence of brain tumors.[29]

It seems likely the majority of familial brain tumors are associated with gene-environment interaction in which susceptible individuals develop cancer after exposure to endogenous or exogenous carcinogenic agents. The term genetic susceptibility often is used to refer to more common genetic alterations that influence oxidative metabolism, carcinogenesis, detoxification, and deoxyribonucleic acid (DNA) stability and repair; this distinguishes them from the highly penetrant genes, rare alterations that lead to genetic predisposition to a disease. The role of genetic polymorphisms (alternative states of genes established in the population) in modulating susceptibility to carcinogenic exposures has been explored in some detail for tobacco-related cancers but much less so for other types, including gliomas. With growth in genetic technology, potentially relevant polymorphisms are only recently available for epidemiologic evaluation. The first study to report the role of polymorphisms and brain tumor risk found cytochrome p450 2D6 (CYP2D6) and glutathione transferase θ (GSTT1) were significantly associated with increased risk of brain tumors.[30] In another study, GSTT1 null genotype was found to be associated only with an increased risk of oligodendroglioma.[31] Trizna and colleagues[32] found no statistically significant associations between the null genotypes of glutathione transferase μ, GSTT1, and CYP1A1 and risk of adult gliomas. However, they observed an intriguing pattern with N-acetyltransferase acetylation status, with nearly twofold increased risk for rapid acetylation and 30 percent increased risk for intermediate acetylation.

A preliminary case-control study suggested that mutagen sensitivity to γ-radiation was significantly associated with risk of gliomas.[33] Capability of DNA repair and predisposition to cancer are related to differences in radiosensitivity, in vitro and in vivo. Clearly much work needs to be done to establish the importance of mutagen sensitivity, radiation exposure, and risk of developing gliomas; however, it is conceivable that individuals sensitive to γ-radiation may have an increased risk for developing brain tumors.

Since it is unlikely that any single polymorphism will predict risk for a substantial proportion of patients, researchers are developing panels of possibly relevant polymorphic genes to integrate with epidemiologic data. It is hoped that such an approach may help to clarify the role of genetic polymorphisms in brain tumor risk.

Ionizing and Nonionizing Radiation

Non-inherited risk factors for brain tumors are summarized in Tables 1–1 and 1–2.

Increased risk of brain tumors due to high-dose therapeutic ionizing radiation has been consistently observed.[4,7] Relatively low doses used to treat ringworm of the scalp (tinea capitis) and skin hemangioma in children or infants also have been associated with increased risk of brain tumors. Relative risks of 18, 10, and 3 have been observed for nerve sheath tumors, meningioma, and glioma, respectively, from an average dose of 1.5 Gy for tinea capitis treatment. A 40 percent increased risk of intracranial tumors was observed for an average dose of 7 cGY for skin hemangioma.[34] One study showed a very high prevalence (17%) of prior therapeutic radiation among patients with glioblastoma, and others have reported increased risk of adult-onset glioma in those who received radiation treatment for acute lymphoblastic leukemia as children. In addition, an elevated risk of subsequent primary or recurrent brain tumors was observed after radiation treatment for childhood cancer (other than leukemia).[35]

Parental exposure to ionizing radiation prior to conception of the affected child has not been shown to be a risk factor for childhood brain tumors.[7] The findings are mixed for exposure in utero. Studies of atomic bomb survivors in Japan have not shown increased risk of brain tumors,[7] whereas other studies have shown a 20 to 60 percent increased risk of childhood brain tumors due to prenatal radiation exposure.

Diagnostic radiation exposures (medical or dental) have not been shown to play any appreciable role in the development of glioma. The evidence is slightly stronger for meningioma, with three studies having a greater than twofold increased relative risk of meningiomas after exposure to dental x-rays.[7] Further studies of this possible association should be conducted in other geographic areas since each of these was conducted in Los Angeles.[7]

A slightly elevated relative risk of 1.2 for brain tumors in employees working in nuclear facilities and materials production has been reported.[36] However, no specific radiation or chemical exposures were implicated. Mortality from brain tumors among airline pilots has been reported to be elevated in one study, but not in another, possibly implicating

Table 1–1. NON-INHERITED RISK FACTORS STUDIED IN RELATION TO ADULT PRIMARY BRAIN TUMORS*

Risk Factors	Relative Risk[†]		
	Glioma	Meningioma	Unspecified or All Brain Tumors
Ionizing radiation			
Therapeutic			++
Diagnostic	+	+	
Industrial			+
Extremely low frequency electromagnetic fields			
Residential			0
Occupational			+
Occupations and industries			
Synthetic rubber			++
Vinyl chloride			++
Petroleum refining/production			++
Pesticides/insecticides			
Chemical manufacturer			–
Licensed pesticide applicator			++
Agricultural worker			0
Formaldehyde			
Professional exposure			+
Industrial exposure			0
Diet and vitamins			
Cured foods	±	++	++
Fruits and vegetables	±		
Vitamins	–		
Nitrates	0		
Nitrites	+		
Nitrosamines	++		
Alcohol	–		
Tobacco			
Active unfiltered	+		
Active filtered	0	+	
Personal medical history			
Head trauma	–	++	++
Epilepsy, seizures, or convulsions	++		++

*Table includes those factors for which sufficient epidemiologic studies have been conducted and does not include every factor studied in relation to adult brain tumors; see text for citations to comprehensive epidemiologic reviews.
[†]Key: ++ positive relative risk—median relative risk of at least three studies exceeds 1.5; + slightly positive relative risk—median relative risk of at least three studies is between 1.1 and 1.5; 0 no association—median relative risk of at least three studies is between 0.9 and 1.1; – slightly negative relative risk—median relative risk of at least three studies is between 0.7 and 0.9; ± two studies with inconsistent results.

Table 1–2. NON-INHERITED RISK FACTORS STUDIED IN RELATION TO CHILDHOOD PRIMARY BRAIN TUMORS*

Risk Factors	Relative Risk[†]
Ionizing radiation	
Therapeutic	++
Diagnostic	+
Parental/prenatal	+
Residential extremely low frequency electromagnetic fields	+
Pesticides/insecticides	++
Diet and vitamins	
Cured foods	
Maternal	++
Child	++
Fruits and vegetables	
Maternal	– –
Child	– –
Vitamins	
Maternal	–
Nitrates—maternal	–
Nitrites—maternal	+
Nitrosamines–maternal	±
Maternal alcohol	+
Maternal tobacco	
Active	0
Passive	0
Personal medical history—head trauma	++

*Table includes those factors for which sufficient epidemiologic studies have been conducted and does not include every factor studied in relation to childhood brain tumors; see text for citations to comprehensive epidemiologic reviews.
[†]Key: ++ positive relative risk—median relative risk of at least three studies exceeds 1.5; + slightly positive relative risk—median relative risk of at least three studies is between 1.1 and 1.5; 0 no association—median relative risk of at least three studies is between 0.9 and 1.1; – slightly negative relative risk—median relative risk of at least three studies is between 0.7 and 0.9; – – negative relative risk—median relative risk of at least three studies is below 0.7; ± two studies with inconsistent results.

exposure to cosmic radiation at high altitudes in brain tumor risk.[4]

Widespread public and scientific interest in potential health effects of electromagnetic fields (EMFs) stems from residential studies that showed increased risks of brain tumors and leukemia in children living in homes with higher EMF exposures. Occupational studies of workers also indicated higher brain tumor mortality and incidence among presumably exposed workers. Recent meta-analyses suggest a nonsignificant 50 percent increased risk of childhood brain tumors with residence in high versus low wire–coded homes[37] and significantly increased risk of 10 to 20 percent for brain cancer among workers in the broad category of electrical workers.[38] Although an effect of EMF on risk of brain tumors has not been definitively disproven, a causal connection also has not been established. The many possible reasons for a failure to definitively resolve the question of whether EMF exposures cause brain tumors are discussed at length in our previous review[3] and in other recent literature.[39,40]

Considerable concern over health effects due to cellular telephones has prompted studies looking to assess whether the use of such phones influences the risk of developing brain tumors. Two case-control studies and a cohort study that were recently published did not detect any meaningful or significant associations between cellular telephone use and brain tumor risk.[41–43] However, additional studies may be needed to determine if any risks are possible from digital phone use since most of the phones used in the previous studies were analog type. Furthermore, because of the relatively low prevalence and intensity of the use of cell phones at the time they were conducted, these studies could not consider the long-term effects of cell phone use, the effects of long-term cell phone use, or whether some small proportion of users might be especially susceptible to developing brain tumors from cell phone use. These are issues that limit the certainty with which a lack of association between cell phone use and brain tumors can be concluded.

Industry and Occupation

People can be exposed to a wide range of potentially carcinogenic chemical, physical, or biologic agents in their workplace. Thomas and Waxweiler[44] reviewed occupational and industrial risk factors for brain tumors in 1986, detailing the conceptual and practical difficulties of linking specific occupational exposures to risk of brain tumors. The controversies and problems they discuss remain relevant, even though there have been many additional studies since it was written.

Despite the likelihood that brain tumors arise from specific workplace exposures, no definitive links have been made even with known or strongly suspected carcinogens. Although animal studies have suggested many likely candidates, pinpointing culprits in occupational studies is especially difficult because workers are rarely exposed to only a single hazardous substance and agents might interact with others to increase or decrease risk. Also, there often are only small numbers of brain tumor cases even in large occupational cohort studies, which precludes the subgroup analyses that would be necessary to identify harmful chemicals, physical agents, work processes, or interactions. Limited understanding of the basic natural history and pathogenesis of brain tumors such as the latency periods between exposure and development of clinical disease also hinders efforts to establish specific causes.

Due to these limitations and the often inconsistent findings observed in epidemiologic studies, moderate to substantial controversy exists for all the occupations and industries listed in Table 1–1 as showing either a slightly positive or positive association with risk of brain tumors. For example, some pesticides and other agricultural chemicals such as organochlorides have a suspected association because these compounds induce cancer in laboratory animals, but brain tumor case-control studies and cohort studies of agricultural workers have about equally often produced negative and positive findings.[45] Also, even though workers involved in manufacturing the pesticides or fertilizers have not exhibited excess risks, most studies of pesticide applicators have shown a nearly threefold median relative risk for brain tumors. A recent meta-analysis of 33 studies of brain cancer and farming showed a statistically significant 30 percent increased risk and suggested that infectious agents or pesticides might be culprits.[46]

The almost twofold increased median relative risk of brain tumors observed in studies of synthetic rubber production and processing workers, combined with the knowledge that synthetic rubber processing produces numerous potentially carcinogenic byproducts (eg, coal tars, carbon tetrachloride, *N*-nitroso compounds, and carbon disulfide), suggests a causal association between work in this industry and increased risk of brain tumors. However, several studies in this industry have shown no increased or a decreased risk of brain tumors.[40,47]

Although vinyl chloride is a known carcinogen and epidemiologic studies of polyvinyl chloride production workers show a median twofold relative risk for death due to brain tumors, some argue that the absence of statistical significance due to small numbers of cases in many individual studies suggest that the positive findings may be due to chance.[40]

A causal role for formaldehyde in human brain tumorigenesis has been rejected because, although those in exposed professional occupations have exhibited increased risks, exposed industrial workers have not.[40] However, it is possible that unknown cofactors conceivably could obscure a true risk in industrially exposed workers and create the false impression of risk in the professionally exposed groups.

The controversy of whether and why petrochemical and oil refinery workers may have an increased brain tumor risk has yet to be resolved in more than 20 years of research. Most studies have shown increased risks of brain tumor mortality among workers in these industries of 20 to 80 percent.[4,7,48] General consistency of findings, despite low statistical power and likely nondifferential exposure misclassification (both of which would tend to conceal true associations), and the multiple possibly carcinogenic exposures support arguments favoring a true causal connection. However, some argue that such a conclusion cannot be made because of the lack of evidence for an important agent or agents to emerge from more detailed industrial hygiene surveys and the possibility that improved diagnostic sensitivity in these workers could artificially elevate brain tumor rates.

Parental Exposures

Some believe that parental occupational exposures may increase the risk of cancer in children. Hypotheses suggest that these exposures may alter the father's DNA prior to conception, or prenatal maternal exposures might directly affect the developing fetus. In addition, parental workplace exposures to infectious agents or to chemicals remaining on the parent's skin or clothing could be transferred to the child and thus result in postnatal exposures. However, no definitive evidence for important pre- or postnatal exposure has emerged because of the usual problems in disease heterogeneity; small sample sizes; multiple, confounded, or rare exposures; and inadequate follow-up.[3,7] Also, results from studies of pre- and postnatal maternal exposures have been inconsistent. Risks of childhood brain tumors have been reported with paternal work with (or in industries of) oil or chemical refining; farming; paper and pulp; solvents; painting, printing, and graphic arts; metallurgy; and air and space. Findings of no association with risk for childhood brain tumors also have been reported for paternal employment in aerospace industries and parental work with hydrocarbons. A recent case-control study concluded that there was an increased risk for childhood astroglial tumors with parental work in a chemical industry.[49] Also, two recent studies found significant elevation in brain tumor incidence in offspring of parents engaged in pig farming or whose parents had exposure to pigs or horses,[50,51] although postnatal exposures may be as or more relevant than prenatal exposures because results were strongest for those subjects who also grew up on a farm. Nonsignificant elevations for chicken farming, grain farming, horticulture, and pesticide use also were observed.

Diet, Vitamins, Alcohol, Tobacco, and Residential Chemicals

Epidemiologic studies of diet, vitamins, alcohol, tobacco, and residential chemicals also are subject to various problems including obtaining accurate exposure measurements and the difficulty in teasing out each compound's individual effects.

N-nitroso compounds have been identified as neurocarcinogens in experimental animal models, and the mechanisms through which *N*-nitroso compounds might operate to cause brain tumors are presented in other reviews.[7,8] Exposure pre- and postnatally to these compounds might contribute to childhood brain tumor development. It also is conceivable that adult tumors could result from prenatal or early postnatal exposures since so little is known about latency of tumor development.

Reliable and comprehensive assessment of exposure to *N*-nitroso compounds has been difficult because they are extremely common and widespread. As summarized elsewhere,[7] about half of human exposure to these chemicals comes from endogenous digestive processes when an amino compound (such as from fish, other foods, and drugs) meets a nitrosating agent (such as nitrites from cured meats) in the right enzymatic milieu. Exogenous sources such as tobacco smoke, cosmetics, and auto interiors also contribute to these exposures. Further complicating the exposure issue is that some sources, such as vegetables that are high in nitrites, also contain vitamins that may block formation of *N*-nitroso compounds—a subject that many studies have tried to examine.

The role of oxidants and antioxidants has become a popular topic in cancer and other degenerative disease research. It is believed that oxidants damage DNA, and this damage accumulates, or is more difficult to repair, with increasing age.[52] Both oxidants and antioxidants derive from an enormous variety of endogenous and exogenous sources. That increased consumption of vegetables and possibly of fruits is associated with decreased cancer risk for most cancer sites studied supports the hypothesis that antioxidants protect against cancer.[53] This observation prompted clinical trials of supplements of β-carotene and vitamin E (two common antioxidants in fruits and vegetables) as cancer preventing agents. These trials were halted upon the surprising and puzzling finding that subjects randomized to β-carotene were more likely to develop lung cancer than those on placebo;[53] these examples painfully demonstrate the perils of ascribing protective factors and designing interventions based on even extremely consistent and biologically plausible associations.

Some studies of dietary *N*-nitroso compounds support associations of these substances to both childhood and adult brain tumors, whereas others do not.[4,7,8,54] For example, greater consumption of cured foods and lower consumption of fruits and vegetables or vitamins that might block nitrosation among brain tumor cases (or their mothers) versus controls have been observed in some studies. However, these findings are also consistent with other hypotheses, such as those of oxidative burden and antioxidant protection discussed above. Also, selection bias favoring participation by controls who consume "healthier" diets could falsely accentuate case-control differences, although the inherent difficulties in accurate dietary assessments lead to misclassification of exposures, which tends to obscure any true differences between cases and controls. In a recent study, vitamin supplementation during all three trimesters of pregnancy appeared to be protective for primitive neuroectodermal, astroglial, and other brain tumors.[55] The finding that maternal dietary folate might be protective for primitive neuroectodermal tumors suggests the continuing need to develop and pursue fresh or understudied hypotheses about brain tumor etiology. New studies examining polymorphisms in genes involved in oxidative metabolism and carcinogen detoxification hope to combine results from environmental exposure assessments with knowledge of individual variation in response to environmental toxins.

Although cigarette smoke is a major environmental source of carcinogens including polycyclic hydrocarbons and nitroso compounds, the many epidemiologic studies examining its role in causing either adult or childhood brain tumors have generally found no evidence to support any important association.[3,4,7,56] However, evidence from two studies suggests that some increased risk of brain tumors might accompany smoking of unfiltered cigarettes.[3,4,7,53]

Maternal alcohol consumption, although it may be associated with impaired cognitive development in offspring, seems to play little role in the risk of childhood brain tumors. Two of three studies showed a median increased risk of about 40 percent among offspring prenatally exposed to alcohol, but only one of the two positive studies was significant.[4,7] Results for adults suggest, if anything, a decreased risk for glioma with consumption of beer and wine.[4]

Most studies of residential chemical exposures have assessed pre- and postnatal pesticide exposures in relation to childhood brain tumors, with inconsistent results.[7] A recent, large population-based study found significantly increased risk of childhood brain tumors with prenatal exposures to flea and tick pesticides.[57] The authors argued that the specificity of the association to flea and tick products suggested it might be real and not due to differential recall by mothers of affected children.

Personal Medical History

Infections

The possible roles of viruses and other infections in causing human brain tumors have not been adequately investigated, despite decades of calls for more research in this area.[4,8] Likely explanations for the paucity of studies in this area are the difficulties of designing meaningful studies and the limited availability of qualified investigators with sufficient cross-training or experience to design and conduct such studies. Retroviruses, papovaviruses, adenoviruses, and polyomaviruses have been shown to cause brain tumors in experimental animal studies, but few epidemiologic studies have examined exposures to these viruses in connection with human brain tumors. Three studies of the effects of simian virus 40 (SV40)–contaminated polio vaccine on cancer incidence have found unconvincing results of a true association with brain tumors.[3,4] With regard to other viruses, one study, but not another, found more mothers of children with medulloblastoma than control mothers were exposed to chickenpox, a herpesvirus, during pregnancy.[4] Adults with glioma in the San Francisco Bay Area were significantly less likely than controls to report having had either chickenpox or shingles.[58] This observation was supported by serologic evidence indicating that cases were less likely than controls to have antibody to varicella-zoster virus, the agent for chickenpox and shingles.

Toxoplasma gondii is another infectious agent investigated with regard to human tumors, at least partly because it is capable of causing gliomas in experimentally exposed animals.[4,8] Although one study convincingly linked astrocytoma with antibodies to *Toxoplasma gondii*, a more recent study found an association with meningioma but not with glioma.

Other studies have shown that people with brain cancer were less likely than controls to report allergies and common infections, and anecdotal reports from neuro-oncologists suggest that many of their patients claim to "have never been sick a day in their lives" before their brain tumor. Therefore, further study of the role of common infections and allergies in preventing brain tumors may be warranted.

Trauma

Serious head trauma has been suspected in the cause of some types of brain tumors, especially meningiomas and acoustic neuroma.[7] Studies of glioma and head trauma have, for the most part, been negative. A large recent Danish cohort study of the incidence of intracranial tumors after hospitalization for head injuries found no increased risk of glioma or meningioma during an average of 8 years of follow-up, except in the first year following the injury.[59] Although the authors attributed the increased risks during the first year postinjury to increased detection of brain tumors from procedures related to the injury, they did not observe the corresponding expected deficit of cases in subsequent years. Studies have often reported increased prevalence of birth trauma or other head injury in children with brain tumors compared to control children.[60] The possibility of differential recall of head injuries by individuals or mothers of children with brain tumors compared to controls prevents confidence in the causal nature of associations of head trauma and brain tumors. To minimize this source of bias, recent studies have asked for severe injuries that most people would not forget or have used a control group that is likely to recall similar events.

Seizures

Brain tumor risk associated with a history of seizures has been observed in several cohort studies of epileptics and in two case-control studies of adult glioma,[25,61] but determination of causality is problematic since it is difficult to determine if the seizures were due to the tumor or the tumor was due to the seizures. Also, even though studies showing an association with seizures occurring many years prior to tumor diagnosis may suggest a true connection, it is difficult to tease out whether the seizures or the medications to control them might increase tumor risk.

Drugs and Medications

Little is known about the effects of medications and drugs on the risk of brain tumors. A nonsignificant protective association was observed for headache, sleep, and pain medications.[7] Diuretics were associated with a nonsignificant association for meningioma but showed the opposite effect for adult glioma.[61] Ryan and colleagues[61] found no association with antihistamine use and adult glioma, but a 60 percent increased relative risk of meningioma with antihistamine use. Prenatal exposures to fertility drugs, oral contraceptives, sleeping pills or tranquilizers, barbiturates, pain medications, antihistamines, neuroactive drugs, or diuretics have been examined in relation to childhood brain tumor risk, but very few significant or consistent findings have been observed. An interesting possibility that needs study is whether nonsteroidal anti-inflammatory drugs known to be protective for some other cancer sites have any association with brain tumors.

SUMMARY

The most consistent features in the descriptive epidemiology of primary brain tumors in adults are gender differences, with glioma showing a preponderance in men and meningioma in women. Etiologic research may eventually explain this provocative clue. Improved registration, more consistently applied histopathologic classification systems, greater use and understanding of molecular and genetic markers to form more similar categories of tumors, incorporating studies of potentially relevant polymorphisms, and further exploration of viral factors or other infectious agents all should help to create a more complete picture of the natural history and pathogenesis of brain tumors. With current knowledge, we know that primary brain tumors have many causes. Since none of the causes thus far identified accounts for a large proportion of cases, many possibilities remain to discover important factors. Moreover, in the continuing search for explanations for this devastating disease, new concepts about neuro-oncogenesis might emerge, making the study of brain tumor epidemiology particularly exciting.

ACKNOWLEDGMENTS

This work was supported by the National Cancer Institute, grant numbers RO1CA52689, RO1CA709-17001, and PO1CA55261.

REFERENCES

1. Central Brain Tumor Registry of the United States. Statistical report: primary brain tumors in the United States, 1992–1997. Chicago (IL): CBTRUS; 2000.
2. American Cancer Society. Cancer facts and figures—2001. Atlanta (GA): American Cancer Society; 2001.
3. Wrensch M, Minn Y, Bondy ML. Epidemiology. In: Bernstein M, Berger M, editors. Essential neuro-oncology. New York: Thieme; 2000. p. 1–17.
4. Wrensch M, Bondy ML, Wiencke J, et al. Environmental risk factors for primary malignant brain tumors: a review. J Neurooncol 1993;17:47–64.
5. Bondy M, Wiencke J, Wrensch M, et al. Genetics of primary brain tumors: a review. J Neurooncol 1994;18:69–81.
6. Inskip PD, Linet MS, Heineman EF. Etiology of brain tumors in adults. Epidemiol Rev 1995;17:382–414.
7. Preston-Martin S, Mack WJ. Neoplasms of the nervous system. In: Schottenfeld D, Fraumeni JF, editors. Cancer epidemiology and prevention. 2nd ed. New York: Oxford University Press; 1996. p. 1231–81.
8. Berleur MP, Cordier S. The role of chemical, physical, or viral exposures and health factors in neurocarcinogenesis: implications for epidemiologic studies of brain tumors. Cancer Causes Control 1995;6:240–56.
9. Surawicz TS, McCarthy BJ, Kupelian V, et al. Descriptive epidemiology of primary brain and CNS tumors: results from the Central Brain Tumor Registry of the United States, 1990–1994. Neurooncology 1999;1:14–25.
10. Counsell CE, Grant R. Incidence studies of primary and secondary intracranial tumors: a systematic review of their methodology and results. J Neurooncol 1998;37:241–50.
11. Davis FG, Malinski N, Haenszel W, et al. Primary brain tumor incidence rates in four United States regions, 1985–1989: a pilot study. Neuroepidemiology 1996;15:103–12.
12. Smith MA, Friedlin B, Gloeckler LA, et. Trends in reported incidence of primary malignant brain tumors in children in the United States. J Natl Cancer Inst 1998;90:1269–77.
13. Davis FG, Bruner JM, Surawicz TS. The rationale for standardized registration and reporting of brain and central nervous system tumors in population-based cancer registries. Neuroepidemiology 1997;16:308–16.
14. Sant M, van der Sanden G, Capocaccia R, and the EUROCARE Working Group. Survival rates for primary malignant brain tumours in Europe. Eur J Cancer 1998;34:2241–47.
15. Davis FG, Freels S, Grutsch J, et al. Survival rates in patients with primary malignant brain tumors stratified by patient age and tumor histological type: an analysis based on Surveillance, Epidemiology, and End Results (SEER) data, 1973–1991. J Neurosurg 1998;88:1–10.

16. Horn B, Heideman R, Geyer R, et al. A multi-institutional restrospective study of intracranial ependymoma in children: identification of risk factors. J Pediatr Hematol Oncol 1999;21:203–11
17. Davis FG, McCarthy BJ, Freels S, et al. The conditional probability of survival of patients with primary malignant brain tumors. Cancer 1999;85:485–91.
18. Cairncross JG, Ueki K, Zlatescu MC, et al. Specific genetic predictors of chemotherapeutic response and survival in patients with anaplastic oligodendrogliomas. J Natl Cancer Inst 1998;90:1473–9
19. Scott JN, Rewcastle NB, Brasher PMA, et al. Long-term glioblastoma multiforme survivors: a population-based study. Can J Neurol Sci 1998;25:197–201.
20. McCarthy BJ, Davis FG, Freels S, et al. Factors associated with survival in patients with meningioma. J Neurosurg 1998;88:831–9.
21. Grovas A, Fremgen A, Rauck, A, et al. The National Cancer Data Base report on patterns of childhood cancers in the United States. Cancer 1997;80:2321–32.
22. Farwell JR, Dohrmann GJ, Flannery JT. Central nervous system tumors in children. Cancer 1977;40:3123–32.
23. Kleihues P, Ohgaki H. Primary and secondary glioblastomas: from concept to clinical diagnosis. Neurooncology 1999;1:44–51.
24. Narod SA, Stiller C, Lenoir GM. An estimate of the heritable fraction of childhood cancer. Br J Cancer 1991;63:993–9.
25. Wrensch M, Lee M, Miike R, et al. Familial and personal medical history of cancer and nervous system conditions among adults with glioma and controls. Am J Epidemiol 1997;145:581–93.
26. Li Y, Millikan RC, Carozza S, et al. p53 mutations in malignant gliomas. Cancer Epidemiol Biomarkers Prev 1998;7:303–8.
27. Gao L, Liu L, van Meyel D, et al. Lack of germ-line mutations of CDK4, p16(INK4A), and p15(INK4B) in families with glioma. Clin Cancer Res 1997;3:977–81.
28. Malmer B, Gronberg H, Bergenheim AT, et al. Familial aggregation of astrocytoma in northern Sweden: an epidemiological cohort study. Int J Cancer 1999;81:366–70.
29. de Andrade M, Barnholtz J, Amos CI, et al. Segregation analysis of cancer in families of glioma patients. Genet Epidemiol 2001;20:258–70.
30. Elexpuru-Camiruaga J, Buxton N, Kandula V, et al. Susceptibility to astrocytoma and meningioma: influence of allelism at glutathione S-transferase (GSTT1 and GSTM1) and cytochrome P-450 (CYP2D6) loci. Cancer Res 1995;55:4237–9.
31. Kelsey KT, Wrensch M, Zuo ZF, et al. A population-based case-control study of the CYP2D6 and GSTT1 polymorphisms and malignant brain tumors. Pharmacogenetics 1997;7:463–8.
32. Trizna Z, de Andrade M, Kyritsis AP, et al. Genetic polymorphisms in glutathione S-transferase mu and theta and N-acetyltransferase, and CYP1A1 and risk of gliomas. Cancer Epidemiol Biomarkers Prev 1998;7:553–5.
33. Bondy ML, Kyritsis AP, Gu J, et al. Mutagen sensitivity and risk of gliomas: a case-control analysis. Cancer Res 1996;56:1484–6.
34. Karlsson P, Holmberg E, Lundell M, et al. Intracranial tumors after exposure to ionizing radiation during infancy: a pooled analysis of two Swedish cohorts of 28,008 infants with skin hemangioma. Radiat Res 1998;150:357–64.
35. Little MP, Vathaire F, Shamsaldin A, et al. Risks of brain tumour following treatment for cancer in childhood: modification by genetic factors, radiotherapy and chemotherapy. Int J Cancer 1998;78:269–75.
36. Loomis DP, Wolf SH. Mortality of workers at a nuclear materials production plant at Oak Ridge, Tennessee, 1947–1990. Am J Ind Med 1996;29:131–41.
37. Meinert R, Michaelis J. Meta-analyses of studies on the association between electromagnetic fields and childhood cancer. Radiat Environ Biophys 1996;35:11–8.
38. Kheifets LI, Afifi AA, Buffler PA, et al. Occupational electric and magnetic field exposure and brain cancer: a meta-analysis. J Occup Environ Med 1995;37:1327–41.
39. National Institute of Environmental Health Sciences. Health effects from exposure to power-line frequency electric and magnetic fields. Research Triangle Park (NC): National Institutes of Environmental Health Sciences; 1999 Publication No.: 99-4493.
40. Wrensch M, Yost, M, Miike R, et al. Adult glioma in relation to residential power frequency electromagnetic field exposures in the San Francisco Bay Area. Epidemiology 1999;10:523–7.
41. Inskip PD, Tarone RE, Hatch EE, et al. Cellular-telephone use and brain tumors. N Engl J Med 2001;344:79–86.
42. Johansen C, Boice JD, McLaughlin JK, Olsen JH. Cellular telephones and cancer—a nationwide cohort study in Denmark. J Natl Cancer Inst 2001;93:203–7.
43. Muscat JE, Malkin MG, Thompson S, et al. Handheld cellular telephone use and risk of brain cancer. JAMA 2000;284:3001–7.
44. Thomas TL, Waxweiler RJ. Brain tumors and occupational risk factors. Scand J Work Environ Health 1986;12:1–15.
45. Bohnen NL, Kurland LT. Brain tumor and exposure to pesticides in humans: a review of the epidemiologic data. J Neurol Sci 1995;132:110–21.
46. Khuder SA, Mutgi AB, Schaub EA. Meta-analyses of brain cancer and farming. Am J Ind Med 1998;34:252–60.
47. Weiland SK, Mundt KA, Keil U, et al. Cancer mortality among workers in the German rubber industry: 1981–91 [comments]. Occup Environ Med 1996;53:289–98.
48. Cooper SP, Labarthe D, Downs T, et al. Cancer mortality among petroleum refinery and chemical manufacturing workers in Texas. J Environ Pathol Toxicol Oncol 1997;16:1–14.
49. McKean-Cowdin R, Preston-Martin S, Pogoda JM, et al. Parental occupation and childhood brain tumors: astroglial and primitive neuro-ectodermal tumors. J Occup Environ Med 1998;40:332–40.
50. Kristensen P, Andersen A, Irgens LM, et al. Cancer in offspring of parents engaged in agricultural activities in Norway: incidence and risk factors in the farm environment. Int J Cancer 1996;65:39–50.
51. Holly EA, Bracci PM, Mueller BA, et al. Farm and animal exposures and pediatric brain tumors: results from the United States West Coast Childhood Brain Tumor Study. Cancer Epidemiol Biomarkers Prev 1998;7:797–802.

52. Ames BN, Shigenaga MK, Hagen TM. Oxidants, antioxidants, and the degenerative diseases of aging. Proc Natl Acad Sci U S A 1993;90:7915–22.
53. Patterson RE, White E, Kristal AR. Vitamin supplements and cancer risk: the epidemiologic evidence. Cancer Causes Control 1997;8:786–802.
54. Lee M, Wrensch M, Miike R. Dietary and tobacco risk factors for adult onset glioma in the San Francisco Bay Area (California, USA). Cancer Causes Control 1997;8:13–24.
55. Preston-Martin S, Pogoda JM, Mueller BA, et al. Results from an international case-control study of childhood brain tumors: the role of prenatal vitamin supplementation. Environ Health Perspect 1998;106(Suppl 3):887–92.
56. Norman MA, Holly EA, Preston-Martin S. Childhood brain tumors and exposure to tobacco smoke. Cancer Epidemiol Biomarkers Prev 1996;5:85–91.
57. Pogoda JM, Preston-Martin S. Household pesticides and risk of pediatric brain tumors. Environ Health Perspect 1997;105:1214–20.
58. Wrensch M, Weinberg A, Wiencke J, et al. Does prior infection with varicella-zoster virus influence risk of adult glioma? Am J Epidemiol 1997;145:594–7.
59. Inskip PD, Mellemkjaer L, Gridley G, et al. Incidence of intracranial tumors following hospitalization for head injuries (Denmark). Cancer Causes Control 1998;9:109–16.
60. Gurney JG, Preston-Martin S, McDaniel AM, et al. Head injury as a risk factor for brain tumors in children: results from a multicenter case-control study. Epidemiology 1996;7:485–9.
61. Ryan P, Lee MW, North JB, et al. Risk factors for tumors of the brain and meninges: results from the Adelaide Adult Brain Tumor Study. Int J Cancer 1992;51:20–7.

Histopathology of Primary Tumors of the Central Nervous System

ADEKUNLE M. ADESINA, MD, PHD
RICHARD W. LEECH, MD
ROGER A. BRUMBACK, MD

Primary central nervous system (CNS) tumors account for 50 to 70 percent of intracranial tumors. Although metastatic solid tumors are frequent in the adult population, they are rare in childhood. There is also a striking difference in the distribution of primary CNS tumors between the adult and childhood populations: 70 percent of CNS tumors are supratentorial in adults whereas 70 percent of childhood tumors are infratentorial. Furthermore, intracranial tumors are second only to leukemia as a cause of childhood cancers.

The classification of CNS tumors is based on the pattern of cell differentiation. This is a reflection of the traditional assumption that the pattern of differentiation reflects the histogenesis of such tumors. Although fairly adequate in providing a working schema for pathologic diagnosis and classification of tumors, this framework is inadequate for explaining the histogenesis of an increasing number of tumors that show divergent or aberrant differentiation. Such aberrant differentiation is consistent with the fact that every tumor cell possesses all of the repertoire of the host's genetic information, and the pattern of differentiation is only a reflection of the set of genes expressed in the tumor cells. In this review, the World Health Organization (WHO) classification for CNS tumors will be used.[1]

In the peripheral organs, histologic classification often implies prognosis. Similarly, in the CNS, there is a strong correlation between the degree of cell differentiation and clinical prognosis. However, the term "benign," when based on histology, does not necessarily determine outcome since outcome is influenced not only by histology (ie, the degree of differentiation) but also by location and relationship to vital centers, surgical resectability, and radio- and chemosensitivity.

MENINGEAL TUMORS

Primary tumors arising in the leptomeninges include meningioma, mesenchymal nonmeningothelial tumors, hemangiopericytoma, and melanocytic tumors.

Meningioma

Meningioma is a tumor composed of neoplastic meningothelial cells and accounts for 13 to 26 percent of intracranial tumors.[2] Meningiomas are most common in middle and advanced age with peak incidence in the sixth and seventh decades. Meningiomas frequently are incidental findings at autopsy. In children, meningiomas are often aggressive. Although most tumors are sporadic, multiple meningiomas can be seen as part of the presentation of neurofibromatosis type 2 (NF2) as well as in genetically predisposed non-NF2 individuals.[3]

Histologic features allow for the division of meningiomas into three grades: (1) benign meningiomas (WHO grade I), accounting for the bulk of meningiomas; (2) atypical meningiomas (WHO grade II), which represent 4.7 to 7.2 percent of all meningiomas; and (3) anaplastic (malignant) meningiomas (WHO grade III), representing 1.0 to 2.8 percent of all meningiomas.

In general, meningiomas occur more commonly in females, with a female-male ratio of 3:2 for intracranial tumors and 10:1 for spinal meningiomas. This female predominance, as well as the positivity of about two-thirds of meningiomas for progesterone receptors, is consistent with a putative role for sex hormones in the development of meningiomas. However, for currently unclear reasons, atypical and anaplastic meningiomas predominate in males.[4] A number of etiologic factors have been proposed for the neoplastic transformation of meningothelial cells. Notable among these is exposure to ionizing radiation. The lag time between exposure to ionizing radiation and clinical diagnosis of meningioma varies from 35 years (as was observed following low-dose [800 rads] scalp radiation for tinea capitis) to 19 to 24 years (following higher-dose [> 2,000 rads] radiotherapy for brain tumors).[5] These observations suggest a positive correlation between lag time and the dose of ionizing radiation.

Another etiologic factor notable among those proposed is a linkage between genetic events involving chromosome 22q and the development of meningiomas, suggested by molecular genetic studies. Loss of heterozygosity at 22q13 is seen in 50 percent of meningiomas.[6] This putative site colocalizes with the NF2 gene site. It is interesting to note that NF2 gene mutation is present in 60 percent of sporadic meningiomas. Analysis of histologic subtypes of meningioma shows the presence of NF2 gene mutations in 70 to 80 percent of fibroblastic and transitional meningiomas and in only 25 percent of meningothelial meningiomas. The lack of linkage to 22q in hereditary non-NF2 families points to the existence of other currently undefined genetic events in subsets of meningioma. 1p, 9q, 10q, 14q and 17p deletions are seen in atypical/malignant meningioma.[7–9]

Meningiomas have been referred to by specific names depending on their location, such as the falx, the sphenoid ridge, the olfactory groove, the foramen magnum, and over the hemispheric convexities. These tumors also have differing clinical presentations related to the functional deficits induced at these specific sites of origin. Grossly, meningiomas are usually firm or rubbery, well-demarcated, round, and occasionally lobulated masses (Figure 2–1). The tumors can occasionally grow as flat masses termed "en plaque" meningioma. The presence of a significant amount of psammoma bodies (concentric calcium containing basophilic to purplish bodies) may impart a gritty texture.

Meningiomas vary in histologic features and have been subtyped according to the predominant histo-

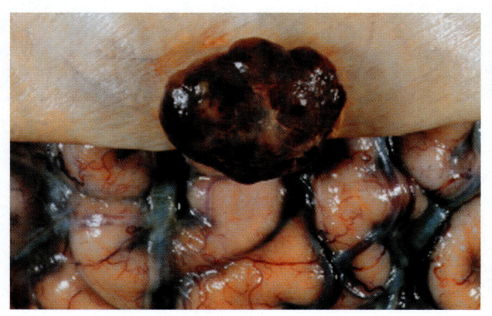

Figure 2–1. A well-demarcated, lobulated meningioma attached to the dura.

logic components. The classic meningothelial or syncytial meningioma is composed of sheets of cells with indistinct cytoplasmic borders and uniform nuclei with frequent intranuclear cytoplasmic pseudoinclusions but no discernible nucleoli (Figure 2–2A). Other subtypes range from the fibroblastic

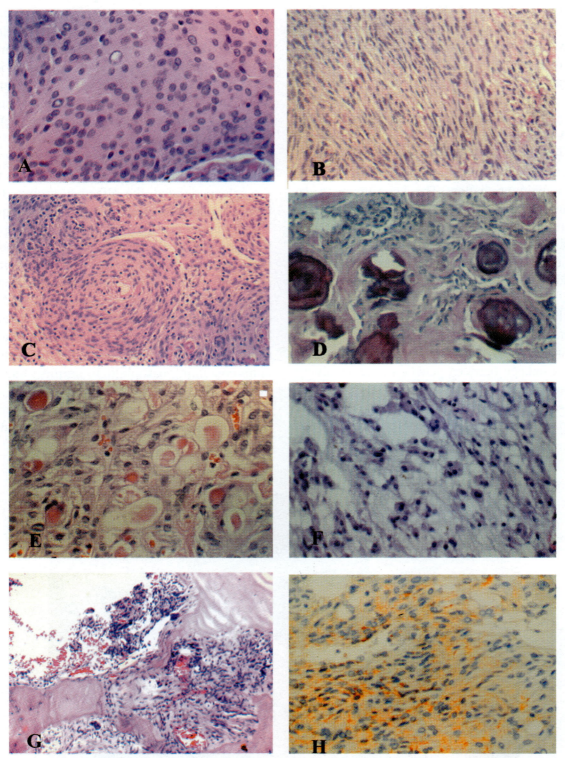

Figure 2–2. Meningiomas. *A,* Syncytial; *B,* fibroblastic; *C,* transitional; *D,* psammomatous; *E,* secretory; and *F,* myxoid meningiomas. *G,* Bone invasion with hyperostosis. *H,* Epithelial membrane antigen positivity in meningioma.

subtype (Figure 2–2B) (with a predominant benign spindle and fibrous component and which, compared to other meningiomas, have an increased frequency of chromosome 22 abnormality[6]) to the transitional form (Figure 2–2C) (with a mixture of the spindle fibroblastic cells of the fibroblastic meningioma and the plump eosinophilic cells of the meningothelial meningioma, arranged in characteristic whorls). Any of the subtypes can have psammoma bodies. However, when psammoma bodies become prominent and represent the bulk of the tumor, the tumors are referred to as psammomatous meningiomas (Figure 2–2D). Angiomatous meningiomas are characterized by the presence of a prominent variably sized benign vasculature. The presence of prominent microcystic degeneration or pale lipid-containing xanthomatous cells identifies other subsets of meningioma. Gland-like structures with lumina containing eosinophilic periodic acid–Schiff (PAS) and epithelial-membrane antigen (EMA)–positive secretion are a feature of the secretory (pseudoglandular) meningioma (Figure 2–2E). Myxomatous or myxoid meningiomas (Figure 2–2F) are characterized by the presence of a diffuse myxoid stroma with stellate cells. The identification of such tumors as meningiomas requires the presence of more classic meningothelial components. Classic meningothelial components can be a minor component requiring generous tissue sampling before identification. In the absence of such a component, the differential diagnosis would include a metastatic mucin-secreting adenocarcinoma. Similarly, the presence of abundant clear cells can raise the differential diagnosis of a metastatic renal cell carcinoma. A diffuse infiltrate of mature benign lymphocytes and plasma cells is a major component of the lymphoplasmacyte-rich meningioma. The mature nature of the cells and their admixture with neoplastic meningothelial cells are key to distinguishing them from non-Hodgkin's lymphoma. Metaplastic meningiomas exhibit focal or sometimes florid differentiation into other mature cell types such as osteoid, chondroid, and adipose tissue. Invasion of dura or dural sinuses is common. Skull invasion is usually associated with hyperostosis (Figure 2–2G).

A major differential diagnosis for meningiomas seen in the cerebellopontine angle or in relation to cranial/spinal nerve roots is schwannoma (neurilemoma). Histologic differentiation can often be done readily on the basis of light microscopic and immunostaining features when the characteristic cellular Antoni A areas with Verocay bodies and the loose myxoid Antoni B areas of typical schwannomas are present. In addition, schwannomas typically show positivity for S-100 protein and negative staining for epithelial-membrane antigen. In contrast, meningothelial cells are positive for epithelial-membrane antigen (Figure 2–2H) and are rarely positive for S-100 protein. These distinguishing features may not be readily obvious in very small biopsy specimens. Therefore, it may be necessary to resort to electron microscopy, in which the demonstration of desmosome junctions, cytoplasmic interdigitations, and a lack of basal lamina in the tumor cells are characteristic of meningioma whereas the presence of a basal lamina and a lack of true desmosome junctions are consistent with Schwann cell differentiation.

In the benign meningioma, there is a distinct demarcation between tumor and brain parenchyma. A demonstrable invasion of underlying brain is indicative of an aggressive meningioma, and careful sampling and analysis will often reveal histologic features of an atypical or malignant meningioma.

Atypical Meningioma

Atypical meningioma represents a subset of meningioma with a slightly higher risk of recurrence when compared with benign meningiomas (29 to 39% vs 7 to 20%). Such tumors are characterized by cellular atypia (cellular pleomorphism), frequent mitotic figures (usually ≥ 5 per 10 high-power [40×] microscopic fields,)[10] proliferation index (MIB-1 index) usually > 5 percent (mean of 2.1% vs mean of 0.7% for benign meningiomas), increased cellularity with sheetlike growth, relatively small areas of spontaneous or geographic necrosis, and invasion of underlying brain (Figure 2–3).

Papillary and Nonpapillary Anaplastic (Malignant) Meningiomas

Papillary meningiomas are malignant meningiomas by definition, and the presence of a distinct papillary pattern is the hallmark of this subset of meningiomas

(Figure 2–4A).[11] They represent a WHO grade II or III. Papillary meningiomas tend to occur more commonly in children. Papillary features in a dural-based lesion should raise the differential diagnosis of a metastatic papillary adenocarcinoma. Local and brain invasion is seen in 75 percent of cases, with a recurrence rate of about 55 percent. Metastases are also seen in about 20 percent of cases.[12]

The diagnosis of anaplastic or malignant meningioma in a nonpapillary tumor requires the presence of overt or frank anaplasia and/or metastases. The more classic lesions are usually characterized by increased cellularity, frequent mitotic figures, and conspicuous necrosis (Figures 2–4B and C). The proliferation index (MIB-1 index) is usually > 10 percent (mean, 11%). The distinction between atypical and malignant meningioma is problematic and varies among individual pathologists. However, there is better agreement among pathologists when there is a strict requirement for the presence of unequivocal anaplasia, extensive necrosis, and brisk mitotic activity (≥ 20 mitosis per 10 high-power [40×] microscopic fields) before a diagnosis of malignant meningioma is made.[13]

Postsurgical recurrence is a common feature of meningiomas and is seen in up to 20 percent of

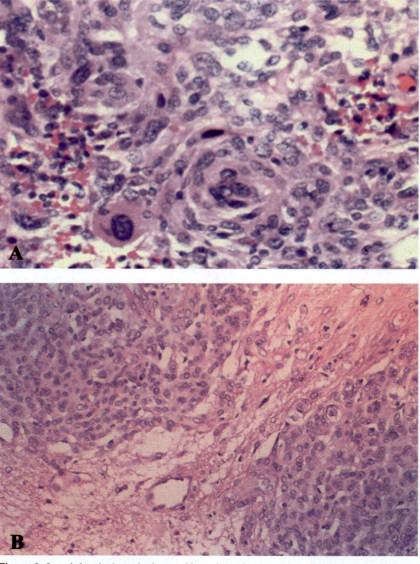

Figure 2–3. A, Atypical meningioma with nuclear pleomorphism. B, Atypical meningioma with brain invasion, indicating aggressive behavior.

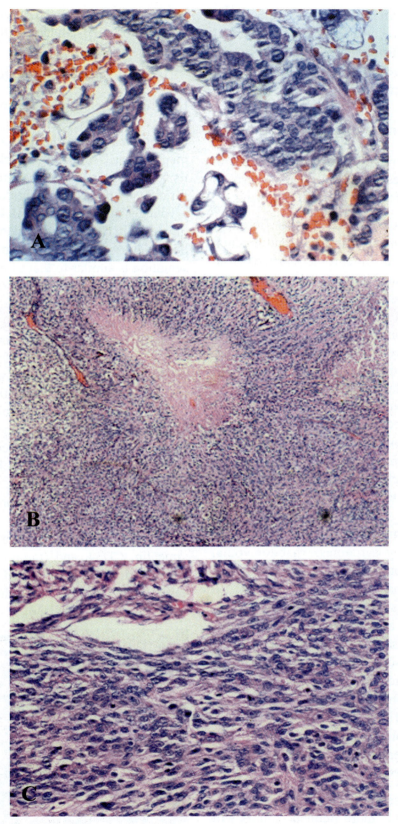

Figure 2–4. Malignant meningioma. *A*, Papillary meningioma. *B*, Increased cellularity and spontaneous tumor necrosis. *C*, Anaplasia with poor meningothelial differentiation.

benign meningiomas after 20 years of follow-up.[14] Indicators of possible recurrence (apart from incomplete resection) are histologic subtype and tumor grade.[10] Anaplastic meningiomas have the highest recurrence rate, about 50 to 78 percent.[13,15]

Mesenchymal Nonmeningothelial Tumors

Mesenchymal nonmeningothelial tumors share similar histologic features with their counterparts in peripheral soft tissues and include the following:

1. Adipose tissue tumors, such as lipomas (fibrolipomatous harmatomas, angiolipomas, and epidural lipomatosis [related to chronic corticosteroid administration]) and intracranial liposarcoma. Lipomas occur most often in the midline and are typically located in the corpus callosum, cerebellar vermis, or mammillary bodies. They may also occur as part of a complex malformation. Mature lipocytes have recently been described as part of a low-grade cerebellar tumor called liponeurocytoma, which is composed of intermixed mature lipocytes and neurocytic cells[16]
2. Fibrohistiocytic tumors, including benign and malignant fibrous histiocytoma
3. Fibrous tumors, including solitary fibrous tumor, hypertrophic intracranial pachymeningitis, and fibrosarcoma
4. Muscle-forming tumors, such as leiomyoma, intracranial leiomyosarcomas, rhabdomyoma, embryonal rhabdomyosarcoma, and malignant ectomesenchymoma
5. Osteocartilaginous tumors, including chondroma, osteoma and osteochondroma, mesenchymal chondrosarcoma, and osteosarcoma
6. Vascular tumors, such as hemangiomas, epithelioid hemangioendotheliomas, angiosarcoma, and Kaposi's sarcoma
7. Tumors of undefined histogenesis, such as hemangiopericytoma, capillary hemangioblastoma, and meningeal sarcoma/sarcomatosis
8. Melanocytic tumors

Since many of these tumors are curiosities in the CNS, only the relatively more frequent tumors will be discussed further. The histologic features of the other tumors are similar to those of their soft-tissue counterparts and are well discussed in the soft-tissue sections of other standard textbooks.

Hemangiopericytoma

Historically, hemangiopericytoma has been referred to by various obsolete names such as "angioblastic meningioma" and "hemangiopericytic variant of meningioma," reflecting a lack of understanding of its true histogenesis. Hemangiopericytoma accounts for only 0.4 percent of all brain tumors and occurs at a younger age (mean age of 43 years) than meningioma.[17–19] Hemangiopericytoma is usually dural based and is rarely intraparenchymal. Clinical presentation is similar to that of meningioma.

Grossly, the tumor is firm, well demarcated, globoid, and slightly lobulated and can bleed profusely during surgical removal. Histologically, it is a highly cellular tumor with monotonous sheets of oval to elongated nuclei (Figure 2–5), variable degrees of nuclear atypia, and prominent mitotic activity. Investment of individual cells by reticulin can be appreciated on reticulin stain. "Staghorn" vessels of variable prominence are also apparent. Invasion of underlying brain can occur. Since many soft-tissue tumors can have hemangiopericytomatous areas, immunostaining and electron microscopy, if available, are important aids in ensuring accurate diagnosis.

Hemangiopericytomas show immunoreactivity for vimentin, CD34, and (rarely) smooth-muscle actin and desmin. The proliferation index (MIB-1 index) varies widely, with median values ranging between 5

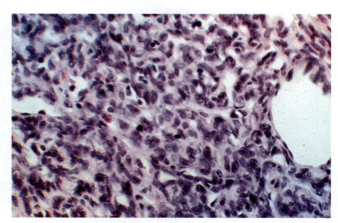

Figure 2–5. Hemangiopericytoma showing a monotonous population of oval cells and dilated vascular channels.

and 10 percent.[20,21] Hemangiopericytomas exhibit a high 15-year local recurrence rate of 85 to 91 percent, and metastases are also seen in about 65 percent of cases followed for more than 15 years.[17,20]

Capillary Hemangioblastoma

Capillary hemangioblastoma is a WHO grade I vasoformative tumor of uncertain histogenesis that commonly occurs in the cerebellum. Spinal and brainstem lesions also occur but less frequently, and supratentorial lesions are very rare. About 25 percent of cases occur in the setting of von Hippel-Lindau disease.[22] von Hippel-Lindau disease–associated tumors occur in younger patients whereas the non–von Hippel-Lindau disease–associated tumors occur in adults. von Hippel-Lindau disease is a neurocutaneous syndrome associated with retinal hemangioblastoma, pheochromocytoma, renal cell carcinoma, and visceral (liver and pancreas) cysts. Hemangioblastomas are slow-growing tumors, often presenting with features of raised intracranial pressure secondary to the blockage of cerebrospinal fluid (CSF) flow. There is often an accompanying secondary polycythemia due to erythropoietin production by the neoplastic stromal cells.

Grossly, capillary hemangioblastoma consists of well-circumscribed red nodules, often in the wall of large cysts. Histologically, the tumors are composed of large vacuolated stromal cells and a rich capillary network (Figures 2–6A and B). The stromal cells show immunopositivity for vimentin, but the tumors

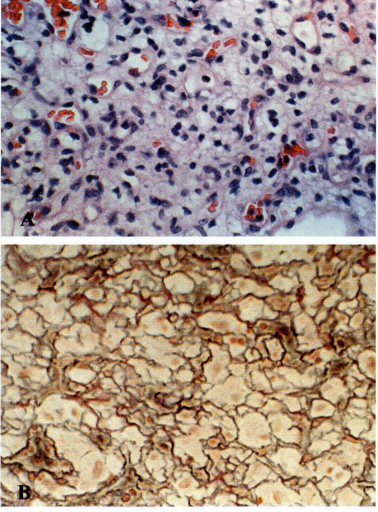

Figure 2–6. Hemangioblastoma. *A*, Capillary proliferation with "clear" stromal cells. *B*, Reticulin stain showing a rich capillary network.

do not show evidence of immunoreactivity for glial fibrillary acidic protein or for endothelial markers such as CD34 or von Willebrand's factor. The "clear cell" appearance of the stromal cells can be confused with metastatic renal cell carcinoma. Rosenthal fibers can be seen in the wall of the cysts. The slow growth of capillary hemangioblastoma is consistent with a low proliferation index (MIB-1 index < 1%). The stromal cells show an increased expression of epidermal growth factor receptor (EGFR), transforming growth factor-α (TGF-α) (which is a ligand for EGFR),[23,24] and vascular endothelial growth factor (VEGF). The endothelial cells express VEGF receptors 1 and 2 (VEGFR-1 and -2) and platelet-derived growth factor (PDGF).[25]

Meningeal Sarcomatosis

Meningeal sarcomatosis is a diffuse leptomeningeal sarcomatous tumor lacking the distinct circumscribed nature characteristic of most meningeal tumors. It is composed of poorly differentiated spindle cells characteristic of undifferentiated sarcomas. Apart from immunostaining for vimentin, the tumor cells are negative for all neuroglial markers.

Mesenchymal Chondrosarcoma

The most common extraosseous site for mesenchymal chondrosarcoma is the CNS. Mesenchymal chondrosarcoma has a distinct small cell tumor component interrupted by islands of atypical hyaline cartilage. The small cell component shares histologic features with hemangiopericytoma and can be confused with it in small biopsy specimens that lack the characteristic chondroid component.

Melanocytic Lesions

Primary melanocytic lesions of the CNS are relatively uncommon, accounting for only 0.06 to 0.1 percent of brain tumors. Melanocytic lesions are more common in Caucasians and arise from melanocytes of the leptomeninges. There are three possible forms of CNS melanocytic lesions: (1) diffuse melanocytosis, (2) melanocytoma, and (3) primary leptomeningeal malignant melanoma.

Diffuse melanocytosis usually presents in childhood with seizures, behavioral disturbances, and hydrocephalus. Histologically, the lesion shows a diffuse proliferation of uniform nevoid polygonal cells within the leptomeninges.

Melanocytomas present as mass lesions composed of a monomorphic population of spindle, fusiform, epithelioid, or polyhedral cells arranged in whorls, sheets, nests, or interlacing bundles of storiform configuration with infrequent mitotic figures (Figure 2–7). Melanin can be present. The tumors are S-100 protein positive and (in our experience)

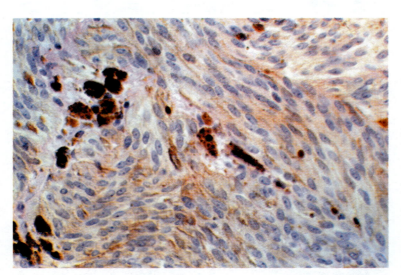

Figure 2–7. Melanocytoma with a monomorphic population of oval to spindle cells arranged in interlacing bundles. Note the abundant melanin pigment and the complete lack of frank anaplasia.

are usually negative for the melanoma antigen marker, HMB-45.

Primary meningeal malignant melanomas also present as mass lesions. They occur classically in the setting of neurocutaneous melanosis, such as in the autosomal dominant Touraine syndrome and in patients with the congenital nevus of Ota. The tumors have an aggressive behavior similar to that seen in cutaneous melanoma and are characterized histologically by marked pleomorphism, high mitotic activity, necrosis, hemorrhage, and invasion of underlying brain (Figure 2–8). The diagnosis of a primary CNS melanoma can be made only after a metastatic melanoma has been excluded. As with cutaneous melanoma, the tumor cells are S-100 protein and HMB-45 positive while being negative for glial fibrillary acidic protein (GFAP), neurofilament protein (NFP), EMA, and cytokeratin. Electron microscopy shows the presence of melanosomes.

ASTROCYTIC TUMORS

Diffuse astrocytomas are infiltrating fibrillary neoplasms with varying degrees of differentiation and tumor grade. They account for 50 percent of primary brain tumors. Astrocytic tumors characteristically have infiltrative margins and range from low-grade diffuse astrocytoma, classified as WHO grade II (peak age of 30 to 39 years), to anaplastic (malignant) astrocytoma, classified as WHO grade III (peak age of 40 to 49 years), to the most aggressive glioblastoma multiforme, classified as WHO grade IV (peak age of 50 to 69 years).

Well-Differentiated (Low-Grade) Astrocytoma

Low-grade astrocytomas represent WHO grade II, are most common in the cerebral white matter, and account for 20 percent of primary brain tumors. Low-grade astrocytomas are composed of a relatively uniform population of proliferating astrocytes in a fibrillary matrix (Figure 2–9A). Mitotic figures are rare. In contrast to reactive gliosis, diffuse astrocytomas have infiltrative poorly defined margins and can have microcystic degeneration (Figure 2–9B). The tumor cells show slight atypia, an important criterion for distinguishing them from reactive gliosis. The tumor cells can have plump eosinophilic cytoplasm. Such cells are referred to as gemistocytes and represent a minor component of most diffuse astrocytomas. However, in the less common gemistocytic astrocytoma (Figure 2–9C), gemistocytes represent > 20 percent of the tumor cells.[26] The tumor cells show cytoplasmic positivity for GFAP (Figure 2–9D).

Pontine glioma represents a diffusely infiltrative low-grade glioma involving the basis pontis. It accounts for 10 percent of childhood brain tumors and is composed of fibrillary astrocytes. The diagnosis is often based on the classic neuroradiologic pre-

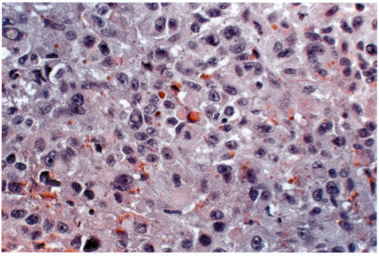

Figure 2–8. Primary leptomeningeal malignant melanoma with cellular pleomorphism, anaplasia, and melanin pigments.

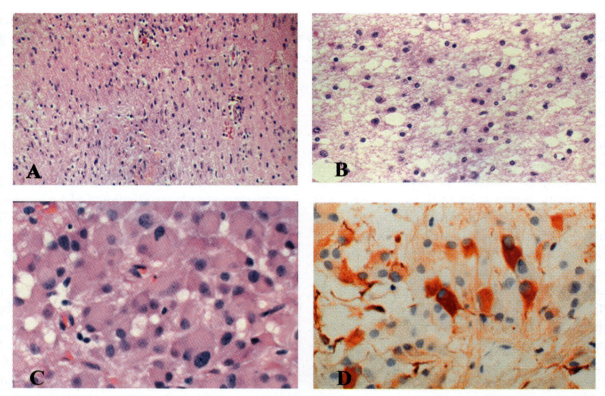

Figure 2–9. Low-grade astrocytoma. *A*, Diffuse fibrillary astrocytoma; *B*, microcystic pattern; *C*, gemistocytic astrocytoma; and *D*, immunopositivity for glial fibrillary acidic protein.

sentation, with no attempts at resection or biopsy. Treatment usually involves radiotherapy, but there is an attendant high propensity of surviving tumor cells to dedifferentiate to a more anaplastic histology including glioblastoma multiforme (Figure 2–10).

Tumor progression from low grade to high grade is not uncommon in other diffuse low-grade astrocytomas and is seen more frequently in the gemistocytic astrocytoma.[27,28] Even in low-grade astrocytomas that do not qualify for designation as gemistocytic astrocytomas, the percentage of gemistocytes present in a given tumor appears to have a negative correlation with the length of time it takes for progression to high-grade gliomas.[28] In addition, the higher the percentage of gemistocytes, the higher the likelihood for a demonstrable p53 mutation in a low-grade astrocytoma.

Predictors of poor prognosis include the presence of a p53 mutation, a proliferation index > 5 percent, and a predominance of the gemistocytic feature in the tumor cells.[26,27] In contrast, a prominent microcystic component and a prominent perivascular lymphocytic infiltrate predict a less aggressive clinical course.[27,29]

Pilocytic astrocytoma represents a slow-growing diffuse fibrillary astrocytoma with a distinctly good prognosis warranting its designation as WHO grade I. It accounts for 20 to 25 percent of all childhood brain tumors, occurring frequently as a cystic cerebellar tumor with a mural nodule (Figure 2–11). Similar tumors may involve the optic nerve, presenting as optic nerve glioma in children and frequently in individuals with neurofibromatosis type 1 (NF1).[30] Supratentorial intra-axial tumors may also involve the hypothalamus or thalamus. The characteristic cells are the GFAP-positive piloid (elongated or "hairlike") astrocytes, which in the juvenile variant are arranged in a biphasic pattern of cellular fibrillary astrocytes with intervening loose microcystic areas (Figure 2–12A). Rosenthal fibers are frequently present, and the abundance of Rosenthal fibers (Figure 2–12B) is a helpful diagnostic feature in frozen sections or crush preparations made during intraoperative consultation. The adult variant does not show the microcystic feature of the juvenile type (Figures 2–12C and D). Unlike in classic astrocytoma, the presence of vascular proliferation and slight pleomorphism does

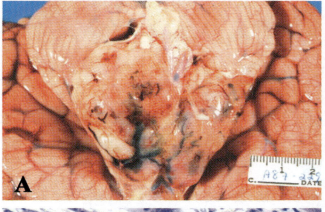
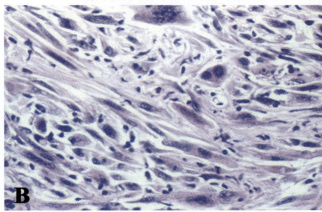
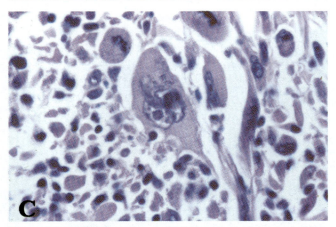

Figure 2–10. Pontine glioma. *A*, Enlargement of the brain stem with infiltration of the cerebellum. *B* and *C*, Marked cellular pleomorphism and anaplastic features.

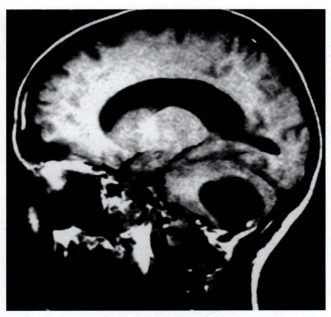

Figure 2–11. Pilocytic astrocytoma. T1-weighted magnetic resonance image of a cystic cerebellar mass with an intramural nodule.

not imply an aggressive high histologic grade. In the rare case, however, the presence of frequent mitotic figures, a significantly increased cellularity, and necrosis justifies the diagnosis of anaplastic (malignant) pilocytic astrocytoma.[31]

Pleomorphic xanthoastrocytoma is a tumor with distinct radiopathologic features, including a superficial meningocerebral location, a common location in the temporal lobe, and frequent association with a long-standing history of seizures. Pleomorphic xanthoastrocytoma accounts for < 1 percent of all astrocytic neoplasms, but two-thirds of cases occur in individuals below the age of 18 years. Histologically, it exhibits significant pleomorphism, with many atypical giant cells and astrocytic cells with slightly prominent nucleoli. Mitotic activity and necrosis are conspicuously absent in the typical pleomorphic xanthoastrocytoma. There is a variably discernible population of foamy (xanthomatous) cells and focal lymphocytic and plasma cell infiltrate in a background of reticulin-positive desmoplasia (Figures 2–13A and B). The astrocytic origin of this tumor has recently come into question because of the demonstration of neuronal markers in subpopulations of tumor cells[32] (Figures 2–13C and D). In addition, the morphologic pattern seen in pleomorphic xanthoastrocytoma may form the glioma component of a ganglioglioma.[33]

Pleomorphic xanthoastrocytoma with anaplastic features is a variant that may represent WHO grade III. These tumors are often seen as part of tumor progression in recurrent lesions. They show features indicative of aggressive behavior, such as increased mitotic activity (> 5 mitosis per 10 high-power [40×] microscopic fields), necrosis, and endothelial proliferation (Figure 2–14).

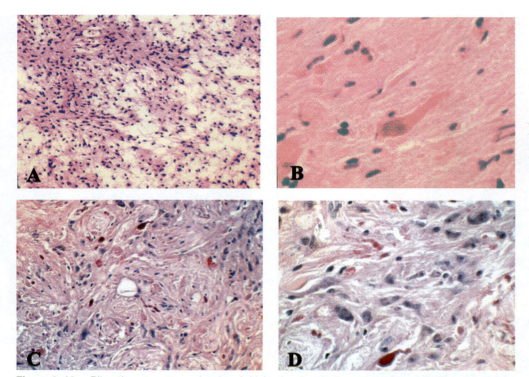

Figure 2–12. Pilocytic astrocytoma showing A, biphasic microcystic pattern of juvenile pilocytic astrocytoma; B, a fibrillary pattern with Rosenthal fibers; and C and D, an adult-type fibrillary pattern. Note the numerous Rosenthal fibers and granular cells.

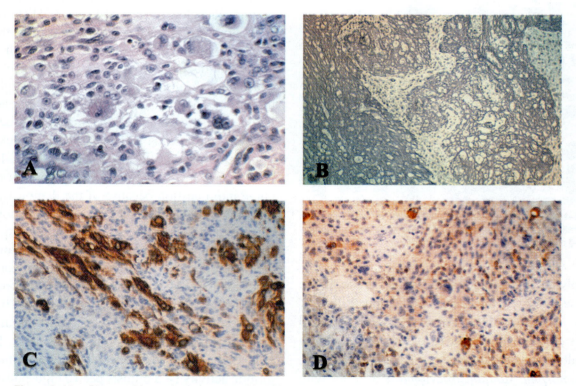

Figure 2–13. Pleomorphic xanthoastrocytoma. Marked cellular atypia with A, xanthomatous cells and lymphocytic infiltrate; B, florid desmoplasia, demonstrated with reticulin stain; C, glial fibrillary acidic protein–positive cells; and D, synaptophysin positivity in tumor cells.

Anaplastic (Malignant) Astrocytoma

Anaplastic astrocytoma represents a high-grade diffuse fibrillary astrocytoma classified as WHO grade III. It has a similar distribution to that of low-grade astrocytoma but is characterized by a greater degree of cellularity and pleomorphism. Mitotic figures are readily discernible (Figure 2–15).

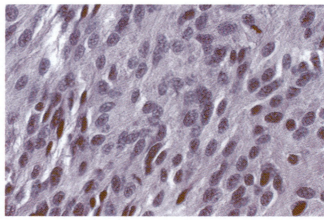

Figure 2–15. Anaplastic astrocytoma with marked cellularity and mitosis.

Glioblastoma Multiforme

Glioblastoma is the most common glioma, accounting for 50 percent of all gliomas. It is clinically the most aggressive glioma and represents an extreme expression of astrocytic anaplasia. Glioblastoma multiforme occurs frequently as a white-matter lesion, is diffusely infiltrative, and can cross the midline by involving the corpus callosum to produce the radiologic "butterfly" pattern. Glioblastoma multiforme is characteristically grossly hemorrhagic and necrotic (Figure 2–16). Histologically, it shows marked cellular pleomorphism, frequent mitotic figures, tumor giant cells, endothelial proliferation, and necrosis with or without pallisading (Figures 2–17A to C). A high proliferation index and immunoposi-

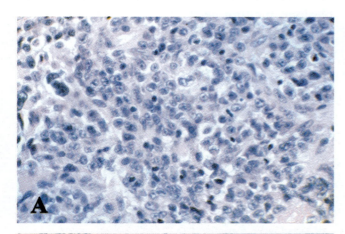
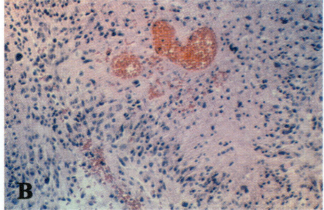
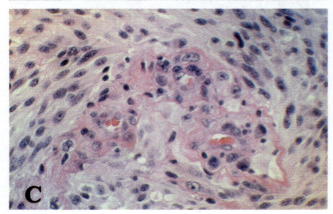

Figure 2–14. Malignant features in a pleomorphic xanthoastrocytoma. A, Increased cellularity; B, necrosis; and C, endothelial proliferation.

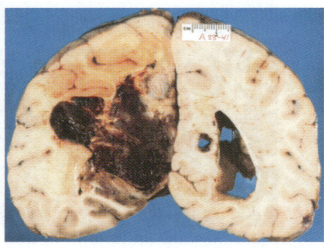

Figure 2–16. Glioblastoma multiforme. Note extensive tumor necrosis, hemorrhage, and edema.

tivity for p53 protein are common features of glioblastoma multiforme (Figures 2–17D and E).

A predominant population of highly proliferative small cells can be seen in the variant form called small cell glioblastoma. The predominance of such cells often raises a differential diagnosis of "small blue cell tumors" including malignant lymphoma. Although cellular pleomorphism is an inherent histologic feature of glioblastoma, an extremely pleomorphic variant with florid multinucleated giant cells constitutes giant cell glioblastoma (Figure 2–17F). A spindle mesenchymal sarcomatous transformation can also be seen in a variant referred to as gliosarcoma (Figure 2–18), which must be differentiated from the secondary diffuse spindle (fibroblastic) cell proliferation that can accompany the invasion of the leptomeninges by glioblastoma multiforme cells. Giant cell glioblastoma has a slightly better prognosis than classic glioblastoma multiforme[34,35] whereas the gliosarcoma has no significantly different outcome from the classic glioblastoma multiforme.[36]

Mutation of the p53 gene has been shown to be especially common in the evolution of low-grade

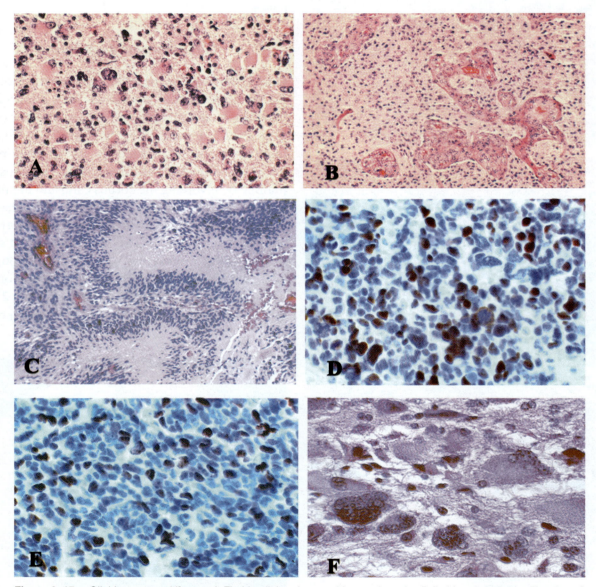

Figure 2–17. Glioblastoma multiforme. A, Florid cellular pleomorphism and atypia; B, florid endothelial proliferation; C, necrosis with pseudopallisading; D, immunopositivity for p53 protein in a large number of cells; and E, a high proliferation index with MIB-1 immunostaining. F, Giant cell glioblastoma.

astrocytoma and in the progression from low-grade to high-grade astrocytoma.[37] Amplification of the mdm2 gene, which provides an alternative pathway for p53 inactivation, occurs only in a minor subset of glioblastomas.[38] The subset of glioblastomas arising secondary to p53 mutation or inactivation has been designated as secondary glioblastoma (see Figure 2–17D). In contrast, de novo or primary glioblastomas are less likely to have mutations of the p53 gene and are more likely to have amplification of the EGFR gene. Therefore, there seems to be at least two largely separate operant pathways in the biologic evolution of the classic types of glioblastoma.[37]

The inactivation of the p53-mdm2-p21cip1 pathway results in increased genomic instability and in the accumulation of other genetic events inactivating other important metabolic pathways.[39] One of the other inactivated pathways is the p16-p15-cdk4-cdk6-RB pathway. The ultimate target for inactivation (by hyperphosphorylation) in this pathway is the retinoblastoma (RB) protein, which is critical in the control of G_1- S phase cell transit. The kinase activity of cdk4 and cdk6 on retinoblastoma protein is controlled by the cdk inhibitors p16/p15. The protein products of p16/p15 are inactivated by deletions within the coding genes rather than by mutations.[40] Hypermethylation of CpG islands in the 5' region of these genes also provides an alternative mechanism for gene inactivation.[41] In tumors lacking p16/p15 inactivation, the inactivation of retinoblastoma pro-

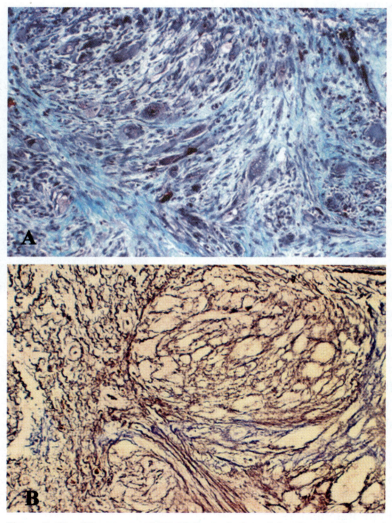

Figure 2–18. Gliosarcoma. *A,* Florid desmoplasia, cellular pleomorphism, and spindle cell transformation of tumor cells (Masson trichrome stain). *B,* Extensive reticulin formation by the sarcomatous component (reticulin stain).

tein (by hyperphosphorylation) is achieved by the amplification of cdk4 or cdk6.[40]

Additional genetic events in the development of high-grade gliomas include epidermal growth factor (EGF) and TGF-α expression providing a loop for autocrine stimulation.[37] Fibroblast growth factor and VEGF overexpression probably plays a major role in the development of angiogenesis, a critical element in the transformation of low-grade astrocytoma to glioblastoma multiforme.[42] Other reported genetic events in astrocytoma progression include loss of the deleted-in-colon-carcinoma (DCC) gene;[43] loss of heterozygosity (LOH) for chromosome 10q23.3 (PTEN gene locus), which is mutated in 30 to 49 percent of high-grade gliomas,[44] or total loss of chromosome 10;[45] loss at chromosome 19q13.3;[46] and loss of chromosome 22q.[45] The giant cell glioblastoma does not appear to share these molecular pathways, thus suggesting that it is a distinctly different biologic entity, a feature consistent with its differing clinical aggressiveness.

EPENDYMAL TUMORS

Ependymal tumors are subdivided into the low-grade *ependymoma* (WHO grade II) and the higher-grade *anaplastic ependymoma* (WHO grade III). Variants include the very low-grade (WHO grade I) *myxopapillary ependymoma*, which occurs almost exclusively in the conus medullosis-cauda equina-filum terminale region, as well as *subependymoma* (Figure 2–19), usually found in the floor of the fourth ventricle and which is also low grade and often an incidental finding at autopsy in elderly persons. Subependymomas can (rarely) undergo spontaneous intratumoral hemorrhage, with associated intraventricular hemorrhage.

Ependymoma (WHO grade II) is a tumor arising from the ependyma of the ventricles and can involve any of the ventricles, the spinal cord, and the filum terminale. It is most frequent in the fourth ventricle, often presenting with obstructive hydrocephalus. Ependymoma is most common in childhood, accounting for 20 percent of childhood brain tumors but only 5 percent of adult brain tumors.

The characteristic feature of ependymoma is the glandlike ependymal rosette (Figures 2–20A and B) with blepharoplasts. However, the perivascular pseudorosette with the central blood vessel and the radiating acellular GFAP-positive processes (Figure 2–20D) is more commonly seen. The tumor cells tend to be round and relatively uniform, with only slight hyperchromasia. Prominent gemistocyte-like cells with fibrillary processes can occasionally be evident, especially in frozen sections, creating a diagnostic dilemma during intraoperative consultation. Immunopositivity can be diffuse for EMA, S-100 protein, and vimentin and focal for cytokeratin. Infrequently, CSF dissemination can occur. A prominent papillary pattern, a predominance of clear cells (Figure 2–20C), evidence of tanycytic (bipolar spindle) cells, lipomatous differentiation, signet-ring cell features, and the presence of melanin

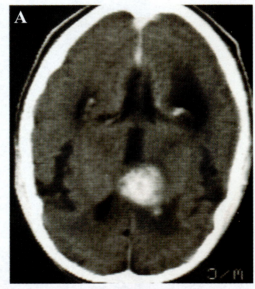

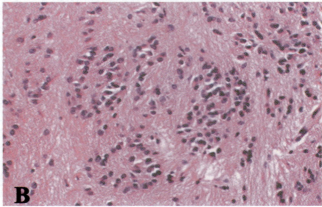

Figure 2–19. Subependymoma. *A,* Contrast enhancing subependymal nodule. *B,* Clusters of proliferating subependymal glia in a fibrillary matrix.

define some of the histologic subsets of ependymoma. Increased cellularity without significant increase in mitotic activity constitutes cellular ependymoma, an entity without any additional adverse prognostic implications. Although most ependymomas have well-demarcated borders, infiltrative tumors can occur in the cerebral hemispheres and spinal cord. Examination of ependymoma with the electron microscope reveals characteristic features of ependymal cells, including cilia, blepharoplasts, luminal microvilli, junctional complexes, and cell processes with intermediate filaments.

Anaplastic ependymoma shows a significantly increased cellularity with anaplasia, frequent mitotic figures, and necrosis (Figure 2–21). This tumor has a propensity for cerebrospinal fluid (CSF) dissemination. The presence of necrosis alone without the other cytologic changes and mitotic activity does not imply aggressive behavior since necrosis can be seen even in low-grade ependymoma. Predictors of poor prognosis in ependymomas include age below 3 years, anaplastic features (high cell density and frequent mitotic figures), incomplete tumor resection, and CSF dissemination. Molecular genetic studies of ependymomas

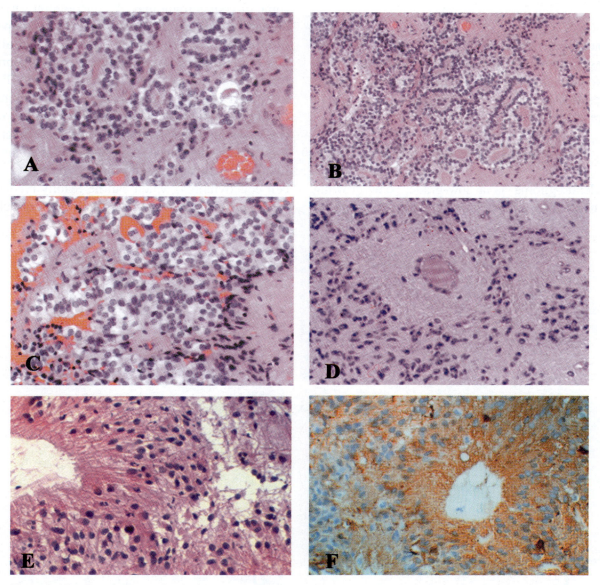

Figure 2–20. Ependymoma, showing *A*, ependymal rosettes; *B*, papillary pattern; *C*, clear cell features; *D*, perivascular pseudorosettes; *E*, prominent fibrillary and astrocytic features on frozen section; and *F*, glial fibrillary acidic protein positivity, which is prominent in an acellular perivascular fibrillary matrix.

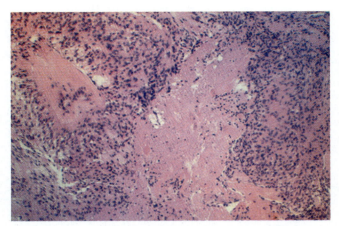

Figure 2–21. Anaplastic ependymoma with increased cellularity and extensive necrosis.

have not identified any of the genetic events associated with astrocytomas. Mutations involving the NF2 have been found only in spinal cord ependymomas, raising the possibility that ependymal tumors of the spinal cord represent a distinct molecular subset.[47]

OLIGODENDROGLIOMA

Oligodendroglioma is a low-grade, slow-growing glial tumor presumably arising from oligodendrocytes of the white matter. A predominant proportion of these tumors involve the frontal lobe. Frequently, there is a long history of poorly controlled seizures. The tumors are composed of uniform round cells with the characteristic delicate capillary vasculature (the so-called chicken-wire vasculature) (Figure 2–22A). Formalin fixation of the tumor produces an antifactual perinuclear halo, giving the so-called fried-egg appearance to the cells of an oligodendroglioma. Calcification is also frequent. A striking pattern of nuclear pallisades is sometimes seen. Staining with antibodies to the Leu-7 (HNK-1) antigen shows membrane positivity of tumor cells in some oligodendrogliomas. An uncommon variant of oligodendroglioma can have a significant component of minigemistocytes (Figure 2–22B). The gliofibrillary oligodendrocyte and minigemistocyes represent transitional forms that express GFAP (Figure 2–22C). Differential diagnosis of classic oligodendroglioma includes (1) central neurocytoma, which can be distinguished by the presence of acellular neuropil islands and positive immunostaining for neuronal antigens such as synaptophysin; and (2) clear cell ependymoma, which can be readily recognized by the presence of focal areas with the more classic

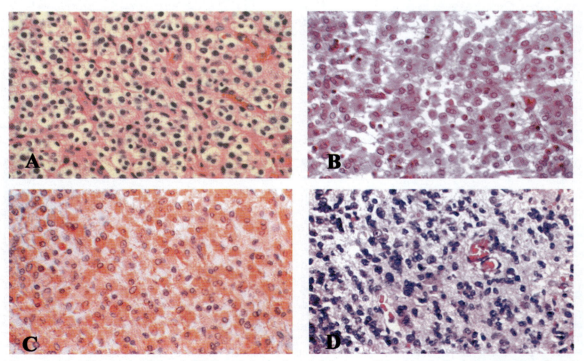

Figure 2–22. Oligodendroglioma. *A*, "Fried-egg" clear cells and delicate capillary network; *B*, minigemistocytes; *C*, glial fibrillary acid protein–positive minigemistocytes; and *D*, anaplastic oligodendroglioma.

ependymal rosettes and positive immunostaining for EMA or cytokeratin. Electron microscopy can also be helpful in making a definitive diagnosis.

Anaplastic oligodendroglioma is characterized by a significantly increased cellularity with nuclear overlap (Figure 2–22D), necrosis, increased mitotic activity, and endothelial proliferation. Increased cellularity and mitotic activity are helpful indicators of anaplastic progression in otherwise classic oligodendrogliomas.

Occasional familial clustering of oligodendroglioma cases has been reported. However, hereditary cancer syndromes involving oligodendrogliomas are rare. Loss of heterozygosity at chromosome 19q represents the most common genetic alteration in low-grade oligodendrogliomas. Loss of heterozygosity of chromosome 1p is the second most common abnormality and appears to occur concurrently with chromosome 19q deletions.[48,49] Chromosome 4q, 11p, and 22q deletions are less common. Anaplastic oligodendrogliomas, while showing chromosome 19q and 1p alterations, also show EGFR overexpression, often without gene amplification. Chromosome 9p and/or 10 deletions have also been implicated in the progression to anaplastic oligodendroglioma. Amplification of cdk4 has been reported in a small subset of anaplastic oligodendroglioma.[50] Chromosome 1p or 19q deletions in anaplastic oligodendrogliomas can be positive predictors of prolonged survival and response to combination chemotherapy with prednisone, cyclophosphamide, and vincristine (PCV).[51]

Mixed Gliomas

Mixed gliomas are being increasingly recognized. Histologically, they are composed of two or more distinct populations of glial elements that can be diffusely mixed or that have predominant cells types in varying proportions in different areas of the tumors. The more common mixed glioma is the oligoastrocytoma (Figure 2–23A), which can present as a WHO grade II tumor or as an anaplastic oligoastrocytoma (Figure 2–23B), which is classified as WHO grade III. The recognition of mixed gliomas and, in particular, the presence of an oligodendroglial component can have therapeutic implications. Ependymoastrocytomas are extremely rare.

Choroid Plexus Tumors

Choroid plexus tumors are intraventricular papillary tumors, ranging from "benign" choroid plexus papilloma (WHO grade I) to malignant choroid plexus carcinoma (WHO grade III). Choroid plexus papillomas occur more commonly in children, with about 10 to 20 percent of cases presenting within the first year of life. Congenital tumors can also occur. Most lateral ventricle tumors are seen in individuals below the age of 20 years. Grossly, choroid plexus papillomas present as well-circumscribed cauliflower-like masses. Histologic features include a distinct papillary pattern with a fibrovascular core and a single layer of cuboidal to columnar epithelium reminiscent of the normal choroid plexus (Figure 2–24).

In contrast, choroid plexus carcinoma is an invasive tumor that can appear solid, hemorrhagic, and necrotic. Histologic features are those of a poorly differentiated anaplastic epithelial-like invasive tumor

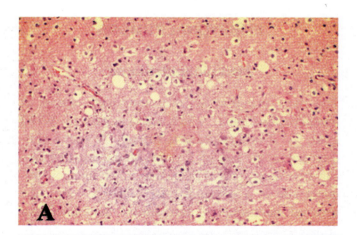

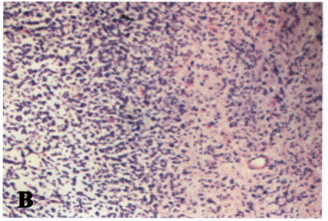

Figure 2–23. Mixed glioma. *A*, Low-grade oligoastrocytoma. *B*, Anaplastic oligoastrocytoma.

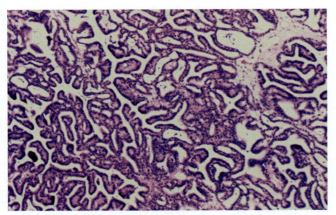

Figure 2–24. Choroid plexus papilloma. Note the resemblance to normal choroid plexus.

with a significant increase in cellularity, brisk mitotic activity, and necrosis. Expression of cytokeratin, vimentin, S-100 protein, and synaptophysin is helpful in distinguishing choroid plexus carcinoma from a metastatic adenocarcinoma since the latter should be negative for S-100 protein and synaptophysin.

EMBRYONAL TUMORS

Medulloepithelioma

The most primitive of the embryonal tumors is medulloepithelioma, which corresponds to WHO grade IV. It occurs characteristically in young children below the age of 5 years. Medulloepithelioma can arise in any part of the neuraxis, but the most frequent site is a periventricular location within the cerebral hemispheres. Intraorbital medulloepitheliomas can also occur. Medulloepithelioma is a primitive neoplastic neuroepithelium mimicking the primitive neural tube. It can be papillary, tubular, or trabecular and represents a distinctive and diagnostic histologic pattern. Aggressive histologic features such as mitotic figures, necrosis, and a population of undifferentiated cells can be present. The tumor cells are positive for nestin and vimentin. Divergent differentiation along neuronal, glial, or mesenchymal elements can also occur.

Medulloblastoma

Medulloblastoma and related primitive neuroectodermal tumors represent another significant group of CNS tumors that occur predominantly in the pediatric population and less frequently in the adult population. They account for 25 percent of childhood intracranial tumors and are the second most common malignant tumors in childhood.

Since morphologic classifications of brain tumors historically were based on the pattern of differentiation and the suspected histogenetic origin of the tumor cells, Bailey and Cushing[52] proposed the name "medulloblastoma" for a specific group of highly aggressive childhood tumors that they presumed arose from the putative stem cell "medulloblast" in the cerebellum (Figure 2–25A and B). Although this name has been widely used for these tumors over the years, the "medulloblast" has remained undefined and has no counterpart in neurogenesis. In recent years, the morphologic similarity between medulloblastoma and other primitive neuroectodermal

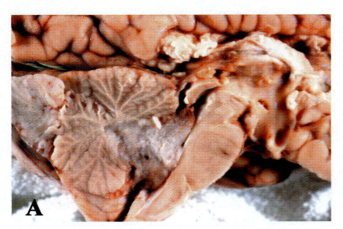
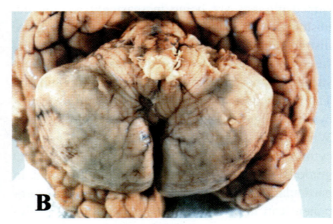

Figure 2–25. Medulloblastoma. *A,* Tumor involving the cerebellar vermis. *B,* Cerebrospinal fluid dissemination.

tumors (PNETs), such as ependymoblastoma, pineoblastoma, and supratentorial PNETs that arise from other sites, has been emphasized. This similarity accounts for the suggested use of the unifying term PNETs for these tumors, irrespective of their primary site of development in the CNS.[53]

The morphologic spectrum of medulloblastoma and related PNETs is varied. It often includes a predominant population of sheets of round to oval (carrot-shaped) undifferentiated and highly proliferative (proliferation index [MIB-1 Index] is usually > 30%) small blue cells (Figure 2–26A). These cells constitute the characteristic histology of the classic medulloblastoma. In a minority of these tumors, neuroblastic differentiation is demonstrated by the formation of Homer Wright rosettes (Figure 2–26B). Focal areas of astrocytic differentiation (Figure 2–26C) can be seen. Divergent differentiation with rhabdomyosarcomatous (medullomyoblastoma) (Figure 2–26D) and melanocytic differentiation (Figure 2–26E) can also be seen. Neuroblastic and astrocytic differentiation, when present, are accompanied by immunopositivity for synaptophysin (Figure 2–26F) (or other neuronal antigens) and GFAP (Figure 2–26G), respectively. This divergent differentiation is consistent with an origin from primitive stem cells that presumably arrested during migration from the germinal matrix. Other distinctive though uncommon histologic features can be seen in subsets of PNETs. These include characteristic ependymoblastic rosettes (multilayered rosettes that merge with surrounding tumor cells) in ependymoblastoma, fleurettes or Flexner-Wintersteiner rosettes in pineoblastomas, and florid desmoplasia (mesenchymal component) in supratentorial PNETs.

Localization of most classic medulloblastomas suggests an origin from proliferative postmigratory precursor cells within the cerebellar vermis whereas the desmoplastic medulloblastoma (Figure 2–26H) subtype (with interspersed pale islands of low proliferative and synaptophysin-positive cells) appears to arise from cells of the external granular layer. The peak incidence for medulloblastoma is within the first two decades. The midline vermis is the frequent site in childhood whereas lateral cerebellar hemispheric tumors (often having desmoplastic features) are seen in adults. Cerebrospinal fluid seeding is common (see Figure 2–25B). Differential positivity for class III β-tubulin, calbindin-D,[54] and neurotrophin receptor trk C[55] has been reported between classic medulloblastoma and desmoplastic medulloblastoma, a finding suggestive of differing histogenetic origins.

Clinical determinants of poor outcome in medulloblastomas include age ≤ 3 years, dissemination at time of presentation, and partial surgical resection.[56] The desmoplastic subtype appears to be associated with a favorable outcome.[57] The large cell variant is associated with shortened survival.[58] Recent molecular studies suggest a correlation between specific genetic events and the prognosis and clinical outcome in medulloblastoma. For example, indicators of poor prognosis include loss of chromosome 17p/17p13[59] and dysregulation of p53 gene expression,[60] either by gene mutation (which is an uncommon event in medulloblastoma)[61] or by other mechanisms such as p53 protein sequestration by SV40 large T antigen.[62] The desmoplastic medulloblastoma subtype shows correlation with chromosome 9q31 deletion[63] (a site that includes the PTCH gene locus), expression of neurotrophin receptor trk C,[55] expression of the cyclin-dependent kinase [cdk] inhibitor p27kip1,[60] and better survival when compared with classic medulloblastoma. Aneuploidy remains an indicator of favorable prognosis.[64]

Atypical Teratoid/Rhabdoid Tumor

The atypical teratoid/rhabdoid tumor is a CNS embryonal tumor with histologic features similar to those of the malignant rhabdoid tumor of the kidney. Even within the same tumor, histologic features can be extremely variable, including rhabdoid, primitive neuroepithelial, epithelial, and mesenchymal components. Irrespective of the spectrum of histologic features, typical rhabdoid cells with eccentric nuclei and prominent nucleoli represent a constant feature (Figure 2–27).[65] The cytoplasm is notably a dense pink and contains whorled bundles of intermediate filaments as seen on electron microscopy. Mitotic activity is very brisk, with areas of necrosis often noted. A germ cell component is notably lacking. The cells show variable immunostaining for vimentin, EMA, GFAP, smooth-muscle actin, and (sometimes) neurofilaments; keratin and desmin can be focally positive. Germ cell tumor markers are usually negative. Molecular studies confirm that this tumor is biologically distinct from the PNETs, with 90 percent of these tumors demonstrating monosomy or loss of heterozygosity or both for chromosome 22. Mutations or deletions in the putative gene

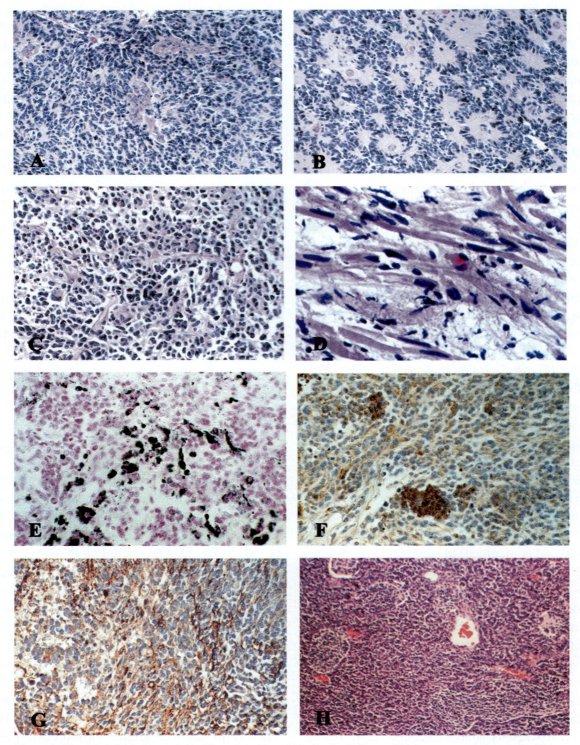

Figure 2–26. Medulloblastoma. *A*, Undifferentiated "small blue" cells. *B*, Homer Wright rosettes. *C*, Astrocytic differentiation. *D*, Skeletal-muscle differentiation with strap cells. *E*, Melanocytic differentiation. *F*, Immunopositivity for synaptophysin. *G*, Immunopositivity for glial fibrillary acidic protein (GFAP). *H*, Desmoplastic variant of medulloblastoma.

hSNF/INI1 have been reported in subsets of CNS and enal rhabdoid tumors.[66]

NEURONAL AND MIXED GLIONEURONAL TUMORS

Gangliocytoma and Ganglioglioma

Gangliocytoma (WHO grade I) and ganglioglioma (WHO grade II) are uncommon tumors that account for only 0.4 to 1.3 percent of all brain tumors at a median age of 8.5 to 25 years. Although these tumors can occur anywhere in the neuraxis, the majority are supratentorial. They are commonly associated with seizures, and most tumors arise in the temporal lobe.

The hallmark of these tumors is the presence of large, multipolar dysplastic neurons (Figure 2–28A). In gangliocytoma, a stroma of non-neoplastic glia cells and reticulin fibers is present whereas there is a neoplastic gliomatous (often pilocytic) component in the ganglioglioma. The gliomatous component can sometimes show anaplastic features (Figures 2–28B to F), warranting a diagnosis of anaplastic ganglioglioma (WHO grade III). Perivascular lymphocytic infiltration is a frequent feature of this tumor. Eosinophilic granular bodies (similar to those in pilocytic astrocytomas), microcysts, and calcification can be seen. A recently described variant of glioneuronal tumors is the papillary glioneuronal tumor characterized by a pseudopapillary histology.[67]

Desmoplastic Infantile Astrocytoma

Desmoplastic infantile astrocytoma (DIA) represents a distinct low-grade (WHO grade I) meningocerebral astocytoma with a prominent desmoplasia (Figure 2–29), characteristically occurring in children below the age of 2 years, although cases occurring in older children have been reported. When a neuronal component is demonstrable, the lesion is referred to as desmoplastic infantile ganglioglioma (DIG). An immature population of neuroepithelial cells can be present. Notable is the frequent attachment of this tumor to dura. Tumors can have a uniloculated or multiloculated cystic component and a solid (often superficial) component. The desmoplastic component can have a prominent storiform pattern and florid reticulin fibers, mimicking a mesenchymal tumor. Immunostaining shows only GFAP and vimentin positivity in desmoplastic infantile astrocytoma or a neuronal component with positivity for synaptophysin and other neuronal antigen markers in desmoplastic infantile ganglioglioma.

Central Neurocytoma

Central neurocytoma is a neuronal tumor that is typically supratentorial. It arises in relation to the lateral and third ventricles, but origin from intraparenchymal sites and the spinal cord has also been described. Peak incidence of the tumor is from 20 to 29 years, and central neurocytoma corresponds to WHO grade II. It is composed of oligodendroglioma-like cells with intervening nucleus-free neuropil (Figure 2–30A). Central neurocytomas show immunopositivity for synaptophysin (Figure

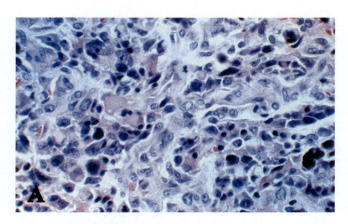
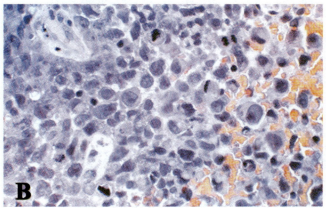

Figure 2–27. Atypical teratoid/rhabdoid tumor. *A,* Anaplastic cells in a mesenchymal stroma. *B,* Characteristic cells with eccentric nuclei and brisk mitotic activity.

2–30B) and other neuronal antigens. Astrocytic differentiation, though rare, has been observed.

Anaplastic variants characterized by increased cellularity and increased mitotic activity can occur. Anaplastic central neurocytomas often have a proliferation index (Ki-67 index) of > 2 percent and demonstrable parenchymal invasion.

Dysembryoplastic Neuroepithelial Tumor

Dysembryoplastic neuroepithelial tumor is a benign WHO grade I tumor arising predominantly in the superficial cortex. This tumor bridges the borderland between hamartoma and neoplasia. Dysembryoplastic neuroepithelial tumor occurs predominantly in children and young adults who often have a long history of poorly controlled partial seizures. Classic complex dysembryoplastic neuroepithelial tumors are multinodular and are characterized by "specific glioneuronal elements" arranged in columns perpendicular to the cortical surface. The columns are formed by bundles of axons with intimately associated oligodendroglia-like (occasionally synaptophysin-positive) cells. Microcystic eosinophilic areas with floating neurons are also present.[68] Cortical dysplasias are often present in adjoining cerebral

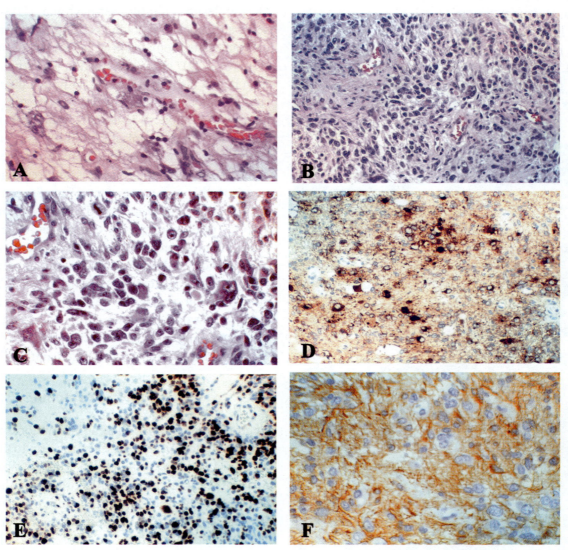

Figure 2–28. Neuroglia tumors. *A*, Gangliocytoma with binucleated neoplastic ganglion cells. *B*, Anaplastic gangliglioma with increased cellularity. *C*, Anaplasia and mitotic activity. *D*, Immunostaining for synaptophysin in anaplastic ganglioma. *E*, MIB-1 immunostaining in an anaplastic ganglioglioma with a high proliferation index. *F*, Glial fibrillary acidic protein immunostaining in an anaplastic ganglioglioma.

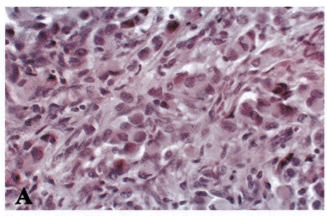
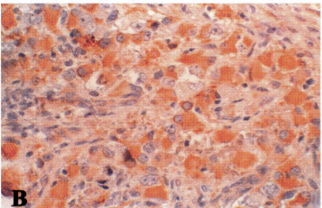

Figure 2–29. Desmoplastic infantile astrocytoma. A, Gemistocyte-like cells in a desmoplastic matrix. B, Immunostain for glial fibrillary acidic protein.

tissue. In the simple form, the histology is less dramatic, can be patchy, and consists of the unique glioneuronal elements only. Although a deep-seated basal ganglia location for this tumor has been reported, the diagnosis of dysembryoplastic neuroepithelial tumor in such a site requires caution because such a diagnosis carries a good prognosis and would result in the deferral of otherwise appropriate therapies. It cannot be overemphasized that combined clinical, radiologic, and pathologic correlations are critical in the accurate diagnosis of dysembryoplastic neuroepithelial tumor.[69,70]

Subependymal Giant Cell Astrocytoma

Subependymal giant cell astrocytoma (WHO grade I) is an intraventricular mass seen in the setting of tuberous sclerosis complex.[71] This complex is characterized by the formation of multiple cortical "tubers" (Figure 2–31A). It appears to evolve from the enlargement of subependymal hamartomatous nodules. It is composed of large eosinophilic astrocyte-like cells with prominent neuron-like nucleoli (Figure 2–31B). The cells classically immunostain for GFAP and have also been reported to be positive for neuronal antigen markers such as synaptophysin.[72]

MISCELLANEOUS TUMORS (INCLUDING TUMORS OF CRANIAL NERVES, LYMPHOID CELLS, AND CELL RESTS)

Schwannoma (Neurilemoma)

Schwannoma is a benign tumor of the peripheral nerve sheath, with a predilection for sensory nerves. It most commonly affects the vestibular portion of the eighth cranial nerve, producing the cerebellopontine-angle mass lesion commonly referred to as acoustic schwannoma (Figure 2–32A). Bilateral acoustic schwannoma is a feature of NF2.

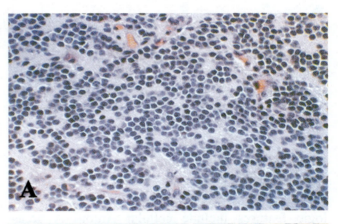
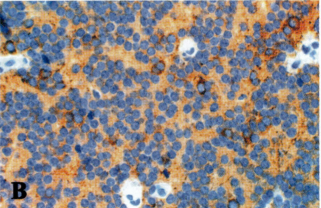

Figure 2–30. Central neurocytoma. A, Monomorphic population of neurocytes with intervening acellular neuropils. B, Perikaryal immunopositivity for synaptophysin.

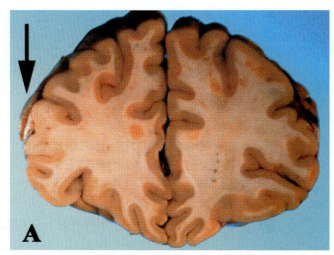
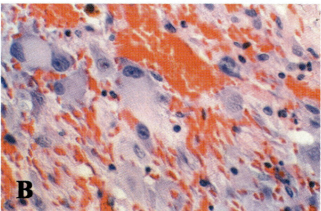

Figure 2–31. *A,* Cortical "tuber" (*arrow*) in tuberous sclerosis. *B,* Subependymal giant cell astrocytoma with large atypical ganglion-like cells.

Although seen less frequently, schwannoma can also involve the fifth cranial nerve, but other cranial nerves are only rarely involved. The classic histologic features include cellular Antoni A areas, Verocay bodies, and loose myxoid Antoni B areas (Figures 2–32B and C). The presence of thick-walled hyalinized vessels is a histologic hallmark of schwannomas. Immunostaining shows positive staining for S-100 protein (Figures 2–32D) and vimentin and negative staining for EMA. Malignant transformation is rare in these tumors.

Primary Central Nervous System Lymphoma

Primary CNS lymphoma is an extranodal lymphoma occurring primarily in the CNS. It must be distinguished from secondary involvement of the CNS by disseminated systemic lymphoma. The frequency of primary CNS lymphoma has increased worldwide, from 1.5 to 6.6 percent of intracranial tumors, primarily due to the acquired immunodeficiency syndrome (AIDS) epidemic. Even in the immune-competent population, there are indications of an increase in the frequency of primary CNS lymphoma, at least in the United States in the past two decades.[73]

More typically, the sporadic (non-AIDS) form of primary CNS lymphoma is seen in elderly individuals and in immunosuppression states such as those following renal transplantation. The epidemic form is associated with AIDS. Tumors are usually located in the cerebral hemispheres and are frequently multicentric and symmetric. Location in the deep basal ganglia may raise the differential diagnosis of toxoplasmosis, especially in the immunodeficiency states. Dissemination to systemic organs is infrequent.

Most CNS lymphomas are non-Hodgkin's lymphomas of B cell origin. Histologically, they appear as a collection of high-grade large cell (Figure 2–33) immunoblastic or small noncleaved-cell lymphomas growing in a diffuse pattern. Extensive coagulative necrosis with isolated islands of viable cells is not uncommon. Neoplastic lymphoid cells often have a perivascular distribution with an increase in perivascular reticulin fibers, an observation leading to the old name of "reticulum cell sarcoma." Although the etiology of primary CNS lymphoma is unknown, more than 95 percent of tumors seen in immunocompromised patients have Epstein-Barr virus (EBV) genome, thus implicating EBV in the induction of B cell proliferation in these individuals.[74,75] Low-grade B cell lymphomas are very uncommon. T cell lymphomas and primary Hodgkin's lymphoma are very rare.[76,77]

Germ Cell Tumors

Germ cell tumors are uncommon in the CNS, accounting for 0.3 to 0.5 percent of all primary intracranial tumors. They present as midline tumors, often in the region of the pineal gland and in the suprasellar region in those below the age of 20 years. Other sites of occurrence include the basal ganglia, the thalamus, and intraventricular, bulbar, and intramedullary spinal cord locations. Histologically, dysgerminoma is similar to gonadal seminoma, with

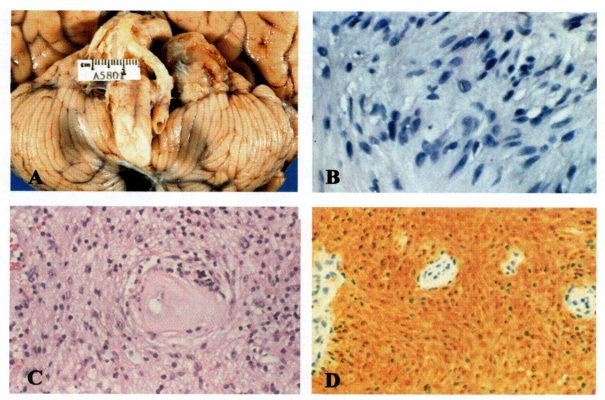

Figure 2–32. Schwannoma. *A,* Cerebellopontine-angle acoustic schwannoma. *B,* Verocay bodies in Antoni A areas. *C,* Loose myxoid Antoni B areas with a hyalinized vessel. *D,* S-100 protein immunostaining.

a uniform population of cells having large vesicular nuclei, prominent nucleoli, and a clear cytoplasm rich in glycogen. Lymphocytic infiltrate and syncytiotrophoblastic giant cells can be seen. Immunostaining for placental alkaline phosphatase (PLAP) is usually positive. The identification of a cytotrophoblastic component is aided by immunostaining for β–human chorionic gonadotropin (β-hCG) and human placental lactogen (HPL). Other germ cell tumors can also occur, showing either a pure histologic subtype or a mixed germ cell tumor composed of any combination of embryonal carcinoma, yolk sac carcinoma, choriocarcinoma, and immature or mature teratomatomatous components.[78]

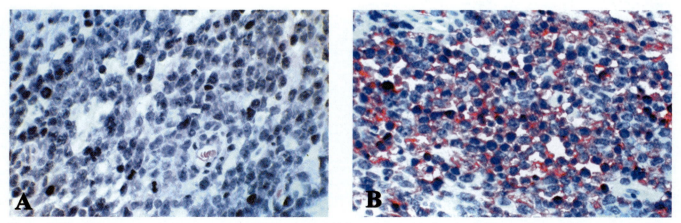

Figure 2–33. Primary central nervous system (CNS) non-Hodgkin's malignant lymphoma. *A,* Diffuse sheet of large cells. *B,* CD20 immunopositivity in tumors, consistent with B cell immunophenotype.

Craniopharyngioma, Colloid Cyst, and Chordoma

Craniopharyngiomas are derived from Rathke's pouch cell rests and present as intrasellar or suprasellar mass lesions with compressive effect on the optic chiasm, third ventricle, hypothalamus, and pituitary. They are usually partly cystic, with prominent calcification. The epithelial component is characterized by keratinizing squamous epithelium with peripheral pallisading (Figure 2–34), sometimes having a close histologic resemblance to adamantinoma.[79] A pseudopapillary pattern is another histologic subtype. A xanthogranulomatous component can also be seen. The cysts often contain oily material (so-called machinery oil), and spillage of this material into CSF causes chemical meningitis. Recurrence is frequent when the tumor is incompletely resected.

A colloid cyst is a mucus-filled epithelial-lined cyst with columnar ciliated cell lining, located typically in

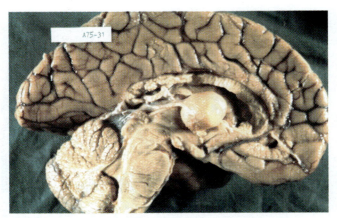

Figure 2–35. A rare sagittal view of a colloid cyst.

the roof of the third ventricle (Figure 2–35). Patients often give a classic history of headache relieved by change of posture. It is not a true neoplasm, but it presents as a mass lesion obstructing the foramen of Monro. Acute obstruction can lead to sudden death.

Chordomas are formed from remnants of the notochord (Figure 2–36A) in the clivus or in the vertebral

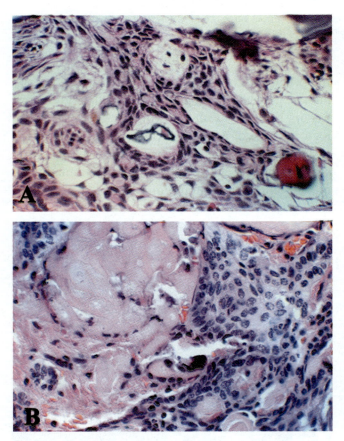

Figure 2–34. Craniopharyngioma. *A*, Adamantinomatous histologic features are characteristic of craniopharyngioma. *B*, Nest of squamoid cells with peripheral pallisading and hyalinized stroma.

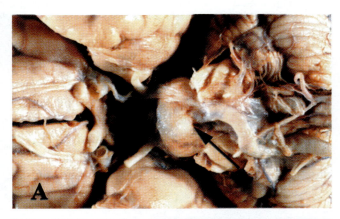

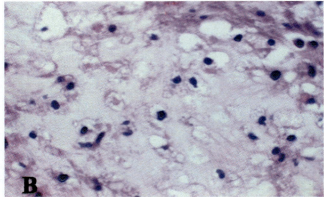

Figure 2–36. Chordoma. *A*, Large notochord remnant "ecchordosis physaliphora" (*arrow*). *B*, Characteristic physaliphorous cells of chordoma.

column, most frequently the sacrum. Chordomas are slow growing and lobulated, with variable cellularity arranged in rows or cords in a myxoid matrix. The typical cell is the vacuolated physaliphorous ("bubble-bearing") cell (Figure 2–36B). Chordomas show positive immunostaining for vimentin, cytokeratin, EMA, and S-100 protein. A histologic subtype with a distinct chondroid component has been referred to as "chondroid chordoma." However, chondroid chordoma possibly represents a low-grade myxoid chondrosarcoma because of its reported lack of staining for epithelial markers and its putative better prognosis.[80,81] This purported better prognosis for chondroid chordoma has been questioned, however, and remains unconfirmed in larger studies.[82]

REFERENCES

1. World Health Organization Classification of Tumors. In: Kleihues P, Cavenee WK, editors. Pathology and genetics, tumors of the nervous system. Lyon: International Agency for Research on Cancer (IARC) Press; 2000. p. 6–7.
2. Lantos PL, VandenBerg SR, Kleihues P. Tumours of the nervous system. In: Graham DI, Lantos PL, editors. Greenfield's neuropathology. 6th ed. London: Arnold; 1996. p. 583–879.
3. Louis DN, Ramesh V, Gusella JF. Neuropathology and molecular genetics of neurofibromatosis 2 and related tumors. Brain Pathol 1995;5:163–72.
4. Matsuno A, Fujimaki T, Sasaki T, et al. Clinical and histopathological analysis of proliferative potentials of recurrent and non-recurrent meningiomas. Acta Neuropathol (Berl) 1996;91:504–10.
5. Harrison MJ, Wolfe DE, Lau TS, et al. Radiation-induced meningiomas: experience at the Mount Sinai Hospital and review of the literature. J Neurosurg 1991;75:564–74.
6. Rutledge MH, Xie YG, Han FY, et al. Deletions on chromosome 22 in sporadic meningioma. Genes Chromosomes Cancer 1994;10:122–30.
7. Lindblom A, Ruttledge M, Collins VP, et al. Chromosomal deletions in anaplastic meningiomas suggest multiple regions outside chromosome 22 as important in tumor progression. Int J Cancer 1994;56:354–7.
8. Simon M, von Deimling A, Larson JJ, et al. Allelic losses on chromosomes 14, 10, and 1 in atypical and malignant meningiomas: a genetic model of meningioma progression. Cancer Res 1995;55:4696–701.
9. Lamszus K, Kluwe L, Matschke J, et al. Allelic losses at 1p, 9q, 10q, 14q, and 22q in the progression of aggressive meningiomas and undifferentiated meningeal sarcomas. Cancer Genet Cytogenet 1999;110:103–10.
10. Maier H, Ofner D, Hittmair A, et al. Classic, atypical, and anaplastic meningioma: three histopathological subtypes of clinical relevance. J Neurosurg 1992;77:616–23.
11. Ludwin SK, Rubinstein LJ, Russell DS. Papillary meningioma: a malignant variant of meningioma. Cancer 1975;36:1363–73.
12. Pasquier B, Gasnier F, Pasquier D, et al. Papillary meningioma. Clinicopathologic study of seven cases and review of the literature. Cancer 1986;58:299–305.
13. Perry A, Scheithauer BW, Stafford SL, et al. "Malignancy" in meningiomas: a clinicopathologic study of 116 patients, with grading implications. Cancer 1999;85:2046–56.
14. Jaaskelainen J. Seemingly complete removal of histologically benign intracranial meningioma: late recurrence rate and factors predicting recurrence in 657 patients. A multivariate analysis. Surg Neurol 1986;26:461–9.
15. Perry A, Stafford SL, Scheithauer BW, et al. Meningioma grading: an analysis of histologic parameters. Am J Surg Pathol 1997;21:1455–65.
16. Soylemezoglu F, Soffer D, Onol B, et al. Lipomatous medulloblastoma in adults: a distinct clinicopathological entity. Am J Surg Pathol 1996;20:413–8.
17. Guthrie BL, Ebersold MJ, Scheithauer BW, Shaw EG. Meningeal hemangiopericytoma: histopathological features, treatment, and long-term follow-up of 44 cases. Neurosurgery 1989;25:514–22.
18. Jaaskelainen J, Servo A, Haltia M, et al. Meningeal hemangiopericytoma. In: Schmidek H, editor. Meningiomas and their surgical treatment. Orlando (FL): WB Saunders; 1991. p. 73–82.
19. Jellinger K, Paulus W, Slowik F. The enigma of meningeal hemangiopericytoma. Brain Tumor Pathol 1991;8:33–43.
20. Vuorinen V, Sallinen P, Haapasalo H, et al. Outcome of 31 intracranial hemangiopericytomas: poor predictive value of cell proliferation indices. Acta Neurochir (Wien) 1996;138:1399–408.
21. Probst-Cousin S, Bergmann M, Schroder R, et al. Ki-67 and biological behaviour in meningeal haemangiopericytomas. Histopathology 1996;29:57–61.
22. Neumann HP, Wiestler OD. Von Hippel-Lindau disease: a syndrome providing insights into growth control and tumorigenesis. Nephrol Dial Transplant 1994;9:1832–3.
23. Bohling T, Hatva E, Kujala M, et al. Expression of growth factors and growth factor receptors in capillary hemangioblastoma. J Neuropathol Exp Neurol 1996;55:522–7.
24. Reifenberger G, Reifenberger J, Bilzer T, et al. Coexpression of transforming growth factor-alpha and epidermal growth factor receptor in capillary hemangioblastomas of the central nervous system. Am J Pathol 1995;147:245–50.
25. Wizigmann V, Breier G, Risau W, Plate KH. Up-regulation of vascular endothelial growth factor and its receptors in von Hippel-Lindau disease-associated and sporadic hemangioblastomas. Cancer Res 1995;55:1358–64.
26. Krouwer HB, Davis RL, Silver P, Prados M. Gemistocytic astrocytomas: a reappraisal. J Neurosurg 1991;74:399–406.
27. Schiffer D, Chio A, Giordana MT, et al. Prognostic value of histologic factors in adult cerebral astrocytoma. Cancer 1988;61:1386–93.
28. Peraud A, Ansari H, Bise K, Reulen HJ. Clinical outcome of supratentorial astrocytoma WHO grade II. Acta Neurochir (Wien) 1998;140:1213–22.
29. Palma L, Di Lorenzo N, Guidetti B. Lymphocytic infiltrates

29. in primary glioblastomas and recidivous gliomas: incidence, fate, and relevance to prognosis in 228 operated cases. J Neurosurg 1978;49:854–61.
30. Lewis RA, Gerson LP, Axelson KA, et al. von Recklinghausen neurofibromatosis. II. Incidence of optic gliomata. Ophthalmology 1984;91:929–35.
31. Tomlinson FH, Scheithauer BW, Hayostek CJ, et al. The significance of atypia and histologic malignancy in pilocytic astrocytoma of the cerebellum: a clinicopathologic and flow cytometric study. J Child Neurol 1994;9:301–10.
32. Powell SZ, Yachnis AT, Rorke LB, et al. Divergent differentiation in pleomorphic xanthoastrocytoma. Evidence for a neuronal element and possible relationship to ganglion cell tumors. Am J Surg Pathol 1996;20:80–5.
33. Perry A, Giannini C, Scheithauer BW, et al. Composite pleomorphic xanthoastrocytoma and ganglioglioma: report of four cases and review of the literature. Am J Surg Pathol 1997;21:763–71.
34. Klein R, Molenkamp G, Sorensen N, Roggendorf W. Favorable outcome of giant cell glioblastoma in a child. Report of an 11-year survival period. Childs Nerv Syst 1998;14:288–91.
35. Burger PC, Vollmer RT. Histologic factors of prognostic significance in the glioblastoma multiforme. Cancer 1980;46:1179–86.
36. Galanis E, Buckner JC, Dinapoli RP, et al. Clinical outcome of gliosarcoma compared with glioblastoma multiforme: North Central Cancer Treatment Group results. J Neurosurg 1998;89:425–30.
37. Watanabe K, Tachibana O, Sato K, et al. Overexpression of the EGF receptor and *p53* mutations are mutually exclusive in the evolution of primary and secondary glioblastomas. Brain Pathol 1996;6:217–24.
38. Reifenberger G, Liu L, Ichimura K, et al. Amplification and overexpression of the MDM2 gene in a subset of human malignant gliomas without p53 mutations. Cancer Res 1993;53:2736–9.
39. Hartwell L. Defects in a cell cycle checkpoint may be responsible for the genomic instability of cancer cells. Cell 1992;71:543–6.
40. Schmidt EE, Ichimura K, Reifenberger G, Collins VP. CDKN2(p16/MTS1) gene deletion or CDK4 amplification occurs in the majority of glioblastomas. Cancer Res 1994;54:6321–4.
41. Costello JF, Berger MS, Huang HJS, Cavenee WK. Silencing of p16/CDKN2 expression in human gliomas by methylation and chromatin condensation. Cancer Res 1996;56:2405–10.
42. Chan AS, Leung SY, Wong MP, et al. Expression of vascular endothelial growth factor and its receptors in the anaplastic progression of astrocytoma, oligodendroglioma, and ependymoma. Am J Surg Pathol 1998;22:816–26.
43. Reyes-Mugica M, Rieger-Christ K, Ohgaki H, et al. Loss of *DCC* expression and glioma progression. Cancer Res 1997;57:382–6.
44. Wang SI, Puc J, Li J, et al. Somatic mutations of PTEN in glioblastoma multiforme. Cancer Res 1997;57:4183–6.
45. James CD, Carlbom E, Dumanski JP, et al. Clonal genomic alterations in glioma malignancy stages. Cancer Res 1988;48:5546–51.
46. von Deimling A, Bender B, Jahnke R, et al. Loci associated with malignant progression in astrocytomas: a candidate on chromosome 19q. Cancer Res 1994;54:1397–401.
47. Ebert C, von Haken M, Meyer-Puttlitz B, et al. Molecular genetic analysis of ependymal tumors: *NF2* mutations and chromosome 22q loss occur preferentially in intramedullary spinal ependymomas. Am J Pathol 1999;155:627–32.
48. Bigner SH, Matthews MR, Rasheed BK, et al. Molecular genetic aspects of oligodendrogliomas including analysis by comparative genomic hybridization. Am J Pathol 1999;155:375–86.
49. Kros JM, van Run PRWA, Alers JC, et al. Genetic aberrations in oligodendroglial tumors: an analysis using comparative genomic hybridization (CGH). J Pathol 1999;188:282–8.
50. Reifenberger G, Reifenberger J, Liu L, et al. Molecular genetics of oligodendroglial tumors. In: Nagai M, editor. Brain tumor research and therapy. Tokyo: Springer-Verlag; 1996. p. 187–209.
51. Cairncross JG, Ueki K, Zlatescu MC, et al. Specific genetic predictors of chemotherapeutic response and survival in patients with anaplastic oligodendrogliomas. J Natl Cancer Inst 1998;90:1473–9.
52. Bailey P, Cushing H. Medulloblastoma cerebelli: a common type of midcerebellar glioma of childhood. Arch Neurol Psychiatry 1925;14:192.
53. Rorke LB, Gilles FH, Davis RL, et al. Revision of the World Health Organization classification of brain tumors for childhood brain tumors. Cancer 1985;56:1869–86.
54. Katsetos CD, Burger PC. Medulloblastoma. Semin Diagn Pathol 1994;11:85–97.
55. Segal RA, Goumnerova LC, Kwon YK, et al. Expression of neurotrophin receptor trk C is linked to a favorable outcome in medulloblastoma. Proc Natl Acad Sci U S A 1994;91:12867–71.
56. Packer RJ. Childhood medulloblastoma: progress and future challenges. Brain Dev 1999;21:75–81.
57. Giangaspero F, Perilongo G, Fondelli MP, et al. Medulloblastoma with extensive nodularity: a variant with favorable prognosis. J Neurosurg 1999;91:971–7.
58. Giangaspero F, Bigner SH, Kleihues P, et al. Medulloblastoma. In: Kleihues P, Cavenee WK, editors. Pathology and genetics, tumors of the nervous system. Lyon: International Agency for Research on Cancer (IARC) Press; 2000. p. 129–37.
59. Batra SK, McLendon RE, Koo JS, et al. Prognostic implications of chromosome 17p deletions in human medulloblastomas. J Neurooncol 1995;24:39–45.
60. Adesina AM, Dunn ST, Moore WE, Nalbantoglu J. Expression of p27kip1 and p53 in medulloblastoma: relationship with cell proliferation and survival. Pathol Res Pract 2000;196:243–50.
61. Adesina AM, Nalbantoglu J, Cavenee WK. p53 gene mutation and mdm2 gene amplification are uncommon in medulloblastoma. Cancer Res 1994;54:5649–51.
62. Krynska B, Del Valle L, Croul S, et al. Detection of human neurotropic JC virus DNA sequence and expression of the viral oncogenic protein in pediatric medulloblastomas. Proc Natl Acad Sci U S A 1999;96:11519–24.
63. Schofield D, West DC, Anthony DC, et al. Correlation of loss

of heterozygosity at chromosome 9q with histologic subtype in medulloblastomas. Am J Pathol 1995;146:472–80.
64. Yasue M, Tomita T, Engelhard H, et al. Prognostic importance of DNA ploidy in medulloblastoma of childhood. J Neurosurg 1989;70:385–91.
65. Rorke LB, Packer RJ, Biegel JA. Central nervous system atypical teratoid/rhabdoid tumors in infancy and childhood: definition of an entity. J Neurosurg 1996;85:56–65.
66. Biegel JA, Zhou JY, Rorke LB, et al. Germ-line and acquired mutations of INI1 in atypical teratoid and rhabdoid tumors. Cancer Res 1999;59:74–9.
67. Komori T, Scheithauer BW, Anthony D, et al. Papillary glioneuronal tumor: a new variant of mixed neuronal-glial neoplasm. Am J Surg Pathol 1998;22:1171–83.
68. Daumas-Duport C, Scheithauer BW, Chodkiewicz JP, et al. Dysembryoplastic neuroepithelial tumor: a surgically curable tumor of young patients with intractable partial seizures. Report of thirty-nine cases. Neurosurgery 1988;23:545–56.
69. Daumas-Duport C. Dysembryoplastic neuroepithelial tumours. Brain Pathol 1993;3:283–95.
70. Honavar M, Janota I. 73 cases of dysembryoplastic neuroepithelial tumour: the range of histological appearances. Brain Pathol 1994;4:428.
71. Roach ES, DiMario FJ, Kandt RS, Northrup H. Tuberous Sclerosis Consensus Conference: recommendations for diagnostic evaluation. National Tuberous Sclerosis Association. J Child Neurol 1999;4:401–7.
72. Lopes MBS, Altermatt HJ, Scheithauer BW, VandenBerg SR. Immunohistochemical characterization of subependymal giant cell astrocytomas. Acta Neuropathol 1996;91:368–75.
73. Eby NL, Grufferman S, Flannelly CM, et al. Increasing incidence of primary brain lymphoma in the US. Cancer 1988;62:2461–5.
74. Camilleri-Broet S, Davi F, Feuillard J, et al. AIDS-related primary brain lymphomas: histopathologic and immunohistochemical study of 51 cases. The French study group for HIV-associated tumors. Hum Pathol 1997;28:367–74.
75. Morgello S. Pathogenesis and classification of primary central nervous system lymphoma: an update. Brain Pathol 1995;5:383–93.
76. Bednar MM, Salerni A, Flanagan ME, Pendlebury WW. Primary central nervous system T-cell lymphoma. Case report. J Neurosurg 1991;74:668–72.
77. Ashby MA, Barber PC, Holmes AE, et al. Primary intracranial Hodgkin's disease. A case report and discussion. Am J Surg Pathol 1988;12:294–9.
78. Rosenblum MK, Matsutani M, Van Meir EG. CNS germ cell tumors. In: Kleihues P, Cavenee WK, editors. Pathology and genetics: tumors of the nervous system. Lyon: IARC Press; 2000. p. 208–14.
79. Paulus W, Stockel C, Krauss J, et al. Odontogenic classification of craniopharyngiomas: a clinicopathological study of 54 cases. Histopathology 1997;30:172–6.
80. Dahlin DC, MacCarty CS. Chordoma: a study of fifty-nine cases. Cancer 1952;5:1170–8.
81. Heffelfinger MJ, Dahlin DC, MacCarty CS, Beabout JW. Chordomas and cartilaginous tumors at the skull base. Cancer 1973;32:410–20.
82. Mitchell A, Scheithauer BW, Unni KK, et al. Chordoma and chondroid neoplasms of the spheno-occiput. An immunohistochemical study of 41 cases with prognostic and nosologic implications. Cancer 1993;72:2943–9.

Familial Brain Tumor Syndromes

EDWARD PAN, MD
JANE H. UYEHARA-LOCK, MD
MARTIN KELLY NICHOLAS, MD, PhD

The familial brain tumor syndromes are a heterogeneous group of disorders characterized by certain systemic clinical manifestations with a concurrent association of a variety of central nervous system (CNS) neoplasms. Some of these syndromes are classified as neurocutaneous syndromes, or phakomatoses, which is derived from the Greek word meaning "birthmark." Phakomatoses have particular skin lesions associated with CNS tumors and other systemic manifestations. Many of these familial brain tumor syndromes have been mapped to specific chromosomes and have identifiable genes and protein products (Table 3–1). Since definitive treatments have not yet been developed, screening and surveillance protocols are crucial for the detection and treatment of the clinical manifestations in their early stages. With further research, the molecular genetics of these syndromes will be completely delineated, which should lead to improved therapies and possibly to their cure and eradication.

NEUROFIBROMATOSIS TYPE 1

Von Recklinghausen's neurofibromatosis type 1 (NF1) is one of the most common genetic syndromes, with a prevalence of approximately 1 in 4,000.[1] Neurofibromatosis type 1 accounts for 90 percent of all of the neurofibromatosis cases and is a completely distinct syndrome from type 2 (NF2).[2] The most common CNS tumors associated with NF1 are low-grade astrocytomas, plexiform neurofibromas, and optic nerve gliomas.[2] It is an autosomal dominant multisystem disorder with 100 percent penetrance and a spontaneous mutation rate of about 50 percent.[3] The NF1 gene is located on chromosome 17q11.2 and codes for a large tumor-suppressor protein called neurofibromin.[4–6] Some studies suggest that some brain tumors in NF1 patients are less aggressive than the corresponding tumors of the same histologic type in patients without NF1.[7] Thus, the treatment of CNS tumors in NF1 warrants conservative management with close clinical and radiologic follow-up.

Clinical Features

Neurofibromatosis type 1 is the most common of the neurocutaneous disorders known as the phakomatoses. The diagnosis is primarily made by clinical criteria (Table 3–2).[8] Occasionally, the diagnosis is made radiographically when the cutaneous signs are subtle or absent. The earliest of the cutaneous lesions are café-au-lait spots (Figure 3–1A), which usually are present at birth and increase in size and number during the first few years of life.[9] Other typical skin lesions of NF1 include axillary freckling (see Figure 3–1B), usually 1 to 3 mm in diameter, and Lisch nodules (see Figure 3–1C), which are asymptomatic pigmented hamartomas of the iris that are pathognomonic for NF1. Since Lisch nodules are often not apparent in early childhood, their absence does not exclude the diagnosis of NF1.[9] Other lesions that appear outside of the CNS are listed in Table 3–3.

Patients with NF1 are at increased risk of developing three distinct clinical groups of benign and malignant neoplasms: CNS tumors, peripheral ner-

Table 3–1. FAMILIAL BRAIN TUMOR SYNDROMES

Syndrome	Characteristic CNS Lesions	Characteristic Skin Lesions	Ophthalmologic Features	Chromosome	Gene	Protein
NF1	Optic pathway glioma Brainstem glioma Neurofibromatosis bright objects (NBO)	Café-au-lait spots Axillary freckling	Lisch nodules	17q11	*NF1*	Neurofibromin
NF2	Bilateral acoustic schwannomas Multiple meningiomas	NF2 plaque Subcutaneous schwannomas		22q12	*NF2*	Merlin
Retinoblastoma	Pineoblastoma (trilateral retinoblastoma)		Leukokoria	13q14	*RB1*	RB1
von Hippel-Lindau	Hemangioblastoma of cerebellum/spine		Retinal angioma (hemangioblastoma)	3p25	*VHL*	VHL
Tuberous sclerosis	Subependymal giant cell astrocytoma Subependymal nodule Cortical tuber	"Ash-leaf" spots Adenoma sebaceum Shagreen patch Ungual fibroma	Retinal astrocytoma ("mulberry lesion")	9q34 16p13.3	*TSC1* *TSC2*	Hamartin Tuberin
Sturge-Weber	Leptomeningeal angiomatosis Cortical calcifications Hemispheric atrophy	Port-wine nevus	Choroidal hemangioma Glaucoma			
Turcot's	Glioblastoma (BTP type 1) Medulloblastoma (BTP type 2)			5q21	*DNA mismatch repair genes* *APC*	
Nevoid basal cell carcinoma (Gorlin's)	Medulloblastoma	Basal cell carcinoma (BCC)		9q22.3	*PTCH*	
Lhermitte-Duclos/Cowden	Dysplastic gangliocytoma of cerebellum	Facial trichilemmoma (Cowden syndrome)		10q23.3 (Cowden syndrome)	*PTEN*	
Li-Fraumeni	Malignant glioma PNET			17q (between exons 5 and 9)	*p53*	

APC = adenomatous polyposis coli; BTP = brain tumor-polyposis; CNS = central nervous system; DNA = deoxyribonucleic acid; NF = neurofibromatosis; PNET = primitive neuroectodermal tumor; PTCH = patched; RB = retinoblastoma; TSC = tuberous sclerosis complex; VHL = von Hippel-Lindau.

Table 3–2. NATIONAL INSTITUTES OF HEALTH DIAGNOSTIC CRITERIA FOR NEUROFIBROMATOSIS TYPE 1*

- ≥ 6 café-au-lait spots
  - >5 mm in greatest diameter in prepubertal patients OR
  - >15 mm in greatest diameter in postpubertal patients
- ≥ 2 neurofibromas (of any type) or ≥ 1 plexiform neurofibromas
- ≥ 2 Lisch nodules (hamartomas of the iris)
- Axillary or inguinal freckling
- Optic pathway glioma
- First-degree relative (parent, sibling, or offspring) diagnosed with NF1
- Distinctive osseous lesion (eg, sphenoid wing dysplasia)

NF1 = neurofibromatosis type 1.
*Diagnosis requires two or more criteria.
Adapted from Ruggieri M, Huson SM. The neurofibromatoses. An overview. Ital J Neurol Sci 1999;20:89–108.

vous system (PNS) solid tumors, and leukemias (particularly in children). The majority of the CNS and PNS tumors in NF1 follow an indolent course.[10] The predominant intracranial tumors associated with NF1 are the optic pathway and brainstem gliomas, with optic nerve gliomas being the most common (see Figures 3–1D and E). Approximately 15 percent of patients with NF1 have unilateral or bilateral optic pathway gliomas (OPGs).[9] The most likely time for a symptomatic OPG to develop is within the first 6 years of life, with a median age of 4.2 years at detection.[11,12] Only about one-third of patients with NF1 and OPG will develop visual symptoms. The most dramatic presentation of a symptomatic optic glioma is rapidly progressive proptosis, which occurs in about 30 percent of symptomatic tumors.[12] Other visual symptoms include decreased visual acuity, afferent pupillary defect, optic nerve atrophy, strabismus, papilledema, and defects in color vision. Unfortunately, significant loss of visual acuity may go unrecognized by the patient.

Pathologically, OPGs are classified as World Health Organization (WHO) grade I astrocytomas, or pilocytic astrocytomas. They are characterized by a biphasic pattern of loose multipolar cells and compact bipolar "piloid" cells with long hairlike processes (see Figure 3–1F). The compact regions may contain Rosenthal fibers, which are eosinophilic hyaline structures within the cytoplasm of astrocytes (see Figure 3–1G). Vascular proliferation is another prominent feature of pilocytic astrocytomas. Histologically, they are identical to pilocytic astrocytomas located elsewhere in the CNS and are indistinguishable from other OPGs not associated with NF1.

About two-thirds of OPGs in children with NF1 affect the optic chiasm. Such children may be at increased risk for developing precocious puberty, with accelerated linear growth often being the first sign. In one series, precocious puberty was found to be the initial complaint in 30 percent of NF1 patients with optic chiasmal tumors.[12] Other symptoms of chiasmal involvement include hypopituitarism, dwarfism, diabetes insipidus, obesity, and increased intracranial pressure. Although symptomatic chiasmal gliomas in NF1 patients are more likely to progress than the intraorbital tumors, most chiasmal gliomas remain quiescent.

Brainstem gliomas in NF1 represent complex entities that differ clinically and radiographically from those not associated with NF1. Molloy and colleagues observed 17 patients with brainstem gliomas and NF1. Only 6 of 17 patients had radiographic tumor progression (mean follow-up of 63 months), and only 3 of those 6 patients had concomitant clinical progression requiring treatment. The pathology of their lesions was consistent with astrocytoma, with 14 of 17 tumors occurring in the medulla.[7] These characteristics differ significantly from brainstem gliomas in patients without NF1, which usually occur in the pons and have very poor long-term outcomes; death from progressive disease usually occurs within 18 months of diagnosis.[7,13] The etiology for the significant difference in the long-term outcomes between brainstem glioma patients with and without NF1 is unclear. There have been reported cases of brainstem gliomas in NF1 that were shown to be low-grade gliomas on biopsy.[14,15] Yet, in many of these cases, the tumor's behavior was even more indolent than that of a typical low-grade glioma since they remained quiescent for years without adjuvant treatment. This raises the intriguing possibility of these brainstem gliomas being more appropriately classified as glial hamartomas.[10]

The typical PNS lesion in NF1 is the plexiform neurofibroma, which is a neoplasm that arises from within a nerve to produce a fusiform mass incorporating the nerve and its axons (see Figure 3–1H). In NF1, they typically involve paraspinal nerves and large peripheral nerve trunks, as well as cranial nerves. Histologically, neurofibromas are composed of a mixture of neoplastic Schwann-like cells and fibroblasts in a background of collagen fibers and myxoid matrix (see Figure 3–1I). In the spine, they appear as intradural extramedullary masses extending out through the neural foramina. The foramina become widened, resulting in the characteristic "dumbbell" shape of the tumors. Other spinal lesions seen in NF1 include intrinsic spinal cord gliomas, dural ectasias, and arachnoid cysts extending out through the exit foramina, particularly in the thoracic region (lateral meningoceles). Malignant peripheral nerve sheath tumors (MPNSTs) are the most common malignancies for which NF1 patients are at increased risk. These tumors are characterized by hypercellularity, increased pleomorphism and mitotic activity, and invasion of surrounding structures. Two-thirds of MPNSTs arise from preexisting plexiform neurofibromas.

Radiographic Features

Magnetic resonance imaging is the neuroimaging modality of choice for tumor evaluation in NF1. In NF1, OPGs and brainstem gliomas are typically isointense to brain on T1-weighted MRI images and hyperintense on T2-weighted images. Optical pathway gliomas often enhance with gadolinium whereas brainstem gliomas are usually non-enhancing. Gliomas in NF1 are radiologically indistinguishable from those not associated with NF1.[16]

Neurofibromatosis bright objects (NBOs) are special neuroradiologic findings specifically associated with NF1 (see Figure 3–1J). They also are typically isointense with gray matter on T1-weighted sequences and hyperintense on T2-weighted sequences. Fluid-attenuated inversion recovery (FLAIR) sequences are particularly sensitive in showing these lesions.[17] The lesions are generally not associated with edema or mass effect, do not enhance with gadolinium, and are not associated with neurologic deficits. Most NBOs are found in the globus pallidus and brain stem, particularly in the midbrain.[2] They occur in early childhood and increase in size until 10 to 12 years of age, and usually disappear by 20 years of age.[3,18] Their precise nature is unclear. Postulated pathologies include heterotopias, hamartomas, dysplasias, or areas of gliosis.[2] However, these pathologies do not fit with the signal characteristics and age-related behavior of NBOs. Although the majority of NBOs follow a benign course with regression by the age of 20 years, the NBOs that do not regress may herald tumor growth.

The role of magnetic resonance spectroscopy (MRS) has recently emerged to potentially enhance noninvasive radiographic monitoring of intracranial lesions in NF1. The principle of spectroscopy is to analyze the choline (CHO)/creatine (CRE) ratios of MRI regions that are suspicious for tumor. Norfray and colleagues followed 24 intracranial lesions in 19 NF1 patients by MRI and MRS. Spectroscopy was able to distinguish three distinct spectra of lesions: a hamartoma spectrum (CHO/CRE < 1.5), a transitional spectrum (CHO/CRE between 1.5 and 2.0), and a glioma spectrum (CHO/CRE > 2.0). Thus, MRS identified those spectra that distinguished hamartomas from gliomas as well as transitional lesions that could progress to gliomas or regress to hamartomas.[19] MRS provided additional imaging value, compared to MRI, by identifying cellularity changes whereas magnetic resonance (MR) images remained stable. Thus, combining MRS with MRI can provide a more accurate characterization of the activity of these NF1 intracranial lesions and can provide further support in determining when appropriate treatment (such as surgery) should be instituted.

Genetics

The linkage of NF1 to chromosome 17q was first described by Barker and colleagues[20] and Seizinger and colleagues.[21] The NF1 gene has been mapped to chromosome 17q11.2 and codes for a protein made up of 2,818 amino acids and called neurofibromin, which has a domain related to mammalian *ras* guanosine triphosphatase (GTPase)–activating protein (GAP) and yeast inhibitor of *ras* activity (IRA) protein, both of which are negative regulators of *ras* protein.[22] The GAP-related domain of neurofibromin catalyzes the conversion of the active GTP-bound form of *ras* p21, a proto-oncogene, to the inactive GDP-bound form.[23] Neurofibromin has also been shown to be involved in the negative control of *ras* in intact cells and in the inhibition of cell prolifera-

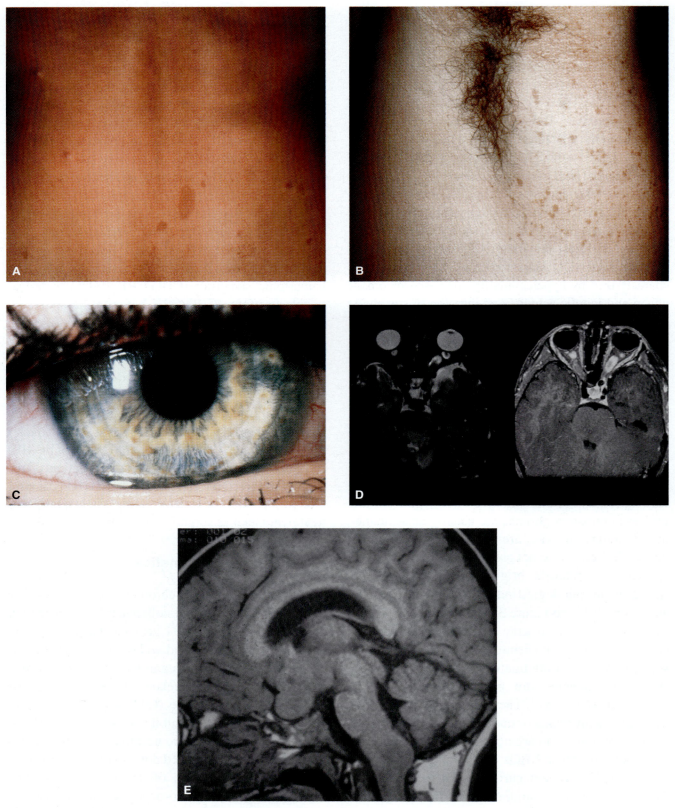

Figure 3–1. *A*, Café-au-lait spots on the midline lower back in a patient with neurofibromatosis type 1 (NF1) *B*, Axillary freckling in a patient with NF1. *C*, Multiple melanocytic hamartomas of the iris (Lisch nodules). *D*, T2-weighted and contrast-enhanced T1-weighted axial magnetic resonance imaging (MRI) of bilateral optic nerve gliomas in NF1. The tumors appear hyperintense on both images. *E*, T1-weighted pre-contrast sagittal MRI demonstrating hypothalamic and brainstem (medullary) gliomas in NF1. The tumors are hypointense to gray matter.

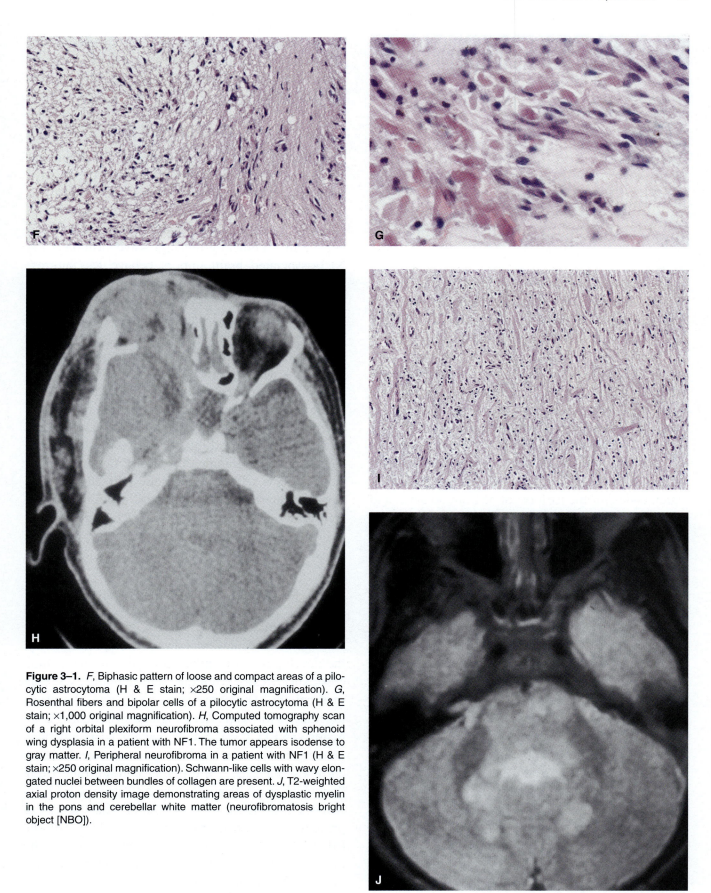

Figure 3–1. *F*, Biphasic pattern of loose and compact areas of a pilocytic astrocytoma (H & E stain; ×250 original magnification). *G*, Rosenthal fibers and bipolar cells of a pilocytic astrocytoma (H & E stain; ×1,000 original magnification). *H*, Computed tomography scan of a right orbital plexiform neurofibroma associated with sphenoid wing dysplasia in a patient with NF1. The tumor appears isodense to gray matter. *I*, Peripheral neurofibroma in a patient with NF1 (H & E stain; ×250 original magnification). Schwann-like cells with wavy elongated nuclei between bundles of collagen are present. *J*, T2-weighted axial proton density image demonstrating areas of dysplastic myelin in the pons and cerebellar white matter (neurofibromatosis bright object [NBO]).

Table 3–3. LESIONS OF NEUROFIBROMATOSIS TYPE 1 THAT OCCUR OUTSIDE THE CENTRAL NERVOUS SYSTEM

Café-au-lait spots
Axillary freckling
Cutaneous neurofibromas
Lisch nodules
Retinal phakomas
Buphthalmos
Bone/vascular dysplasias
Endocrine tumors
Renal artery stenosis

Adapted from Romanowski CA, Cavallin LI. Neurofibromatosis types I and II: radiological appearance. Hosp Med 1998;59:134–9.

tion.[23] Loss of neurofibromin results in increased p21-*ras* activity and increased astrocyte proliferation, leading to tumor formation. Hence, the NF1 gene is considered to be a tumor-suppressor gene.

The NF1 gene produces multiple transcripts generated by alternative splicings that encode neurofibromin and its isoforms.[23] These isoforms include type I messenger ribonucleic acid (mRNA), which codes for neurofibromin of 2,818 amino acids; type II mRNA, which codes for neurofibromin containing the insertion of 21 amino acids in the GAP-related domain;[24–26] and an N-isoform mRNA, which codes for the isoform of 551 amino acids and that shares the same N-terminal 547 residues with neurofibromin but lacks the GAP-related domain.[27] The type II isoform has lower GAP activity than the type I isoform.[23] Astrocytic tumors have been found to predominantly express the type II NF1 mRNA whereas normal tissues predominantly express the type I mRNA isoform.[28] The N-isoform mRNA is similarly expressed in both brain tumors and normal brain tissues.[23] Thus, it appears that increased type II NF1 protein may play an important role in the growth of astrocytic tumors.[28]

Loss of NF1 expression at the ribonucleic acid (RNA) and protein level has been demonstrated in MPNSTs, pheochromocytomas, and myeloid leukemic cells. Also, loss of heterozygosity (LOH) in the NF1 region and NF1 gene mutations have been identified in NF1-associated malignant tumors.[29] In a study by Gutmann and colleagues, immunohistochemistry demonstrated loss of neurofibromin expression in 8 of 8 pilocytic astrocytomas.[29] Thus, not only does NF1 play a critical role in the molecular pathogenesis of NF1-associated malignant tumors, but it also appears to be an important primary event in the pathogenesis of nonaggressive NF1-associated pilocytic astrocytomas.

Management

The essential guiding principle of the treatment approach for gliomas in NF1 patients is conservative management. This is based on several factors: (1) the vast majority of NF1-associated tumors are optic pathway pilocytic astrocytomas, which tend to behave in a clinically nonaggressive fashion;[29] (2) NF1-associated brain tumors behave less aggressively than tumors not associated with NF1 in similar locations;[7,10,30,31] (3) both optic pathway[32,33] and tectal gliomas[34] have been reported to spontaneously regress (partially or nearly completely) without treatment; and (4) many radiographic abnormalities in patients with NF1 (eg, NBO) are benign and usually not associated with tumor progression.[2,19] Therefore, treatment with a combination of surgery, chemotherapy, and radiation should be reserved for those patients who exhibit clinically symptomatic or significant radiographic evidence of tumor progression. Patients with asymptomatic NF1 should have periodic physical and neurologic examinations as well as serial neuroimaging by MRI. Patients with known OPGs should also have frequent eye evaluations by an experienced ophthalmologist.

NEUROFIBROMATOSIS TYPE 2

Neurofibromatosis type 2 (NF2) is an autosomal dominant neurocutaneous disorder characterized by the development of tumors derived from the neural crest, specifically vestibular schwannoma (VS) and meningioma. For many years, NF2 was classified together with von Recklinghausen's neurofibromatosis (NF1). It was finally recognized as a distinct genetic entity when the NF2 gene was localized to chromosome 22q12, a different chromosome from that which is the location of the NF1 gene (17q11.2). It has a prevalence of 1 in 50,000[1] and encodes a protein called moesin-ezrin-radixin–like protein (MERLIN) (or schwannomin),[35,36] which is thought to be a unique tumor-suppressor protein with an undefined mechanism of action.[37]

Clinical Features

The diagnostic criteria for NF2 are listed in Table 3–4. Patients with unilateral VS or multiple meningiomas in addition to some of the other features of NF2 should be considered as possibly having NF2 and should be evaluated more thoroughly. The hallmark of NF2 is the development of bilateral VS, which may not be synchronous (Figure 3–2A). Neurofibromatosis type 2 may be clinically divided into mild (Gardner) and severe (Wishart) subtypes. Patients with the Gardner subtype usually present after the age of 25 years, develop fewer and more indolent tumors (often only bilateral VS), and generally survive beyond the fifth decade.[8] However, patients with the Wishart subtype usually present before 25 years of age, develop three or more tumors, require repeated surgeries, and often do not survive beyond 50 years of age.[38] Vestibular schwannomas in NF2 patients usually become symptomatic in the second or third decades of life. This is in contrast to patients without NF2 (including those with NF1), whose VSs typically become symptomatic in the fifth or sixth decades. Other clinical manifestations of NF2 are listed in Table 3–5.

The first presenting symptom in most NF2 patients is hearing loss, which is often initially unilateral. Hearing loss may be preceded or accompanied by tinnitus, vertigo, and imbalance. These symptoms are attributed to VS affecting the eighth (vestibulocochlear) cranial nerve. Among NF2 patients, 20 to 30 percent present with non-VS tumors, which may herald a more severe disease course.

Histologically, schwannomas are spindle cell neoplasms composed of compact elongated cells (with occasional palisading nuclei [Antoni A areas]) alternating with loosely arranged areas of decreased cellularity containing lipid-laden cells (Antoni B areas) (see Figure 3–2B). Verocay bodies (regions of nuclear palisades separated by anucleate areas) are present in Antoni A areas and are seen more often in schwannomas not associated with the eighth cranial nerve (see Figure 3-2C). The neoplastic process involves only the Schwann cells whereas neurofibromas involve both Schwann cells and nerve fibers and consequently have axons running through the tumor.

The meningiomas in NF2 patients present similarly to those occurring sporadically, except that in NF2, they occur at an earlier age and are frequently multiple.[3] They typically occur supratentorially in the falx and around the frontal, parietal, and temporal regions, as well as intraspinally (see Figure 3–2A). As many as 10 percent of patients presenting with an isolated meningioma in childhood go on to develop NF2.[39] The most common subtypes are fibrous, meningothelial, and transitional meningiomas. Histologically, they have a lobular architecture with formations of concentric whorls of cells (see Figure 3–2D). Malignant progression of meningiomas is occasionally associated with radiation treatment.[40]

Other lesions associated with NF2 include spinal schwannomas and neurofibromas. Low-grade ependymomas and gliomas in NF2 patients occur mostly in the cervical spine and brain stem and are usually very indolent.[41] Thus, management of these lesions is controversial.

The cutaneous features of NF2 are more subtle and occur less frequently than those of NF1. Only 10 percent of NF2 patients with skin tumors have more than 10 lesions.[41] There are several different types of skin tumors, the most common being an intracutaneous, slightly raised, pigmented plaque-like lesion often containing excess hair. Other lesions occur as deep subcutaneous nodular tumors on large peripheral nerves. The majority of these subcutaneous lesions are schwannomas and are not neurofibromas; however, neurofibromas do occasionally occur in NF2.

Ophthalmologic features are also prominent in NF2. Cataracts, the most common eye finding in NF2, are developed by 60 to 80 percent of NF2 patients;[41] they are presenile posterior subcapsular opacities that rarely require excision. Other ophthal-

Table 3–4. DIAGNOSTIC CRITERIA FOR NEUROFIBROMATOSIS TYPE 2	
Either	Bilateral vestibular schwannoma (VS) or Family history (1st-degree relative) of NF2 PLUS unilateral VS diagnosed earlier than 30 years of age Or
Two of	Meningioma Schwannoma Glioma Juvenile posterior subcapsular lens opacities Juvenile cortical cataract

NF2 = neurofibromatosis type 2.
Adapted from Ruggieri M, Huson SM. The neurofibromatoses. An overview. Ital J Neurol Sci 1999;20:89–108.

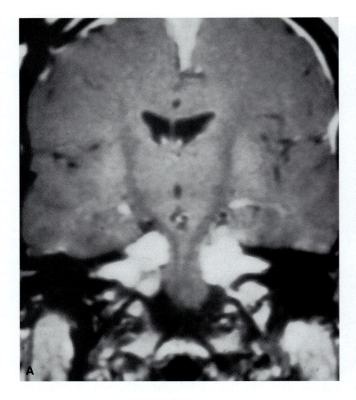
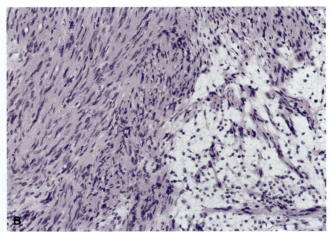
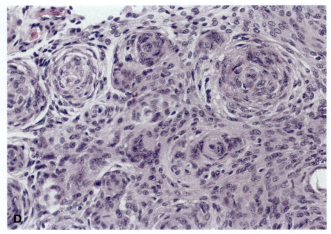
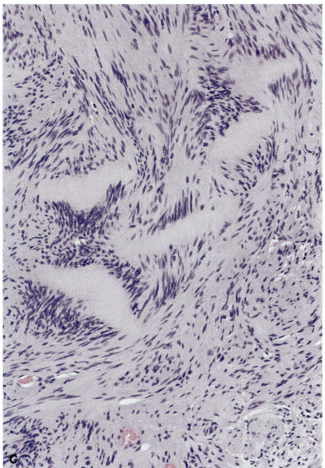

Figure 3–2. *A*, T1-weighted coronal postcontrast magnetic resonance imaging (MRI) of bilateral vestibular schwannomas and midline falcian meningiomas. The lesions enhance brightly with gadolinium. *B*, Biphasic pattern of a schwannoma with compact (Antoni A) and loose (Antoni B) areas (H & E stain; ×500 original magnification). *C*, Verocay bodies in a schwannoma (H & E stain; ×250 original magnification). *D*, Transitional meningioma. Note the lobular architecture and concentric whorls of cells (H & E stain; ×500 original magnification).

Table 3–5. CLINICAL FEATURES OF NEUROFIBROMATOSIS TYPE 2

- Bilateral vestibular schwannomas
- Multiple meningiomas
- Spinal cord meningiomas
- Spinal cord ependymomas
- Café-au-lait spots
- Nerve root schwannomas
- Cataracts

Adapted from Romanowski CA, Cavallin LI. Neurofibromatosis types I and II: radiological appearance. Hosp Med 1998;59:134–9.

mologic features include optic nerve meningiomas and retinal hamartomas, both of which can cause visual disturbances and can be misdiagnosed as retinoblastomas. Optic nerve meningiomas can cause visual loss in the first years of life.

Genetics

In 1993, detailed deletion mapping analyses pinpointed the location of the NF2 gene to chromosome 22q12.[35,36] The NF2 complimentary deoxyribonucleic acid (cDNA) encodes a protein of 595 amino acids, with homology to a highly conserved protein family that is thought to connect the cytoskeleton to plasma membrane components.[41] Members of this band-4.1 superfamily of proteins include ezrin, moesin, and radixin. The NF2 gene product exhibits its most extensive homology (63%) to these specific proteins, which gives rise to the name of the NF2 gene product, MERLIN (from *m*oesin-*e*zrin-*r*adixin–*l*ike-prote*in*).[35,41] This gene product has two predominant isoforms that are generated by the inclusion or exclusion of exon 16: isoform I lacks exon 16 and has 595 amino acids; isoform II includes exon 16 and a premature stop codon, has 590 amino acids, and has a modified C-terminus.[42] These isoforms appear to be tissue specific; in cranial nerve VIII, only isoform I is detectable whereas the cerebellum almost exclusively contains isoform II.[42] In experimental models, only isoform I is associated with the potential to inhibit cell growth, suggesting that protein conformation may be relevant for tumor-suppressor function.[39]

The role of the NF2 gene as a tumor suppressor was demonstrated by Lutchman and colleagues when they found that transfection into National Institutes of Health (NIH) 3T3 cells resulted in growth suppression.[43] Conversely, adding blocking antisense oligodeoxynucleotides to MERLIN led to the suppression of its synthesis and to increased cell proliferation.[44] The NF2 protein has been shown to impair cell adhesion, motility, and spreading properties, all of which are essential for tumor formation.[39] Like neurofibromin, MERLIN has also been found to have an anti-*ras* function.[45]

There is evidence that mutations of the NF2 gene may contribute to the development of sporadic tumors typically associated with NF2, such as VS and meningiomas.[45–48] Studies of LOH have demonstrated the absence of chromosome 22 in approximately 60 percent of sporadic meningiomas. Both NF2 gene mutations and the allelic loss of chromosome 22q were found in > 70 percent of fibrous and transitional meningiomas but in < 30 percent of the meningothelial subtypes.[49] Most meningiomas in NF2 patients are of the fibrous subtype. Mutations of the NF2 gene were found to be present in 20 to 60 percent of sporadic schwannomas.[47] One study found NF2 gene alteration in only 1 of 8 sporadic ependymomas.[45] Thus, loss of MERLIN appears to be critical to the formation of both sporadic and NF2-associated schwannomas as well as fibrous and transitional meningiomas. However, it appears that tumor-suppressor genes on chromosome 22q (other than MERLIN) may be more central to the pathogenesis of ependymomas and other CNS tumors.

Although the transmission rate is 50 percent in second and subsequent generations, the risk of transmission in an apparent sporadic case of NF2 is < 50 percent because of mosaicism.[39] Mosaic NF2 disease, in which only a proportion of cells contains the mutated NF2 gene, results in milder cases of NF2. Up to 20 percent of NF2 cases without a family history of NF2 are mosaic.[39] Only a subset of germ cells will carry the mutation, thus resulting in a milder disease course and a risk of transmission of < 50 percent. However, if the offspring inherit the mutations, their disease course will be more severe since the offspring will carry the mutations in all of their cells. Mosaicism may be more likely in NF2 if the VSs are predominantly unilateral.[39]

Management

Since there is no present cure, the treatment of NF2 patients is directed toward the symptomatic relief of

NF2-associated neoplasms, particularly VS. The treatment approach must be individualized to each patient, depending on the size of the tumor, the unilateral or bilateral nature of its involvement, and the degree of hearing loss caused by the tumor. Treatment modalities for VS and meningioma include surgical resection and stereotactic radiosurgery in selected patients.

Although preservation of hearing and other cranial-nerve function is the goal of surgery for VS whenever possible, it is often not achieved, and the primary goal then becomes the decompression of the brain stem to relieve CSF obstruction. Because there are many difficult management issues, NF2 patients optimally should be cared for by an experienced multidisciplinary team, and a comprehensive treatment plan must be carefully outlined to optimize functional hearing, facial nerve function, and preservation of life.

Screening Protocol

For family members of patients with known NF2, formal screening for VS should begin at 10 years of age, as it is rare for tumors to become symptomatic before that age, even in severely affected families.[39] The standard imaging for identifying VS is MRI of the head, with 3-mm cuts and fat-suppression images in both the axial and coronal views, with and without gadolinium, through the internal auditory canals. For asymptomatic patients with a family history of NF2, MRI screening every 2 years is recommended for patients younger than 20 years of age and every 3 years for those older than 20 years of age.[39] Since cataracts can affect vision in early life, patients at high risk for developing NF2 should have a formal ophthalmologic evaluation in the first or second year of life.[8] Also, special attention should be directed to signs and symptoms referable to the spinal cord. Asymptomatic spinal tumors are found frequently on screening whole-spine MRIs. Audiologic tests are used as adjuncts to MRI and are more critical once VSs are detected. The risk of developing NF2 in an unaffected patient over 30 years of age with a normal MRI scan and favorable DNA linkage analysis is extremely small.[44]

A brain and whole-spine MRI scan and both ophthalmologic and otolaryngologic assessments (including audiometry and brainstem evoked potential studies) should be performed and repeated annually for newly diagnosed NF2 patients.[8,39] In families with more than one affected member, linkage analysis is the test of choice because it can give > 99 percent certainty of affected status.[39] However, mutation detection is expensive and time-consuming, which limits its value as a widespread practical screening tool at this time. The prospects for NF2 treatment appear encouraging due to the relative paucity of phenotypic variation in patients with the same mutation, as well as to the lack of involvement of other genes in the tumors themselves.

RETINOBLASTOMA

Retinoblastoma (RB) is the most common primary intraocular tumor in children, with an incidence of 1 in 20,000 live births.[50] It occurs as sporadic and familial forms. The latter is an autosomal dominant condition with a nearly 100 percent penetrance. As with NF1 and NF2, RB serves as a prototype of a group of neoplasms that arise from the inactivation of tumor-suppressor genes. The presence of bilateral RB combined with an intracranial midline tumor is a distinct syndrome called trilateral retinoblastoma (TRB). The presence of the intracranial lesion in TRB patients results in a significantly decreased survival compared to patients who have only RB. With their varied patterns of metastases and poor prognoses even with treatment, RB and TRB present complex and difficult challenges for evaluation and treatment.

Clinical Features

The most common presenting sign of RB is leukokoria, which occurs in about 60 percent of patients.[51] This is a white, yellow-white, or pink-white pupillary finding ("cat's eye") that results from any intraocular abnormality that reflects light back through the pupil (Figure 3–3A). In RB, leukokoria is due to the opacification of the vitreous by the tumor cells themselves or by an associated retinal detachment. The second most common presenting sign of RB is strabismus, or misalignment of the eyes. This is caused by tumor involvement of the macula, initially resulting in visual loss and then sensory strabismus. Other presenting signs are listed in Table 3–6.

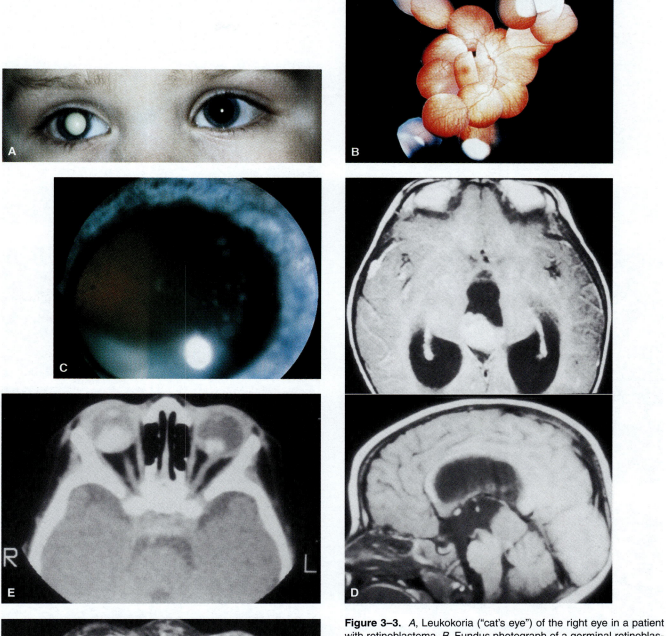
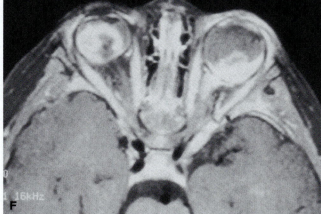

Figure 3–3. *A*, Leukokoria ("cat's eye") of the right eye in a patient with retinoblastoma. *B*, Fundus photograph of a germinal retinoblastoma. There are four tumor lesions. *C*, Fundus photograph of vitreous seeding by retinoblastoma. *D*, T1-weighted postcontrast axial and sagittal magnetic resonance imaging (MRI) of a pineoblastoma in a patient with a history of retinoblastoma. *E*, Computed tomography scan of bilateral retinoblastomas. They are hyperdense on CT due to their calcifications. *F*, T1-weighted axial MRI of bilateral retinoblastomas. There is probable extension of the tumor into the left sclera and optic nerve.

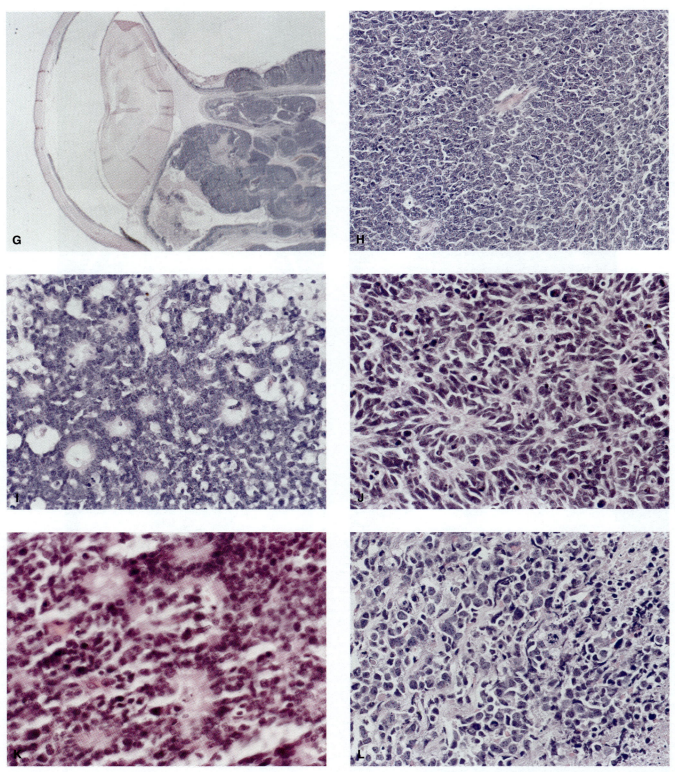

Figure 3–3. *G,* Sagittal section of a retinoblastoma within the vitreous chamber of the eye (H & E stain; ×25 original magnification). *H,* Region of retinoblastoma with poorly differentiated cells (H & E stain; ×250 original magnification). *I,* Flexner-Wintersteiner rosettes in a retinoblastoma. Note the central lumens lined by tall cuboidal cells (H & E stain; ×500 original magnification). *J,* Homer-Wright rosettes in a retinoblastoma. The cuboidal cells are arranged around a central tangle of cytoplasmic processes rather than a lumen (H & E stain; ×700 original magnification). *K,* Multiple fleurettes in a retinoblastoma (H & E stain; ×500 original magnification). Note the eosinophilic bulbous extension of processes into the lumen. *L,* Highly cellular sheets of primitive-appearing cells in a pineoblastoma (H & E stain; ×500 original magnification). Numerous mitotic figures and areas of necrosis are featured.

Table 3–6. PRESENTING SIGNS OF RETINOBLASTOMA
Leukokoria
Strabismus
Glaucoma
Iris heterochromia
Proptosis
Vision loss
Pseudo-orbital cellulitis
Pain

Adapted from Kaufman LM, Mafee MF, Song CD. Retinoblastoma and simulating lesions. Role of CT, MR imaging and use of Gd-DTPA contrast enhancement. Radiol Clin North Am 1998;36:1101–17.

On ophthalmologic examination, small RB lesions are usually seen as gray-white intraretinal foci (see Figure 3–3B). Intraocular tumor spread results from small portions of the tumor breaking off and floating freely in the vitreous or subretinal space (see Figure 3–3C). Tumors can grow within the vitreous cavity even if they lack blood supply. Thus, RB may present in one of several manifestations: (1) a retinal or subretinal mass with or without an associated retinal detachment or vitreous opacity, (2) a nonspecific retinal detachment, (3) an opaque vitreous obscuring the retinal structures, or (4) a combination of the above.[51] Retinoblastomas are categorized into five groups by their size, location, and seeding, to provide useful information regarding the prognosis for orbital globe salvage (Table 3–7).[52,53]

Metastatic Disease

Patients with familial RB are at increased risk for developing other non-ocular cancers. These include osteosarcomas as well as other tumors both at and outside the fields of prior radiation therapy. The incidence of second tumors after initial diagnosis is 20 percent at 10 years, 50 percent at 20 years, and 90 percent at 30 years.[51]

Metastasis occurs in < 10 percent of patients with RB. The mean age of metastatic presentation is approximately 3 years, with an average time of 12 months from initial diagnosis to presentation.[54] The most common sites for extension and metastases are the orbital and cranial bones. Disease can also spread to the lymph nodes, long bones, and viscera (eg, liver, kidney, pancreas, and gonads). Curiously, the lungs are a rare site for RB metastases.[54] Messmer and colleagues found that three particular risk factors were calculated as high-risk variables for metastasis: choroidal involvement, optic nerve involvement at the transection line, and late enucleation.[55] Histopathologic evidence of tumor invasion into the sclera, optic nerve, and orbit is the most highly predictive risk factor for metastasis and poor survival.[54] The median time to death in one study was 6.4 months in unilateral cases and 14.2 months in bilateral cases.[56] Positive bone marrow aspirates and abnormal bone scans have significant correlations with both advanced stages of RB (defined as extraocular disease within adnexal structures or as extraocular disease with distant metastases) and choroidal involvement in enucleated eyes.[54] Hence, bone marrow aspirates and bone scans are recommended tests for the initial diagnostic work-up of advanced-stage metastatic RB.

Trilateral Retinoblastoma

Trilateral retinoblastoma is a rare syndrome in which bilateral RBs occur in association with an ectopic (nonmetastatic) midline intracranial malignancy. This association was first described by Jako-

Table 3–7. REESE-ELLSWORTH CLASSIFICATION OF RETINOBLASTOMAS	
Group and Prognosis*	Location, Size, Seeding
I-Very favorable	Solitary tumor <4 disc diameters in size located at or behind the equator OR Multiple tumors (none >4 disc diameters) located at or behind the equator
II-Favorable	Solitary or multiple tumors (4–10 disc diameters) located at or behind the equator
III-Doubtful	Any tumor located anterior to the equator OR Solitary tumor >10 disc diameters located behind the equator
IV-Unfavorable	Multiple tumors, some > 10 disc diameters OR Any lesion extending anteriorly to the ora serrata
V-Very unfavorable	Massive tumors involving over half the retina OR Vitreous seeding

*For preservation of eye.
Adapted from Shields CL, Shields JA. Recent developments in the management of retinoblastoma. J Pediatr Ophthalmol Strabismus 1999;36:8–18.

biec and colleagues[57] in 1977 and was subsequently termed trilateral retinoblastoma by Bader and colleagues in 1980.[58] The incidence of TRB is approximately 4 percent in patients with RB.[59] The following characteristic patterns have been observed: (1) nearly all TRB patients have hereditary bilateral RB, (2) the midline lesion is most commonly a primitive neuroectodermal tumor (PNET) in the pineal region (pineoblastoma), (3) the mean age at diagnosis of the bilateral ocular RB in TRB is 7 months (earlier than the usual 15 months for classic bilateral RBs),[60] (4) the intracranial mass is discovered approximately 24.6 months after diagnosis of the ocular RB,[61] and (5) patients die soon after diagnosis of TRB. Mean time from diagnosis to death is 6.6 months, and this figure decreases to 1.3 months if TRB is untreated.[60] The most common cause of death is metastatic seeding of TRB throughout the neuraxis and spinal column.

The most common initial symptoms of TRB involve signs of increased intracranial pressure (ICP), such as headache, nausea, vomiting, loss of appetite, lethargy, and somnolence. Other signs and symptoms include seizures, ataxia, progressive weakness, personality changes, cranial nerve VI palsies, decreased visual acuity, upgaze paralysis, fever, ophthalmoplegia, and meningismus. Patients occasionally are asymptomatic, and their intracranial mass is detected on screening neuroimaging. About 89 percent of patients have bilateral ocular tumors, whereas only 11 percent have unilateral RB. The average age at diagnosis of the intracranial neoplasm of TRB is 30.7 months.[61]

Several presentations of TRB have been documented. In one variant, a unilateral RB occurs concurrently with a solitary intracranial neoplasm, often in the pineal region (see Figure 3–3D). This variant is considered to be the forme fruste of TRB.[62] Other variants differ with respect to the location of the intracranial mass (such as in the sellar/parasellar region,[62] cerebellum,[60] or the fourth ventricle).[60] Patients with "sellar" TRB appear to have characteristics that differ from those with TRB in the pineal region. The sellar mass presents initially more often and at an earlier age than the pineal-mass variant of TRB. It also occurs more frequently in females and is more often associated with unilateral RB tumors.[62]

Radiographic Features

The presence of intraocular calcification in children younger than 3 years of age is highly suggestive of RB.[51] Over 90 percent of cases demonstrate calcifications by computed tomography (CT), although calcifications are much less likely to be present in diffuse infiltrating RB and are rarely present in the extraocular spread of RB.[51] On CT, the tumor appears isodense or mildly hyperdense and enhances with contrast (see Figure 3–3E). Retinoblastomas are slightly or moderately hyperintense relative to normal vitreous on T1-weighted MR images and enhance significantly (see Figure 3–3F). They appear as areas of marked to moderate low-signal intensity on T2-weighted MR images.

Calcifications in the pineal region are generally nonspecific. However, any calcification of the pineal gland in a child less than 6 years old is likely to be abnormal and should prompt an MRI to exclude a pineal neoplasm.[59] Also, any pineal neoplasm presenting in the first 4 years of life should prompt consideration of TRB and result in a thorough ophthalmologic examination. Hence, any pineal or parasellar neoplasm in a child with bilateral or familial RB should be considered to represent TRB.[59]

Histopathology

The majority of cells in RB resemble the undifferentiated retina of the embryo (embryonic medullary epithelium), prompting Verhoeff and Jackson to give the tumor its present name[63] (see Figure 3–3G). Retinoblastoma is derived from primitive embryonal retinal cells (either neuronal or photoreceptor). On light microscopy, the undifferentiated areas of RB are composed of round to ovoid cells with large hyperchromatic nuclei, scanty cytoplasm, and numerous mitotic figures (see Figure 3–3H). The histologic features may show marked variability as some tumors may demonstrate prominent foci of calcification or significant necrosis. Some tumors may also exhibit areas of glial differentiation.[51]

There are several differentiated structures within RBs (see Figures 3–3I to K). The most characteristic structure is the Flexner-Wintersteiner rosette, which consists of tall cuboidal cells arranged around a central lumen. Other structures include Homer

Wright rosettes, which appear as radial arrangements of cells around a central tangle of cytoplasmic processes, and fleurettes, which are large cells with smaller nuclei and abundant eosinophilic cytoplasm arranged in fleur-de-lis formations. Fleurettes and Flexner-Wintersteiner rosettes represent an attempt at photoreceptor differentiation. Variability in immunoreactive protein expression patterns has led to the hypothesis that the likely cell of origin of ocular RB is a primitive neuroepithelial cell with the potential to undergo varying differentiation.[61]

The pineal organ and the retina express common immunologic antigens, such as S-antigen and interphotoreceptor retinoid–binding protein.[64] This is not unexpected; phylogenetically, the pineal organ has been observed to develop from a photoreceptor organ in lower vertebrates to a secretory gland in humans that is involved in diurnal rhythm and in melatonin secretion. Also, pineal photoreceptor differentiation, such as cilia with 9+0 array of microtubules, has been observed in human pineal tumors,[61] leading to the characterization of the pineal gland as the "third eye." Initially, it was thought that the cell of origin for the midline intracranial neoplasm in TRB was restricted to pinealoblasts. However, given the variation of its location, it is more accurate to consider the third mass in TRB as being within the spectrum of PNETs, of which pineoblastoma is one category. Primitive neuroectodermal tumors are thought to be undifferentiated tumors that resemble germinal matrix cells of the embryonic neural tube and that maintain the capacity to undergo differentiation along glial or neuronal lines.[61] Histologically, pineoblastomas are highly cellular neoplasms composed of cells with small round to oval nuclei, scant cytoplasm, and numerous mitotic figures (see Figure 3–3L). They may demonstrate neuronal (eg, Homer Wright rosettes) or glial differentiation and immunoreactivity. Pineoblastomas may also exhibit photoreceptor differentiation with fleurettes and Flexner-Wintersteiner rosettes.[61] Trilateral retinoblastoma is considered to represent a second primary tumor, rather than the metastatic spread of ocular RB.

Genetics

Retinoblastoma is a prototype of the group of cancers caused by the loss of tumor-suppressor genes. Knudson and colleagues proposed a "two-hit" model to explain the basis for bilateral hereditary RB.[65] In this model, at least two mutational genetic events must occur before RB develops, suggesting that the loss of one copy of the protein product of the RB gene (pRB) is insufficient for RB development. The first event occurs prezygotically and affects all cells in the body. The second event affects only a subset population of susceptible cells, resulting in the genesis of specific neoplasms. In the case of hereditary RB, the first mutational retinal event occurs either by the inheriting of a mutant allele from a carrier parent or as a new germinal mutation. The second event in the retina is somatic. In contrast, sporadic nonfamilial RB results from acquiring two sequential mutational somatic events, leading to the loss or inactivation of both RB alleles. These RBs present as unilateral solitary tumors and are biologically identical to hereditary RBs.

The RB locus has been mapped to the long arm of chromosome 13 (13q14) by linkage studies and deletion analysis.[50] Hereditary RB presents as a mendelian autosomal dominant trait with nearly 100 percent penetrance. The RB protein (pRB) spans 928 bases and exerts its tumor-suppressor effects by positively or negatively regulating transcription to block cell division and promote differentiation. The RB gene is expressed in all adult tissues, but specific cell types initiate RB expression at specific developmental times.[50] For example, pRB expression in the retina coincides with its terminal differentiation. The absence of pRB in the developing retina results in apoptosis, or programmed cell death. Apoptosis normally balances the continued cell proliferation caused by the loss of pRB. However, another genetic mutational event that disrupts the apoptosis pathway could initiate the formation of RB.[50]

Inactivation of the RB gene has also been demonstrated in other tumor types, including sarcomas and breast, bladder, small cell, and non–small cell lung carcinomas.[66] In addition, LOH of 13q14 has been shown to contribute to the formation of high-grade astrocytomas, thus implicating the RB gene (in addition to the p53 gene) as another tumor-suppressor gene in astrocytoma tumorigenesis.[66] The roles of p53 and RB in astrocytoma formation appear to be distinct; p53 mutations are detected in astrocytomas of all grades whereas RB inactivation is found to be restricted only to high-grade astrocytomas.[66] Thus, p53 mutation may be critical in the formation of astrocytomas whereas RB inactivation may contribute to the malignant progression of astrocytomas.

Management

The treatment for RB is complex and requires a multidisciplinary approach by a team consisting at least of an ophthalmologist, a pediatric oncologist, a pediatric neurologist, a neurosurgeon, and a radiation oncologist. The management plan should be tailored to each individual patient, with the primary goal being preservation of life, followed by preservation of vision if possible. The treatment for RB may include enucleation, radiation therapy, and chemotherapy.[67] Management becomes more complicated in cases of TRB, where neurosurgical involvement becomes more essential, because it is the lethality of the intracranial tumor that significantly affects outcome and survival. Successful treatment of TRB with a combination of systemic chemotherapy, intrathecal chemotherapy, and craniospinal-axis (CSA) radiation has been documented.[68]

Screening

Moll and colleagues found that the mean age at diagnosis in familial RB patients from birth onward was 4.9 months with fundoscopic screening, as opposed to 17.2 months for those diagnosed without fundoscopic screening.[69] The latest onset of familial RB presentation was about 4 years of age. Thus, ophthalmologic screening of high-risk children and their siblings is recommended until at least the age of 4 years in order to detect RB as early as possible.[69]

The low incidence of TRB makes routine screening with MRI a controversial issue. Meadows argued that screening with neuroimaging should be done every 3 months to diagnose TRB in an early and treatable stage, but this is not cost-effective.[70] However, longer survival has been observed in patients with TRB diagnosed prior to the onset of symptoms than in TRB patients who were symptomatic at their time of diagnosis.[68] In a meta-analysis of 106 children with TRB, Kivelä noted that median survival was significantly longer if the intracranial tumor was ≤ 15 mm by largest diameter.[71] Also, the majority of intracranial tumors in TRB develop within the first 4 years of diagnosis. Nelson and colleagues proposed the following neuroimaging screening regimen: MRI every 3 months for the first 2 years after diagnosis of RB, MRI every 4 months for the next 2 years, and then MRI every 6 months for the next 5 years.[68] Screening should also be considered for siblings of patients with TRB as their risk for developing TRB themselves varies between 1 to 7 percent, depending on the presence of a family history of TRB.[62] Thus, given the poor prognosis of TRB, the above screening regimen is probably a reasonable protocol to improve survival by earlier diagnosis and aggressive treatment.

VON HIPPEL-LINDAU DISEASE

Von Hippel-Lindau (VHL) disease is an autosomal dominant disorder caused by deletions or mutations to the VHL gene, which is a tumor-suppressor gene mapped to chromosome 3p25-26. Hallmark features of VHL disease include vascular tumors of the retina and CNS, pheochromocytomas, and renal cell carcinomas (RCCs). Von Hippel-Lindau disease is seen in all ethnic groups, and both genders are affected equally. The birth incidence in eastern England is 1 in 36,000, penetrance is approximately 80 to 90 percent by the age of 65 years, and expressivity is highly variable.[72] Of interest, the type of VHL gene mutation appears to significantly determine the clinical profile of VHL disease's manifestations. Such genotype-phenotype correlation studies have been useful in patient counseling, especially with regard to the risk of developing a pheochromocytoma.

Clinical Features

The characteristic features of VHL disease include CNS hemangioblastoma, retinal angioma, and RCC. The average life expectancy of VHL disease patients in one series was approximately 46 years of age, with the usual range being 40 to 50 years of age.[73] Hemangioblastomas and RCCs were noted to be equal in their frequency as the leading causes of death.[73] A list of clinical features of VHL disease appears in Table 3–8.[74]

The earliest manifestation of VHL disease is hemangioblastoma of the retina or retinal angioma. They are found at a mean age of 25 years at diagnosis. Retinal angiomas occur in more than half of all patients with VHL disease.[72] These tumors are typically benign, multiple, bilateral, and recurrent. Untreated, they can cause blindness due to retinal detachment and hemorrhage, but they are often asymptomatic until such serious damage occurs. Their classic appearance on ophthalmologic examination is as reddish spherical masses of varying sizes, with a dilated feeding artery and a draining vein (Figure 3–4A).

The next manifestation of VHL disease is the CNS hemangioblastoma, which presents at a mean age of 30 years.[75] In comparison to patients with sporadic hemangioblastoma, this age is significantly lower. As well, sporadic hemangioblastomas tend to occur as solitary masses. Central nervous system hemangioblastoma is the most common manifestation of VHL disease and occur in 21 to 72 percent of VHL disease patients.[72] They often occur bilaterally, and 75 percent of CNS hemangioblastomas occur in the posterior fossa whereas 25 percent occur in the spinal cord (see Figures 3–4B and C). Of the infratentorial CNS hemangioblastomas, 95 percent occur in the cerebellum while the rest occur in the brain stem; supratentorial hemangioblastomas are rare. Symptoms of cerebellar hemangiomas (such as headache, nausea, vomiting, vertigo, gait ataxia, papilledema, dysarthria, nystagmus, somnolence, and limb ataxia) are caused by local disruption of neurologic function and/or by increased ICP. Spinal cord hemangioblastomas may cause syringomyelia. Erythrocytosis occurs in 5 to 20 percent of VHL disease patients and is due to tumor production of erythropoietin (Epo).[76]

Renal lesions in VHL disease include cysts and carcinomas. Renal cysts occur in 50 to 70 percent of VHL disease patients and are often multiple and bilateral. The predominant histology of the renal tumor in VHL disease is that of clear cell carcinoma. The mean age of presentation of RCC in VHL disease patients is 37 years,[75] and RCC is the cause of death in 15 to 50 percent of VHL disease patients.[72]

The incidence of pheochromocytomas in VHL disease is approximately 20 percent. Pheochromocytomas may cause palpitations, diaphoresis, headaches, and uncontrolled hypertension, and they may be life threatening for patients undergoing surgery or pregnancy. Pheochromocytomas in VHL disease differ from those in sporadic cases in that they (a) occur in younger patients; (b) are often bilateral, multiple, and extra-adrenal; and (c) metastasize infrequently.[72] They are diagnosed by establishing increased catecholamine levels (epinephrine, norepinephrine, and metanephrine) in 24-hour urine collections; this is combined with the results of imaging studies such as CT, MRI, and ultrasonography (US).

Endolymphatic sac tumors (ELSTs) are very rare lesions that have only recently been recognized as a complication of VHL disease.[77] They are low-grade papillary adenocarcinomas arising from a duplication of the dura of the posterior aspect of the petrous pyramid (see Figure 3–4D). They can grow into the cerebellopontine (CP) angle and/or the middle ear and can destroy the temporal bone; they can also occur bilaterally. On MRI, they appear as markedly enhancing heterogeneous lesions displaying high signal intensity on T2-weighted images (see Figure 3–4E). Presenting symptoms include tinnitus, sudden or progressive hearing loss, and vertigo. These symptoms can present from several months to up to 30 years before the diagnosis is made.[78]

Table 3–8. CHARACTERISTIC LESIONS IN VON HIPPEL-LINDAU DISEASE

System	Lesion
CNS	Hemangioblastoma*
	Syringomyelia
Retina	Angioma (hemangioblastoma)
Kidney	Clear cell carcinoma
	Cysts
Pancreas	Cysts
	Neuroendocrine tumors
Adrenal medulla	Pheochromocytoma
Internal auditory canal	Endolymphatic sac tumors
Epididymus/broad ligament	Cystadenomas

CNS = central nervous system.
*Almost always involves the posterior fossa and/or spinal cord.
Adapted from Hardwig P, Robertson DM. Von Hippel-Lindau disease: a familial, often lethal, multi-system phakomatosis. Ophthamology 1984;91:263–70.

Diagnostic Criteria

The diagnosis of VHL disease is based primarily on clinical findings. In a patient with a positive family history of VHL disease, the documentation of one retinal or cerebellar hemangioblastoma, pheochromocytoma, or RCC is sufficient to make the diagnosis of VHL disease. The diagnosis can also be made in a patient with two or more retinal or CNS hemangioblastomas, or with a single hemangioblastoma and a characteristic visceral tumor.[72] It has been argued that the presence of multiple pancreatic cysts and a positive family history of VHL disease should also be sufficient to make the diagnosis. Multiple renal or epididymal cysts alone are not sufficient because of their fairly frequent occurrence in the general population; however, one must suspect VHL disease if they occur in children or young adults as such cysts are uncommon (especially if multiple) in that age group.[72]

Histopathology

Hemangioblastoma, the hallmark tumor of VHL disease, is characterized by sheets of large vacuolated stromal cells and a rich network of capillary vessels.

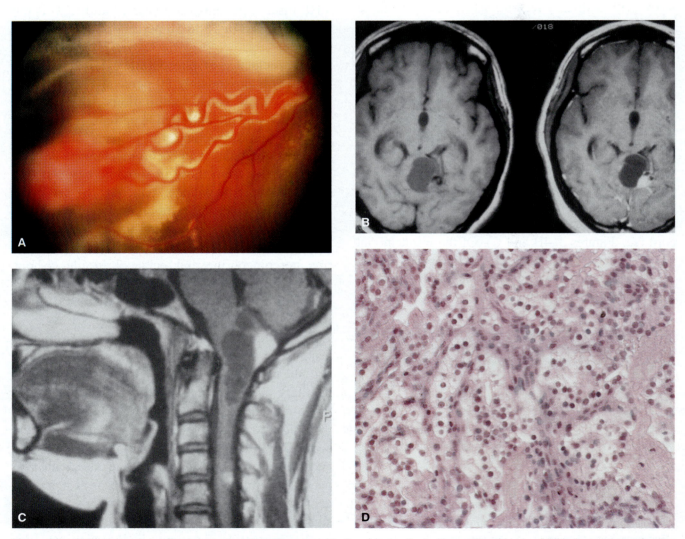

Figure 3–4. *A*, Fundoscopic image of a retinal angioma (hemangioblastoma) in a patient with von Hippel-Lindau (VHL) disease. Large feeding and draining vessels are visible. *B*, Pre- and postcontrast T1-weighted axial MRI images of a cerebellar hemangioblastoma in VHL disease. The solid portion of the lesion enhances brightly after contrast administration. *C*, Postcontrast T1-weighted sagittal MRI of a lower brainstem/upper cervical hemangioblastoma, with a second tumor at the C4-5 spinal level in a patient with VHL disease. *D*, Endolymphatic sac tumor in a patient with VHL (H & E stain; ×500 original magnification). Note the papillary and glandular architecture.

The stromal cells have a polygonal shape and relatively small uniform nuclei with numerous lipid-filled vacuoles within the cytoplasm, which gives this neoplasm a clear cell appearance (see Figure 3–4F). Stromal cells have been shown to be the neoplastic cell type in hemangioblastomas although their histologic origin has not yet been defined.[79,80]

Because of its clear cell appearance, the hemangioblastoma may be very difficult to distinguish from a metastatic RCC on routine hematoxylin-eosin (H and E) stains[81] (see Figure 3–4G). Immunohistochemistry can be of value when H and E stains are insufficient for distinction. Positive staining by anti–epithelial-membrane antigen (EMA) is consis-

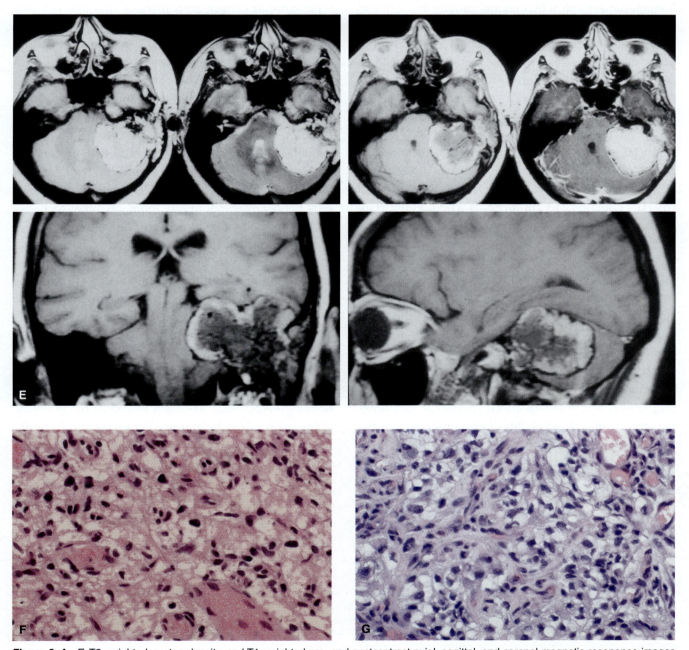

Figure 3–4. *E,* T2-weighted, proton density, and T1-weighted pre- and postcontrast axial, sagittal, and coronal magnetic resonance images of an endolymphatic sac tumor arising along the left posterior petrous ridge at the level of the endolymphatic sac in a patient with VHL disease. *F,* Clear lipid-filled stromal cells of a hemangioblastoma in a patient with VHL disease (H & E stain; ×500 original magnification). Note the rich network of capillaries. *G,* Metastatic renal cell carcinoma (H & E stain; ×500 original magnification). Note the rich vascular network and clear cell cytologic features, which are histologically similar in appearance to hemangioblastomas.

tent with metastatic RCC whereas uniform absence of staining with anti-EMA favors the diagnosis of cerebellar hemangioblastoma.[81] Electron microscopy demonstrating microvilli on the tumor cells also supports the diagnosis of metastatic RCC and excludes cerebellar hemangioblastoma.[81] The importance of their differentiation is obvious in the implications for diagnosis, prognosis, and management. A solitary hemangioblastoma is benign and usually amenable to surgical resection and cure whereas a metastatic RCC lesion is malignant and heralds a dismal prognosis even with treatment, as metastatic spread to other sites may be concurrently found.

Genetics

The VHL gene has been mapped to the chromosome region 3p25-26.[82] This region is frequently deleted or altered in sporadic RCC.[72] Its protein product (pVHL) contains 213 amino acids with no important homology to other proteins; pVHL binds to two proteins, elongin B and C, creating the protein complex CBC^{VHL}. This binding is often mutated in VHL disease.[72] The protein complex CBC^{VHL} prevents the formation of a complex called elongin (SIII), which activates mRNA transcription by blocking the binding of the B/C complex with its catalytic subunit, elongin A. Hence, binding of elongin B/C with pVHL competitively inhibits elongin A, thereby downregulating the mRNA transcription rate of certain genes. Mutations of pVHL that alter this binding ability may disrupt the tumor-suppressor function of the VHL gene by preventing transcription regulation.[72] At least two target substrates that bind to the CBC^{VHL} complex are now known: hypoxia-inducible factors 1α and 2α (HIF-1α and HIF-2α).[83] A model of VHL gene–mediated vascularization has been proposed in which inactivation of the VHL gene leads to the binding of the elongin A/B/C complex, which upregulates some target genes such as HIF-1α and HIF-2α.[82] Under hypoxic conditions, they are stable and form a heterodimer that binds to specific hypoxia-regulated response elements and activates genes such as vascular endothelial growth factor (VEGF), transferrin receptors, and inducible nitric oxide synthetase. However, under normoxic (normal oxygen level) conditions, the alpha subunits of HIF are rapidly degraded by proteolysis mediated by pVHL. Mutations in the VHL gene result in the stabilization of HIF-α subunits and the activation of HIF-1α in normoxia. Consequently, VEGF is constitutively upregulated to levels that typically occur only under hypoxic conditions.[82] Hypoxia-inducible mRNA stability of VEGF results in increased vascularization. The association of VHL gene mutations with familial cancer demonstrates that this is a key pathway in tumorigenesis.[83]

A striking feature of VHL disease is the strong correlation between mutation type and clinical phenotype presentation. The clinical types are divided into VHL disease patients without pheochromocytomas (type 1) and those with pheochromocytomas (type 2). Patients with type 2 VHL disease are further subdivided by the additional presence of hemangioblastomas without RCC (type 2A) and hemangioblastomas with RCC (type 2B); patients who have only pheochromocytomas without any other manifestations are classed as type 2C. Truncation and deletion mutations are strongly associated with type 1 and (occasionally) type 2B VHL disease whereas missense mutations resulting in amino acid substitutions are associated with a high risk of developing all of the type 2 VHL disease subtypes.[78] Truncation mutations are more common in sporadic RCC (Table 3–9).

Angiogenesis is an important underlying feature in the clinical manifestations of VHL disease. The hypervascular nature of typical VHL lesions such as hemangioblastomas has been linked to the overproduction of VEGF by tumors; VEGF is significantly overexpressed in RCC, sporadic and VHL-associated hemangioblastomas, and glioblastomas.[72] Thus, treatment for VHL disease is being directed toward blocking VEGF receptors, which (it is hoped) would decrease the formation of these highly vascular VHL-associated tumors. Erythropoietin is also highly expressed in hemangioblastomas, suggesting that loss of pVHL function may also upregulate Epo expression in hemangioblastomas.[84]

Management

Surgery is the treatment of choice for CNS hemangioblastomas as these tumors can be cured by complete resection.[78] Studies have indicated that stereo-

Table 3–9. CLINICAL AND MOLECULAR CLASSIFICATIONS OF VON HIPPEL-LINDAU DISEASE LESIONS				
Lesion	Type I	Type IIA	Type IIB	Type IIC
Pheochromocytoma	No	Yes	Yes	Yes
CNS hemangioblastoma	Yes	Yes	Yes	No
Retinal hemangioblastoma	Yes	Yes	Yes	No
Endolymphatic sac tumors	Yes	Yes	Yes	No
Renal cell carcinoma	Yes	No	Yes	No
Pancreatic tumors	Yes	No	Yes	No
Molecular characteristics				
Protein truncation (%)	73–96	—	8–31	—
Amino acid substitution (%)	4–27	100	69–92	100
Mutation loci	Multiple	Codon 98	Codon 167	—

CNS = central nervous system.
Adapted from Richard S, David P, Marsot-Dupuch K, et al. Central nervous system hemangioblastomas, endolymphatic sac tumors, and von Hippel-Lindau disease. Neurosurg Rev 2000;28:1–22.

tactic radiosurgery is also effective in controlling the majority of primary and recurrent hemangioblastomas.[85,86] Retinal angiomas are treated by cryotherapy or laser therapy, depending on the size, location, and number of tumors.[87] Endolymphatic sac tumors require immediate surgical resection by ear, nose, and throat (ENT) specialists to prevent significant hearing loss; because of their slow-growing nature, radiation therapy is not indicated.[78]

Thus far, there is no effective medical therapy for the clinical manifestations of VHL disease. One new strategy is to create drugs designed to block the VEGF signaling pathway. The effect of SU-5416, a VEGF-mediated tyrosine kinase inhibitor, is being evaluated in VHL disease patients in a phase I trial.[83] It is hoped that antiangiogenic therapy will provide significant long-term benefits for patients with VHL disease.

Screening and Surveillance

Genetic testing should be used for patients with family members who have VHL disease. Deleterious mutations in the VHL gene can be identified in greater than 80 percent of families with VHL disease.[72] Family members with asymptomatic VHL disease who are found to have the causal mutation should undergo careful screening, whereas family members who do not have the specific mutation do not require further clinical follow-up. In patients with sporadic pheochromocytomas, a germline mutation was found to occur in 3.0 to 8.8 percent of VHL disease patients in large series and in up to 80 percent in those with bilateral pheochromocytomas.[78] Thus, VHL-gene testing may be offered to patients with pheochromocytoma, especially if it is bilateral or familial or if the patient is a child.

Close clinical follow-up is important for early diagnosis and treatment of the manifestations of VHL disease. The minimum age for the diagnosis of VHL disease is 5 years because the earliest potentially debilitating lesions are detectable at that age.[78] Regular surveillance tests should include periodic brain and spine MRI, abdominal CT or US, 24-hour collection of urinary metanephrines to detect pheochromocytomas, and thorough ophthalmologic examinations. The frequency of the specific examinations depends on the age, number, and types of manifestations at diagnosis in each patient.

TUBEROUS SCLEROSIS COMPLEX

Tuberous sclerosis (TS), previously called Bourneville's disease, is an autosomal dominant neurocutaneous syndrome with a low penetrance, involving various types of benign systemic tumors, including cerebral subependymal giant cell astrocytomas, cardiac rhabdomyomas, and renal angiomyolipomas. Approximately 68 percent of TS cases occur as a result of new mutations, and there is no predilection for race or gender.[88] Two different genes, one each on chromosomes 9 and 16, can cause phenotypically identical TS.[89,90] This syndrome affects an estimated 1 in 10,000 births[91] and is the second most common neurocutaneous syndrome (NF1 is the most common).[88]

Clinical Features

The diagnostic criteria for TS are divided into major and minor features (Table 3–10). The diagnosis of TS requires the presence of either two major features or one major and two minor features; TS should also be suspected in patients with one major and one minor feature. The classic clinical triad of TS (seizures, mental retardation, and facial angiofibromas) occurs infrequently and is seen only in patients with more severe disease courses. At some point, 80 percent of patients with TS experience seizures. The seizures usually begin before 2 years of age and may present at birth as infantile spasms. Intelligence is normal in one-fourth of TS seizure patients, but nearly all TS patients with mental retardation have seizures.[88] Controlling the secondary generalization of infantile spasms appears to be important for maximizing the cognitive development of a child with TS.[92]

Cerebral lesions associated with TS include cortical tubers, subependymal glial nodules, and subependymal giant cell astrocytomas. Cortical tubers are benign potato-like growths occurring along the gyri and sulci, most commonly in the frontal lobe. They are regions of cortical dysplasia that likely result from aberrant neuronal migration during corticogenesis. Cortical tubers are best detected by MRI and are associated with seizures. They can cause hydrocephalus and death by blocking the foramen of Monro in the third ventricle. The number of calcified tubers increases with age; by 10 years of age, 50 percent of TS patients have calcified tubers.[88]

Subependymal nodules ("candle gutterings") are calcified lesions that line the ventricles, and they are best demonstrated by CT. Hosoya and colleagues found that TS patients with eight or more subependymal nodules found at their initial or subsequent scans had an increased incidence of infantile spasms and mental retardation (ie, intelligence quotient [IQ] < 70).[93] This suggests that the number of ventricular subependymal nodules might be predictive of the severity of a TS patient's course.

Subependymal giant cell astrocytomas occur in 5 to 10 percent of TS patients.[94] They are diagnosed at a mean age of 13 years. Although typically benign, they are a major cause of death in TS, due to their frequent occurrence near the foramen of Monro. As these tumors grow, they can obstruct cerebrospinal fluid (CSF) flow and result in brainstem herniation. The natural history of the systemic tumors in TS varies: astrocytomas may grow whereas cardiac rhabdomyomas tend to regress and renal angiomyolipomas often degenerate. Giant cell astrocytomas rarely undergo malignant transformation.[88] Such progression appears to be associated with the presence of mitotic figures and necrotic zones on histologic examination.

"Ash-leaf" spots are the earliest skin manifestation (Figure 3–5A). They occur at birth or in early infancy in 87 percent of TS patients. They appear as hypomelanotic macules most easily visible with Wood's light. Facial angiofibromas (adenoma

Table 3–10. DIAGNOSTIC CRITERIA FOR TUBEROUS SCLEROSIS	
Major Features	**Minor Features**
Facial angiofibroma (adenoma sebaceum)	Multiple randomly distributed dental enamel pits
≥ 3 Hypomelanotic macules (ash-leaf spots)	Gingival fibromas
Shagreen patch	Bone cysts
Nontraumatic ungual or periungual fibroma	Nonrenal hamartomas
Multiple retinal hamartomas ("mulberry lesions")	"Confetti" skin lesions
Cortical tuber	Multiple renal cysts
Subependymal nodule ("candle gutterings")	Retinal achromic patch
Subependymal giant cell astrocytoma	Hamartomatous rectal polyps
Cardiac rhabdomyoma	
Renal angiomyolipoma*	
Pulmonary lymphangiomyomatosis*	

*Other features should be documented before a definitive diagnosis is made.
Adapted from Hurst JS, Wilcoski S. Recognizing an index case of tuberous sclerosis. Am Fam Physician 2000;61:703–8, 710.

sebaceum) appear after 4 years of age and occur in 75 percent of TS patients (see Figure 3–5B). They can be mistaken for acne and may require repeated dermal abrasions for cosmetic treatment. Other common dermatologic manifestations include the shagreen patch, which is a connective-tissue hamartoma characterized by thickened skin with an "orange peel" texture and most often found on the middle to lower back, and the ungual fibroma, which is a flesh-colored papule that can distort the nail bed (see Figures 3–5C and D). Unlike ash-leaf spots, which are relatively common in the general population, ungual fibromas are fairly specific to TS.[88]

Multiple systemic features are associated with TS. Cardiac rhabdomyomas are frequently asymptomatic but can cause heart failure due to outflow obstruction of one or both ventricles. Renal cysts occur in mostly children whereas renal angiomyolipomas occur more often in adults. Retinal "mulberry lesions" are astrocytomas of the retina and occur in 50 to 75 percent of TS patients.[88] They appear as large whitish multinodular (mulberry-like) lesions that can be mistaken for RBs (see Figure 3–5E).

Radiographic Features

Parenchymal cortical tubers appear as low- or intermediate-signal areas on T1-weighted MRI and as high-signal areas on T2-weighted MRI (see Figure 3–5F). Typically, only 10 percent of tubers demonstrate enhancement. Subependymal nodules have an intensity similar to that of white matter, but approximately 30 percent of these lesions enhance.[95] One-third of subependymal giant cell astrocytomas exhibit serpentine flow voids due to dilated vessels. Their MRI appearance is variable, and they may be very difficult to distinguish from subependymal nodules either by signal intensity or by contrast enhancement (see Figure 3–5G). It is the change in the size of these nodules that is the most important aspect to carefully monitor.

Nabbout and colleagues observed 24 TS patients by serial brain CT and MRI to evaluate for any radiologic features that would predict the evolution of subependymal nodules into giant cell astrocytomas.[94] The subependymal nodules of > 5 mm in diameter that were incompletely calcified and enhanced with gadolinium were found to have a higher probability of evolving into giant cell astrocytomas, particularly in those patients with familial TS.[94] These radiologic risk factors (size, calcification, and enhancement) can be detected on MRI as early as 1 year of age. Thus, sequential brain MRI starting at an early age may be of value in predicting the development of giant cell astrocytomas, especially since clinical examinations alone would not yield any such significant predictive value. Nonspecific white-matter lesions, which are thought to be islets of disordered neurons and glial cells, are also seen on the MRI scans of TS patients.

Histopathology

Tubers contain a heterogeneous population of cellular elements, such as giant cells, normal and abnormal neurons, and astrocytes. Giant cells, which are the hallmark histologic cell type of TS, are distributed from the pial surface to the subcortical white matter, without clear radial orientation, and appear as large (80 to 150 μm in diameter) polygonal or ovoid eosinophilic cells that extend processes of unclear identity (axons or dendrites).[91] Microscopically, the normal structure of the cerebral cortex is lost within the tuber, and the junction between gray and white matter is often blurred. However, the cytoarchitecture of the cortex surrounding the tubers is often normal.

Subependymal giant cell astrocytomas are microscopically similar to subependymal nodules and tubers. They consist of large cells resembling astrocytes and smaller elongated cells within a fibrillary background. They tend to cluster, exhibit cellular pleomorphism, and may demonstrate perivascular pseudopalisading. Multinucleated giant cells are frequently seen (see Figure 3–5H). These tumors are classified as grade 1 astrocytomas by WHO criteria. Their low mitotic index, using the Ki-67 marker MIB-1, supports the benign histologic nature of these tumors.[91] They have been shown to arise from subependymal nodules.[93] The pathogenesis of the CNS lesions in TS is unclear as the cell precursor for the giant cells seen in tubers, subependymal nodules, and giant cell astrocytomas is not clearly defined. Most likely, the giant cells are derived from a mixed glioneuronal precursor cell, which would give rise to a clonal cellular line with varied differentiation.[91]

Genetics

Genetic studies have linked TS to two different loci: the TS complex-2 (*TSC2*) gene on chromosome 16p13.3 and the TS complex-1 (*TSC1*) gene on chromosome 9q34. Approximately 50 percent of TS families exhibit genetic linkage to *TSC1*, and 50 percent exhibit linkage to *TSC2*.[91] At least two-thirds of TS patients have no prior family history of TS and probably represent sporadic mutations rather than familial pedigrees.[91] The *TSC2* gene codes for a protein of 1,807 amino acids, called tuberin,[89] whereas the *TSC1* gene encodes a protein of 1,164 amino acids, called hamartin.[90] Recently, tuberin and hamartin were found to interact directly, which suggests that they are components of a single cellular pathway. This may explain the essentially identical clinical syndromes caused by *TSC1* and *TSC2* mutations.[91] The function of hamartin is currently not known. Tuberin has GAP activity specific for rap-1, which functions in the regulation of DNA synthesis and cell cycle transition. Loss of tuberin induces quiescent cells to enter the S phase.[96] Observed differences in the subcellular distribution of tuberin and hamartin cultured in vivo and in vitro suggest that tuberin and hamartin have varied functions and contribute in different ways to the formation of CNS lesions in TS.[97]

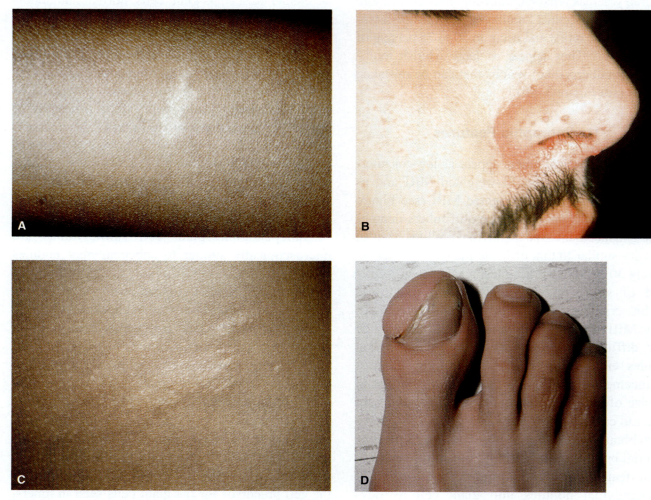

Figure 3–5. *A*, "Ash-leaf" lesion on the skin of a patient with tuberous sclerosis. *B*, Facial angiofibromas (adenoma sebaceum) on the right side of the face of a patient with tuberous sclerosis. *C*, Shagreen patch lesion on the skin of a patient with tuberous sclerosis. *D*, Ungual fibroma under the nail bed of the right first toe in a patient with tuberous sclerosis.

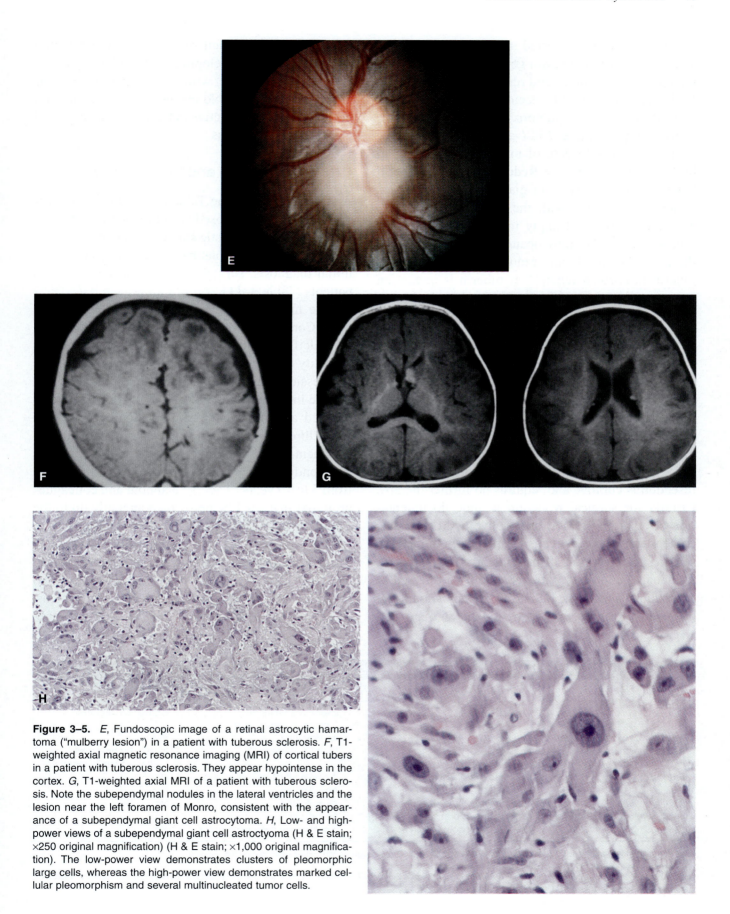

Figure 3–5. *E*, Fundoscopic image of a retinal astrocytic hamartoma ("mulberry lesion") in a patient with tuberous sclerosis. *F*, T1-weighted axial magnetic resonance imaging (MRI) of cortical tubers in a patient with tuberous sclerosis. They appear hypointense in the cortex. *G*, T1-weighted axial MRI of a patient with tuberous sclerosis. Note the subependymal nodules in the lateral ventricles and the lesion near the left foramen of Monro, consistent with the appearance of a subependymal giant cell astrocytoma. *H*, Low- and high-power views of a subependymal giant cell astroctyoma (H & E stain; ×250 original magnification) (H & E stain; ×1,000 original magnification). The low-power view demonstrates clusters of pleomorphic large cells, whereas the high-power view demonstrates marked cellular pleomorphism and several multinucleated tumor cells.

Studies have suggested that both *TSC1* and *TSC2* are tumor-suppressor genes. In subependymal giant cell astrocytomas and renal angiomyolipomas, LOH has been found to occur, which supports the two-hit model for TS tumors.[91,98] In a given tumor, LOH occurs at either *TSC1* or *TSC2*;[91] there have been no reports to date of mutations occurring in both loci simultaneously. Reduced or absent tuberin has been demonstrated in giant cell astrocytomas, which is consistent with the two-hit model.[96,98,99] This model may not apply to the pathogenesis of tubers since LOH rarely occurs in them[98] and since there is no significant reduction or absence of tuberin in cortical tubers.[96] If tuberin is in fact an important tumor-suppressor protein, then the loss of tuberin may be a marker for the deletion of both alleles of *TSC1* or *TSC2*.[96]

Management

The primary treatment modality for CNS manifestations of TS is surgery, which is used primarily for enlarging cerebral lesions such as subependymal giant cell astrocytomas that become symptomatic. Since these lesions are grade 1 tumors, a complete resection is curative and requires no further therapy. Criteria for surgical resection include documentation of enlarging tumor, obstructive hydrocephalus, and epileptogenic foci causing medically intractable seizures. Seizures in TS patients are often difficult to manage, and these patients should be referred to an epilepsy specialist. Radiation therapy should not be given routinely for the treatment of giant cell astrocytomas since their recurrence rate is low and the potential for developing a second malignancy (such as glioblastoma) within the radiation field has been documented.[100] No chemotherapy regimen has been shown to be effective in treating subependymal giant cell astrocytomas.

Screening and Surveillance

A subcommittee at the Tuberous Sclerosis Consensus Conference proposed recommendations for the rational use of diagnostic studies in patients with TS. These recommendations have been targeted for the initial diagnosis, surveillance, and screening of TS patients (Table 3–11).

The mainstay of diagnostic evaluation in TS is MRI. Computed tomography is excellent for detecting calcified lesions, but MRI is the neuroimaging modality of choice, particularly for documenting the progression of giant cell astrocytoma. Magnetic resonance imaging of the brain with contrast is recommended at initial diagnosis and then every 1 to 3 years through adolescence, depending on clinical judgment. The peak age range for symptomatic subependymal giant cell astrocytomas to occur is from 5 to 10 years of age.[101] Nabbout and colleagues proposed that MRI be performed annually up to the age of 10 years in TS patients with radiographic risk factors for giant cell astrocytoma transformation.[94] Magnetic resonance imaging has not been found to be highly predictive of TS in family members of TS patients who show no clinical signs or symptoms. There are nonspecific abnormalities that are more

Table 3–11. SCREENING AND SURVEILLANCE RECOMMENDATIONS FOR TUBEROUS SCLEROSIS

Diagnostic Test	Initial Testing	Surveillance	Family Screening*
MRI	At diagnosis	Every 1–3 years in children/adolescents	Cranial CT preferred
Ophthalmologic examination	At diagnosis	As indicated	Yes
Renal ultrasonography	At diagnosis	Every 1–3 years	Initially for potentially affected family members
Echocardiography	If cardiac symptoms occur	If cardiac dysfunction occurs	No
EKG	At diagnosis	As indicated	No
EEG	If seizures occur	As indicated	No
Neurodevelopmental testing	At diagnosis and at school entry	As indicated	No
Chest CT	At adulthood (women only)	If pulmonary symptoms occur	No

CT = computed tomography; EEG = electroencephalogram; EKG = electrocardiogram; MRI = magnetic resonance imaging.
*For asymptomatic family members of patients with tuberous sclerosis.
Adapted from Roach ES, DiMario FJ, Kandt RS, Northrup H. Tuberous Sclerosis Consensus Conference: recommendations for diagnostic evaluation. National Tuberous Sclerosis Association. J Child Neurol 1999;14:401–7.

disease specific to TS that are better detected on CT. Thus, head CT is the recommended test in these family members because it costs less and is more specific than MRI.[102]

Ophthalmologic, dermatologic, cardiac, and renal evaluations should be performed at initial diagnosis and subsequently as indicated for the patient, as well as to potentially affected family members. Neurodevelopmental testing should be performed in children at initial diagnosis and also prior to school entry. Electrocardiography should be performed when clinically indicated, but it is not indicated as a screening test for non-epileptic TS patients or their family members. Pulmonary lymphangiomyomatosis occurs almost exclusively in women and is rare in children. Chest CT should be performed in female TS patients at initial diagnosis once they have reached adulthood and should be repeated if pulmonary symptoms develop.[102]

Molecular testing for TS is not yet commercially available. Genetic counseling should inform families with one affected child that there is a 1 to 2 percent possibility of recurrence, even when parents show no evidence of TS.[102] Gene characterization may eventually identify TS patients at risk for developing certain complications, which would improve the individualization of diagnostic studies and reduce the number of unnecessary tests.

TURCOT'S SYNDROME

Turcot's syndrome, also known as brain tumor–polyposis (BTP) syndrome, is a heritable disorder characterized by the association of primary neuroepithelial neoplasms of the CNS with colorectal cancer. Crail[103] first described this disorder in 1949. In 1969, Turcot described two siblings who both were afflicted with adenomatous colorectal polyposis and a CNS tumor, suggesting a common etiology for seemingly disparate manifestations.[104] Turcot's syndrome encompasses a heterogeneous group of patients with varied presentations and clinical courses. Its genetic mode of transmission is still controversial.

Clinical Features

Mastronardi and colleagues initially hypothesized that Turcot's syndrome could be classified into two distinct syndromes.[105] Subsequently, Paraf and colleagues delineated two clinical syndrome types (BTP types 1 and 2) on the basis of several criteria: (1) the phenotype of the colonic polyps, (2) the genetic defects, (3) the type of CNS neoplasm, (4) the presence of skin lesions, and (5) consanguinity (Table 3–12).[106] The mean age at manifestation is 18.5 years, and the syndrome is mostly restricted to the second and early third decades of life.[107] More than 70 percent of patients present with intestinal symptoms initially; neurologic symptoms develop in the following 1 to 5 years. In contrast, when cerebral symptoms manifest initially, the colonic polyps become symptomatic mostly during the first year (with an average of 1.4 years).[107] Although Turcot's syndrome is typically associated with glioblastoma or medulloblastoma, concurrent associations with colonic adenocarcinoma and ganglioglioma, as well as malignant ependymomas, have been reported.[108,109] In addition to cerebral and colonic manifestations, congestive hypertrophy

Table 3–12. FEATURES OF BRAIN TUMOR–POLYPOSIS SYNDROMES		
Feature	BTP Type 1*	BTP Type 2
Brain tumor type	Glioma	Medulloblastoma
Associated hereditary colorectal syndromes	HNPCC	FAP
Family history of polyposis	Present	Absent
Number of colonic polyps	20–100	100–1,000
Skin lesions (eg, café-au-lait spots)	Frequent	Occasional
Consanguinity	Frequent	None
Mode of inheritance	Multifactorial autosomal recessive	Autosomal dominant
Gene mutation	Mismatch repair genes	APC (chromosome 5q21)

HNPCC = hereditary nonpolyposis colorectal cancer; FAP = familial adenomatous polyposis; APC = adenomatous polyposis coli; BTP = brain tumor–polyposis syndromes.
*Classic Turcot's syndrome.
Adapted from Paraf F, Jothy S, Van Meir EG. Brain tumor-polyposis syndrome: two genetic diseases? J Clin Oncol 1997;15:2744–58.

of the retinal-pigment epithelium (CHRPE) has been noted in patients with Turcot's syndrome.[110]

The type 1 syndrome is characterized by the presence of gliomas and colorectal adenomas without polyposis. Most patients with this type have colorectal phenotypes similar to that of patients in group 1 of the Itoh classification system: 20 to 100 colorectal polyps, some polyps > 3 cm in diameter, and a tendency to develop colorectal cancer at a young age (ie, 20 to 30 years of age).[111] In their study, Paraf and colleagues found that 98 percent of the CNS neoplasms were gliomas, 81 percent of which were malignant astrocytomas (Figure 3–6A). Of the patients with malignant gliomas, 81 percent were younger than 20 years of age. There is also a higher incidence of skin lesions (especially café-au-lait spots) in type 1 patients.[106] Type 1 BTP is considered to be the true Turcot's syndrome as originally described by Turcot in 1969.[106]

Type 2 BTP syndrome patients typically harbor a CNS neoplasm (usually a medulloblastoma rather than a glioblastoma) with a colorectal polyposis pattern similar to that seen in families with familial adenomatous polyposis (FAP)[106] (Figure 3–6B), an autosomal

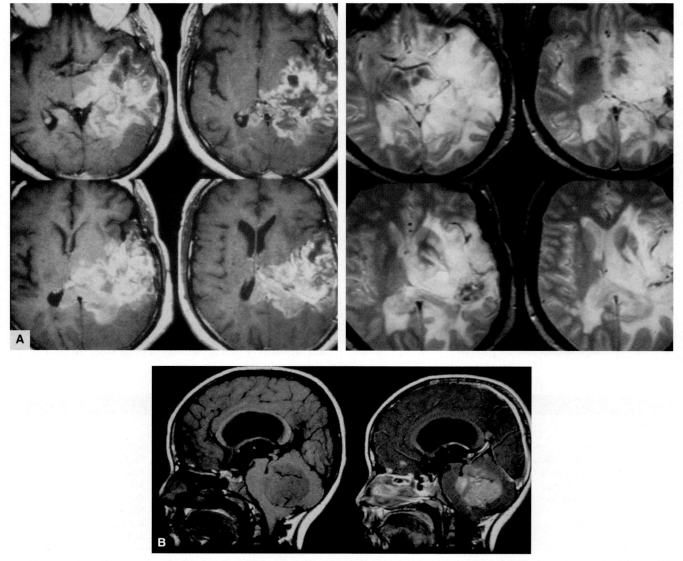

Figure 3–6. *A,* T1-weighted postcontrast and T2-weighted axial magnetic resonance imaging (MRI) of a left temporoparietal glioblastoma multiforme. *B,* T1-weighted pre- and postcontrast sagittal MRI of a child with a posterior fossa medulloblastoma. The lesion is hypointense on the precontrast image and enhances on the postcontrast image.

dominant syndrome in which affected families develop hundreds to thousands of adenomatous colorectal polyps. Colorectal adenocarcinomas inevitably occur if affected portions of the bowel are not resected. In contrast to type 1 patients, the occurrence of colorectal cancer without polyposis is rare in type 2 patients, and skin lesions are infrequent. There is a 92-fold increase in the relative risk of developing a medulloblastoma among FAP families, suggesting a direct association between FAP and the development of CNS neoplasms.[112] Type 2 BTP syndrome is not considered to be true Turcot's syndrome but may perhaps be a variant phenotypic manifestation of FAP[112] (ie, classic FAP with concomitant brain neoplasms).

Genetics

The controversy over whether Turcot's syndrome is a separate entity or another variant of FAP, as well as over its mode of inheritance, has not been fully resolved. Lewis and colleagues divided reported cases into three types based on family history and concluded that BTP syndrome is autosomal dominant and represents another variant of FAP.[113] However, Itoh and Ohsato divided the cases into three groups based on the size and number of the colonic polyps. They concluded that BTP syndrome is a separate entity, distinct from FAP.[114] The latter conclusion was further supported by Tops and colleagues, who described patients with brain tumors and colonic polyposis in families with FAP. Involvement of the FAP gene was excluded by linkage analysis, suggesting that Turcot's syndrome is not allelic to FAP.[115] Subsequent studies have identified germline mutations either in the adenomatous polyposis coli (APC) gene or in the DNA mismatch repair genes in Turcot's syndrome.[112]

Patients with BTP syndrome type 1 include patients who have one or more siblings with colorectal adenomas and/or gliomas, as well as patients with nonfamilial cases of Turcot's syndrome.[106] Consanguinity occurs more often in type 1 families. Neoplasms in these patients exhibit DNA replication errors. Mutations in DNA mismatch repair genes such as human mutation S homologue 2 (*hMSH2*), human mutation L homologue 1 (*hMLH1*), and human postmeiotic segregation 1 and 2 (*hPMS1* and *hPMS2*) have been noted.[108] Mutations in these groups of genes have been linked to the pathogenesis of hereditary nonpolyposis colorectal cancer (HNPCC), suggesting its relationship to BTP syndrome type 1, or Turcot's syndrome. The mode of inheritance for BTP syndrome type 1 is probably multifactorial autosomal recessive.[106]

In contrast, patients with type 2 BTP syndrome have a family history of polyposes (FAP or FAP kindred) and are not consanguinous. The inheritance mode is autosomal dominant. These patients have a germline mutation in the APC gene,[112] which is on chromosome 5q21 and which is detected in up to 80 percent of families affected with FAP.[106] This suggests that the type 2 (non-Turcot) syndrome is related to FAP and that it may represent a variant manifestation of the APC gene defect.

Management

The CNS tumors in Turcot's syndrome are managed as they would be in the general population. Depending on the tumor type, a combination of surgery, radiotherapy, and chemotherapy is often used. Patients with a history of familial hereditary colon cancer (either HNPCC or FAP) are at risk for developing a CNS malignancy, depending on the syndrome type. In a family with FAP and one member with a CNS neoplasm, other members in that family are at significantly higher risk of harboring a CNS tumor. Conversely, a previously healthy patient diagnosed with a brain tumor and having a family history of FAP should undergo screening and surveillance colonoscopy because CNS lesions can precede gastrointestinal (GI) symptoms in Turcot's syndrome.[109] Patients diagnosed with Turcot's syndrome should undergo genetic testing to identify the potential gene defect in order to provide further data on the genetic association between Turcot's syndrome and the hereditary colon cancer syndromes, as well as to possibly provide useful prognostic information.

STURGE-WEBER SYNDROME

Sturge-Weber syndrome (SWS), also called encephalotrigeminal angiomatosis, is a neurocutaneous disorder characterized by abnormal vascular lesions of the face, meninges, brain, and eye. Unlike most other phakomatoses, SWS does not have a familial, gender, or racial predilection.[116] The classic form of SWS consists of a cutaneous angioma (port-wine nevus) involving the part of the face innervated by the ophthalmic division of the trigeminal nerve with ipsilateral leptomeningeal angiomatosis.[116] In contrast to the other neurocutaneous disorders, SWS does not have an obvious genetic cause, and its etiology is still unknown.

Clinical Features

In addition to the unilateral port-wine nevus and ipsilateral leptomeningeal angiomatosis, the clinical features of SWS also include partial seizures (the clinical manifestations of which are often contralateral to the port-wine nevus) as well as occipital-region calcifications, glaucoma, and intellectual impairment (Table 3–13). Cases of SWS without the facial nevus have also been reported.[117,118]

The facial port-wine nevus is usually present at birth. As the child grows, the nevus typically thickens and changes in color, from pink to red to deep purple.[116] It is usually unilateral and located over the cutaneous distribution of the trigeminal division, thereby involving the forehead and upper eyelid (Figure 3–7A). Patients with a port-wine nevus that does not involve the ophthalmic division are unlikely to have SWS.[119] The nevus results from ectasia of cutaneous venules; these vary in size, from a few millimeters to several centimeters, and are irregularly shaped. They occur in about 0.3 percent of live births.[116,119] The nevus may be extensive, and on occasions may involve the scalp, palate, and neck. The extent of the nevus does not correlate with the extent of leptomeningeal disease[120] but does have positive correlation with the presence of choroidal hemangiomas.[119]

Patients with bilateral SWS have considerably worse outcomes than those with unilateral disease. Predictably, SWS patients with bilateral involvement have more neurologic deficits, earlier onset of seizure, and poorer prognoses for mental development.[121] Bilateral SWS is relatively uncommon (7.5% of SWS cases)[120] and is diagnosed by demonstrating bihemispheric leptomeningeal angiomatoses on MRI. Despite the intractable seizures, bilateral SWS is a contraindication to hemispherectomy or other types of surgery for epilepsy.

The most common clinical symptoms in SWS are seizures, which are most often focal and contralateral to the port-wine nevus. Other focal neurologic deficits result from the anatomic location of angiomatosis involvement. For example, contralateral hemianopias occur often due to calcifications commonly over the occipital lobe whereas angiomatosis that affects the central sulcus results in hemiparesis. Developmental delay and poor intellectual function are also seen commonly in SWS. In a study by Pascual-Castroviejo and colleagues, 24 (60%) of 40 SWS patients had mental retardation (IQ < 75), and 13 (32.5%) of 40 patients had severe mental retardation (IQ < 40).[120] The age of seizure onset may correlate with the severity of intellectual impairment. Keith and colleagues found that the incidence of mental retardation was 65 percent in patients whose onset of seizure was before the age of 6 months, 49 percent in those whose seizure onset occurred between the ages of 6 months and 2 years, and 34 percent for those whose seizure onset was between the ages of 2 and 4 years.[122] In addition to neuropathologic aspects causing decreased intellectual development, the psychopathology of the visible cutaneous stigmata of SWS must not be overlooked. Several cases of psychiatric disorders that develop in patients with SWS and that also contribute to intellectual impairment have been documented.[123]

Ocular defects occur commonly in SWS. Glaucoma is found in 30 to 50 percent of SWS patients

Table 3–13. CLINICAL FEATURES OF STURGE-WEBER SYNDROME

System	Lesion
CNS	Leptomeningeal angiomatosis
	Cortical calcification ("railroad track" appearance)
	Hemispheric atrophy
	Choroid plexus enlargement
Skin	Port-wine nevus (encephalofacial angiomatosis)
Eye	Choroidal hemangioma
	Glaucoma
	Dilation and tortuosity of intraocular vessels
	Retinal detachment
	Strabismus
	Buphthalmos

CNS = central nervous system.

and is almost always ipsilateral to the port-wine nevus.[116] In one study,[124] choroidal hemangiomas were noted to occur in 71 percent of SWS cases. They may present in early childhood, with visual loss and visual field defects due to continuous exudation causing compression of melanocytes and hyperplasia of retinal-pigment epithelium. If this process continues unabated, retinal or choroidal detachment requiring surgery may occur. Choroidal hemangiomas in SWS patients are typically diffuse, occur near the posterior pole, appear as a bright red "tomato catsup" fundus on fundoscopic examination, and can be bilateral[125] (see Figure 3–7B).

Radiographic Features

The diagnosis of SWS is made on clinical grounds, combined with supportive radiologic findings. The classic neuroradiologic finding in SWS is the "railroad track" appearance of calcifications underlying the angiomatosis (see Figure 3–7C). They appear in a dense gyriform pattern, usually located in the posterior parietal and occipital lobes. The calcifications are thought to be due to chronic intraparenchymal hypoxia secondary to the lack of superficial cortical venous drainage. In a review by Griffiths, calcifications were present in 84 percent of SWS patients who were 4 years of age or younger; all of the patients without calcifications were under 9 months of age.[119] Classic railroad track calcifications can be detected as early as 6 months of age and are best observed by CT. However, gradient echo T2-weighted MRI may be superior to CT in demonstrating microcalcifications in SWS, which appear diffusely in the superficial and deep white matter as well as in the cortex.

Leptomeningeal enhancement on T1-weighted MR contrast images is the "gold standard" for assessing the extent of disease in SWS (see Figure 3–7D) because the extent of leptomeningeal enhancement is usually greater than the area of calcification seen on noncontrast MRI or CT.[119] Atrophy is also a common finding that is best demonstrated by MRI and that can be even more extensive than calcifications or leptomeningeal enhancement. When atrophy is extensive, there may be compensatory enlargement of the skull base and vault, which is best demonstrated on CT. This enlargement manifests on CT as paranasal sinus and mastoid hypertrophy and as elevation of the petrous apex.

Magnetic resonance imaging of the orbits with contrast and fat-suppression images is important in evaluating such ocular manifestations of SWS as glaucoma, which can cause buphthalmos (globe enlargement) and choroidal hemangiomas (see Figure 3–7E). Unless vascular pathologies such as dural arteriovenous fistulas or arteriovenous malformations are suspected by sectional imaging, the routine use of cerebral angiography in the initial diagnosis of SWS is not recommended.[119]

Histopathology

The neuropathology of SWS consists of leptomeningeal and choroid plexus angiomatosis, as well as venous engorgement and tortuosity.[116] The fundamental abnormality in SWS is the lack of superficial cortical venous drainage of the affected hemispheric areas. The blood is redirected into the developing meninges, causing the development of abnormal vascular channels. The primary neuropathology of SWS, angiomatosis of the trigeminal and leptomeningeal regions, may be the result of incomplete degeneration of the vascular plexus formed at the cephalic end of the neural tube during the sixth week of gestation.[117] The relationship of the cerebral angioma and the facial nevus is not entirely clear but can be partially explained embryologically by the common ectodermal origins of the skin and CNS.

Leptomeningeal angiomas consist of thin-walled veins confined within the pia mater and cause the meninges to thicken and darken from increased vascularity[116] (see Figure 3–7F). The port-wine nevus is a benign congenital ectasia of cutaneous venules. Since it has no endothelial proliferation, it is not a hemangioma. Antibodies to S-100 protein demonstrate a decrease in the number of neurons surrounding the superficial venules, perhaps resulting in decreased vascular tone and subsequent progressive dilation of the cutaneous superficial vascular plexi. This neuronal loss (probably of sympathetic autonomic origin) may be the pathologic basis of the progressive ectasias in SWS.[116]

Management

The management of SWS is directed primarily toward the medical control of seizures, which cause most of the morbidity in SWS.[116] Carbamazepine (Tegretol) or valproate (Depakote) is often used as a first-line therapeutic agent. Vigabatrin is also used as an effective adjunctive agent. The role of surgery is to stop or control seizure activity. Surgical options, which include hemispherectomy, partial lobectomy, and corpus callosotomy, are contraindicated in bilateral SWS. Port-wine nevi can be coagulated and destroyed by laser surgery, with minimal scarring.[116] External beam radiation therapy (EBRT) and scattered photocoagulation have been used to treat choroidal hemangiomas.[116] Trabeculotomy in infants and the guarded-filtration procedure used in older children have been shown to decrease glaucomatous complications.[126]

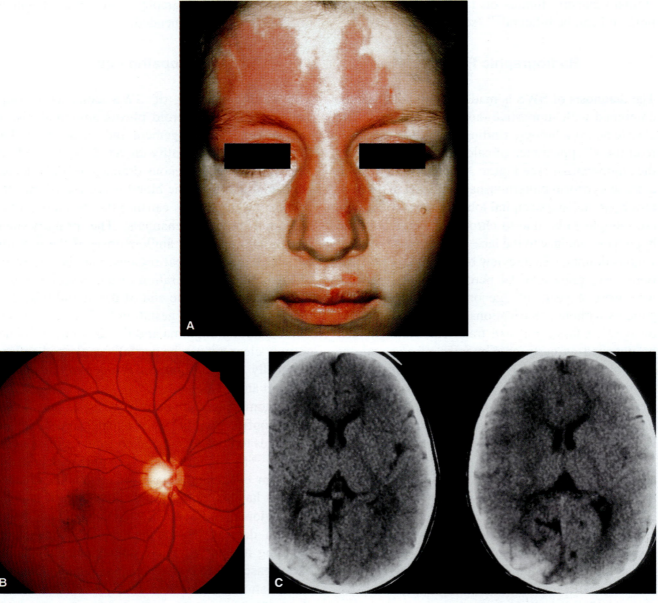

Figure 3–7. *A*, Bilateral port-wine nevi in a patient with Sturge-Weber syndrome. The involvement corresponds with the ophthalmic division of the trigeminal nerve bilaterally. *B*, Fundoscopic image of a diffuse choroidal hemangioma in a patient with Sturge-Weber syndrome. Note the "tomato catsup" appearance of the fundus. *C*, Computed tomography (CT) of leptomeningeal "railroad track" calcifications of the right occipital cortex in a patient with Sturge-Weber syndrome.

NEVOID BASAL CELL CARCINOMA (GORLIN'S) SYNDROME

Nevoid basal cell carcinoma syndrome (NBCCS), also known as Gorlin's syndrome, is an autosomal dominant disorder characterized by the development of basal cell carcinoma (BCC) at a young age, jaw keratocysts, skeletal abnormalities, and an increased risk of developing medulloblastomas. This syndrome was first described by Gorlin and Goltz in 1960 and has an estimated prevalence of 1 in 60,000.[127] It is characterized by a high rate of penetrance, spontaneous mutation rates ranging from 35 to 50 percent, and highly variable clinical phenotypes.[127] The responsible gene has been mapped to chromosome 9. The estimated incidence of medulloblastomas in patients with Gorlin's syndrome is approximately 5 to 20 percent.[128]

Clinical Features

There are five major features of Gorlin's syndrome: (1) multiple BCCs from the third decade of life onward (Figure 3–8A), (2) pits at the palms and/or

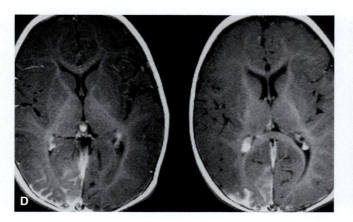

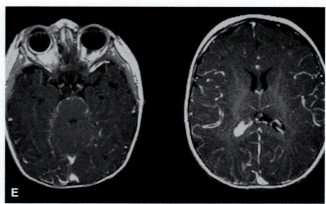

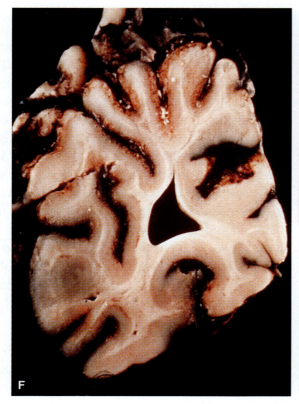

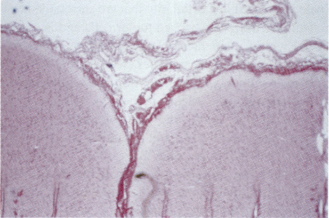

Figure 3–7. *D,* T1-weighted postcontrast axial magnetic resonance imaging (MRI) in a patient with Sturge-Weber syndrome. Note the right hemispheric atrophy and the leptomeningeal enhancement in the right occipital cortex. *E,* T1-weighted postcontrast axial MRI demonstrating enhancement of a right retinal hemangioma and enlarged right choroid plexus in a patient with Sturge-Weber syndrome. *F,* Gross coronal and microscopic sections through the occipital lobes of a patient with Sturge-Weber syndrome (H & E stain; ×50 original magnification). Note the darkened surface of the brain due to extensive leptomeningeal angiomatoses on the gross section. The microscopic section demonstrates leptomeningeal angiomatosis and calcifications in the superficial cortex of a patient with Sturge-Weber syndrome.

soles, (3) congenital skeletal anomalies, (4) odontogenic keratocysts, and (5) ectopic calcification of the falx cerebri.[129] Other manifestations associated with Gorlin's syndrome are divided into major and minor features (Table 3–14).[130] Diagnosis is made when two major features or one major and two minor features are present.

Medulloblastoma is the most common posterior fossa tumor in children, accounting for about 20 percent of all childhood brain tumors. The mean age at diagnosis is 6.3 years, with male children affected more often than female children.[131] The 5-year survival rate is 60 to 80 percent; treatment involves surgery, radiation, and chemotherapy. Less than 5 percent of children with medulloblastomas also have Gorlin's syndrome.[131] Medulloblastomas associated with Gorlin's syndrome present at an average age of 2 years, which is earlier than in sporadic cases.[132] Also, patients with medulloblastomas associated with Gorlin's syndrome tend to survive longer than patients with sporadic medulloblastoma. Case studies have reported survival rates > 10 years after resection;[132,133] this may be partly explained by the observation that patients with Gorlin's syndrome have the "desmoplastic" medulloblastoma phenotype.[128] The desmoplastic type is characterized by nodular reticulin-free areas (pale islands) of low cellularity that are surrounded by reticulin-rich densely packed tumor cells and is associated with a more favorable prognosis than that of other medulloblastoma subtypes (see Figure 3–8B).

Less commonly, Gorlin's syndrome is associated with meningiomas. Most are benign, but the two patients in one study who had malignant meningiomas had received cranial irradiation to treat BCCs.[133,134] Although one may infer from these cases that prior irradiation leads to an increased risk of developing malignant meningiomas, no definitive conclusions should be drawn from such a small number of cases.

Genetics

Gorlin's syndrome results from mutations that inactivate the patched gene (*PTCH*), a homologue of the *Drosophila* segment polarity gene.[135] The patched gene is a tumor-suppressor gene located on chromosome 9q22.3.[128] It functions as a cell-cycle regulator in the absence of its ligand, *sonic hedgehog* (Hh-N), and is part of the "hedgehog signaling pathway."[136] Although LOH on *PTCH* has been demonstrated in medulloblastoma patients with Gorlin's syndrome,[135,137,138] *PTCH* is probably not the classic tumor-suppressor gene to which Knudson's two-hit model applies. This conclusion is based on the observation that several congenital manifestations of Gorlin's syndrome (such as macrocephaly, bifid ribs, and cleft lip and palate) may result solely from the initial (germline) "hit," unlike BCCs and medulloblastomas, which require two hits to form and develop.[139]

In the hedgehog signaling pathway, *PTCH* without its ligand Hh-N inhibits the *smoothed* gene (another transmembrane gene), thereby preventing the expression of downstream genes that control cell proliferation. Thus, mutations in the *PTCH* gene would inactivate its ability to inhibit *smoothed*, leading to downstream gene transcriptional activation, resulting in increased cell proliferation. Mutations in Hh-N and *smoothed*, either alone or in combination with a germline (first-hit) mutation of *PTCH*, have been proposed as possible explanations for the variable clinical presentations of a minority of Gorlin's syndrome patients who do not exhibit all of the classic manifestations.[139]

Management

The management approach is similar for both sporadic medulloblastomas and for those medulloblastomas associated with Gorlin's syndrome. Standard treatment involves surgical resection, followed by CSA irradiation and adjuvant chemotherapy. In patients with Gorlin's syndrome, radiation-induced BCCs have been documented to develop 1 to 4 years after radiation treatment.[129] Thus, special attention must be paid to areas of irradiated skin. Cutaneous lesions in Gorlin's syndrome patients are best treated with photodynamic therapy and not with radiation.[129] Oral retinoid therapy has been found to be successful in preventing the emergence of new BCCs in patients with Gorlin's syndrome but does not significantly affect the existing lesions.[129]

LHERMITTE-DUCLOS DISEASE

Lhermitte-Duclos disease (LDD) is a rare and unusual hamartoma involving the cerebellum. It was

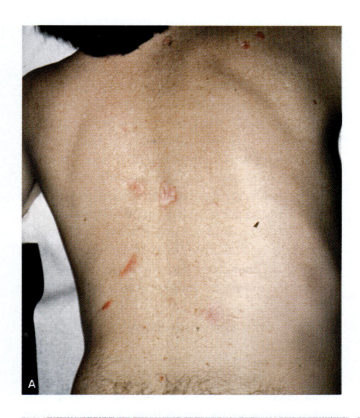
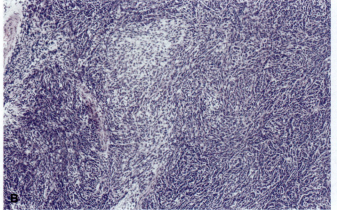
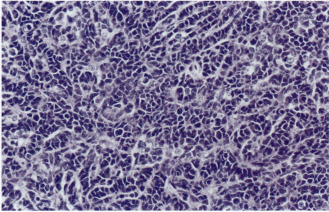

Figure 3–8. *A*, Multiple basal cell carcinomas of the middle and lower back. *B*, Low- and high-power views of medulloblastoma (H & E stain; ×160 original magnification) (H & E stain; ×500 original magnification). Note the pale island surrounded by a dense population of neoplastic cells. The higher-power view demonstrates many mitotic figures and apoptotic cells.

first described by Lhermitte and Duclos in 1920.[140] It is also known as dysplastic gangliocytoma of the cerebellum and is more consistent with dysplasia than neoplasia. Its association with Cowden syndrome (CS), or multiple hamartoma-neoplasia syndrome, may represent a single disease complex that may be categorized as a unique phakomatosis.

Clinical Features

Lhermitte-Duclos disease (LDD) is believed to be a hamartomatous overgrowth arising from the cerebellar cortex. The age of clinical manifestation ranges widely, from the neonatal period to the age of 74 years, but most cases are diagnosed in the third and fourth decades.[141] The duration of symptoms ranges from a few months up to 30 years prior to developing severe clinical symptoms.[142] Recurrences several years after resection have been described,[143,144] but malignant transformation has not been reported.

Patients with LDD typically present with signs and symptoms of increased ICP and hydrocephalus, as well as cerebellar signs (eg, limb/trunk/gait ataxia, vertigo, nystagmus). Less commonly,

Table 3–14. DIAGNOSTIC CRITERIA FOR NEVOID BASAL CELL CARCINOMA (GORLIN'S) SYNDROME

Major Criteria
    Multiple BCC OR one BCC under age of 30 years OR >10 basal cell nevi
    Any odontogenic keratocyst* or polyostotic bone cyst
    Ectopic calcification: lamellar or early (< 20 years of age) calcification of falx
    ≥ 3 palmar or plantar pits
    Family history of Gorlin's syndrome
Minor Criteria
    Congenital skeletal anomaly (bifid or fused rib/vertebra)
    Medulloblastoma
    Cardiac or ovarian fibroma
    Congenital malformation†
    Lymphomesenteric cysts
    OFC > 97% tile with frontal bossing

BCC = basal cell carcinoma; OFC = occipitofrontal head circumference.
*Proven histologically.
†Cleft lip/palate, polydactyly, cataract, microphthalmia, coloboma.
Adapted from Evans DGR, Ladusans EJ, Rimmer S, et al. Complications of the naevoid basal cell carcinoma syndrome: results of a population based study. J Med Genet 1993;30:460–4.

patients can present with cranial-nerve dysfunction, motor weakness and spasticity, Babinski's sign, hyperreflexia, tremors, orthostatic hypotension, and apneic spells. About one-third of LDD cases are associated with the development of congenital malformations such as megalencephaly.

Cowden syndrome is an autosomal dominant condition characterized by mucocutaneous lesions that are usually apparent by 20 years of age, systemic hamartomas, and a high incidence of systemic carcinoma, particularly breast cancer. The pathognomonic skin lesion of CS is the trichilemmoma,[141] which appears as facial papules clustered around the orifices (Figure 3–9A). They can be similar to the adenoma sebaceum lesions typical of patients with TS. Neurologically, CS has been associated with megalencephaly, low intelligence, coordination disturbances, and seizures. Of note, patients with CS have been found to have a 1,000-fold increased risk of developing meningiomas.[145]

Radiographic Features

Kulkantrakorn and colleagues outlined the typical radiologic features of LDD.[146] There is a characteristic nongyriform pattern with enlargement of the cerebellar folia (see Figure 3–9B). The inner portion of the cerebellar folia (consisting of the white matter, the abnormal granule cell layer, and the deep molecular layer) appears hypointense and hyperintense on T1- and T2-weighted MR images, respectively. The outer portion of the folia, consisting of the outer molecular layer and leptomeninges within the effaced sulci, appears isointense with the normal cerebellum on MR images. Vascular proliferation in the pia mater may be associated with calcifications or (rarely) contrast enhancement. Enlargement of the folia can produce enough mass effect to efface the sulci, rendering them radiographically indistinct. Within the folia, there appears to be a contorted laminar pattern that is much less evident on CT compared to MRI. Therefore, MRI is the neuroimaging modality of choice for the diagnosis and surveillance of the dysplastic gangliocytoma of LDD.

Histopathology

Lhermitte-Duclos disease has previously been called diffuse ganglioneuroma of the cerebellar cortex and hamartoblastoma and is currently called dysplastic gangliocytoma of the cerebellum. This reflects the uncertainty about whether the lesion represents a congenital malformation, a hamartoma, or a true neoplasm.[145] The pathogenesis and cell of origin are still unclear although some evidence favors the Purkinje cell (rather than an extreme form of hypertrophic dysplastic granule cell) as the progenitor cell type.[142] Many of the known characteristics of this lesion do not support a neoplastic process: the lesion does not invade surrounding brain tissue or metastasize, there is an absence of significant mitotic activity, progression is extremely slow, and there is little or no proliferative activity.[142]

The essence of LDD is a thickened zone of abnormal cells that replaces the normal granule cell layer in the affected areas of the cerebellar cortex. Macroscopically, LDD lesions are poorly circumscribed, firm masses that may appear immediately beneath the normal-appearing surface of the cerebellum. The cerebellum exhibits thick and enlarged folia, with multiple foci of myelination in the outer zone, thick underlying gray matter, and decreased white matter. Cerebellar folia can enlarge up to a width of 7 mm.[146] Microscopically, there is widening of the molecular layer, absence of the Purkinje cell layer, and hypertrophy of the granule cell layer.

The molecular layer is replaced by an upper layer of abnormally myelinated axons in parallel arrays (see Figure 3–9C) while the normal Purkinje cell and internal granule cell layers are replaced by a wide lower layer of dysplastic disorganized neurons (inverted cerebellar cortex) (see Figure 3–9D). This lesion is believed to be derived from a hamartomatous (non-neoplastic) process. The phenotype of these dysplastic cells is confirmed by immunohistochemistry as being neuronal in origin.[142]

The association between LDD and CS was first recognized by Padberg and colleagues, who proposed that the two syndromes represented a single phakomatosis.[147] Subsequently, there have been more than 20 documented cases of patients with both LDD and CS.[145] There has been no established genetic locus for LDD although some associations with trisomy 13, 15, and 18 have been noted.[141] The susceptibility gene for CS was designated PTEN (phosphatase and tensin homologue deleted on chromosome 10) by Li and colleagues[148] and has been mapped to a locus on chromosome 10q23.3.[149] It acts as a tumor-suppressor gene by inactivating signal transduction pathways that regulate critical processes such as cell division.[145] Sutphen and colleagues reported a patient with both LDD and CS who had missense mutations in the region of the active site in PTEN, suggesting a genetic connection between the two syndromes.[150] Robinson and Cohen concurred with the initial hypothesis of Padberg and colleagues that LDD and CS are a single complex representing a true phakomatosis and have designated it the Cowden and Lhermitte-Duclos disease (COLD) complex.[145] However, Murata and colleagues suggested that CS and LDD do not make up a single disease entity since they felt that the occurrence of CS results from a germline mutation whereas LDD is a result of additional somatic mutations on either the remaining PTEN allele or another unknown gene.[151] To definitively characterize the relationship between LDD and CS, the molecular genetics must be better delineated, particularly for LDD.

Management

The primary treatment modality for dysplastic gangliocytoma is surgical resection. A preoperative diagnosis can be made on the basis of MRI findings.[146] Lhermitte-Duclos disease that is discovered incidentally by MRI should be managed conservatively with annual MRI, more frequently if patients become symptomatic.[142] Due to its protracted and nonmalignant clinical course, surgery is recommended only for patients who become symptomatic from obstructive hydrocephalus. Long-term follow-up is recommended after resection as recurrences as late as 12 years postoperatively have been reported.[145] Ventriculoperitoneal shunting relieves the symptoms of hydrocephalus but does not relieve the symptoms arising from cerebellar compression by the lesion. There is no known role for chemotherapy, and the routine use of radiation in these patients is not recommended.[145] Given the association of LDD and CS, patients diagnosed with CS (as well as family members of patients with LDD who have megalencephaly) should be assessed by screening MRI.[146]

LI-FRAUMENI SYNDROME

Li-Fraumeni syndrome (LFS) is a rare autosomal dominant familial disorder characterized by the early occurrence of sarcomas, breast carcinomas, leukemias, adrenocortical carcinomas, and brain tumors in affected family members. Li-Fraumeni syndrome results from mutations in the p53 tumor-suppressor gene, which is located on chromosome 17p. Although p53 mutations occurring in tumor tissues are common in many malignant gliomas, germline p53 mutations occur only in a small fraction of these tumors in the general population.[152] However, germline p53 mutations occur in up to 80 percent of LFS families.[153]

Clinical Features

The diagnosis of LFS requires a patient to have (a) a sarcoma diagnosed before the age of 45 years, (b) a first-degree relative diagnosed with cancer before the age of 45 years, and (c) another first- or second-degree relative with either sarcoma diagnosed at any age or any cancer diagnosed before 45 years of age.[154] Soft-tissue sarcomas usually develop in the first 5 years of life, whereas CNS tumors and acute leukemias develop throughout childhood and young adulthood. Breast cancer is the most common malignancy in adults with LFS. The brain tumors associated with LFS are malignant neuroepithelial tumors, such as anaplastic gliomas and glioblastomas, and are less commonly PNETs.[154] It is these types of brain tumors that occur at a higher incidence in association with mutations of the p53 gene. Histologically, glioblastomas are characterized by the following: hypercellularity, marked nuclear and cytoplasmic pleomorphism, high mitotic activity, microvascular proliferation, and/or pseudopalisading necrosis (Figures 3–10A to C). Li-Fraumeni syndrome has also been reported to occur concurrently in a patient with SWS, but it is not clear whether this case represents a coincidence or a forme fruste of LFS.[152]

Genetics

The area between exons 5 and 9 of the p53 gene on chromosome 17p is the region that harbors the LFS mutation.[153] The p53 gene acts as a tumor-suppressor gene in a manner consistent with Knudson's two-hit model. Mutations of the p53 gene are one of the most common molecular alterations in a large variety of tumors, including those of the CNS. The p53 gene regulates cell growth by mediating a cell-cycle checkpoint so that cells with DNA damage are suspended from the cell cycle so that the damage can be repaired prior to completion of the cycle and replication.[155] Overexpression of mutant p53 has been shown to

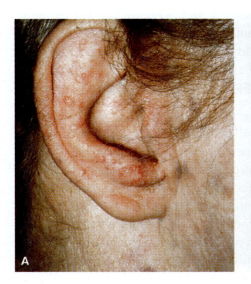
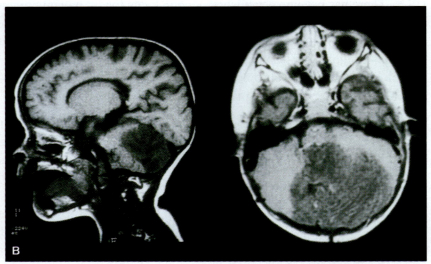

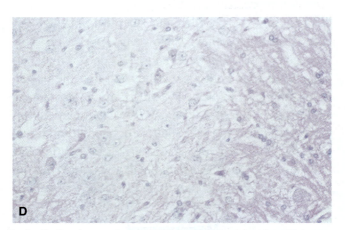

Figure 3–9. *A*, Trichilemmoma lesions on the right external ear of a patient with Cowden syndrome. *B*, T1-weighted axial and sagittal magnetic resonance imaging (MRI) in a child with Lhermitte-Duclos disease. There is a large hypointense non-enhancing posterior fossa mass lesion consistent with the appearance of a dysplastic gangliocytoma of the cerebellum. *C*, Parallel arrays of abnormally myelinated axons in a dysplastic gangliocytoma in a patient with Lhermitte-Duclos disease (H & E stain; ×50 original magnification). *D*, Dysplastic gangliocytoma in a patient with Lhermitte-Duclos disease (H & E stain; ×1,000 original magnification). Large ganglion cells have replaced the Purkinje cell and internal granule cell layers in the cerebellum.

extend the life span of human diploid fibroblasts past the point of senescence,[156] which may facilitate the immortalization observed in the fibroblasts of patients with LFS.[157] Recently, a germline mutation in the human checkpoint kinase 2 *(hCHK2)* gene has been found in some members of LFS families. It encodes a protein controlling the checkpoints in the signal transduction pathways associated with tumorigenesis, suggesting that the *hCHK2* gene may also be a tumor-suppressor gene associated with LFS.[158]

Although mutations of the p53 gene have been established as a causal event for LFS, the molecular genetics of LFS are still not completely understood. Patients with a glioma and a family history of cancers should have genetic testing in order to develop individualized screening, surveillance, and treatment strategies for the purposes of earlier diagnosis and management, with the goal being the improvement of the patient's outcome and quality of life.

CONCLUSION

This chapter has discussed various hereditary brain tumor disorders and has highlighted their important CNS manifestations. Each syndrome exhibits distinctive clinical features and characteristic genetic profiles associated with higher incidences of brain and spinal cord neoplasms than occurs in the general population. The specific treatment guidelines for these syndromes are beyond the scope of this chapter. Potential management modalities in development include somatic gene therapy (which involves replacing the tumor-suppressor product directly into the tumors through viral vectors or by direct recombination) as well as antiangiogenesis medications and improved genetic screening methods. Future advances in genetic research to further characterize the molecular characteristics of these debilitating familial brain tumor syndromes will be critical for the development of effective treatments.

ACKNOWLEDGMENTS

The authors wish to gratefully acknowledge the following individuals for their invaluable contributions: A. James Barkovich, MD, and Nancy Fishbein, MD, for the radiographic images; Timothy Berger, MD, for the dermatologic images; David Clay and Devron Char, MD, for the ophthalmologic images; Richard L. Davis, MD, for the pathology images; and Agnes Villamin for her assistance with slide preparations.

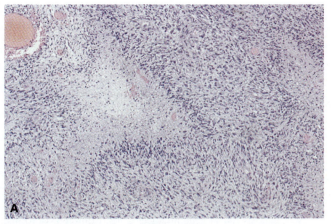
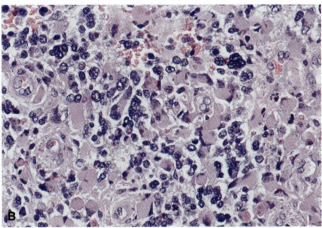
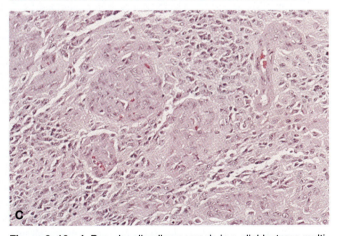

Figure 3–10. *A,* Pseudopalisading necrosis in a glioblastoma multiforme (×100 original magnification). *B,* High cellularity and marked nuclear and cytoplasmic pleomorphism of astrocytes in a glioblastoma multiforme (×1,000 original magnification). *C,* Marked microvascular proliferation in a glioblastoma multiforme (×250 original magnification). (H & E stain)

REFERENCES

1. Neurofibromatosis. Conference statement. National Institutes of Health Consensus Development Conference. Arch Neurol 1988;45:575–78.
2. Mukonoweshuro W, Griffiths PD, Blaser S. Neurofibromatosis type 1: the role of neuroradiology. Neuropediatrics 1999;30:111–9.
3. Romanowski CA, Cavallin LI. Neurofibromatosis types I and II: radiological appearance. Hosp Med 1998;59:134–9.
4. Cawthorn RM, Weiss R, Xu GF, et al. A major segment of the neurofibromatosis type 1 gene: cDNA sequence, genomic structure, and point mutations. Cell 1990;62:193–201.
5. Viskochil D, Buchberg AM, Xu G, et al. Deletions and translocation interrupt a cloned gene at the neurofibromatosis type 1 locus. Cell 1990;62:187–92.
6. Wallace MR, Marchuk, DA, Andersen LB, et al. Type 1 neurofibromatosis gene: identification of a large transcript disrupted in three NF1 patients. Science 1990;249:181–6.
7. Molloy PT, Bilaniuk LT, Vaughan SN, et al. Brainstem tumors in patients with neurofibromatosis type 1: a distinct clinical entity. Neurology 1995;45:1897–902.
8. Ruggieri M, Huson SM. The neurofibromatoses. An overview. Ital J Neurol Sci 1999;20:89–108.
9. Miller VS, Roach ES. Neurofibromatosis. In: Bradley WG, Daroff RB, Fenichel GM, Marsden CD, editors. Neurology in clinical practice. 3rd ed. Woburn (MA): Butterworth-Heinemann; 2000. p. 1665–2000.
10. Pollack IF, Mulvihill JJ. Special issues in the management of gliomas in children with neurofibromatosis. J Neurooncol 1996;28:257–68.
11. Listernick R, Charrow J, Greenwald MJ, Esterley NB. Optic gliomas in children with neurofibromatosis type 1. J Pediatr 1989;114:788–92.
12. Listernick R, Charrow J, Greenwald MJ, Mets M. Natural history of optic pathway tumors in children with neurofibromatosis type 1: a longitudinal study. J Pediatr 1994;125:63–6.
13. Reddy AT, Mapstone TB. Brainstem tumors. In: Bernstein M, Berger MS, editors. Neuro-oncology: the essentials. 1st ed. New York: Thieme; 2000. p. 352–62.
14. Cohen ME, Duffner PK, Heffner RR, et al. Prognostic factors in brainstem gliomas. Neurology 1986;36:602–5.
15. Raffel C, McComb JG, Bodner S, Gilles FE. Benign brainstem lesions in pediatric patients with neurofibromatosis: case reports. Neurosurgery 1989;25:959–64.
16. Griffiths PD, Blaser S, Mukonoweshuro W, et al. Neurofibromatosis bright objects in children with neurofibromatosis type 1: a proliferative potential? Pediatrics 1999;104(4):e49.
17. Yamanouchi H, Kato T, Matsuda H, et al. MRI in neurofibromatosis type 1: using fluid-attenuated inversion recovery pulse sequences. Pediatr Neurol 1995;12:286–90.
18. Itoh T, Magnaldi S, White RM, et al. Neurofibromatosis type 1: the evolution of deep grey and white matter abnormalities. AJNR Am J Neuroradiol 1994;15:1513–9.
19. Norfray JF, Darling C, Byrd S, et al. Short TE proton MRS and neurofibromatosis type 1 in intracranial lesions. J Comput Assist Tomogr 1999;23:994–1003.
20. Barker D, Wright E, Nguyen K, et al. Gene for von Recklinghausen neurofibromatosis is in the pericentric region of chromosome 17. Science 1987;236:1100–2.
21. Seizinger BR, Rouleau GA, Ozelius LJ, et al. Genetic linkage of von Recklinghausen neurofibromatosis to the nerve growth factor receptor gene. Cell 1987;49:589–94.
22. Nishi T, Saya H. Neurofibromatosis type I (NF1) gene: implications in neuroectodermal differentiation and genesis of brain tumors. Cancer Metastasis Rev 1991;10:301–10.
23. Takahashi K, Suzuki H, Kayama T, et al. Multiple transcripts of the neurofibromatosis type 1 gene in human brain and in brain tumors. Clin Sci (Colch) 1994;87:481–5.
24. Nishi T, Lee PSY, Oka K, et al. Differential expression of two types of neurofibromatosis type 1 (NF1) gene transcripts related to neuronal differentiation. Oncogene 1991;6:1555–9.
25. Suzuki Y, Suzuki H, Kayama T, et al. Brain tumors predominantly express the neurofibromatosis type 1 gene transcripts containing the 63 base insert in the region coding for GTP-ase activating protein-related domain. Biochem Biophys Res Commun 1991;181:955–61.
26. Andersen LB, Ballester R, Marchuk DA, et al. A conserved alternative splice in the von Recklinghausen neurofibromatosis (NF1) gene produces 2 neurofibromin isoforms, both of which have GTPase activating protein activity. Mol Cell Biol 1993;13:487–95.
27. Suzuki H, Takahashi K, Kubota Y, Shibahara S. Molecular cloning of a cDNA coding for neurofibromatosis type 1 protein isoform lacking the domain related to *ras* GTPase-activating protein. Biochem Biophys Res Commun 1992;187:984–90.
28. Tokuyama T, Uemura K, Fujita M. The 2 types of mRNAs for neurofibromin isoforms produced by von Recklinghausen neurofibromatosis (NF1) gene: analysis in human astrocytic tumors. Neurosci Lett 1995;196:189–92.
29. Gutmann DH, Donahoe J, Brown T, et al. Loss of neurofibromatosis 1 (NF1) gene expression in NF1-associated pilocytic astrocytomas. Neuropathol Appl Neurobiol 2000;26:361–7.
30. Bilaniuk LT, Molloy PT, Zimmerman RA, et al. Neurofibromatosis type 1: brain stem tumors. Neuroradiology 1997;39:642–53.
31. Listernick R, Charrow J, Gutmann DH. Intracranial gliomas in neurofibromatosis type 1. Am J Med Genet 1999;89(1):38–44.
32. Perilongo G, Moras P, Carollo C, et al. Spontaneous partial regression of low-grade glioma in children with neurofibromatosis 1: a real possibility. J Child Neurol 1999;14:352–6.
33. Parazzini C, Triulzi F, Bianchini E, et al. Spontaneous involution of optic pathway lesions in neurofibromatosis type 1: serial contrast MR evaluation. AJNR Am J Neuroradiol 1995;16:1711–8.
34. Kim G, Mehta M, Kucharczyk W, Blaser S. Spontaneous regression of a tectal mass in neurofibromatosis 1. AJNR Am J Neuroradiol 1998;19:1137–9.
35. Trofatter JA, MacCollin MM, Rutter JL, et al. A novel moesin-, ezrin-, radixin-like gene is a candidate for the neurofibromatosis 2 tumor suppressor. Cell 1993;72:791–800.
36. Rouleau GA, Merel P, Lutchman M, et al. Alteration in a new gene encoding a putative membrane-organizing protein causes neuro-fibromatosis type 2. Nature 1993;363:515–21.

37. Tsukita S, Yonemura S. Cortical actin organization: lessons from ERM (ezrin/radixin/moesin) proteins. J Biol Chem 1999;274:34507–10.
38. Mautner VF, Tatagiba M, Guthoff R, et al. Neurofibromatosis 2 in the pediatric age group. Neurosurgery 1993;33(1):92–6.
39. Evans DGR, Sainio M, Baser ME. Neurofibromatosis type 2. J Med Genet 2000;37:897–904.
40. Baser ME, Evans DGR, Jackler RK, et al. Malignant peripheral nerve sheath tumors, radiotherapy, and neurofibromatosis 2. Br J Cancer 2000;82:998.
41. Evans DGR, Birch JM, Ramsden R. Paediatric presentation of type 2 neurofibromatosis. Arch Dis Child 1998;81:496–9.
42. Kley N, Whaley J, Seizinger BR. Neurofibromatosis type 2 and von Hippel-Lindau disease: from gene cloning to function. Glia 1995;15:297–307.
43. Lutchman M, Rouleau GA. The neurofibromatosis type 2 gene product, schwannomin, suppresses growth of NIH 3T3 cells. Cancer Res 1995;55:2270–4.
44. Huynh DP, Pulst SM. Neurofibromatosis 2 antisense oligodeoxynucleotides induce reversible inhibition of schwannomin synthesis and cell adhesion in STS26T and T98G cells. Oncogene 1996;13:73–84.
45. Hitotsumatsu T, Iwaki T, Kitamoto T, et al. Expression of neurofibromatosis 2 protein in human brain tumors: an immunohistochemical study. Acta Neuropathol (Berl) 1997;93:225–32.
46. Huynh DP, Mautner V, Baser ME, et al. Immunohistochemical detection of schwannomin and neurofibromin in vestibular schwannomas, ependymomas, and meningiomas. J Neuropathol Exp Neurol 1997;56:382–90.
47. Gutmann DH, Giordano MJ, Fishback AS, Guha A. Loss of merlin expression in sporadic meningiomas, ependymomas, and schwannomas. Neurology 1997;49(1):267–70.
48. Merel P, Haong-Xuan K, Sanson M, et al. Predominant occurrence of somatic mutations of the NF2 gene in meningiomas and schwannomas. Genes Chromosomes Cancer 1995;13:211–6.
49. Maxwell M, Shih S, Galanopoulos T, et al. Familial meningioma: analysis of expression of neurofibromatosis 2 protein Merlin. Report of two cases. J Neurosurg 1998;88:562–9.
50. DiCiommo D, Gallie BL, Bremner R. Retinoblastoma: the disease, gene and protein provide critical leads to understand cancer. Semin Cancer Biol 2000;10:255–69.
51. Kaufman LM, Mafee MF, Song CD. Retinoblastoma and simulating lesions. Role of CT, MR imaging and use of Gd-DTPA contrast enhancement. Radiol Clin North Am 1998;36:1101–17.
52. Reese AB, Ellsworth RM. Evaluation and current concept of retinoblastoma therapy. Trans Am Acad Ophthalmol Otolaryngol 1963;67:164.
53. Shields CL, Shields JA. Recent developments in the management of retinoblastoma. J Pediatr Ophthalmol Strabismus 1999;36:8–18.
54. Karcioglu ZA, al-Mesfer SA, Abboud E, et al. Workup for metastatic retinoblastoma. A review of 261 patients. Ophthalmology 1997;104:307–12.
55. Messmer EP, Heinrich T, Höpping W, et al. Risk factors for metastases in patients with retinoblastoma. Ophthalmology 1991;98:136–41.
56. Kopelman JE, McLean IW, Rosenberg SH. Multivariate analysis of risk factors for metastasis in retinoblastoma treated by enucleation. Ophthalmology 1987;94:371–7.
57. Jakobiec FA, Tso MO, Zimmerman LE, Danis P. Retinoblastoma and intracranial malignancy. Cancer 1977;39:2048–58.
58. Bader JL, Miller RW, Meadows AT, et al. Trilateral retinoblastoma. Lancet 1980;2:582–3.
59. Bagley LJ, Hurst RW, Zimmerman RA, et al. Imaging in the trilateral retinoblastoma syndrome. Neuroradiology 1996;38:166–70.
60. Finelli DA, Shurin SB, Bardenstein DS. Trilateral retinoblastoma: two variations. AJNR Am J Neuroradiol 1995;16:166–70.
61. Marcus DM, Brooks SE, Leff G, et al. Trilateral retinoblastoma: insights into histogenesis and management. Surv Ophthalmol 1998;43(1):59–70.
62. Bejjani GK, Donahue DJ, Selby D, et al. Association of a suprasellar mass and intraocular retinoblastoma: a variant of pineal trilateral retinoblastoma? Pediatr Neurosurg 1996;25:269–75.
63. Verhoeff FJ, Jackson E. Minutes of the proceedings, 62nd annual meeting. Trans Am Ophthalmol Soc 1926;24:34–43.
64. Rodrigues MM, Bardenstein DS, Donoso LA, et al. An immunohistopathologic study of trilateral retinoblastoma. Am J Ophthalmol 1987;103:776–81.
65. Knudson AG, Meadows AT, Nichols WW, Hill R. Chromosomal deletion and retinoblastoma. N Engl J Med 1976;295:1120–3.
66. Henson JW, Schnitker BL, Correa KM, et al. The retinoblastoma gene is involved in malignant progression of astrocytomas. Ann Neurol 1994;36:714–21.
67. Finger PT, Czechonska G, Demirci H, Rausen A. Chemotherapy for retinoblastoma: a current topic. Drugs 1999;58:983–96.
68. Nelson SC, Friedman HS, Oakes WJ, et al. Successful therapy for trilateral retinoblastoma. Am J Ophthalmol 1992;114(1):23–9.
69. Moll AC, Imhof SM, Meeteren AY, Boers M. At what age could screening for familial retinoblastoma be stopped? A register based study 1945–98. Br J Ophthalmol 2000;84:1170–2.
70. Meadows A. Trilateral retinoblastoma. Med Pediatr Oncol 1986;14:323–6.
71. Kivelä T. Trilateral retinoblastoma: a meta-analysis of hereditary retinoblastoma associated with primary ectopic intracranial retinoblastoma. J Clin Oncol 1999;17:1829–37.
72. Couch V, Lindor NM, Karnes PS, Michels VV. von Hippel-Lindau disease. Mayo Clin Proc 2000;75:265–72.
73. Niemelä M, Lemeta S, Summanen P, et al. Long-term prognosis of haemangioblastoma of the CNS: impact of von Hippel-Lindau disease. Acta Neurochir (Wien) 1999;141:1147–56.
74. Hardwig P, Robertson DM. von Hippel-Lindau disease: a familial, often lethal, multi-system phakomatosis. Ophthalmology 1984;91:263–70.
75. Friedrich CA. von Hippel-Lindau syndrome: a pleomorphic condition. Cancer 1999;86:2478–82.

76. Choyke PL, Glenn GM, McClennan MW, et al. von Hippel-Lindau disease: genetic, clinical, and imaging features. Radiology 1995;194:629–42.
77. Manski TJ, Heffner DK, Glenn GM, et al. Endolymphatic sac tumors: a source of morbid hearing loss in von Hippel-Lindau disease. JAMA 1997;277:1461–6.
78. Richard S, David P, Marsot-Dupuch K, et al. Central nervous system hemangioblastomas, endolymphatic sac tumors, and von Hippel-Lindau disease. Neurosurg Rev 2000;23: 1–22.
79. Stratmann R, Krieg M, Haas R, Plate KH. Putative control of angiogenesis in hemangioblastomas by the von Hippel-Lindau tumor suppressor gene. J Neuropathol Exp Neurol 1997;56:1242–52.
80. Vortmeyer AO, Gnarra JR, Emmert-Buck MR, et al. von Hippel-Lindau gene deletion detected in the stromal cell component of a cerebellar hemangioblastoma associated with von Hippel-Lindau disease. Hum Pathol 1997;28: 540–3.
81. Clelland CA, Treip CS. Histological differentiation of metastatic renal cell carcinoma in the cerebellum from cerebellar hemangioblastoma in von Hippel-Lindau disease. J Neurol Neurosurg Psychiatry 1989;52:162–6.
82. Decker HJH, Weidt EJ, Brieger J. The von Hippel-Lindau tumor suppressor gene. A rare and intriguing disease opening new insight into basic mechanisms of carcinogenesis. Cancer Genet Cytogenet 1997;93:74–83.
83. Harris AL. von Hippel-Lindau syndrome: target for anti-vascular endothelial growth factor (VEGF) receptor therapy. Oncologist 2000;5(Suppl 1):32–6.
84. Krieg M, Marti HH, Plate KH. Coexpression of erythropoetin and vascular endothelial growth factor in nervous system tumors associated with von Hippel-Lindau tumor suppressor gene loss of function. Blood 1998;92: 3388–93.
85. Patrice SJ, Sneed PK, Flickinger JC, et al. Radiosurgery for hemangioblastoma: results of a multiinstitutional experience. Int J Radiat Oncol Biol Phys 1996;35:493–9.
86. Chang SD, Meisel JA, Hancock SL, et al. Treatment of hemangioblastomas in von Hippel-Lindau disease with linear accelerator-based radiosurgery. Neurosurgery 1998;43:28–35.
87. Schmidt D, Natt E, Neumann HP. Long-term results of laser treatment for retinal angiomatosis in von Hippel-Lindau disease. Eur J Med Res 2000;5(2):47–58.
88. Hurst JS, Wilcoski S. Recognizing an index case of tuberous sclerosis. Am Fam Physician 2000;61:703–8, 710.
89. The European Chromosome 16 Tuberous Sclerosis Consortium. Identification and characterization of the tuberous sclerosis gene on chromosome 16. Cell 1993;75:1305–15.
90. Van Slegtenhorst M, de Hoogt R, Hermans C, et al. Identification of the tuberous sclerosis gene TSC1 on chromosome 9q34. Science 1997;277:805–8.
91. Crino PB, Henske EP. New developments in the neurobiology of the tuberous sclerosis complex. Neurology 1999;53:1384–90.
92. Jambaque I, Chiron C, Dumas C, et al. Mental and behavioural outcome of infantile epilepsy treated by vigabatrin in tuberous sclerosis patients. Epilepsy Res 2000;38: 151–60.
93. Hosoya M, Naito H, Nihei K. Neurological prognosis correlated with variations over time in the number of subependymal nodules in tuberous sclerosis. Brain Dev 1999;21:544–7.
94. Nabbout R, Santos M, Rolland Y, et al. Early diagnosis of subependymal giant cell astrocytoma in children with tuberous sclerosis. J Neurol Neurosurg Psychiatry 1999; 66:370–5.
95. Evans JC, Curtis J. The radiological appearances of tuberous sclerosis. Br J Radiol 2000;73:91–8.
96. Arai Y, Ackerley CA, Becker LE. Loss of the TSC2 product tuberin in subependymal giant-cell tumors. Acta Neuropathol (Berl) 1999;98:233–9.
97. Gutmann DH, Zhang Y, Hasbani MJ, et al. Expression of the tuberous sclerosis complex gene products, hamartin and tuberin, in central nervous system tissues. Acta Neuropathol (Berl) 2000;99:223–30.
98. Henske EP, Wessner LL, Golden J, et al. Loss of tuberin in both subependymal giant cell astrocytomas and angiomyolipomas supports a two-hit model for the pathogenesis of tuberous sclerosis tumors. Am J Pathol 1997;151:1639–47.
99. Mizuguchi M, Kato M, Yamanouchi H, et al. Loss of tuberin from cerebral tissues with tuberous sclerosis and astrocytoma. Ann Neurol 1996;40:941–4.
100. Matusumura H, Takimoto H, Shimada N, et al. Glioblastoma following radiotherapy in a patient with tuberous sclerosis. Neurol Med Chir (Tokyo) 1998;38:287–91.
101. Torres OA, Roach ES, Delgado MR, et al. Early diagnosis of subependymal giant cell astrocytoma in patients with tuberous sclerosis. J Child Neurol 1998;13:173–7.
102. Roach ES, DiMario FJ, Kandt RS, Northrup H. Tuberous Sclerosis Consensus Conference: recommendations for diagnostic evaluation. National Tuberous Sclerosis Association. J Child Neurol 1999;14:401–7.
103. Crail HW. Multiple primary malignancies arising in the rectum, brain, and thyroid. Report of a case. US Nav Med Bull 1949;49:123–8.
104. Turcot J, Despres JP, St Pierre F. Malignant tumors of the central nervous system associated with familial polyposis of the colon. Report of 2 cases. Dis Colon Rectum 1959; 2:465–8.
105. Mastronardi L, Ferrante L, Lunardi P, et al. Association between neuroepithelial tumor and multiple intestinal polyposis (Turcot's syndrome): report of a case and critical analysis of the literature. Neurosurgery 1991;28: 449–52.
106. Paraf F, Jothy S, Van Meir EG. Brain tumor-polyposis syndrome: two genetic diseases? J Clin Oncol 1997;15: 2744–58.
107. Jamjoon ZA, Sadiq S, Mofti AB, et al. Turcot syndrome: report of a case and review of the literature. Int Surg 1989;74(1):45–50.
108. Tamiya T, Hanazaki S, Ono Y, et al. Ganglioglioma in a patient with Turcot syndrome. Case report. J Neurosurg 2000;92(1):170–5.
109. Mullins KJ, Rubio A, Myers SP, et al. Malignant ependymomas in a patient with Turcot's syndrome. Case report and management guidelines. Surg Neurol 1998;49:290–4.
110. Munden PM, Sobol WM, Weingeist TA. Ocular findings in Turcot syndrome (glioma-polyposis). Ophthalmology 1991;98(1):111–4.

111. Itoh H, Hirata K, Ohsato K. Turcot's syndrome and familial adenomatous polyposis associated with brain tumor: review of related literature. Int J Colorectal Dis 1993; 8:87–94.
112. Hamilton SR, Liu B, Parsons RE, et al. The molecular basis of Turcot's syndrome. N Engl J Med 1995;332:839–47.
113. Lewis JH, Ginsberg AL, Toomey KE. Turcot's syndrome. Evidence for autosomal dominant inheritance. Cancer 1983;51:524–8.
114. Itoh H, Ohsato K. Turcot syndrome and its characteristic colonic manifestations. Dis Colon Rectum 1985;28:399–402.
115. Tops CM, Vasen HF, van Berge Henegouwen G, et al. Genetic evidence that Turcot syndrome is not allelic to familial adenomatous polyposis. Am J Med Genet 1992; 43:888–93.
116. Kihiczak NI, Schwartz RA, Józwiak S, et al. Sturge-Weber syndrome. Pediatr Dermatol 2000;65:133–6.
117. Aydin A, Cakmaki H, Kovanlikaya A, Dirik E. Sturge-Weber syndrome without facial nevus. Pediatr Neurol 2000; 22:400–2.
118. Ambrosetto P, Ambrosetto G, Michelucci R, Bacci A. Sturge-Weber syndrome without port-wine nevus: report of 2 cases studied by CT. Childs Brain 1983;10:387–92.
119. Griffiths PD. Sturge-Weber syndrome revisited: the role of neuroradiology. Neuropediatrics 1996;27:284–94.
120. Pascual-Castroviejo I, Diaz-Gonzalez C, Garcia-Melian RM, et al. Sturge-Weber syndrome: study of 40 patients. Pediatr Neurol 1993;9:233–8.
121. Bebin EM, Gomez MR. Prognosis in Sturge-Weber disease: comparison of unihemispheric and bihemispheric involvement. J Child Neurol 1988;3:181–4.
122. Keith HM, Ewert JC, Green MW, Gage RP. Mental status of children with convulsive disorders. Neurology 1955;5:419–25.
123. Lee S. Psychopathology in Sturge-Weber syndrome. Can J Psychiatry 1990;35:674–8.
124. Sullivan TJ, Clarke MP, Morin JD. The ocular manifestations of the Sturge-Weber syndrome. J Pediatr Ophthalmol Strabismus 1992;29:349–56.
125. Sucac JO, Smith JL, Sceleo RJ. "Tomato catsup" fundus in Sturge-Weber syndrome. Arch Ophthalmol 1974;92:69–70.
126. Irkec M, Kiratli H, Bilgic S. Results of trabeculotomy and guarded filtration procedure for glaucoma associated with Sturge-Weber syndrome. Eur J Ophthalmol 1999;9:99–102.
127. Gorlin RJ. Nevoid basal cell carcinoma (Gorlin) syndrome: unanswered issues. J Lab Clin Med 1999;134:551–2.
128. Schofield D, West DC, Anthony DC, et al. Correlation of loss of heterozygosity at chromosome 9q with histological subtype in medulloblastomas. Am J Pathol 1995;146:472–80.
129. Walter AW, Pivnick EK, Bale AE, Kun LE. Complications of the nevoid basal cell carcinoma syndrome: a case report. J Pediatr Hematol Oncol 1997;19:258–62.
130. Evans DGR, Ladusans EJ, Rimmer S, et al. Complications of the naevoid basal cell carcinoma syndrome: results of a population based study. J Med Genet 1993;30:460–4.
131. Stavrou T, Dubovsky EC, Reaman GH, et al. Intracranial calcifications in childhood medulloblastoma: relation to nevoid basal cell carcinoma. AJNR Am J Neuroradiol 2000;21:790–4.
132. Evans DGR, Farndon PA, Burnell LD, et al. The incidence of Gorlin syndrome in 173 consecutive cases of medulloblastoma. Br J Cancer 1991;64:959–61.
133. Albrecht S, Goodman JC, Rajagopolan S, et al. Malignant meningioma in Gorlin's syndrome: cytogenetic and p53 gene analysis. Case report. J Neurosurg 1994;81:466–71.
134. Dawber RPR, Ryan TJ. Basal cell naevus syndrome and malignant meningioma. Br J Dermatol 1991;5(Suppl 18): 643–6.
135. Vortmeyer AO, Stavrou T, Selby D, et al. Deletion analysis of the adenomatous polyposis coli and PTCH gene loci in patients with sporadic and nevoid basal cell carcinoma syndrome-associated medulloblastoma. Cancer 1999; 85:2662–7.
136. Ming JE, Roessler E, Muenke M. Human developmental disorders and the sonic hedgehog pathway. Mol Med Today 1998;4:343–9.
137. Cowan R, Hoban P, Kelsey A, et al. The gene for the naevoid basal cell carcinoma syndrome acts as a tumour-suppressor gene in medulloblastoma. Br J Cancer 1997;76:141–5.
138. Wolter M, Reifenberger J, Sommer C, et al. Mutations in the human homologue of the *Drosophila* segment polarity gene patched (PTCH) in sporadic basal cell carcinomas of the skin and primitive neuroectodermal tumors of the central nervous system. Cancer Res 1997;57:2581–5.
139. Cohen MM. Nevoid basal cell carcinoma syndrome: molecular biology and new hypotheses. Int J Oral Maxillofac Surg 1999;28:216–23.
140. Lhermitte J, Duclos P. Sur un ganglioneurome diffus du cortex du cervelet. Bull Assoc Franc Cancer 1920;9:99.
141. Koch R, Scholz M, Nelen MR, et al. Lhermitte-Duclos disease as a component of Cowden's syndrome. Case report and review of the literature. J Neurosurg 1999;90:776–9.
142. Tuli S, Provias JP, Bernstein M. Lhermitte-Duclos disease: literature review and novel treatment strategy. Can J Neurol Sci 1997;24:155–60.
143. Marano SR, Johnson PC, Spetzler RF. Recurrent Lhermitte-Duclos disease in a child. J Neurosurg 1988;69:599–603.
144. Williams DW, Elster AD, Ginsberg LE, Stanton C. Recurrent Lhermitte-Duclos disease: report of two cases and association with Cowden's disease. AJNR Am J Neuroradiol 1992;13:287–90.
145. Robinson S, Cohen AR. Cowden disease and Lhermitte-Duclos disease: characterization of a new phakomatosis. Neurosurgery 2000;46:371–83.
146. Kulkantrakorn K, Awwad EE, Levy B, et al. MRI in Lhermitte-Duclos disease. Neurology 1997;48:725–31.
147. Padberg GW, Schot DL, Vielvoye GJ, et al. Lhermitte-Duclos disease and Cowden disease: a single phakomatosis. Ann Neurol 1991;29:517–23.
148. Li J, Yen C, Liaw D, et al. PTEN, a putative protein tyrosine phosphatase gene mutated in human brain, breast, and prostate cancer. Science 1997;275:1943–7.
149. Nelen MR, Padberg GW, Peeters EAJ, et al. Localization for the gene in Cowden disease to chromosome 10q22-23. Nat Genet 1996;13:114–6.

150. Sutphen R, Diamond TM, Minton SE, et al. Severe Lhermitte-Duclos disease with unique germline mutation of PTEN. Am J Med Genet 1999;82:290–3.
151. Murata J, Tada M, Sawamura Y, et al. Dysplastic gangliocytoma (Lhermitte-Duclos disease) associated with Cowden disease: report of a case and review of the literature for the genetic relationship between the two diseases. J Neurooncol 1999;41:129–36.
152. Lynch HT, McComb RD, Osborn NK, et al. Predominance of brain tumors in an extended Li-Fraumeni (SBLA) kindred, including a case of Sturge-Weber syndrome. Cancer 2000;88:433–9.
153. Brown LTR, Sexsmith E, Malkin D. Identification of a novel PTEN intronic deletion in Li-Fraumeni syndrome and its effect on RNA processing. Cancer Genet Cytogenet 2000;123:65–8.
154. Dockhorn-Dworniczak B, Wolff J, Poremba C, et al. A new germline TP53 gene mutation in a family with Li-Fraumeni syndrome. Eur J Cancer 1996;32A:1359–65.
155. Kastan MB, Onyekwere O, Sidransky D, et al. Participation of p53 protein in the cellular response to DNA damage. Cancer Res 1991;51:6304–11.
156. Bond JA, Wyllie FS, Wynford-Thomas D. Escape from senescence in human diploid fibroblasts induced directly by mutant p53. Oncogene 1994;9:1885–9.
157. Bischoff FZ, Yim SO, Pathak S, et al. Spontaneous abnormalities in normal fibroblasts from patients with Li-Fraumeni cancer syndrome: aneuploidy and immortalization. Cancer Res 1990;50:7979–84.
158. Bell DW, Varley JM, Szydlo TE, et al. Heterozygous germ line hCHK2 mutations in Li-Fraumeni syndrome. Science 1999;286:2528–31.

4

Molecular Genetics of Malignant Glioma

AKIO MANTANI, MD, PHD
PENGCHIN CHEN, PHD
ANDREW W. BOLLEN, DVM, MD
MARK A. ISRAEL, MD

Cancer arises as a somatic disorder of genes controlling the cellular processes that contribute to malignancy. Genetic damage to genes critical for such processes as cell division and cell migration leads to the disordered regulation of these processes. The result is that cells proliferate at times in the life of the organism when they should not be dividing, and they migrate at times when they should remain quiescent. The genetic changes in cells that give rise to primary brain tumors have been widely catalogued. In adults, approximately 85 percent of all such tumors are tumors of cells in the astrocytic lineage; these are also the most common tumors of childhood.

Diffuse astrocytic tumors of adults arise most commonly in the cerebral hemispheres and manifest a wide range of histopathologic features that are organized as tumor grades, most frequently according to a classification schema outlined by the World Health Organization (WHO). This classification includes astrocytoma (WHO grades I and II), anaplastic astrocytoma (AA) (WHO grade III), and glioblastoma multiforme (GBM) (WHO grade IV), in order of increasing malignancy.[1] These designations generally reflect the tumor's degree of cellularity, mitotic activity, and cellular anaplasia as marked by nuclear and cytoplasmic atypia and pleomorphism.[2] Additionally, microvascular proliferation and necrosis are important indicators on which current grading is based (Figure 4–1).

A focus of current research elucidating the origins of astrocytic tumors is the determination of how specific genetic alterations contribute to the characteristic pathology of specific grades of tumors.[3] There is increasing evidence that the progression from low-grade astrocytoma to AA and GBM is associated with a cumulative acquisition of multiple genetic alterations (Figure 4–2). The types of molecular alterations that contribute to the development of cancers including primary brain tumors fall into two general classes. One type of genetic change typically results in the loss of cellular activities that operate physiologically to restrain growth. Genes that are altered in this manner are known as *tumor-suppressor genes*. Since each cell contains two copies of all genes that are located on the non-sex chromosomes, loss of both normal alleles generally is necessary to promote neoplasia. The second class of mutations results in the inappropriate activation of genes that typically enhance cellular proliferation or other features of malignancy. These genes are known as *proto-oncogenes*. Proto-oncogenes encode proteins such as growth factors or growth factor receptors, mediators of signaling pathways, or regulators of gene expression. Activating mutations convert proto-oncogenes to oncogenes; oncogenes have a variety of functions promoting the neoplastic phenotype.

PATHOGENESIS OF ASTROCYTIC TUMORS

A key aspect of the development of malignant tumors is the occurrence of genetic alterations in cellular pathways important for the regulation of genetic instability. Cells use a variety of different strategies to protect the integrity of their genomes, and it is thought that one or more such safeguards must be compromised for the cell to collect a sufficient number of genetic alterations to grow as a malignant tumor. Astrocytic tumors are an important example of tumors in which it is sometimes possible to observe the evolution of an aggressive malignancy from a less malignant one in association with the accumulation of genetic alterations in the most rapidly growing cells of the tumor[4] (Figure 4–3). Some patients who initially present with low-grade, diffuse, astrocytic tumors are not cured by surgical resection and develop recurrent lesions, which are sometimes of higher pathologic grade than the original lesions. These tumors typically are associated with additional genetic alterations; studies that have surveyed specific genetic alterations in many tumors of different pathologic grades have led to a model that describes the pathogenesis of high-grade astrocytic tumors (see Figure 4–3).[5] Grade IV astrocytic tumors that arise as the result of this pattern of sequential genetic change have been dubbed "sec-

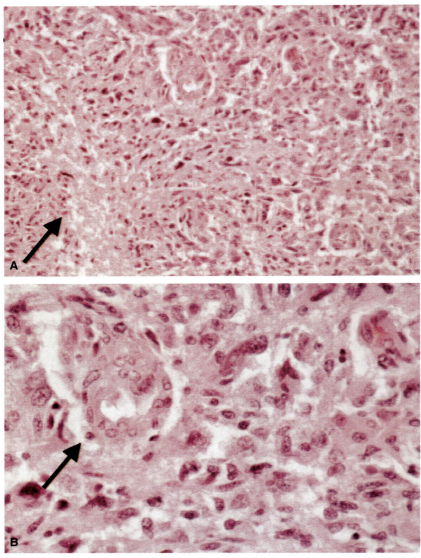

Figure 4–1. Histopathology of glioblastoma multiforme. *A*, Low magnification (×100) of this neoplasm stained with hematoxylin and eosin demonstrates the increased cellularity, necrosis with pseudopalisading, and vascular endothelial proliferation that is typical of advanced-grade astrocytic neoplasms. *B*, Higher magnification (×400) better demonstrates the vascular endothelial proliferation and nuclear atypia that are present.

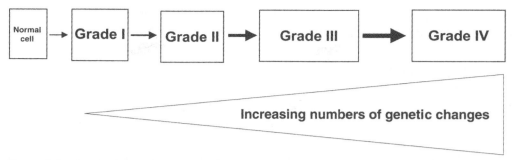

Figure 4–2. Accumulation of genetic alterations is associated with progression from low-grade to high-grade tumors.

ondary GBM." The most prominent genetic alteration in these tumors is the inactivation of *P53*. Secondary GBMs constitute only a small proportion of all GBMs.

Although it is believed that all tumors arise as the result of sequential genetic alterations, which confer increasingly malignant characteristics on tumor behavior, some tumors may not be detected until numerous alterations have occurred. This may occur (1) because the sequential accumulation of the specific genetic alterations that give rise to this subgroup of tumors occurs over a very short period of time or (2) because cells that acquire this particular pattern of genetic alterations grow rapidly. It is of interest that grade IV astrocytic tumors presenting without an evident precursor lesion generally are characterized by a somewhat different group of genetic alterations than those observed in secondary GBM (see Figure 4–3).[6] The most prominent alteration in these tumors is amplification of the epidermal growth factor receptor gene (EGFR). These tumors are sometimes called de novo or primary GBM and constitute a large majority of all grade IV astrocytic tumors.

An important strategy for the identification of genes of importance in the development of brain tumors has been the determination of genes responsible for several different inherited cancer predisposition syndromes, which include brain tumors. Although some genes recognized in this manner, such as *P53*, clearly play a role in the development of sporadically occurring primary brain tumors,[7] the importance of other such genes, for example *NF1*, remains largely unknown.[8] Additionally, genomic surveys have revealed many other putative sites of deoxyribonucleric acid (DNA) rearrangement, which seem likely to include genes of importance for the pathogenesis of these tumors. For astrocytic tumors, these alterations include (among others) the gain of DNA from chromosome 7 and loss of DNA from chromosomes 10, 19, and 22 (see below).[9] Emerging data have made it possible to recognize that some genes altered in the pathogenesis of astrocytic tumors encode functions that are important within the same cell regulatory pathway. We interpret these findings as indicating the particular importance of these pathways, and below

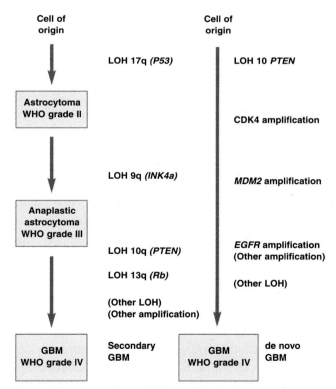

Figure 4–3. Genetic alterations associated with the development of astrocytic tumors. WHO = World Health Association; GBM = glioblastoma multiforme; LOH = loss of heterozygosity; CDK4 = cyclin-dependent kinase 4; EGFR = epidermal growth factor receptor. (Adapted from von Deimling A, Louis DN, Wiestler OD. Molecular pathways in the formation of gliomas. Glia 1995;15:328–38.)

we have outlined pathways that the most commonly altered genes in astrocytic tumors appear to function.

SPECIFIC GENETIC ALTERATIONS IN ASTROCYTIC TUMORS

P53/MDM2/ARF Pathway

The *P53* gene is located on chromosome 17p13.1 and encodes a 53-kDa protein, p53, that plays a role in several key cellular processes, including regulation of the cell cycle, the response of cells to DNA damage, genomic instability, cell death, cell differentiation, and neovascularization.[10] Inheritance of one mutant allele of *P53* can cause a well-described cancer predisposition syndrome, the Li-Fraumeni syndrome. The predominant tumor types in humans who are heterozygous for *P53* mutation are soft tissue and bone sarcomas, carcinomas of the breast, and astrocytic tumors of the brain.[11]

p53 may have multiple functions, but it is best characterized as a transcription factor to induce or repress the transcription of multiple genes through sequence-specific interaction with DNA. Little is known of the precise determinants that regulate p53 function as a transcription factor; however, there is considerable evidence that the loss of *P53*, which has been described in a variety of tumor types, affects the transcription of many different genes, including some recognized as being critical for cellular processes that contribute to the dysregulated growth and malignant characteristics of brain tumors. These include genes that are involved in the cell cycle, tumorigenesis, neoangiogenesis, and apoptosis.

As mentioned, usually the biologic effects of the inactivation of a tumor-suppressor gene are recognizable only after both copies of the gene are inactivated by a mutational mechanism. Inactivation of one copy typically would lead to a loss of 50 percent of the protein encoded by the two copies, and this might not affect its normal, physiologic cellular activities. A prominent exception to this rule is the occurrence of mutations in one copy of a gene whose protein products function as multimers. If the genetic alteration in one copy results in a protein that renders the multimeric complexes in which it functions unstable, mutations in only a single allele can cause a loss of gene function that results in altered cell behavior. Such mutations are called dominant negative mutations, and they have been reported to occur in *P53*. However, inactivation of the *P53* locus more commonly involves inactivating point mutations in the DNA of one allele and loss of the normal allele by deletion of the region of the chromosome on which it is located.

Often, the loss of this second *P53* allele can easily be recognized by studying polymorphic sites on the chromosome in the vicinity of the *P53* gene (Figure 4–4). Silent alterations in primary DNA structure, polymorphisms, occur frequently, and if different polymorphic alleles are inherited from each parent, normal tissue will have both alleles. That individual can be said to be heterozygous at that locus. If a deletion occurs in a chromosome containing one of these polymorphic alleles, the individual will have a loss of

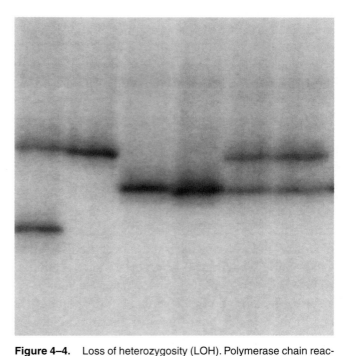

Figure 4–4. Loss of heterozygosity (LOH). Polymerase chain reaction primers flanking simple repeat regions in intron 1 of *P53* were used to amplify normal (N) and tumor (T) DNA pairs from three different glioma patients. Tumor DNA in case 1 had LOH in the *P53* gene, case 2 was non-informative, and tumor DNA in case 3 did not show loss of alleles in the *P53* region.

heterozygosity (LOH) in that particular region. When this loss occurs in the region of a tumor-suppressor gene that has already been inactivated on the paired chromosome, usually by the random occurrence of a mutational event, the locus is totally inactivated and is likely to contribute to the phenotype of the tumor.

A variety of molecular technologies have been developed to identify LOH and point mutations that occur in tumor-suppressor genes. Polymerase chain reaction (PCR)-based strategies (see Figure 4–4), single-strand conformation polymorphism (SSCP)-based approaches (Figure 4–5), and DNA sequencing (Figure 4–6) are among the most popular and have been widely exploited for the evaluation of *P53*, as well as other tumor-suppressor genes important for the pathogenesis of astrocytic tumors. Because *P53* mutation reduces degradation of the abnormal protein product, immunohistochemical assays will detect mutant *P53* accumulation, though this can sometimes be difficult to distinguish from the expression of apparently wild-type *P53* in some tumors. Immunohistochemistry is a standard method available in most diagnostic pathology laboratories and is therefore well suited for clinical research using routinely processed archival tissue. *P53* mutations have been reported in approximately 30 to 40 percent of astrocytic tumors. They occur in approximately 40 percent of grade I and II astrocytoma, in 30 percent of AA, and in 30 percent of GBM. This suggests that *P53* mutations are associated principally with the change from normal tissue to low-grade neoplasia, rather than with the progression from low-grade to high-grade tumors.[12] *P53* mutations are found most commonly in gliomas occurring in young adults. In contrast, *P53* mutations have not been as frequently observed in supratentorial astrocytic tumors of children, although they do occur in childhood brainstem gliomas. The prognostic implication of *P53* mutations has not yet been clearly defined. It remains a strong candidate for being clinically significant, however, since *P53* mediates the response of tumors to irradiation, an important modality of treatment for these tumors.[13] Mice with homozygously deleted *P53* or one deleted allele are phenotypically normal, but they develop spontaneous tumors at a higher frequency than do heterozygotes. Brain tumors occur

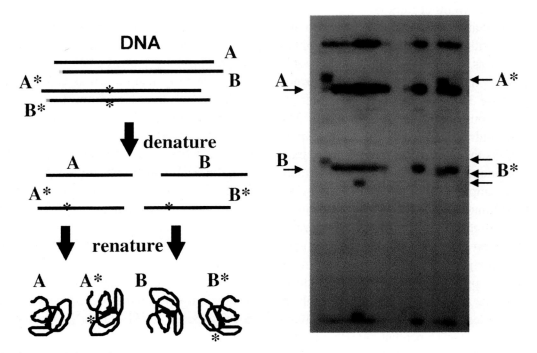

Figure 4–5. Use of single-strand conformation polymorphism to detect small DNA changes (point mutations or small deletions) in the *P53* gene. Single-stranded DNA with mutations (A* and B*) assumes different conformation and migrates differently in nondenaturing gel compared with DNA with wild-type sequences (A and B). Arrows next to A and B point to the migration of DNA with wild-type sequences; arrows next to A* and B* point to aberrant migration as a result of mutations.

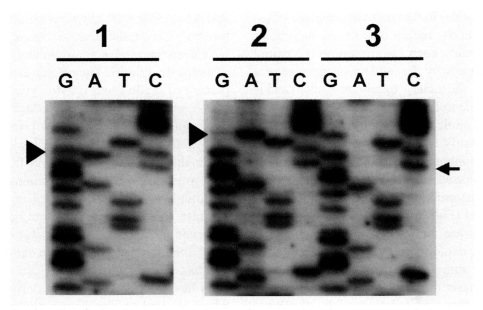

Figure 4–6. DNA sequencing analysis on exon 5 of the *P53* gene. Tumor DNA in case 3 had normal DNA sequences for codons 175 and 176, cgc-tgc (bottom to top starting from location of *arrow*). Tumor DNA in cases 1 and 2 had point mutations (indicated by *solid triangles*). The patient in case 1 had a cgc to c(G/A)c change at codon 175 resulting in an amino acid change of arginine to histidine/arginine. The patient in case 2 had a tgc to tAc change at codon 176 resulting in an amino acid change of cysteine to tyrosine. G = guanosine; A = adenosine; T = thymidine; C = cytosine.

infrequently in such animals, perhaps because they die so early in life from other tumors.

MDM2 is found at chromosome 12q14.3–q15 and encodes a protein with a predicted molecular weight of 54 kDa. *MDM2* was discovered by cloning a highly amplified gene from a spontaneously transformed derivative of mouse 3T3 cells that displayed *m*ultiple *d*ouble *m*inute chromosomes—hence its name. The MDM2 protein binds to the acidic activation domain of P53 and inhibits the ability of *P53* to promote transcription. In addition, MDM2 promotes the degradation of P53. This amplification of *MDM2* and dysregulation of MDM2 function are alternative mechanisms for escaping *P53*-regulated control of cell growth. MDM2 can function as an oncogene, and in contrast to tumor-suppressor gene mutations that result in the loss of function of proteins key for the inhibition of cell proliferation, the activation of oncogenes results in enhanced function leading to increased cell proliferation. Approximately 10 to 15 percent of GBM and AA and 7 percent of glioblastoma cell lines have been reported to display amplification of *MDM2*[14] (Figure 4–7). Overexpression of *MDM2* has been observed immunohistochemically in more than 50 percent of primary glioblastomas, but the fraction of immunoreactive cells varies considerably.

The human *INK4a* locus maps to chromosome 9p21 and contains an alternative reading frame encoding two proteins, human p19^{ARF} and p16^{INK4a} (Figure 4–8). *INK4a* is also known as CDKN2, MTS-1, and CDK4I. Each transcript from the p16^{INK4a} locus has a different promoter and a different specific 5' exon, E1α or E1β, that is spliced into common exons E2 and E3. The E1α-containing transcript encodes p16^{INK4a}, and the E1β-containing transcript encodes p19^{ARF} from a different reading frame initiated in *E2*.[15] Recent studies provide evidence that ARF modulates P53 function as a checkpoint in response to proliferative signals but not in response to DNA damage. Overexpression of *MYC*, *E1A*, or *E2F1* in primary mouse embryo fibroblasts upregulates *ARF* expression and results in apoptosis that is *P53* dependent. Apoptosis does not occur in *ARF*-null or *P53*-null cells. ARF can directly bind to MDM2 and inhibit MDM2-mediated *P53* degradation and transactivational silencing. Deletion of the *ARF* locus as shown in Figure 4–8 (sample 1) can result in the enhanced degradation of p53 and the loss of *P53* function. Interestingly, expression of

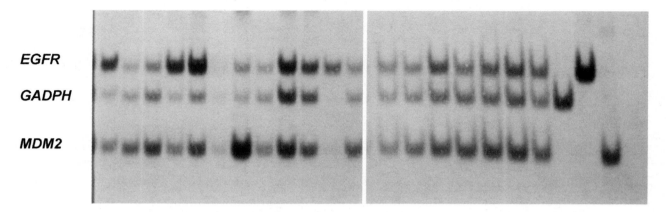

Figure 4–7. Multiplex polymerase chain reaction (PCR) assay for gene amplification of *EGFR* and *MDM2*. Lanes 1–19 and 23: multiplex PCR with primers that simultaneously amplify fragments of *EGFR*, *GAPDH*, and *MDM2* genes. Lanes 20–22 were control PCR with primers used to amplify individual gene fragments (lane 20: *GAPDH*; lane 21: *EGFR*; and lane 22: *MDM2*). Lanes 1–12: tumor DNA samples; lanes 13–19: normal DNA controls; lane 23: water. Lanes 1, 4, 5, and 11 had amplifications of *EGFR*; lane 7 had amplification of the *MDM2* gene.

ARF is negatively regulated by p53 and in some human tumor cell lines correlates inversely with *P53* function.

Ectopic expression of the ARF protein can induce an arrest in both the G1 and G2 phases of the cell cycle in a variety of cells, including those derived from glioblastoma. This arrest is p16 and p53 independent. Thus, the two distinct tumor suppressors, p16 and ARF, encoded by the single genetic p16^{INK4a} locus regulate both the *Rb1* and *P53* pathways. Approximately 25 to 50 percent of AA and 40 to 70 percent of GBM carry homozygous deletions of *INK4a* (Figure 4–9).

Rb1/INK4a/CDK4/CDK6 Pathway

The retinoblastoma gene, *Rb1*, is a well-characterized tumor-suppressor gene located on chromosome 13q14. Patients with hereditary retinoblastoma have a germline mutation in one *Rb1* allele. Both copies of the *Rb1* gene are mutated or deleted in tumor tissue from these patients as well as in sporadic retinoblastomas. The cytogenetic observation that some glioblastomas are associated with loss of 13q and the observation that some hereditary retinoblastoma patients also develop brain tumors have prompted speculation that this gene may be important in the pathogenesis of sporadic glial tumors.

The human *Rb1* gene encodes a 110-kDa protein, pRb. pRb is a nuclear phosphoprotein that contains a bipartite nuclear localization signal. pRb also has two globular domains (A and B) that bind viral oncoproteins, including SV40 T antigen, adenovirus E1A, and human papillomavirus E7, when pRb is in its unphosphorylated form. These regions are also critical for

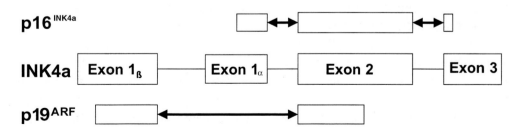

Figure 4–8. Structural organization of the *INK4a* locus. The human *INK4a* locus encodes not only p16^{INK4a}, but as the result of alternative splicing and an alternative reading frame, it also encodes the unrelated protein human p19^{ARF}. (Adapted from Quelle DE, Zindy F, Ashmun RA, Sherr CJ. Alternative reading frames of the INK4a tumor-suppressor gene encode two unrelated proteins capable of inducing cell cycle arrest. Cell 1995;83:993–1000.)

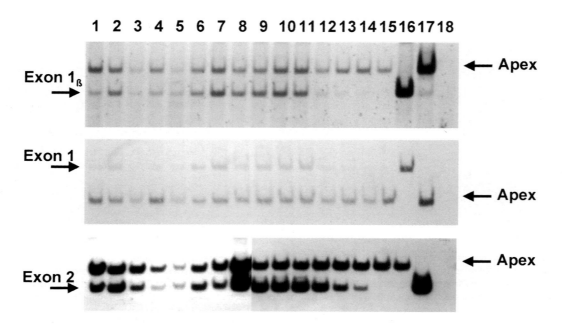

Figure 4–9. Deletion analyses of the *INK4a* gene in glioma; polymerase chain reaction (PCR) amplifications of exon 1ß, exon 1, and exon 2 of *INK4a*, respectively. Primers that amplify apex nuclease (apex) were included in each PCR as an internal control for presence of DNA and the PCR reaction. Lanes 1–5: tumor DNA samples; lanes 6–8: normal DNA controls; lanes 9–15: a series of mixed DNA between normal DNA and DNA with *INK4a* deletion at different ratios (lane 9: 100% normal DNA; lane 10: 90% normal DNA; lane 11: 75% normal DNA; lane 12: 50% normal DNA; lane 13: 25% normal DNA; lane 14: 10% normal DNA; lane 15: 0% normal DNA). Deletion (samples with target to apex ratios that are less than that of samples with less than 50% normal DNA) for exon 1ß was detected in sample 1; deletions for exon 1 were detected in samples 1, 3, 4, and 5; deletions for exon 2 were detected in samples 1, 3, and 4.

binding to transcription factors such as E2F. The ability of pRb to regulate cell growth is tightly linked to its ability to bind to and inhibit E2F, an important mediator of cellular proliferation (Figure 4–10).

Although the frequency of *Rb1* inactivation in primary astrocytic tumors has not been well defined, other genes that influence *Rb1* function are frequently altered in these tumors (see Figure 4–10). Most prominent among these is the tumor-suppressor gene *INK4a*.[16,17] p16^{INK4a} functions as an inhibitor of CDK4, a cyclin-dependent kinase whose normal action is to promote cell division by mediating the phosphorylation of pRb. Phosphorylation of pRb decreases the inhibitory effects of pRb on the E2F transcription factor with which it complexes and thereby leaves E2F unopposed in stimulating cell proliferation.

The CDK4 gene encodes a 33-kDa protein and maps to chromosome 12q13–14. CDK6, another cyclin-dependent kinase that phosphorylates pRb and is inhibited by p16^{INK4a}, encodes a 38-kDa protein and maps to chromosome 7q21–22. Both CDK4 and CDK6 require interaction with their regulatory subunits, members of the cyclin D family, to achieve activation. Overexpression of either of these kinases or deletion of the genes encoding their inhibitors such as p16^{INK4a} leads to inappropriate phosphorylation of pRb, which results in a loss of growth suppression. The CDK4 gene is amplified in nearly 15 percent of high-grade gliomas, particularly in those without *INK4a* alterations. Additionally, a few tumors without *INK4a* mutations or CDK4 amplification have been shown to have CDK6 amplification (see Figure 4–10).

PTEN

PTEN, a tumor-suppressor gene also known as *MMAC* or *TEP1*, is located at 10q23. Deletion of chromosome 10 occurs frequently in astrocytic tumors, and there is considerable evidence for the presence of multiple tumor suppression genes on this chromosome. In addition to its predicted involvement in brain tumors, germline *PTEN* mutations have been detected in the autosomal dominant cancer predisposition syndromes, Cowden disease, and Bannayan-Zonana syndrome. These syndromes are notable for hamartomas—benign tumors consisting of normally differentiated cells within highly disorganized tissue architectures.

The protein product of the *PTEN* gene contains a central domain closely homologous to the catalytic region of protein tyrosine phosphatases. The *PTEN* protein has an amino-terminal domain with extensive homology to tensin and auxilin, which are cytoplasmic proteins that interact with actin filaments at focal adhesions and on clathrin-coated vesicles, respectively. Also, *PTEN* functions as a lipid phosphatase, dephosphorylating one of the three phosphates on PIP3, an important component of a regulatory pathway that acts both to stimulate proliferation and inhibit apoptosis. When *PTEN* is functional, it decreases cellular PIP3 levels, which in turn decreases the activity of protein kinase B (PKB/Akt) releasing the suppression of proliferation and inhibition of cell death that is normally mediated by this pathway.

Loss of heterozygosity at 10q23 has been reported to occur in as many as 70 percent of GBM, and *PTEN* has been found to be mutated in 30 to 44 percent of high-grade gliomas.[18] *PTEN* is also altered in a variety of other tumors, including carcinomas of the prostate, endometrium, lung and renal parenchyma; melanoma; and meningeal tumors.

EGFR

The epidermal growth factor receptor is a proto-oncogene implicated in the pathogenesis of astrocytic tumors (see Figure 4–3). Amplification is a frequent mechanism by which proto-oncogenes are activated. Gene amplification is a manifestation of genetic instability, an important characteristic of many, if not all, cancers. The protein product of EGFR is a 170-kDa transmembrane receptor responsible for transducing growth stimulatory signals following interaction with its extracellular ligands, EGF and transforming growth factor α (TGF-α). *EGFR* has been shown to be amplified in several tumor types, with an increased copy number that is directly correlated to an increase in the number of receptors on the cell surface. EGFR is composed of four major domains: the ligand-binding extracellular domain; the transmembrane, anchoring domain; the catalytic tyrosine kinase domain; and the carboxyl terminus, which contains five tyrosines that are both target substrates for the kinase and motifs responsible for ligand-activated endocytosis. *EGFR* was first implicated in the pathogenesis of tumors as the cellular homologue of the *v-erbB* oncogene found in an acutely transforming avian erythroblastosis virus. In some tumors, *EGFR* is not only amplified but also carries mutations that lead to the constitutive activation of an EGFR-mediated autocrine growth stimulatory loop.

The *EGFR* gene is the most frequently amplified oncogene in astrocytic tumors; it is amplified in about half of GBMs and in a few AAs.[19] Figure 4–7 demonstrates experimental evidence for this amplification. Amplification of *EGFR* occurs in approximately 40 percent of astrocytomas and correlates with advanced disease.[20] Moreover, there is also evidence that gliomas express the *EGFR* ligands, EGF and TGF-α, suggesting the potential for these tumor cells to have autocrine growth stimulatory loops.

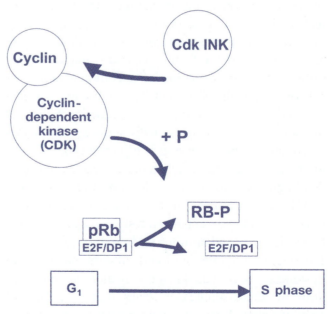

Figure 4–10. pRb function is regulated by phosphorylation. pRb complexes with members of the E2F transcription factor family and binds to DNA, inhibiting the gene transcription that is critical for cell-cycle progression into S phase. Phosphorylation of pRb by cyclin-dependent kinases (such as CDK4) and their regulatory cyclins (such as cyclin D) inactivates pRb and allows cell-cycle progression. Cyclin-dependent kinase inhibitors (Cdk INK) such as p16[INK4a] inhibit this process and thereby inhibit progression through the cell cycle.

OTHER GENETIC ALTERATIONS IN ASTROCYTIC TUMORS

Regions of chromosomal gain or loss in astrocytic tumors are thought to be strong candidates for marking the presence of currently unknown tumor-suppressor genes and oncogenes. Such regions have been identified in astrocytic tumors using comparative genomic hybridization.[21] Comparative genomic hybridization surveys the entire genome for copy number aberrations. Tumor-specific alterations have been reported from several laboratories for astrocytic tumors, and these include frequent gains on chromosomes 17q, 19, and 20. Frequently involved areas of loss include chromosomes 9q21, 10p, and 10q25. Other chromosomal copy number aberrations include +3q (13.3–29), –4q, +5q, –9q34, +12, –13q, –15, –16p, +17qter, –18, –21, and –22.

PATHOGENESIS OF OLIGODENDROGLIOMA

Oligodendrogliomas occur less commonly than astrocytic tumors and account for only about 5 to 10 percent of primary intracranial tumors. Most frequently oligodendrogliomas occur supratentorially and display various histologic grades of malignancy. Many gliomas have mixtures of cells with both astrocytic and oligodendroglial features, and it is unclear if this reflects the transformation of a common precursor cell or simply the divergent histopathologic appearance of these tumor types. Cytogenetic studies of oligodendrogliomas occasionally show a loss of chromosomes 9p and 22 or a gain of chromosome 7, but the most characteristic cytogenetic findings in oligodendrogliomas are loss of chromosomes 1p36 and 19q13.3. The presence of these alterations is thought to correspond to an enhanced responsiveness to cytotoxic therapies and an improved prognosis.[22] Loss of 1p36 occurs not only in oligodendrogliomas but also in some astrocytomas. Presumably these are the locations of tumor-suppressor genes that have not yet been isolated. Loss of heterozygosity for chromosome 9p loci, observed in some oligodendrogliomas, corresponds to deletions at the *INK4a* locus, and these have been associated with a poor prognosis for patients with this tumor type. Other molecular genetic events common in astrocytic tumors seem to be rare in oligodendrogliomas. *P53* mutations and *EGFR* amplification are almost never present, although high levels of *EGFR* expression have been reported in up to 40 percent of these tumors.

PATHOPHYSIOLOGY OF ANGIOGENESIS IN GLIOMAS

An important event that accompanies glioma development and progression is the formation of a blood vessel system supplying the tumor with oxygen and nutrients. The vasculature of low-grade gliomas closely resembles that of normal brain, whereas high-grade gliomas show prominent microvascular (eg, smooth muscle/pericyte and endothelial cell) proliferation and often contain areas with a much higher vascular density than low-grade gliomas and normal brain (see Figure 4–1). Indeed, GBMs are among the most highly vascularized tumors in humans.

Angiogenesis in gliomas is regulated by endothelial cell receptor tyrosine kinases including vascular endothelial growth factor (VEGF) receptor-1, VEGF receptor-2, Tie-1, Tie-2, PDGF receptor-b, c-met, and integrins such as $a_v\beta_3$. Typically, these receptors are not expressed in quiescent endothelium such as that found in the normal adult brain. Each of these receptors, however, is typically upregulated in proliferating tumor vessels, suggesting a role in tumor progression. The ligands for these receptors typically are expressed in the tumor cells, arguing in favor of a paracrine pathway (glioma cell–endothelial cell) mediating angiogenesis in these tumors. Current evidence suggests that VEGF, which binds to the VEGF receptor-1 and VEGF receptor-2, is the most important regulator of vascular proliferation in glioma-induced angiogenesis. Vascular endothelial growth factor is a secreted dimeric glycoprotein that specifically acts on endothelial cells and induces angiogenesis and vascular permeability in vivo. During glioma progression, VEGF expression is upregulated in tumor cells.[23] Its expression is particularly high in GBM where it is abundantly expressed in the perinecrotic palisading cells. Expression of VEGF is hypoxia inducible, and a major trigger of angiogenesis in gliomas appears to be cellular hypoxia. Functions of VEGF not only mediate tumor neoangiogenesis but also enhance vascular permeability of the established vasculature. Due to this dual function, VEGF may be responsible for both the microvascular proliferation and the peritumoral edema that is routinely found in malignant gliomas. This model is consistent with the finding that dexamethasone, a drug widely used for the management of peritumoral edema, downregulates the expression of VEGF.

Vascular remodeling, including both proliferation and recruitment of smooth muscle pericytes, is regulated by TGF-β and an additional group of receptors, including receptors for TGF-β, the PDGF receptor-b, and Tie-2. The Tie-2 receptor is specifically upregulated on endothelial cells during glioma progression. The agonist for this receptor, angiopoietin-1, is constitutively expressed in glioma cells. Interestingly, its antagonistic ligand, angiopoietin-2, is also upregulated, suggesting a role for this ligand in some other pathophysiologic pathway.

ACKNOWLEDGMENTS

The authors thank Ms. Lucy Avila for her editing of this manuscript. The preparation of this work was supported by the Nissen Family and the Preuss Foundation.

REFERENCES

1. Kleihues P, Cavenee WK, editors. Pathology and genetics of tumors of the nervous system. Lyon: International Agency for Research on Cancer (IARC) Press; 2000. p. 314.
2. Barker FI, Israel M. The gliomas. In: Berger MS, Wilson C, editors. Molecular genetics of gliomas. Philadelphia (PA): WB Saunders; 1999. p. 39–51.
3. Hanahan D, Weinberg RA. The hallmarks of cancer. Cell 2000;100:57–70.
4. Bögler O, Huang HJ, Kleihues P, Cavanee WK. The *p53* gene and its role in human brain tumors. Glia 1995;15:308–27.
5. von Deimling A, Louis DN, Wiestler OD. Molecular pathways in the formation of gliomas. Glia 1995;15:328–38.
6. Tortosa A, Ino Y, Odell N, et al. Molecular genetics of radiographically defined de novo glioblastoma multiforme. Neuropathol Appl Neurobiol 2000;26:544–52.
7. Ichimura K, Bolin MB, Goike HM, et al. Deregulation of the p14ARF/MDM2/p53 pathway is a prerequisite for human astrocytic gliomas with G1-S transition control gene abnormalities. Cancer Res 2000;60:417–24.
8. Jensen S, Paderanga DC, Chen P, et al. Molecular analysis at the NF1 locus in astrocytic brain tumors. Cancer 1995;76:674–7.
9. Smith JS, Alderete B, Minn Y, et al. Localization of common deletion regions on 1p and 19q in human gliomas and their association with histological subtype. Oncogene 1999;18:4144–52.
10. Fulci G, Ishii N, Van Meir EG. p53 and brain tumors: from gene mutations to gene therapy. Brain Pathol 1998;8:599–613.
11. Nichols KE, Malkin D, Garber JE, et al. Germ-line p53 mutations predispose to a wide spectrum of early-onset cancers. Cancer Epidemiol Biomarkers Prev 2001;10:83–7.
12. Watanabe K, Sato K, Biernat W, et al. Incidence and timing of p53 mutations during astrocytoma progression in patients with multiple biopsies. Clin Cancer Res 1997;3:523–30.
13. Haas-Kogan DA, Kogan SS, Yount G, et al. p53 function influences the effect of fractionated radiotherapy on glioblastoma tumors. Int J Radiat Oncol Biol Phys 1999;43:399–403.
14. Reifenberger G, Reifenberger J, Ichimura K, et al. Amplification of multiple genes from chromosomal region 12q13-14 in human malignant gliomas: preliminary mapping of the amplicons shows preferential involvement of CDK4, SAS, and MDM2. Cancer Res 1994;54:4299–303.
15. Quelle DE, Zindy F, Ashmun RA, Sherr CJ. Alternative reading frames of the INK4a tumor supressor gene encode two unrelated proteins capable of inducing cell cycle arrest. Cell 1995;83:993–1000.
16. Ueki K, Ono Y, Henson JW, et al. CDKN2/p16 or RB alterations occur in the majority of glioblastomas and are inversely correlated. Cancer Res 1996;56:150–3.
17. He J, Olson JJ, James CD. Lack of p16INK4 or retinoblastoma protein (pRb), or amplification-associated overexpression of cdk4 is observed in distinct subsets of malignant glial tumors and cell lines. Cancer Res 1995;55:4833–6.
18. Zhou XP, Li YJ, Hoang-Xuan K, et al. Mutational analysis of the PTEN gene in gliomas: molecular and pathological correlations. Int J Cancer 1999;84:150–4.
19. Sauter G, Maeda T, Waldman FM, et al. Patterns of epidermal growth factor receptor amplification in malignant gliomas. Am J Pathol 1996;148:1047–53.
20. Galanis E, Buckner J, Kimmel D, et al. Gene amplification as a prognostic factor in primary and secondary high-grade malignant gliomas. Int J Oncol 1998;13:717–24.
21. Nishizaki T, Ozaki S, Harada K, et al. Investigation of genetic alterations associated with the grade of astrocytic tumor by comparative genomic hybridization. Genes Chromosomes Cancer 1998;21:340–6.
22. Cairncross JG, Ueki K, Zlatescu MC, et al. Specific genetic predictors of chemotherapeutic response and survival in patients with anaplastic oligodendrogliomas. J Natl Cancer Inst 1998;90:1473–9.
23. Plate KH, Risau W. Angiogenesis in malignant gliomas. Glia 1995;15:339–47.

5

Magnetic Resonance Imaging of Central Nervous System Tumors

CYNTHIA T. CHIN, MD
WILLIAM P. DILLON, MD

GENERAL IMAGING CONSIDERATIONS

Magnetic resonance imaging (MRI) has become the imaging modality of choice in the evaluation of intracranial and spinal cord tumors. The major advantages of MRI include its inherent superb tissue contrast and its ability to image directly in multiple planes. Magnetic resonance imaging has been shown to be more sensitive than computed tomography (CT) for both detection and determining the extent of tumor.[1]

Hydrogen protons in water are of low signal intensity on T1-weighted images (T1WIs) and high signal intensity on T2-weighted images (T2WIs). Pathologic processes such as tumors, infections, and infarcts all produce an increase in extracellular water. Compared to normal brain tissue, these pathologic regions show decreased signal on T1WIs and increased signal on T2WIs. Tissue contrast is usually most apparent on T2WIs, which show a high signal intensity from pathologic processes in contrast to the intermediate signal intensity of normal brain parenchyma.

Although intracranial neoplasms are generally hypointense on T1WIs and hyperintense on T2WIs, they also frequently contain heterogeneous regions of high signal on T1WIs and low-signal foci on T2WIs. This heterogeneous signal may be the result of calcification, hemorrhage, necrosis, proteinaceous debris, fibrous stroma, and signal voids from rapid flow. In general, heterogeneous signal intensity is seen in higher-grade neoplasms.

Sensitivity and Lesion Localization

Magnetic resonance imaging has been shown to be clearly superior to CT scanning in the detection of intracranial neoplasms. Due to MRI's inherent superb contrast resolution, small lesions can be detected that would otherwise be missed on a contrast-enhanced CT scan. In addition to being more sensitive than CT for the detection of primary brain tumors, MRI has been found to show the extent of the tumor more completely. T2-weighted abnormalities usually extend well beyond the corresponding low-attenuation lesions on CT scan.[2] In addition to the increased area of T2-weighted signal abnormalities, the region of MRI contrast enhancement is equal to or greater than that present on CT scan.[3]

One of the major drawbacks of CT scanning is its insensitivity to lesions of the temporal lobes and posterior fossa due to the beam-hardening artifact from the adjacent skull. Unaffected by bone artifact, MRI is able to demonstrate temporal lobe and posterior fossa anatomy with superior detail.

One of the advantages of MRI is its ability to image directly in multiple planes. This usually permits the distinction of peripheral intra-axial masses from extra-axial lesions such as meningiomas. Features favoring an extra-axial mass include broad attachment to the dura, buckling of white matter, and a cerebrospinal fluid (CSF) cleft adjacent to the mass (Figure 5–1). Enhancement of the adjacent dura (the so-called dural tail,) can be seen with, but is not pathognomonic of, a meningioma.

Pitfalls

Lack of Specificity

Despite the exquisite sensitivity of MRI for the detection of cerebral neoplasms, multiple pathologic processes can demonstrate low signal intensity on T1WIs and high signal intensity on T2WIs. The MRI examination lacks specificity, and infarcts, inflammatory lesions, demyelination, and radiation necrosis are common processes that can simulate intracranial neoplasms.

Infarcts, especially in the subacute phase, may demonstrate focal hyperintensity on T2WIs and contrast enhancement that can simulate a neoplasm. An accurate clinical history often aids in distinguishing infarction from neoplasm. Features of MRI that favor an infarct include location in a vascular territory, gyral involvement, and well-defined borders. MR diffusion weighted imaging is helpful for confirming acute infarction within the first 7 to 10 days, demonstrating reduced diffusion typical of acute ischemic injury (Figure 5–2). If diffusion imaging is

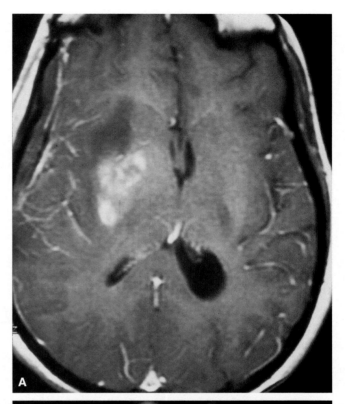

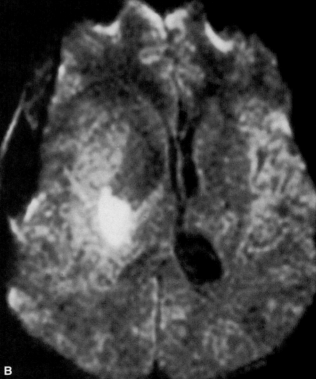

Figure 5–2. *A*, Axial postgadolinium T1-weighted sequence in a patient status post right frontal craniotomy for glioma resection demonstrates enhancement within the tumor bed involving the right basal ganglia. *B*, Axial diffusion weighted sequence in the same patient demonstrates reduced diffusion within the right basal ganglia corresponding to the area of enhancement, compatible with acute infarction.

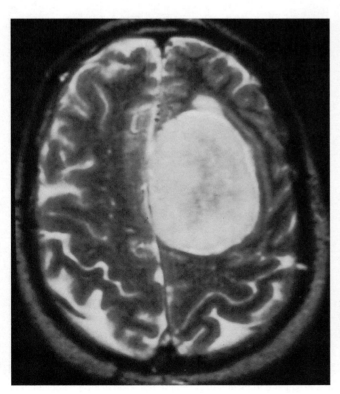

Figure 5–1. Axial T2-weighted sequence demonstrates a large left frontal meningioma with associated gray-white matter buckling and adjacent cerebrospinal fluid (CSF) cleft, features of an extra-axial mass.

unavailable, a follow-up MRI in 10 days can be extremely helpful. With infarction, there is usually a rapid change in the enhancement pattern and mass effect as the infarct evolves from subacute to chronic stages. In general, most tumors will not exhibit much change over a period of 1 to 2 weeks.

Cerebral abscesses typically have a thin rim of enhancement, compared to the thick and nodular enhancement seen in gliomas. Other features of cerebral abscesses include high-intensity rim on precontrast T1WIs and on satellite images. However, there is enough imaging overlap between the two processes that the clinical history is usually vital in making the distinction (Figure 5–3).

Occasionally, demyelinating disease such as multiple sclerosis may sometimes present in a tumefactive fashion. The acute plaque may demonstrate mass effect, enhancement, and vasogenic edema similar to that of primary brain tumors. Short-term follow-up MRI scans within 6 to 8 weeks usually demonstrate resolution of mass effect and enhancement. Other signal-intensity abnormalities in the periventricular white matter and corpus callosum would support a diagnosis of multiple sclerosis. In addition, a "leading-edge," incomplete ring of enhancement around a demyelinating plaque has been described (Figure 5–4).

Enhancement Does Not Equate with Histologic Grade

The introduction of MRI contrast agents in 1988 had a tremendous impact on the evaluation of tumors of the central nervous system (CNS). The most commonly used MRI contrast agent is gadopentetate dimeglumine. Gadolinium is a rare earth metal with seven unpaired electrons. These unpaired electrons enable nearby protons to re-align more quickly with the main magnetic field and thus shorten T1 relaxation time. On a T1WI, molecules that re-align

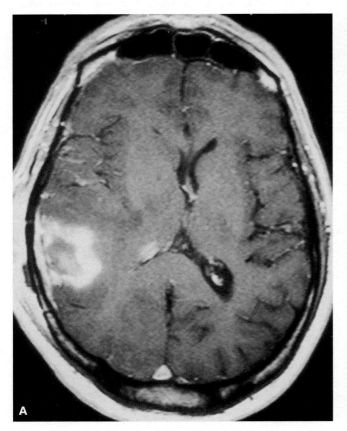
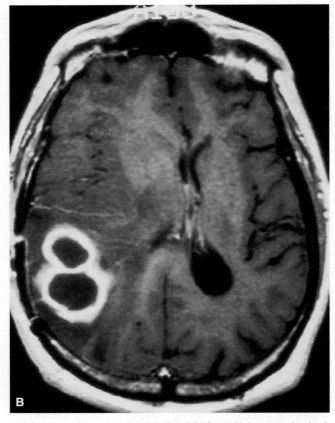

Figure 5–3. *A*, Axial postgadolinium T1-weighted sequence demonstrates irregular enhancement within the right frontal lobe resection bed, compatible with recurrent glioma. The recurrent tumor was subsequently resected. *B*, Axial postgadolinium T1-weighted sequence in the same patient (who returned with fever several months after the resection) demonstrates development of masses within the resection bed that have a thin uniform peripheral rim of enhancement compatible with abscesses.

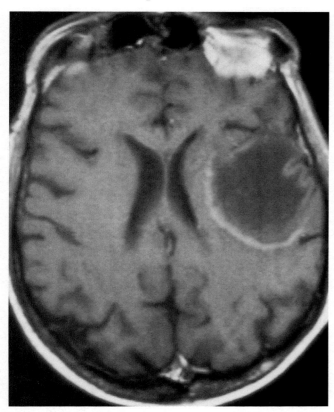

Figure 5–4. Axial postgadolinium T1-weighted sequence demonstrates a large left frontal lobe lesion with an "incomplete ring" of enhancement compatible with demyelination.

rapidly with a magnetic field will have higher signal intensity than those that re-align slowly. Thus, gadolinium enhancement results in an increase in the signal intensity on T1WIs. Although gadolinium shortens both T1 and T2 relaxation times, the effect on T1 relaxation time is much greater, accounting for the exclusive use of T1-weighted sequences after the administration of contrast material.

Normal brain capillaries with an intact blood-brain barrier are impermeable to gadolinium complexes because of tight endothelial junctions. Regions of the brain that normally lack a blood-brain barrier, such as the pituitary gland, pineal gland, choroid plexus, and dura, will enhance normally and should not be mistaken for pathology. Neoplasm-induced angiogenesis, especially in more malignant gliomas, results in capillaries with a discontinuous basic membrane that lacks a blood-brain barrier. These abnormal capillaries allow diffusion of gadolinium into adjacent brain parenchyma, which demonstrates enhancement on T1WIs. These regions of enhancing tumor generally correspond to the areas of greatest concentration of the capillaries. Enhancement can help guide stereotactic biopsy and surgical resections; however, it does not necessarily reflect the most metabolically active portion of a tumor as necrosis may also occur within the region of contrast enhancement.

In general, higher-grade gliomas generally enhance more frequently than lower-grade gliomas. Nevertheless, benign or low-grade tumors, such as juvenile pilocystic astrocytoma, typically show intense enhancement, reflecting their prominent vascularity. Likewise, higher-grade malignant tumors may occasionally demonstrate minimal (if any) enhancement.[4]

Enhancement does not delineate the exact border of tumors. Stereotactic biopsies have demonstrated viable tumor cells outside the region of contrast enhancement on MRI. In addition, tumor cells have also been found in regions of the brain that were normal on the T2WIs.[2]

Effect of Steroids on Contrast Enhancement

Corticosteroids may alter the enhancement pattern of tumors, reducing both the extent and the intensity of contrast enhancement as well as the amount of peritumoral edema.[5] Lymphoma is particularly sensitive to steroids, and significant decreases in mass effect and enhancement can occur rapidly after steroids are administered.[6,7]

Radiation Necrosis

Radiation injury to the brain is becoming increasingly recognized because of the sensitivity of MRI. Radiation injury is classified as acute and late radiation injury. Late radiation injury usually occurs months to years after therapy and is irreversible. Two patterns of late radiation injury are diffuse and focal injury. Diffuse injury of white matter is seen on MRI as a non-enhancing high T2-weighted signal within white matter.

Focal late radiation injury usually manifests as a region of localized contrast enhancement on MRI. When necrosis develops after irradiation for cerebral tumors, it usually occurs in the region of the original tumor. This is thought to be secondary to vascular compromise by peritumoral vasogenic edema. When one encounters a patient with clinical deterioration and a prior history of radiation therapy, the distinction between late radiation necrosis and recurrent tumor is difficult on MRI. Unfortunately, late radiation necrosis and recurrent tumor share many similar MRI features. Both present as a region of decreased T1 signal and increased T2 signal with significant enhancement and extensive vasogenic edema. Positron emission tomography (PET) or magnetic resonance (MR) spectroscopy may be helpful in evaluating intracranial tumors and distinguishing recurrent tumor from radiation necrosis (Figure 5–5)

IMAGING FEATURES OF TUMORS OF NEUROEPITHELIAL TISSUE

Astrocytic Tumors

There are two classes of astrocytic tumors, based on overall growth pattern and capacity for brain invasion as well as progressive malignant potential.[8] The more common astrocytic tumors are the diffuse astrocytic tumors designated "astrocytomas," which are characterized by the significant potential to undergo anaplastic progression and diffuse infiltration. These tumors are graded according to the World Health Organization (WHO) designations of astrocytoma: astrocytoma (WHO grade II), anaplastic astrocytoma (WHO grade III), and glioblastoma (WHO grade IV) (Figure 5–6).

Astrocytomas represent the majority of all primary brain tumors and are the most common intracranial neoplasms. They can occur throughout the brain but most often involve the cerebral hemispheres.

The second class of astrocytic tumors is made up of pilocytic astrocytoma, pleomorphic xanthoastrocytoma, and subependymal giant cell astrocytoma. These relatively dissimilar tumors exhibit a more favorable prognosis due to a limited infiltration of the brain and a more circumscribed growth pattern.

Astrocytoma

Astrocytomas (WHO grade II) are diffusely infiltrating tumors composed of well-differentiated neo-

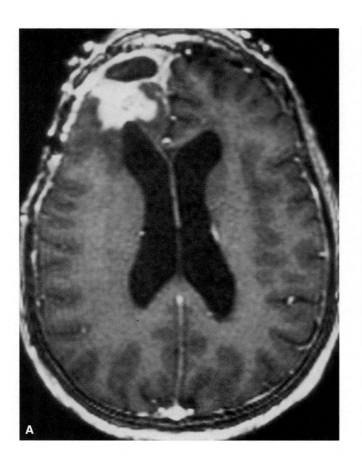
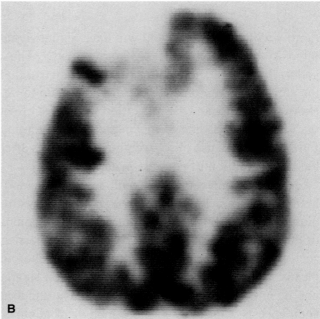

Figure 5–5. *A*, Axial postgadolinium T1-weighted sequence demonstrates nodular enhancement within the right frontal lobe resection bed concerning tumor recurrence. *B*, Positron emission tomography (PET) scan in the same patient demonstrates decreased glucose uptake in the right frontal lobe corresponding to the area of enhancement compatible with necrosis.

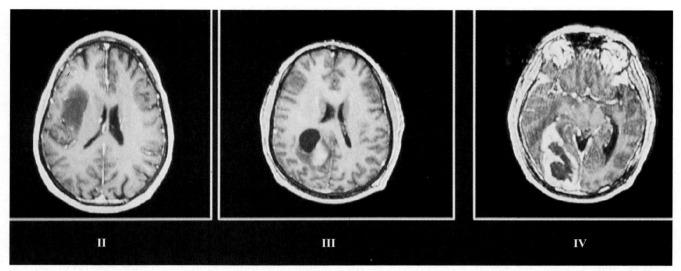

Figure 5–6. Postgadolinium axial T1-weighted sequences in three different patients with grades II, III, and IV gliomas, respectively. In general, higher-grade gliomas may enhance more frequently than lower-grade gliomas. Low-grade gliomas tend to be more well defined and homogeneous. Anaplastic astrocytomas tend to be more heterogeneous, with possible cysts and calcifications. Glioblastomas are heterogeneous, reflecting a combination of cysts, hemorrhage, and necrosis, with mass effect and vasogenic edema. These are general principles, and variations from these observations are not uncommon.

plastic astrocytes. They account for approximately 25 percent of hemispheric gliomas and typically occur in early adult life, with a peak incidence in the fourth and fifth decades.

Microscopically, astrocytomas are ill defined and tend to diffusely infiltrate the surrounding brain, resulting in enlargement and distortion of the structures involved. Mild pleomorphism and hypercellularity may be present although necrosis and endothelial proliferation are not seen. Calcification may be present in approximately 50 percent of cases although this is rarely appreciated on MRI. The three major histopathologic variants are fibrillary, gemistocytic, and protoplasmic.

On MRI, astrocytomas are typically well-defined homogeneous masses that are hypointense on T1WIs and hyperintense on T2WIs. Mass effect and associated edema are usually minimal for the size of the tumor although mass effect is always present to some degree. Astrocytomas are usually superficial in location, and there may be involvement of the overlying gray matter. Enhancement is variable. At the present time, it is not possible to predict with certainty the histologic grade of a glioma, based on its MRI appearance. Higher-grade glial tumors can appear radiographically identical to lower-grade gliomas (see Figure 5–6).

Anaplastic Astrocytoma

Anaplastic astrocytomas (WHO grade III) occur later in life than astrocytomas although they share a similar regional distribution. Pathologically, they can have increased hypercellularity, pleomorphism, and mitosis. The absence of necrosis and endothelial proliferation distinguishes anaplastic astrocytomas from glioblastomas.

Anaplastic astrocytomas tend to be more heterogeneous on MRI than astrocytomas. Characteristically, they have less well-defined borders and a greater degree of mass effect, vasogenic edema, and enhancement.[9] Cysts and calcification can also be seen. Hemorrhage may be present although it is more commonly seen in the higher-grade glioblastoma multiforme. On noncontrast T1- and T2-weighted images, heterogeneous signal intensity is usually present. The frequency of contrast enhancement is generally greater than in lower-grade gliomas. It must be stressed, however, that these are general principles and that variations from these observations are not uncommon (see Figure 5–6).

Glioblastoma Multiforme

Glioblastoma multiforme (GBM) (WHO grade IV) is the most common astrocytic tumor, representing

50 percent of astrocytic tumors and 15 to 20 percent of all intracranial tumors. Its peak incidence is at the age of 45 to 60 years. It occurs most commonly in the frontal lobes but can also be seen in the cerebellum, brain stem, and spinal cord. A characteristic pattern of GBM is spread across the white-matter tracts of the corpus callosum to involve the contralateral cerebral hemisphere (the so-called butterfly appearance). Pathologically, GBM is often a heterogeneous tumor, typically with areas of necrosis, hemorrhage, and endothelial proliferation (Figure 5–7).

The MRI appearance of GBM reflects the heterogeneous pathologic features. Generally, GBMs exhibit heterogeneous signal intensity on both T1WIs and T2WIs, reflecting a combination of cysts, hemorrhage, and necrosis (see Figure 5–6). Linear, serpiginous punctate regions of low signal on T1WIs and T2WIs may represent flow voids from tumor vascularity. The tumors are usually poorly defined, with extensive mass effect and vasogenic edema. Hemorrhage is common in GBM and is helpful in distinguishing glioblastoma from lower-grade astrocytomas.

Contrast enhancement is more frequent in GBM than with other astrocytic tumors and occurs in up to 95 percent of all glioblastomas. The enhancement pattern is typically irregular or nodular, with multiple foci extending throughout the lesion. It is not uncommon to see rests of contrast enhancement connected by non-enhancing regions of abnormal T2 signal intensity.

Glioblastoma multiforme is almost always associated with a large region of high signal seen on T2WIs. This region is composed of both vasogenic edema and microscopic tumor infiltration of the white- and gray-matter tracts and cannot be differentiated on MRI. In most cases, the extent of microscopic invasion is limited to a 2-cm margin surrounding the enhancing tumor although malignant cells may extend several centimeters beyond the enhancing-tumor margins. Tumor may be visualized on T2 fluid-attenuated inversion recovery (FLAIR) sequences coursing down white-matter tracts such as the internal capsule and into the brain stem.

Glioblastoma is the most common of the glial tumors to spread to the subarachnoid space. Contrast-enhanced MRI is far more sensitive than contrast CT in detecting leptomeningeal spread. An early indication of leptomeningeal spread is abnormal enhancement surrounding cranial nerves, most commonly seen along the fifth, seventh, and eighth cranial nerves.

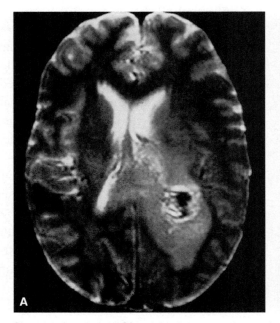 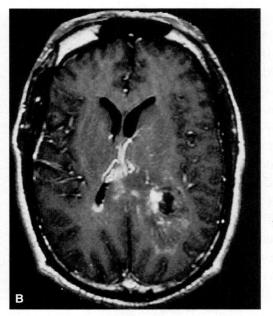

Figure 5–7. *A*, Axial T2-weighted sequence in a patient with glioblastoma multiforme demonstrates abnormal signal and enhancement involving the splenium of the corpus callosum, crossing to the right of midline. *B*, Post-gadolinium T1-weighted sequence, demonstrating same.

Gliomatosis Cerebri

Recognized as a rare, specific entity among the neuroepithelial tumors, gliomatosis cerebri is the diffuse infiltration of white and gray matter with neoplastic glial cells of varying levels of differentiation. Patients usually present between the third and fourth decades, often with headaches, insidious onset of personality changes, or seizures.

The cerebral hemispheres are more commonly affected, with involvement of the cerebellum, brain stem, and medulla being less common. Typically, there is a relative lack of mass effect, with characteristic preservation of the underlying neuroanatomic architecture. Histologically, there is diffuse proliferation of glial elements infiltrating normal tissue, with destruction of myelin sheath and only slight neuronal and axonal damage. Perineuronal and perivascular tumor spread is also seen.[10,11]

Magnetic resonance imaging is more sensitive than CT for detecting lesions and for demonstrating the extent of disease. Characteristically on MRI, there is poorly defined subtle diffuse high T2 signal involving at least two lobes and usually involving both gray and white matter. Lesions are isointense to hypointense relative to normal brain on T1WIs. Focal parenchymal and meningeal enhancement can occur, usually late in the disease course.[12–14]

Pilocytic Astrocytoma

Pilocytic astrocytomas are designated as WHO grade I. They are well-circumscribed tumors that are less biologically aggressive than the diffuse astrocytomas, displacing rather than infiltrating adjacent brain, and therefore resulting in a more favorable prognosis.[15,16]

Pilocytic astrocytomas occur primarily in children and young adults and are typically located in the midline, involving the cerebellum, optic pathways, third ventricle, thalamus, median temporal lobes, and brain stem.

Cerebellar astrocytomas represent the most common type of posterior fossa tumors in children in most series. Approximately 75 to 85 percent of cerebellar astrocytomas are juvenile pilocytic astrocytomas (JPAs) with a peak incidence in the first decade. Most cerebellar JPAs occur in the midline, with approximately 15 percent involving only the cerebellar hemispheres. These tumors can be cystic, solid, or solid with a necrotic center[17] (Figure 5–8).

Approximately 50 percent of JPAs are cystic, with a solid tumor nodule in the wall of the cyst. Approximately 40 percent are predominantly solid tumor with a cystic center. The cyst walls in these tumors are comprised of tumor cells that generally show enhancement. A well-defined mural nodule will not be seen. Fewer than 10 percent of JPAs are completely solid tumors. These are usually round to oval, lobulated, well-defined masses that show heterogeneous to homogeneous enhancement.

Juvenile pilocytic astrocytomas in a supratentorial compartment occur most frequently in the diencephalon, chiasm, hypothalamus, floor of the third ventricle, and (less commonly) cerebral hemispheres. There is an equal male-female ratio, with a peak age of approximately 2 years. Although microcysts are commonly seen at pathology, macrocysts are less commonly seen when compared with infratentorial JPAs.[17]

Pathologically, JPA is typically a sharply marginated lobular mass with abundant Rosenthal

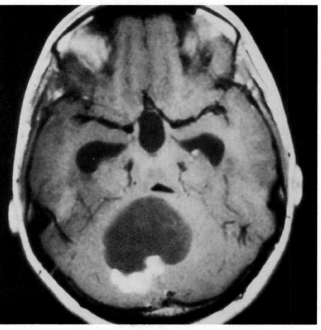

Figure 5–8. Axial postgadolinium T1-weighted sequence demonstrates a well-defined cystic mass within the cerebellum with an intensely enhancing mural tumor nodule, characteristic of juvenile pilocytic astrocytomas. There is mass effect effacing the fourth ventricle, resulting in obstructive hydrocephalus.

fibers, vascular proliferation, and cyst formation. There is often a vascular tumor nodule within the cyst wall. In contrast to most low-grade astrocytomas, the endothelial cells within a JPA have open tight junctions and fenestrations, allowing for profound enhancement. This may also result in high activity on fluorine-18-fluoro-2-deoxyglucose (FDG) PET studies. Unlike in other astrocytomas, however, the extensive contrast enhancement does not indicate an unfavorable prognosis.

On MRI, the tumor nodule generally shows intense enhancement whereas the remaining cyst wall generally does not show evidence of enhancement. The cyst is hypointense on T1WIs and hyperintense on T2WIs. The cyst fluid may have higher signal on T1WIs relative to CSF due to increased protein content. In addition, it should be emphasized that a tumor should not be described as cystic because it shows low signal on T1WIs and high signal on T2WIs. Solid tumors can have a similar appearance. Other features, such as a fluid level and motion artifact from fluid pulsations, can help in this distinction.[18]

Subependymal Giant Cell Astrocytoma

Subependymal giant cell astrocytoma (SEGA) is almost exclusively seen in the setting of tuberous sclerosis. Tuberous sclerosis is a phakomatosis with cutaneous, intracranial, cardiac, and renal manifestations. The four major intracranial abnormalities are cortical tubers, subependymal nodules, white-matter lesions, and SEGAs. These lesions all share similar histopathologic features, with giant cells surrounded by areas of gliosis and demyelination. Cortical tubers, subependymal nodules, and white-matter lesions are seen in more than 90 percent of patients whereas SEGAs are seen in approximately 10 percent of patients. The peak age is between 8 and 18 years, with no gender predilection. These benign tumors are slow growing and noninvasive and rarely recur after excision. They most commonly present with obstructive hydrocephalus.

These tumors occur in a subependymal location and project into the ventricle. They almost always occur at the foramen of Monro and are much less frequently found in the regions of atria and temporal horns. On MRI, they are predominantly hypointense to white matter on T1WIs and heterogeneously hyperintense on T2WIs. Heterogeneous signal on T2WIs most likely reflects calcification and hemorrhage. Serpentine flow voids most likely represent tumor vessels. Contrast enhancement is usually marked. Peritumoral edema is very uncommon[19] (Figure 5–9).

The most common explanation of the pathogenesis of SEGAs is that they arise from subependymal nodules. Radiologically, the distinction between the two entities may be difficult. However, benign subependymal nodules tend to be small, most ranging in size between 1 and 10 mm, whereas SEGAs are usually larger than 2 cm. Enhancement can be seen in both lesions although it tends to be greater in SEGAs. Finally, linear signal voids, interval growth, and obstructive hydrocephalus all favor a diagnosis of SEGA.

Pleomorphic Xanthoastrocytoma

Pleomorphic xanthoastrocytoma (PX) is a rare, usually benign tumor that is primarily located in the supratentorial cortex of the temporal lobes. The most common presenting symptoms are seizures and headaches. Males and females are equally affected. Although it occurs at any age, it is a tumor primarily of children and young adolescents. On gross examination, PX usually consists of a largely cystic mass with a mural nodule adjacent to a dural surface. At surgery, leptomeningeal involvement is commonly seen and may account for occasional tumor recurrence.

On MRI, PX typically appears as a cortically based mass, primarily in the temporal lobes. The tumor mass shows nonspecific low signal intensity on T1WIs and high signal on T2WIs, with marked enhancement of the tumor nodule. Cysts are frequently seen and may comprise the bulk of the tumor mass.

Leptomeningeal and gyral enhancement have been reported. Mass effect and edema are usually minimal, and extensive peritumoral edema may indicate more aggressive lesions. Calcification is rarely seen.

Brainstem Glioma

Brainstem gliomas account for approximately 10 percent of pediatric CNS neoplasms and 25 percent of posterior fossa neoplasms in children. The peak incidence is between the ages of 3 and 10 years, and there is no sex predilection. Presenting symptoms usually result from involvement of cranial nerves, corticospinal tracts, and cerebellum. The majority of brainstem astrocytomas are of the diffuse fibrillary type whereas 20 percent resemble JPAs on histology. The pons is the most common site of origin of brainstem gliomas (60% of cases).[20]

Magnetic resonance imaging has greatly facilitated the diagnosis of brainstem gliomas. The MRI appearance is typically an expansile mass that is hypointense on T1WIs and hyperintense on T2WIs. Contrast enhancement has been reported in about 50 percent of cases and is usually irregular and heterogeneous. The brain stem may enlarge diffusely or exophytically. Exophytic pontine gliomas grow ventrally into the pre-pontine cistern surrounding the basilar artery and less commonly into the cerebellopontine angle.[21] Longitudinal extension into the midbrain and medulla and axial extension into the middle cerebellar peduncle and cerebellum are common. Hemorrhage or cysts have been reported in less than 5 percent of patients[21] (Figure 5–10).

Brainstem gliomas, especially those originating in the pons, are best appreciated on midline sagittal T2WIs. Sagittal images demonstrate the pontine enlargement, undulating contour of the ventral surface of the pons, and mass effect on the fourth ventricle. It is important that patients being evaluated for brainstem tumors be imaged in both the axial and sagittal planes.

Brainstem gliomas occur less frequently in the midbrain or medulla. Similar to pontine gliomas, they frequently show diffuse expansion, exophytic growth, and extension into adjacent parenchyma. Midbrain lesions frequently extend rostrally into the thalamus. Survival varies significantly according to the primary site, with lesions occurring in the midbrain and medulla having a better prognosis com-

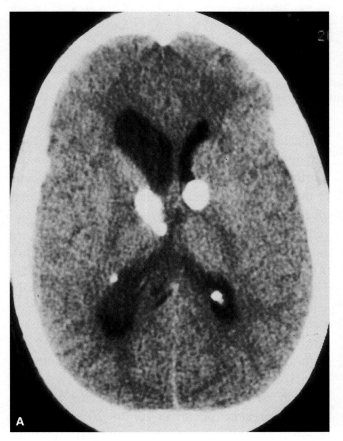
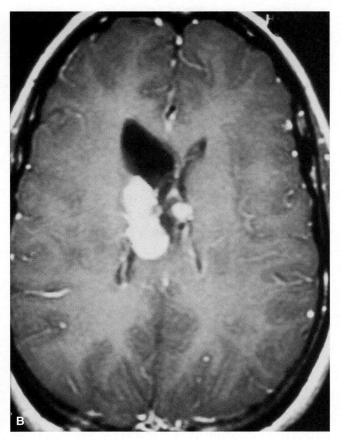

Figure 5–9. *A*, Axial non-enhanced computed tomography demonstrates multiple calcified subependymal hamartomas in a patient with tuberous sclerosis. *B*, Axial postgadolinium T1-weighted sequence in the same patient demonstrates an enhancing subependymal giant cell astrocytoma, located characteristically at the foramen of Monro, with resultant trapping of the right frontal horn.

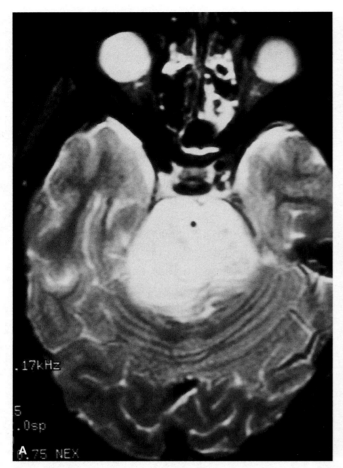
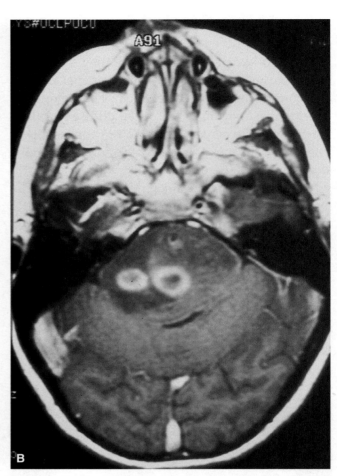

Figure 5–10. *A*, Axial T2-weighted sequence and, *B*, postgadolinium T1-weighted sequence demonstrate an expansile heterogeneously enhancing mass diffusely involving the pons and encasing the basilar artery, compatible with a brainstem glioma.

pared to pontine tumors. In addition, an inverse relationship exists between the extent of brainstem enlargement and survival.[22] Dorsally exophytic brainstem gliomas have a relatively better prognosis compared to the diffuse pontine gliomas, with a predominance of pilocytic histology demonstrated in one series.[23]

The differential diagnosis of focal signal-intensity abnormalities in the brain stem includes encephalitis, infarct, hematoma, and demyelinating disease.

Oligodendrogliomas

Oligodendrogliomas are uncommon brain tumors representing approximately 4 to 7 percent of intracranial gliomas. It is a relatively slow-growing tumor, and the presenting symptoms are usually a long history of seizures and (less commonly) headaches. Males are affected slightly more than females, and the peak incidence occurs between the fourth and sixth decades. These tumors tend to occur in the peripheral aspects of the frontal and parietal lobes. It is rare for these tumors to occur within the ventricles, cerebellum, and spinal cord.[24,25]

Macroscopically, oligodendrogliomas are solid, infiltrative lesions with well-defined borders. They frequently contain other glial cells, usually astrocytes, and are mixed in up to half of the cases. These tumors are generally round or oval and are rarely multilobulated. Oligodendrogliomas are the intra-axial tumor with the highest frequency of calcification; calcification has been reported in up to 30 to 70 percent of cases. Cystic degeneration and hemorrhage occur in up to 20 percent of lesions. There is no correlation of calcification, hemorrhage, or cyst formation with tumor purity or grading.[26]

On MRI, oligodendrogliomas are usually heterogeneous in signal intensity but are predominantly isointense with gray matter on T1WIs and hyperintense on T2WIs. The heterogeneous signal seen in these tumors reflects a combination of calcification, hemorrhage, and cystic change. Gradient echo imaging is far more sensitive to calcification and hemorrhage than spin echo sequences and is a very useful sequence in imaging oligodendrogliomas. Approximately half of oligodendrogliomas will demonstrate faint, patchy enhancement whereas the remainder may show no evidence of enhancement. Peritumoral edema is usually mild or absent. Overlying calvarial erosion has been seen with peripherally located oligodendrogliomas.[27]

Ependymomas

Ependymomas represent 2 to 6 percent of all gliomas. They arise from ependymal cells that are usually related to the ventricular system or the central canal of the spinal cord. Ependymomas are common tumors in children, in whom they account for 10 percent of all CNS neoplasms. Intracranial ependymomas usually occur in children whereas intraspinal ependymomas are most often seen in adults. Seventy percent of intracranial ependymomas are infratentorial in location, arising from the floor of the fourth ventricle. The peak age is 1 to 5 years, and males and females are equally affected.[28] Infratentorial ependymomas have a tendency to extend through the outlet foramen of the fourth ventricle into the vallecula, cerebellopontine angle, foramen magnum, and upper cervical subarachnoid space. Other tumors (especially the primitive neuroectodermal tumor [PNET]) can exhibit a similar morphology. Sagittal and coronal MRI are particularly suited for the evaluation of extraventricular extension of tumor.

The majority of supratentorial ependymomas are parenchymal in location rather than intraventricular, with the reported frequency of parenchymal origin ranging from 56 to 85 percent. These parenchymal tumors are thought to arise from ependymal rests. They are most frequent in the frontal and parietal lobes although any portion of the cerebral hemispheres can be affected. These lesions tend to be larger than the infratentorial ependymomas (in one series, 94% of the tumors were larger than 4 cm) and may undergo cystic degeneration more frequently.[29]

On gross pathology, ependymomas are extremely heterogeneous, with areas of calcification, cysts, and occasional hemorrhage.

Magnetic resonance imaging reflects the heterogeneous pathology. The solid portions of the tumor are hypointense on T1WIs and hyperintense to white matter on proton density and T2-weighted images. Foci of signal heterogeneity within solid tumors represent methemoglobin, hemosiderin, necrosis, calcification, and encased native vessels. Enhancement is usually patchy and irregular, unlike the more homogeneous enhancement of a medulloblastoma.[30,31]

The tumor often grows through the foramina of Luschka into the cerebellopontine angles (15% of cases), through the foramen of Magendie into the cisterna magna (up to 60% of cases), and through the foramen magnum and into the spinal cord. Invasion into cerebellar parenchyma occurs in 30 to 40 percent of cases. Heterogeneous signal characteristics make the diagnosis of ependymoma difficult on the basis of signal characteristics alone. Extension through foramina is well demonstrated and is one of the more important imaging findings (Figure 5–11).

Ependymoma is the most common of the childhood posterior fossa tumors to calcify. Calcification may be missed on spin echo sequences but will be apparent on gradient echo pulses. Cysts are more common in supratentorial ependymomas and will usually have slightly higher intensity than CSF on T1-weighted and proton density images due to protein. Almost all ependymomas enhance with contrast.

Subarachnoid spread of benign ependymoma is uncommon (10 to 12% of cases). If subarachnoid seeding is present, anaplastic ependymoma or ependymoblastoma should be suspected.

Subependymoma

Subependymomas are rare benign neoplasms that contain both astrocytes and ependymal cells. They are generally sharply marginated, lobulated tumors arising beneath the ventricular lining and extending

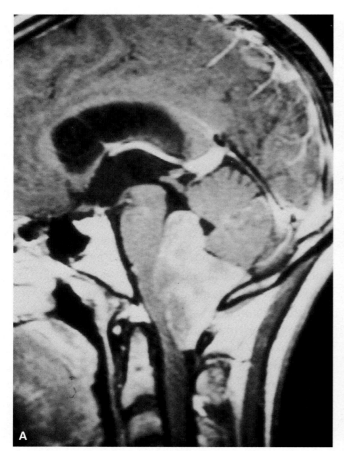 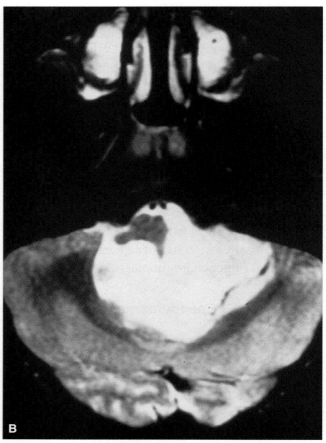

Figure 5–11. *A*, Sagittal postgadolinium T1-weighted sequence demonstrates tumor extension through the foramen magnum. *B*, Axial T2-weighted sequence in a different patient demonstrates tumor extension through the foramen of Luschka. Both extensions are characteristic of ependymomas.

into the ventricle. These benign lesions are usually asymptomatic, even when large, and do not undergo malignant degeneration or subarachnoid spread. Subependymomas are more common in men and occur at a mean age of approximately 60 years. The most frequent location for subependymomas is in the fourth ventricle (75% of cases), but they can occur in other sites, including the lateral ventricles and the spinal cord. Solid tumors tend to be homogeneous whereas larger lesions can have focal areas of cysts, calcification, and hemorrhage. Symptomatic subependymomas are related to ventricular outflow obstruction.

On MRI, subependymomas demonstrate nonspecific T1-weighted hypointense and T2-weighted hyperintense signals. The T2-weighted signal tends to be heterogeneous, especially in larger lesions. Contrast enhancement is variable; when present, it may range from patchy to homogeneous. The key to preoperative diagnosis of a subependymoma depends on identifying its intraventricular location, the most common site being the fourth ventricle. Lesions in the lateral ventricle are usually adjacent to the septum pellucidum (Figure 5–12). The differential diagnosis includes other intraventricular neoplasms, such as ependymoma, neurocytoma, meningioma, choroid plexus papilloma, and astrocytoma.[32,33]

Choroid Plexus Tumors

Choroid plexus papillomas and choroid plexus carcinomas are rare tumors arising from the epithelium of the choroid plexus. They account for less than 1 percent of all primary brain tumors but constitute 10 to 20 percent of tumors in the first year of life and 5 percent of supratentorial tumors of childhood. Most present at fewer than 5 years of age, with a male predominance.

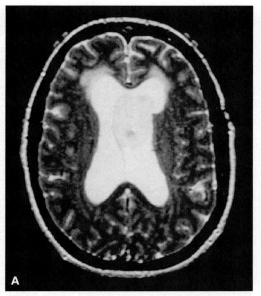 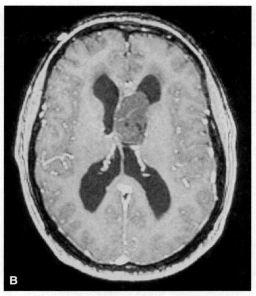

Figure 5–12. A, Axial T2-weighted sequence and, B, postgadolinium T1-weighted sequence demonstrate a non-enhancing heterogeneous intraventricular mass within the left lateral ventricle adjacent to the septum pellucidum, compatible with a subependymoma.

The lateral ventricle, especially the trigone, is the most common location in children (vs the fourth ventricle in adults). Left-sided predominance is reported, and choroid plexus tumors are rarely bilateral. Calcification occurs in 20 percent of cases.[34,35]

Papillomas are well-defined tumors, compared to carcinomas, which have a more irregular contour and which are often heterogeneous. Carcinomas nearly always invade the ventricular wall into the adjacent parenchyma and may disseminate along CSF pathways. Vasogenic edema is a helpful distinguishing sign. Malignant change is seen in less than 10 to 20 percent of cases.

Hydrocephalus is usually associated with these tumors and results from CSF overproduction, pathway obstruction of CSF by tumor, or impaired CSF absorption due to hemorrhage.

On CT, choroid plexus papilloma is an often slightly hyperdense mass with calcification and enhancement (Figure 5–13A). Carcinomas tend to have mixed densities, with cysts and hemorrhage and with prominent variable enhancement.

On MRI, benign papilloma demonstrates homogeneous iso- and hypointense signal on T1WIs, hyperintense signal on T2WIs, and homogeneous enhancement (see Figure 5–13B). Carcinomas tend to have a heterogeneous appearance on T1WIs and T2WIs with irregular enhancement, hemorrhage, and cyst formation, commonly invading the surrounding brain with associated edema.[36,37]

Gangliogliomas and Ganglioneuromas

Ganglioglioma and ganglioneuroma represent 3 percent of brain tumors in children, with an equal male-female ratio. They are composed of glial cells and neuronal elements. A predominance of neural elements results in ganglioneuroma (or gangliocytoma); a predominance of glial cells results in ganglioglioma. Ganglioglioma is more common in children and young adults. Although gangliogliomas are often associated with a relatively favorable prognosis and long survival, the presence of anaplastic features predicts a worse outcome.[38,39]

Gangliogliomas are usually cortically based in the cerebrum, the temporal lobes being the most common site. The frontal and parietal lobes, third ventricle, and hypothalamus are other common sites. The peripheral location of the mass within a cerebral hemisphere associated with adjacent calvarial erosion is helpful in establishing the diagnosis. On imaging, gangliogliomas are well defined and are usually without a large amount of mass effect. Characteristics on MRI consist of iso- and

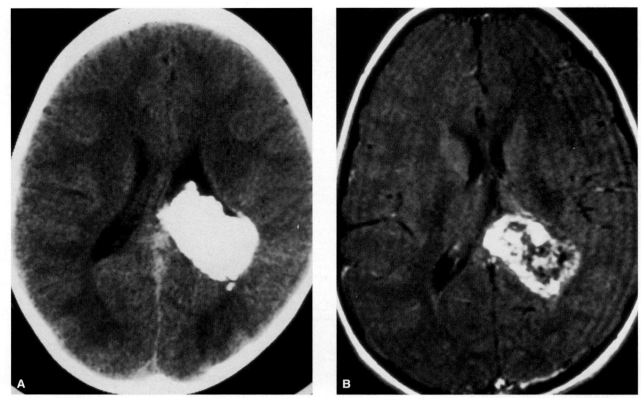

Figure 5–13. *A*, An unenhanced computed tomography scan and, *B*, axial postgadolinium T1-weighted sequence demonstrate a heavily calcified enhancing choroid plexus papilloma within the left lateral ventricle.

hypointense T1-weighted signal and iso- and hyperintense T2-weighted signal. Cysts are seen in 38 to 50 percent of cases, and calcification is seen in 35 percent of cases. Enhancement is variable[40,41] (Figure 5–14).

Dysembryoplastic Neuroepithelial Tumors

Dysembryoplastic neuroepithelial tumors (DNETs) are benign intra- or subcortical tumors that nearly always present with partial complex seizure disorders in children. Over 60 percent are located within the temporal lobes, and 30 percent are within the frontal lobes. They tend to be solid, with microcystic or macrocystic components, and usually demonstrate minimal contrast enhancement.

On MRI, DNETs are hypointense on T1WIs, are hyperintense on T2WIs, and demonstrate a characteristic gyral configuration, often with small "satellite" cystic-appearing lesions. They may have an MRI appearance identical to those of gangliogliomas, oligodendrogliomas, or low-grade astrocytomas.[42]

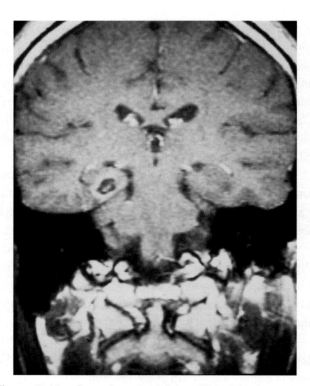

Figure 5–14. Coronal postgadolinium T1-weighted sequence demonstrates a well-defined enhancing calcified mass, cortically based within the left temporal lobe, characteristic of a ganglioglioma.

Desmoplastic Infantile Gangliogliomas

Desmoplastic infantile gangliogliomas are rare glial tumors occurring in patients 2 months to 4 years of age. They are massive cystic tumors typically superficially located within the cerebral hemispheres and attached to the dura. Despite their large size, they tend to have a relatively benign course. The superficial solid components often enhance. Histologically, the tumor shows evidence of glial and ganglionic differentiation accompanied by extreme desmoplastic reaction.[43]

Pineoblastomas and Pineocytomas

Pineoblastomas and pineocytomas constitute 20 to 40 percent of tumors in the pineal region. Pineoblastomas are highly malignant primitive small round cell tumors seen primarily within the first decade of life and primarily in males. There is an association between pineoblastoma and bilateral retinoblastoma.

Pineocytomas are composed of relatively mature cells and can be seen during the first decade of life although they are more common in adults.

These tumors tend to be enhancing lobular masses, often containing calcifications. Pineoblastomas tend to be larger and more irregular than pineocytomas. Pineoblastomas may also have nonenhancing foci due to focal necrosis, hemorrhage, and cyst formation. The appearance is nonspecific on MRI (iso- and hypointense on T1WIs and iso- and hyperintense on T2WIs)[44,45] (Figure 5–15).

Medulloblastomas (Primitive Neuroectodermal Tumors of the Posterior Fossa)

Medulloblastoma is a highly malignant tumor composed of primitive undifferentiated small round cells. It represents 30 to 40 percent of posterior fossa tumors and 20 percent of pediatric CNS tumors; 75 percent present within the first decade of life, and there is a male predominance.

In approximately two-thirds of cases, tumors are located within the vermis. In adults, however, medulloblastomas are more often found in the cerebellar hemispheres. They usually arise from the fetal granular layer of the cerebellum or inferior

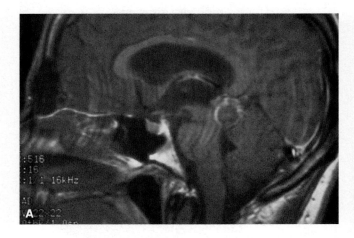
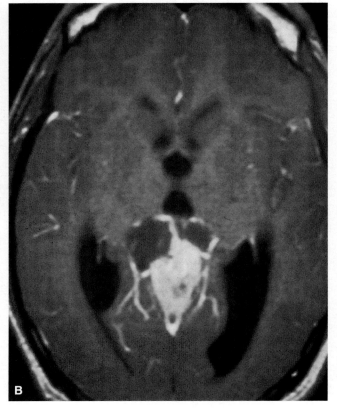

Figure 5–15. *A,* Postgadolinium sagittal T1-weighted sequence demonstrates a small well-defined, calcified, peripherally enhancing pineal mass compatible with a pineocytoma. *B,* Postgadolinium axial T1-weighted sequence in a different patient demonstrates a large solid, cystic, heterogeneously enhancing pineal mass consistent with a pineoblastoma.

medullary velum, growing anteriorly into the fourth ventricle. Brainstem invasion occurs in one-third of cases, and leptomeningeal invasion is frequent. Cysts or necrosis are seen in 50 percent of cases, and hemorrhage is uncommon.

These tumors also occur in patients with basal cell nevus syndrome (Gorlin's syndrome), Turcot's syndrome, ataxia-telangiectasia, xeroderma pigmentosum, and blue rubber bleb nevus syndromes.

On CT, medulloblastomas are iso- and hyperdense secondary to a high nuclear-cytoplasmic ratio. There is mild to moderate edema, with calcification seen in 10 to 20 percent of cases. Enhancement is usually uniform. Hydrocephalus is present in 95 percent of patients.

The MRI appearance of medulloblastoma is variable and nonspecific: hypointense on T1WIs and heterogeneously iso- and hypointense on T2WIs. Marked and variable enhancement is typical. It is important to evaluate for CSF tumor spread in the vermian cisterns, subependyma, and subfrontal region and along the spinal cord and cauda equina[46,47] (Figures 5–16 and 5–17).

Primitive Neuroectodermal Tumors

Primitive neuroectodermal tumors (PNETs) are rare tumors representing less than 5 percent of supratentorial neoplasms. They are malignant and primarily undifferentiated tumors within the cerebral hemispheres and also include primitive tumors with common neuroepithelial precursors in the brain stem, cerebellum, spinal cord, and extra-CNS locations. This tumor is also described as cerebral or central neuroblastoma, PNET of the cerebrum, and cerebral medulloblastoma. The peak incidence of PNET is up to 5 years of age, with an equal male-female ratio. The majority of PNETs occur within the cerebral hemispheres.

Primitive neuroectodermal tumors are characteristically large, expansile, sharply marginated, and markedly heterogeneous masses with a cystic component often present; 50 percent demonstrate necrosis and calcification, and hemorrhage is seen in 10 percent.

On CT, PNETs are hyperdense, presumably secondary to a high nuclear-cytoplasmic ratio, and exhibit variable enhancement. Calcification, calvarial asymmetry, and bone erosion are occasionally demonstrated. On MRI, PNETs are hypointense on T1WIs and iso- and hyperintense on T2WIs.[48]

IMAGING FEATURES OF MENINGIOMAS

Meningiomas are the most common extra-axial tumors and the most common CNS tumors induced by radiation. Ninety percent of meningiomas are located supratentorially in the parasagittal location (arising from the wall of the sagittal sinus), over the convexities, sphenoid wing, cerebellopontine angle, olfactory groove, and planum sphenoidale. Twenty percent of cases will demonstrate bony changes, either hyperostotic or osteolytic.

On CT, 60 percent of these tumors are hyperdense, and 20 percent demonstrate calcification. Cystic and fatty degeneration are rare features. Homogeneous

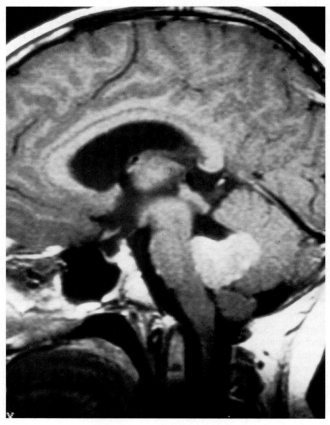

Figure 5–16. Sagittal postgadolinium T1-weighted sequence demonstrates an enhancing mass arising from the cerebellar vermis and growing into the fourth ventricle with resultant hydrocephalus, compatible with medulloblastoma (primitive neuroectodermal tumor [PNET] of the posterior fossa).

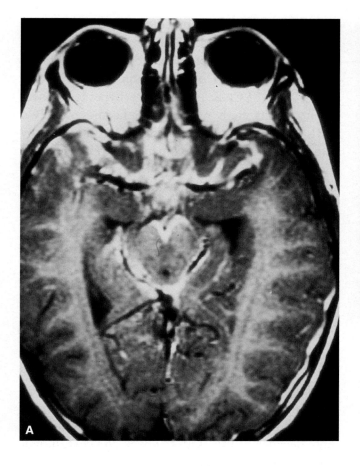
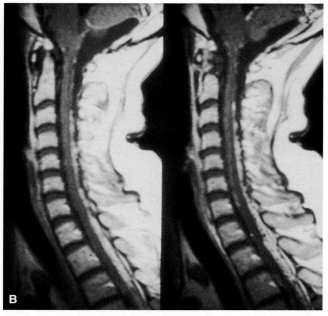

Figure 5–17. *A,* Postgadolinium T1-weighted sequence of the head demonstrates abnormal enhancement within the subarachnoid spaces and basilar cisterns as well as coating of the spinal cord, *B,* compatible with diffuse cerebrospinal fluid spread of tumor in this patient with medulloblastoma (primitive neuroectodermal tumor [PNET] of the posterior fossa).

and intense enhancement is typical. On MRI, the tumors are iso- and hypointense on T1WIs and iso- and hyperintense on T2WIs. Associated dural enhancement ("dural tail") is seen in approximately 72 percent of cases (representing neoplasm or reactive proliferation) (Figure 5–18). On angiography, a characteristic tumor blush with dural and pial blood supply may be seen early during the capillary phase and staying late into the venous phase.[49–51]

Meningiomas are rare in childhood and there is a high association with type 2 neurofibromatosis (25% of cases). The most common location is within the lateral ventricles and posterior fossa. They are usually multiple and are frequently associated with multiple schwannomas.

IMAGING FEATURES OF HEMANGIOBLASTOMAS

Hemangioblastoma is the most common primary infratentorial tumor in adults. Eighty-three percent of cases occur in the cerebellum, with the remainder arising within the spinal cord, medulla, and cerebrum. Hemangioblastomas are relatively benign vascular endothelial tumors consisting characteristically of a cystic mass with a solid mural nodule (55% of cases); 40 percent of the tumors are purely solid masses.

The tumors are highly vascular, and associated flow voids are seen on MRI in 72 percent of cases. The mural nodule demonstrates intense enhancement whereas the cyst wall does not enhance. These tumors do not calcify and are not associated with significant edema (Figure 5–19).

Twenty percent of hemangioblastomas are associated with the von Hippel-Lindau syndrome; 40 percent of patients have polycythemia secondary to increased erythropoietin production.[52]

IMAGING FEATURES OF LYMPHOMA

Primary lymphoma of the central nervous system (PLCNS) is often associated with immunodeficiency and frequently occurs in patients with acquired immunodeficiency syndrome (AIDS), Sjögren's syndrome,

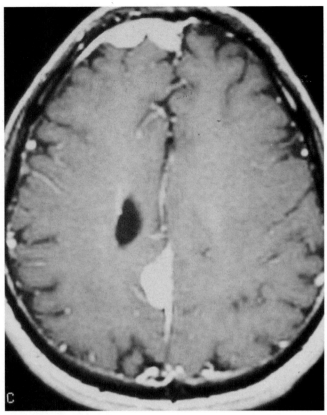

Figure 5–18. Postgadolinium axial T1-weighted sequence of the head demonstrates multiple meningiomas with associated enhancing "dural tails."

and Wiskott-Aldrich syndrome and in organ transplantation patients who are undergoing immunosuppressive therapy. It can also occur in immunocompetent adults.

The tumor is typically located in the deep gray matter and periventricular white matter. Subependymal spread is seen in 38 percent of cases. Secondary involvement of the CNS by extracerebral lymphomas is usually a leptomeningeal process and may be less visible on CT or MRI scans.

On CT, PLCNS is typically hyperdense secondary to its high nuclear-cytoplasmic ratio. On MRI, its appearance is variable, but it typically demonstrates avid enhancement and relatively low signal on T2WIs (Figure 5–20). In AIDS patients, smaller lesions may demonstrate ring enhancement more commonly[53–55] (Figure 5–21).

IMAGING FEATURES OF GERM CELL TUMORS

Germinomas

Germinoma is the most common intracranial germ cell tumor and the most common pineal-region tumor, accounting for more than 50 percent of the neoplasms in this region. Males are affected 10 times more frequently than females. Pineal-region germinomas occur most frequently during the first three decades of life, with the peak age corresponding to the onset of puberty.

On CT, germinomas are typically iso- and hyperdense. On MRI, they are iso- and hypointense on T1WIs and hyperintense on T2WIs. Occasionally, they exhibit low signal on T2WIs, probably due to a high nuclear-cytoplasmic ratio. The mass uniformly enhances.[56–58]

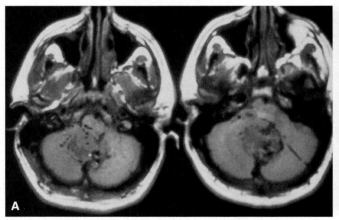 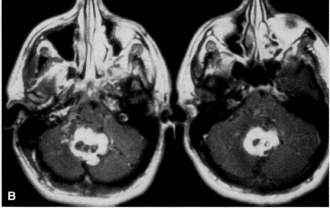

Figure 5–19. *A*, Non-enhanced axial T1-weighted sequences of the head in a patient with von Hippel-Lindau syndrome demonstrate a cerebellar hemangioblastoma with associated prominent flow voids. *B*, Enhanced axial T1-weighted sequences in the same patient demonstrate intense enhancement characteristic of these highly vascular tumors.

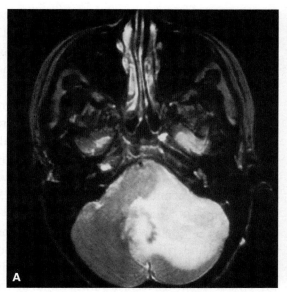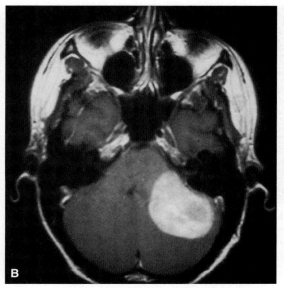

Figure 5–20. A, Axial T2-weighted sequence and, B, postgadolinium T1-weighted sequence in a patient with lymphoma demonstrate the characteristic avid enhancement and relatively low T2 signal due to the high nuclear-cytoplasmic ratio within these tumors.

Teratomas

Teratoma is the second most common germ cell tumor of the pineal region (15% of pineal masses) and may also be found in the suprasellar region, pituitary fossa, and third ventricle. It occurs almost exclusively in males. Most teratomas are well circumscribed and benign.

On CT and MRI, teratomas are typically lobulated and variegated midline masses with marked heterogeneity due to the presence of cysts, blood, fat, calcification, and bone. Enhancement is not typically seen unless malignant degeneration is present[56,57] (Figure 5–22).

IMAGING FEATURES OF EMBRYONIC TUMORS (EPIDERMOIDS AND DERMOIDS)

Epidermoids and dermoids are believed to arise from congenital cell rests that remain intracranial

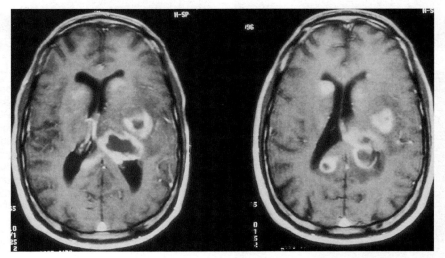

Figure 5–21. Axial postgadolinium T1-weighted sequence in an acquired immunodeficiency syndrome (AIDS) patient with lymphoma demonstrates small periventricular lesions with peripheral ring enhancement, a pattern that can be seen in patients with AIDS.

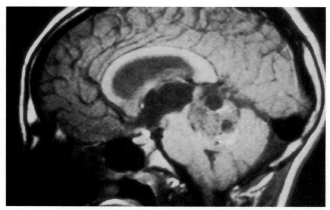

Figure 5–22. Non-enhanced sagittal T1-weighted sequence demonstrates a pineal-region teratoma displaying typical marked heterogeneity due to the presence of cysts, blood, fat, calcification, and bone.

presumably due to incomplete separation of neuroectoderm from cutaneous ectoderm at the time of neural-tube closure. These lesions are slow-growing tumors that are lined by stratified squamous epithelium. They are the most common embryonic tumor, most often located in the cerebellopontine angle; the parasellar region and the middle cranial fossa are other common locations.

On imaging, epidermoids are lobular extra-axial masses that do not enhance and that deform surrounding structures with densities and signal intensities identical to those of CSF. On MRI, diffusion and FLAIR imaging may help differentiate these tumors from arachnoid cysts[59,60] (Figure 5–23).

Dermoids are inclusion ectodermal and mesodermal cysts lined with stratified squamous cell epithelium and filled with hair follicles and sebaceous and sweat glands. They can be located within the spinal canal as well as intracranially. Intracranially, they are located most frequently within the posterior fossa, especially in the fourth ventricle and vermis.

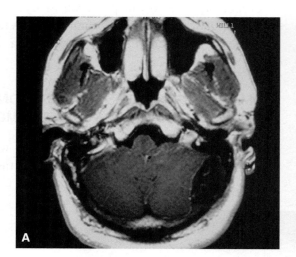

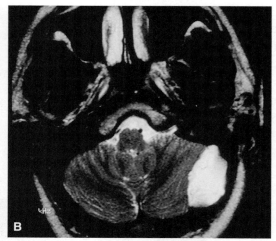

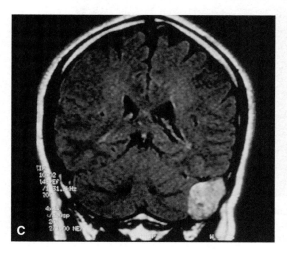

Figure 5–23. *A*, Axial postgadolinium T1-weighted sequence demonstrates a well-defined non-enhancing extra-axial mass within the left posterior fossa, identical to cerebrospinal fluid intensity on the axial T2-weighted sequence shown in *B*. *C*, Coronal-fluid attenuated inversion recovery (FLAIR) imaging in the same patient demonstrates a corresponding high signal intensity within the mass, compatible with an epidermoid. This high signal distinguishes the mass from an arachnoid cyst, which would demonstrate low signal intensity identical to that of the cerebrospinal fluid within the subarachnoid spaces and in the ventricles.

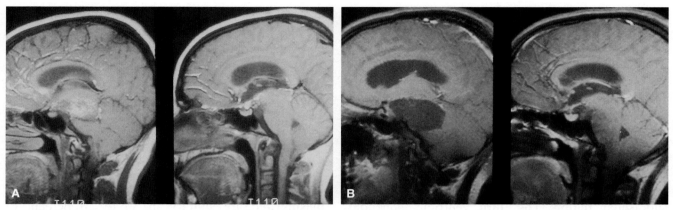

Figure 5–24. *A*, Non-enhanced sagittal T1-weighted sequence demonstrates a cerebellopontine-angle dermoid, which is intrinsically bright on the T1-weighted sequence due to the presence of fat. Hyperintense signal is also seen in the adjacent subarachnoid spaces consistent with rupture and the spread of fatty contents. There is also an associated chemical shift artifact, manifest as hypointense signal shadowing the hyperintense fat signal within the subarachnoid spaces. *B*, The lipid content of the mass and within the subarachnoid spaces can be verified by the loss of intrinsic hyperintensity on T1-weighted sequences with the use of fat saturation techniques.

On MRI, dermoids are non-enhancing extra-axial masses that contain fat, hair, and calcifications. The fat exhibits a hyperintense signal on T1WIs and a hypointense signal on T2WIs. Fat saturation and chemical shift artifacts may be helpful in verifying the lipid content.

Rupture of dermoids may occur, resulting in the spread of fatty contents throughout the subarachnoid space. This may result in chemical meningitis and communicating hydrocephalus[61] (Figure 5–24).

IMAGING FEATURES OF PITUITARY ADENOMAS

Pituitary adenomas are classified by size and function. Microadenomas are ≤ 10 mm in size and often secrete prolactin, growth hormone, or adrenocorticotropic hormone (ACTH). Microadenomas may demonstrate focal convexity of the superior border of the gland and deviation of the infundibular stalk away from the lesion. Dynamic imaging during gadolinium injection is preferred for optimal detection. Microadenoma presents as a focal hypointensity that is more apparent on MRI immediately after gadolinium injection (Figure 5–25). After 2 to 3 minutes, the adenoma begins to trap sufficient contrast, rendering it isointense to the remainder of the normal gland.

Macroadenomas are > 1 cm in size, are generally nonfunctioning, and may compress the optic chiasm, erode the sellar floor, or invade the cavernous sinus. Macroadenomas are isodense and isointense to brain parenchyma and usually enhance homogeneously.[62]

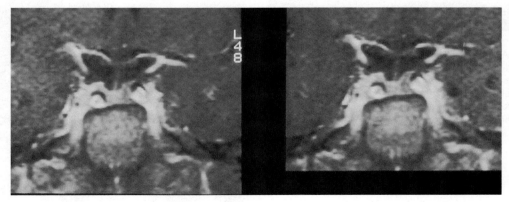

Figure 5–25. Dynamic coronal T1-weighted imaging of the sella and pituitary gland during gadolinium injection demonstrates a small hypointense focus of relatively slower gadolinium uptake within the left pituitary gland, consistent with a microadenoma.

IMAGING FEATURES OF CRANIOPHARYNGIOMA

Craniopharyngioma is the most common suprasellar mass in the pediatric age group. Peak age is 10 to 14 years, with a second peak in the fourth to sixth decades. Craniopharyngioma arises from embryonic squamous cell rests believed to be remnants of Rathke's craniopharyngeal pouch and may occur anywhere along the hypothalamus, pituitary stalk, and pituitary gland. The vast majority arise in the suprasellar region. The third ventricle, sphenoid sinus, and clivus are rare sites. They can be divided into three groups based on location: sellar, prechiasmatic, and retrochiasmatic. In 25 percent of patients, the tumor may extend into the anterior, middle, or posterior cranial fossae.

Craniopharyngiomas can be solid or cystic or both and can vary greatly in size. Typically, they have a multilobular and multicystic appearance on CT and MRI. Ninety percent demonstrate a cystic component, 90 percent are partially calcified, and 90 percent enhance. The solid components are iso- and hypointense on T1WIs and iso- and hyperintense on T2WIs, with enhancement of the solid tumor and cyst wall. Cysts may have high signal on all sequences due to the presence of aqueous cholesterol, hemorrhage, or proteinaceous fluid[63–66] (Figure 5–26).

METASTASES

Metastases represent 40 percent of intracranial neoplasms and are solitary in 30 to 50 percent of patients. The lung (30% of cases) and breast (18 to 30% of cases) are the most common primary sites. Melanoma, renal cell tumors, and thyroid tumors also commonly metastasize intracranially. Metastases tend to be well-defined enhancing lesions with moderate surrounding edema and are typically located peripherally at the gray-white junction.

Significantly more lesions are detected when triple doses of gadolinium are administered.[67,68]

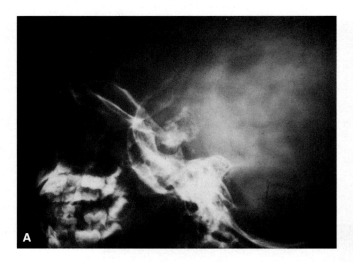
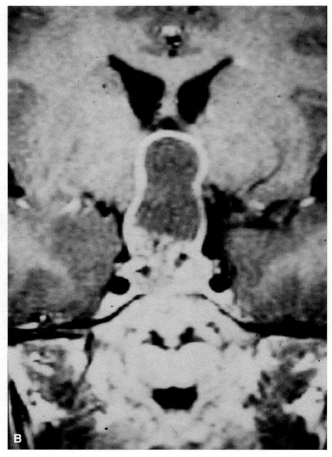

Figure 5–26. *A,* Lateral plain film of the skull demonstrates enlargement of the sella with calcifications in the sellar and suprasellar regions in this patient with craniopharyngioma. *B,* Coronal post-gadolinium T1-weighted sequence in the same patient demonstrates the sellar and suprasellar, solid and cystic, enhancing mass typical of a craniopharyngioma.

REFERENCES

1. Lee BC, Kneeland JB, Cahill PT, Deck MD. MR recognition of supratentorial tumors. AJNR Am J Neuroradiol 1985; 6:871–8.
2. Kelly PJ, Daumas-Duport C, Kispert DB, et al. Imaging-based stereotaxic serial biopsies in untreated intracranial glial neoplasms. J Neurosurg 1987;66:865–74.
3. Earnest FT, Kelly PJ, Scheithauer BW, et al. Cerebral astrocytomas: histopathologic correlation of MR and CT contrast enhancement with stereotactic biopsy. Radiology 1988;166:823–7.
4. Kondziolka D, Lunsford LD, Martinez AJ. Unreliability of contemporary neurodiagnostic imaging in evaluating suspected adult supratentorial (low-grade) astrocytoma. J Neurosurg 1993;79:533–6.
5. Cairncross JG, Macdonald DR, Pexman JH, Ives FJ. Steroid-induced CT changes in patients with recurrent malignant glioma. Neurology 1988;38:724–6.
6. DeAngelis LM, Yahalom J, Heinemann MH, et al. Primary CNS lymphoma: combined treatment with chemotherapy and radiotherapy. Neurology 1990;40:80–6.
7. Hochberg FH, Miller DC. Primary central nervous system lymphoma. J Neurosurg 1988;68:835–53.
8. Kleihues P. Histological typing of tumours of the central nervous system. New York: Springer-Verlag; 1993.
9. Dean BL, Drayer BP, Bird CR, et al. Gliomas: classification with MR imaging. Radiology 1990;174:411–5.
10. Artigas J, Cervos-Navarro J, Iglesias JR, Ebhardt G. Gliomatosis cerebri: clinical and histological findings. Clin Neuropathol 1985;4:135–48.
11. Ponce P, Alvarez-Santullano MV, Otermin E, et al. Gliomatosis cerebri: findings with computed tomography and magnetic resonance imaging. Eur J Radiol 1998;28:226–9.
12. Yanaka K, Kamezaki T, Kobayashi E, et al. MR imaging of diffuse glioma. AJNR Am J Neuroradiol 1992;13: 349–51.
13. Shin YM, Chang KH, Han MH, et al. Gliomatosis cerebri: comparison of MR and CT features. AJR Am J Roentgenol 1993;161:859–62.
14. Kim DG, Yang HJ, Park IA, et al. Gliomatosis cerebri: clinical features, treatment, and prognosis. Acta Neurochir (Wien) 1998;140:755–62.
15. Clark GB, Henry JM, McKeever PE. Cerebral pilocytic astrocytoma. Cancer 1985;56:1128–33.
16. Forsyth PA, Shaw EG, Scheithauer BW, et al. Supratentorial pilocytic astrocytomas. A clinicopathologic, prognostic, and flow cytometric study of 51 patients. Cancer 1993; 72:1335–42.
17. Maroldo TV, Barkovich AJ. Pediatric brain tumors. Semin Ultrasound CT MR 1992;13:412–48.
18. Lee YY, Van Tassel P, Bruner JM, et al. Juvenile pilocytic astrocytomas: CT and MR characteristics. AJR Am J Roentgenol 1989;152:1263–70.
19. Braffman BH, Bilaniuk LT, Naidich TP, et al. MR imaging of tuberous sclerosis: pathogenesis of this phakomatosis, use of gadopentetate dimeglumine, and literature review. Radiology 1992;183:227–38.
20. Faerber EN, Roman NV. Central nervous system tumors of childhood. Radiol Clin North Am 1997;35:1301–28.
21. Barkovich AJ, Krischer J, Kun LE, et al. Brain stem gliomas: a classification system based on magnetic resonance imaging. Pediatr Neurosurg 1990;16:73–83.
22. Packer RJ, Vezina G. Pediatric glial neoplasms including brain-stem gliomas. Semin Oncol 1994;21:260–72.
23. Khatib ZA, Heideman RL, Kovnar EH, et al. Predominance of pilocytic histology in dorsally exophytic brain stem tumors. Pediatr Neurosurg 1994;20:2–10.
24. Peterson K, Cairncross JG. Oligodendrogliomas. Neurol Clin 1995;13:861–73.
25. Brandes AA, Fiorentino MV. Clinical, pathological and therapeutic aspects of oligodendroglioma. Cancer Treat Rev 1998;24:101–11.
26. Kros JM. Oligodendrogliomas: clinicopathological correlations. J Neurooncol 1995;24:29–31.
27. Lee YY, Van Tassel P. Intracranial oligodendrogliomas: imaging findings in 35 untreated cases. AJR Am J Roentgenol 1989;152:361–9.
28. Naidich TP, Zimmerman RA. Primary brain tumors in children. Semin Roentgenol 1984;19:100–14.
29. Armington WG, Osborn AG, Cubberley DA, et al. Supratentorial ependymoma: CT appearance. Radiology 1985; 157:367–72.
30. Barkovich AJ. Neuroimaging of pediatric brain tumors. Neurosurg Clin N Am 1992;3:739–69.
31. Spoto GP, Press GA, Hesselink JR, Solomon M. Intracranial ependymoma and subependymoma: MR manifestations. AJR Am J Roentgenol 1990;154:837–45.
32. Hoeffel C, Boukobza M, Polivka M, et al. MR manifestations of subependymomas. AJNR Am J Neuroradiol 1995; 16:2121–9.
33. Chiechi MV, Smirniotopoulos JG, Jones RV. Intracranial subependymomas: CT and MR imaging features in 24 cases. AJR Am J Roentgenol 1995;165:1245–50.
34. Tomita T, McLone DG, Flannery AM. Choroid plexus papillomas of neonates, infants and children. Pediatr Neurosci 1988;14(1):23–30.
35. Sarkar C, Sharma MC, Gaikwad S, et al. Choroid plexus papilloma: a clinicopathological study of 23 cases. Surg Neurol 1999;52(1):37–9.
36. Coates TL, Hinshaw DB Jr, Peckman N, et al. Pediatric choroid plexus neoplasms: MR, CT, and pathologic correlation. Radiology 1989;173:81–8.
37. Ellenbogen RG, Winston KR, Kupsky WJ. Tumors of the choroid plexus in children. Neurosurgery 1989;25: 327–35.
38. Hakim R, Loeffler JS, Anthony DC, Black PM. Gangliogliomas in adults. Cancer 1997;79:127–31.
39. Rumana CS, Valadka AB, Contant CF. Prognostic factors in supratentorial ganglioglioma. Acta Neurochir (Wien) 1999;141:63–8.
40. Luo CB, Teng MM, Chen SS, et al. Intracranial ganglioglioma: CT and MRI findings. Kao Hsiung I Hsueh Ko Hsueh Tsa Chih 1997;13:467–74.
41. Matsumoto K, Tamiya T, Ono Y, et al. Cerebral gangliogliomas: clinical characteristics, CT and MRI. Acta Neurochir (Wien) 1999;141:135–41.
42. Kuroiwa T, Bergey GK, Rothman MI, et al. Radiologic appearance of the dysembryoplastic neuroepithelial tumor. Radiology 1995;197:233–8.

43. Tenreiro-Picon OR, Kamath SV, Knorr JR, et al. Desmoplastic infantile ganglioglioma: CT and MRI features. Pediatr Radiol 1995;25:540–3.
44. Tien RD, Barkovich AJ, Edwards MS. MR imaging of pineal tumors. AJR Am J Roentgenol 1990;155:143–51.
45. Smirniotopoulos JG, Rushing EJ, Mena H. Pineal region masses: differential diagnosis. Radiographics 1992;12:577–96.
46. Nelson M, Diebler C, Forbes WS. Paediatric medulloblastoma: atypical CT features at presentation in the SIOP II trial. Neuroradiology 1991;33:140–2.
47. Meyers SP, Kemp SS, Tarr RW. MR imaging features of medulloblastomas. AJR Am J Roentgenol 1992;158:859–65.
48. Robles HA, Smirniotopoulos JG, Figueroa RE. Understanding the radiology of intracranial primitive neuroectodermal tumors from a pathological perspective: a review. Semin Ultrasound CT MR 1992;13:170–81.
49. Spagnoli MV, Goldberg HI, Grossman RI, et al. Intracranial meningiomas: high-field MR imaging. Radiology 1986;161:369–75.
50. Aoki S, Sasaki Y, Machida T, Tanioka H. Contrast-enhanced MR images in patients with meningioma: importance of enhancement of the dura adjacent to the tumor. AJNR Am J Neuroradiol 1990;11:935–8.
51. Wilms G, Lammens M, Marchal G, et al. Thickening of dura surrounding meningiomas: MR features. J Comput Assist Tomogr 1989;13:763–8.
52. Ho VB, Smirniotopoulos JG, Murphy FM, Rushing EJ. Radiologic-pathologic correlation: hemangioblastoma. AJNR Am J Neuroradiol 1992;13:1343–52.
53. Koeller KK, Smirniotopoulos JG, Jones RV. Primary central nervous system lymphoma: radiologic-pathologic correlation. Radiographics 1997;17:1497–526.
54. Schwaighofer BW, Hesselink JR, Press GA, et al. Primary intracranial CNS lymphoma: MR manifestations. AJNR Am J Neuroradiol 1989;10:725–9.
55. Johnson BA, Fram EK, Johnson PC, Jacobowitz R. The variable MR appearance of primary lymphoma of the central nervous system: comparison with histopathologic features. AJNR Am J Neuroradiol 1997;18:563–72.
56. Zimmerman RA. Pediatric supratentorial tumors. Semin Roentgenol 1990;25:225–48.
57. Hoffman HJ, Otsubo H, Hendrick EB, et al. Intracranial germ-cell tumors in children. J Neurosurg 1991;74:545–51.
58. Salzman KL, Rojiani AM, Buatti J, et al. Primary intracranial germ cell tumors: clinicopathologic review of 32 cases. Pediatr Pathol Lab Med 1997;17:713–27.
59. Tsuruda JS, Norman D, Dillon W, et al. Three-dimensional gradient-recalled MR imaging as a screening tool for the diagnosis of cervical radiculopathy. AJR Am J Roentgenol 1990;154:375–83.
60. Kallmes DF, Provenzale JM, Cloft HJ, McClendon RE. Typical and atypical MR imaging features of intracranial epidermoid tumors. AJR Am J Roentgenol 1997;169:883–7.
61. Wilms G, Casselman J, Demaerel P, et al. CT and MRI of ruptured intracranial dermoids. Neuroradiology 1991;33:149–51.
62. Elster AD. Modern imaging of the pituitary. Radiology 1993;187:1–14.
63. Pusey E, Kortman KE, Flannigan BD, et al. MR of craniopharyngiomas: tumor delineation and characterization. AJR Am J Roentgenol 1987;149:383–8.
64. Ahmadi J, Destian S, Apuzzo ML, et al. Cystic fluid in craniopharyngiomas: MR imaging and quantitative analysis. Radiology 1992;182:783–5.
65. Hoffman HJ, De Silva M, Humphreys RP, et al. Aggressive surgical management of craniopharyngiomas in children. J Neurosurg 1992;76(1):47–52.
66. Tsuda M, Takahashi S, Higano S, et al. CT and MR imaging of craniopharyngioma. Eur Radiol 1997;7:464–9.
67. Healy ME, Hesselink JR, Press GA, Middleton MS. Increased detection of intracranial metastases with intravenous Gd-DTPA. Radiology 1987;165:619–24.
68. Yuh WT, Fisher DJ, Runge VM, et al. Phase III multicenter trial of high-dose gadoteridol in MR evaluation of brain metastases. AJNR Am J Neuroradiol 1994;15:1037–51.

Positron Emission Tomography Imaging of Brain Tumors

SUDHA CHALLA, MD
RANDALL A. HAWKINS, MD, PhD
GARY R. CAPUTO, MD

Because brain tumors characteristically have a high glucose metabolic rate, positron emission tomography (PET) imaging with the glucose analogue 2-[F-18]fluoro-2-deoxy-D-glucose (FDG) has had success in grading tumors, assessing prognosis, and differentiating necrosis (encephalomalacia) from recurrent metabolically active tumor. Additionally, research investigations with PET have demonstrated the ability of the method to image and quantify a wide variety of neurochemical and physiologic processes relevant to brain tumors, such as blood flow, protein synthesis, and hypoxic cell density.

RADIOPHARMACEUTICALS COMMONLY USED FOR POSITRON EMISSION TOMOGRAPHY BRAIN IMAGING

Radiopharmaceuticals of significance for PET brain tumor imaging can be categorized into (1) agents used to measure the permeability of the blood-brain barrier, (2) cerebral perfusion agents, (3) cerebral metabolic agents, (4) cerebral neurotransmitter agents, and (5) cerebral receptor-binding agents.

Characteristics of brain tumors such as tumor grade and response to radiotherapy and chemotherapy are important prognostic indicators that can be measured with PET imaging. Table 6–1 lists PET imaging radiotracers.

Blood-Brain Barrier Agents

Blood-brain barrier (BBB) agents used for PET imaging include gallium-68 ethylenediaminetetraacetic acid (EDTA) and rubidium-82 chloride. These agents cannot normally cross the BBB in appreciable quantities but do so when the permeability surface area product (PS) is increased. In 1982, Ericson and colleagues showed the accumulation of gallium-68 (Ga-68) EDTA within brain lesions.[1,2] The permeability of the BBB can be numerically measured by using Ga-

Table 6–1. RADIOPHARMACEUTICALS USED IN CEREBRAL TUMOR IMAGING

Type of Agent	Pharmaceutical
Cerebral metabolic	F-18 FDG C-11 glucose C-11 leucine C-11 L-methylmethionine C-11 tyrosine
Blood-brain barrier	Ga-68 EDTA Rb-82 chloride
Hypoxia	F-18 misonidazole
Cerebral perfusion, O_2 metabolism	O-15 O_2 and O_2-labeled water N-13 ammonia F-18 fluoromethane Cu-62 (PTSM)
Miscellaneous	^{3}H-labeled pBDZR/ligand PK11195

C = carbon; Cu-62 (PTSM) = copper-62–labeled bis-N4-methylthiosemicarbazone; F = fluorine; Ga = gallium; ^{3}H = tritium; N = nitrogen; O = oxygen; O_2 = molecular oxygen; pBDZR = peripheral benzodiazepine receptor; PK = pyruvate kinase; Rb = rubidium; EDTA = ethylenediaminetetraacetic acid; FDG = 2-[F-18] fluoro-2-deoxy-D-glucose.

68 EDTA, and this was demonstrated by Hawkins and colleagues using a two-compartment model.[3] In a similar fashion, rubidium-82 (Rb-82) has been used to measure the permeability of the BBB in patients with primary and metastatic brain lesions.[4] The measurement of the BBB is useful for estimating the degree to which radiotherapy of brain lesions can alter the permeability of the BBB, an alteration that may lead to cerebral edema, a potentially life-threatening complication. The optimization of chemotherapy delivery may also require the estimation of BBB permeability in patients with brain tumors. Although lipid-mediated transport plays the major role in delivering soluble molecules of < 400 to 600 Da, other molecules that are not lipid soluble and peptide-based drugs have virtually no transport across the BBB. Apart from molecular size, another factor seen to play a possible role in the movement of molecules across the BBB is the naturally present efflux systems in the BBB, such as P-glycoprotein. Similarly, there are influx-mediating agents, namely, nutrient transport systems such as DOPA and glucose transporter (GLUT1). Such influx systems can be potentially exploited for delivering adequate amounts of necessary drugs to the brain and the spinal cord.[5] Positron emission tomography imaging with various radiotracers labeled to such systems or dependent on these transporters can help measure not only the BBB permeability but also the drug dose being delivered to the interstitial space within the brain matter.

Using Ga-68 EDTA in normal volunteers, Hawkins and colleagues estimated the forward transport designated as K_1 to be 0.0029 ± 0.0016 mL/min/g and the reverse movement of the tracer designated as k^2 to be 0.0310 ± 0.0156 mL/min/g^3. In 1985, Jarden and colleagues measured the blood-to-brain and blood-to-tumor transport of Rb-82.[4] In their study, consisting of patients with primary and metastatic brain tumors, it was found that steroid administration had profound effects on BBB permeability. In 8 patients who had been administered dexamethasone, there was a 9 to 48 percent decrease in the tumor K_1 and a 21 percent decrease in the tumor plasma water volume from the baseline values within 24 to 72 hours whereas the patients who underwent radiation therapy with 200 to 600 rads after the administration of steroids did not show this change.

Another potential technique is the combining of FDG and Rb-82 or Ga-68 PET scans to differentiate radiation necrosis from recurrent tumors. Studies have shown a rapid accumulation of Rb-82 in tumors compared to areas of necrosis whereas FDG showed increased accumulation in tumors and a decreased uptake in areas of radiation necrosis.

Cerebral Perfusion Agents

Most cerebral perfusion studies with PET have been carried out for the evaluation of ischemic and infarcted brain tissue and to assess misery and luxury perfusion.[1]

Different investigators have found a correlation between cerebral tumor glucose metabolism, blood flow, and oxygen extraction fraction and the survival of the patients.[6–8] It has been found that brain tumors exhibit regional abnormal tissue perfusion. Although the tumor cerebral blood flow (CBF) varies widely among patients and tumors, the oxygen extraction fraction is usually markedly reduced. Cerebral blood flow is expressed as blood flow per unit volume of tumor or brain tissue (such as milliliters per minute per 100 mL). Similarly, the vascularity of tumors (which is the volume of vascular space in relation to the total tissue) is expressed as cerebral blood volume (CBV). In normal brain, CBF and CBV correlate, but in tumor tissue, this is altered. Leenders studied CBF and CBV in normal white and gray matter and in tumor tissue.[8] In his study, the CBF was 42.8 ± 8.4 mL/min/100 mL in the gray matter, 24.0 ± 4.3 mL/min/100 mL in the normal white matter, and 24.2 ± 14.8 mL/min/100 mL in tumor tissue. The percentage values of CBV for gray matter, white matter, and tumor tissues were 3.8 ± 0.5, 2.5 ± 0.3, and 3.4 ± 1.3, respectively. Similarly, the oxygen extraction rate (OER) of brain tumors has consistently been found to be low despite an adequate oxygen supply. This has been suggested as partly due to an altered metabolism of the tumor cells, which appear to shift their metabolic pathways to an anaerobic pathway. This hypothesis has been validated by PET studies measuring CBF and CBV after steroid administration. Using this protocol, Jarden and colleagues demonstrated that the steroids, while decreasing CBV and CBF in gliomas and brain metastases, increased the

OER.[4] Another measurement usually used in cerebral tumor perfusion studies is the cerebral metabolic rate of oxygen consumption (CMRO$_2$), which is derived from the OER, the CBF, and the molecular oxygen (O$_2$) concentration in the plasma.

Cerebral Metabolic Agents

Positron emission tomography FDG imaging of brain tumors is based on Otto Warburg's observation in the 1930s that the malignant transformation of cells is associated with an acceleration of the glycolytic rate. Investigators have shown that some tumor types, such as juvenile pilocytic astrocytoma, appear to be exceptions to this rule in that they exhibit an unusually high avidity for FDG despite slow progression.[9,10]

Cerebral metabolic agents used for PET imaging may be classified into those that can reflect tumor glucose metabolism, such as FDG; agents that reflect the protein synthesis within tumors, such as carbon (C)-11 leucine, or amino acid incorporation, such as C-11 methionine and C-11 tyrosine; dopaminergic tracers such as fluorine-18–labeled DOPA; those agents that depict deoxyribonucleic acid (DNA) synthesis, such as C-11 putrescine; and ligands for peripheral benzodiazepine receptors, such as tritium (^{3}H)-labeled pyruvate kinase (PK) 11195.[11–16] 2-[F-18] fluoro-2-deoxy-D-glucose has found the widest application, followed by C-11 methionine for studying the metabolism of brain tumors. 2-[F-18] fluoro-2-deoxy-D-glucose is a glucose analogue that permits the measurement of the regional cerebral or tumor glucose metabolic rate. The transmethylation rate in tumor cells has been found to be high, and C-11 L-methionine measures the rate of amino acid transport in the brain. The primary role of C-11 L-methionine is in the detection of various tumors.

Recently, other radiopharmaceuticals such as carbon-11 choline, C-11 L-tyrosine, fluorine (F)-18–labeled fluoroborono-phenylalanine, and F-18 fluoromisonidazole have been used for brain tumor imaging successfully. Carbon-11 putrescine has been studied with PET to measure the polyamine uptake in brain tumors. Tissue concentration of glucose in gray and white matter and in tumors is measured by using the Sokoloff equation and is expressed as the glucose metabolic rate, or MRGl.[9]

K$_1$ and k$_2$ are rate constants for the transport rates of glucose between the plasma and the tissue, and k3 is the rate constant of the phosphorylation reaction, catalyzed by hexokinase. The end product of this reaction is FDG-6-phosphate, which undergoes no further metabolism and which remains trapped in the tumor tissue for several hours. This metabolic trapping effect facilitates imaging with FDG.

IMAGING OF GLIOMAS

Gliomas are the most common primary brain tumors that have been widely studied with PET imaging. Although computed tomography (CT) and magnetic resonance imaging (MRI) are the primary modalities used for the initial diagnosis of cerebral tumors, magnetic resonance spectroscopy (MRS) and PET imaging have both proven useful in detecting tumor recurrence and in differentiating viable tumor from encephalomalacia. The cerebral blood volume of gliomas can be mapped by MRI and PET FDG.[8,9,17]

It is well known that gliomas can be very heterogeneous tumors, exhibiting various degrees of dedifferentiation within the same tumor. Consequently, they tend to present the neurosurgeon with a dilemma when it comes to obtaining an adequate biopsy sample from the most representative area within the tumor. Contrast-enhanced CT and MRI have been found to provide limited information regarding the ideal sampling area within the tumor. On the other hand, other parameters such as blood volume/vascularity and metabolism appear to reflect the heterogeneity inherent within gliomas as well as illustrate the spectrum of the least malignant and most malignant areas within a tumor.[18–21] Cerebral perfusion by PET is measured with oxygen-15–labeled tracers using either constant infusion (steady state) or bolus injection methods. The oxygen extraction fraction (OEF) and the CMRO$_2$ are measured with this method in addition to the CBV.

In 1993, Mineura and colleagues studied tumor perfusion and metabolism in 23 patients with gliomas, using PET, with the oxygen (O)-15 steady-state inhalation technique and FDG, respectively. They found that not only did the tumor glucose metabolism help predict the survival rate but that the tumor circulation also proved to be a strong indicator of patient response to treatment.[18] In 1994, Leenders postulated that perhaps changes in oxygen metabolism of cerebral tumors are a better indicator of tumor response than tumor blood flow. Leenders and colleagues also noted that although dexamethasone treatment of patients with gliomas and brain metastases decreased the CBF and CBV of the tumors and contralateral brain tissue, the OER increased.[19] Sasajima and colleagues used PET perfusion and metabolic studies in one patient with a malignant astrocytoma before and after the intracarotid injection of human tumor necrosis factor-α and found that response could be detected after a shorter interval with PET imaging than with MRI or CT.[20]

For metabolic studies, 185 MBq of FDG are injected intravenously and the images of the brain are obtained parallel to the orbitomeatal line at 40 minutes post injection.

Axial, coronal, and sagittal images of the brain are essential for the accurate mapping of any given lesion and for correlation with anatomic studies. Analyses of PET images may be visual (qualitative) or semiquantitative, with comparison of the FDG uptake within the lesion with that of the surrounding gray and white matter. Normal gray matter (cortical as well as subcortical gray-matter structures such as the basal ganglia and thalamus) has about five times the glucose metabolic rate as white matter. Partial volume averaging of gray- and white-matter regions will make the measured ratio of gray to white matter somewhat less than this. With the visual analysis, moderate- to high-grade gliomas (grades III to IV) have an FDG uptake in the range of that of normal to gray matter, whereas low-grade gliomas have indices between those of gray and white matter.[9] Di Chiro and colleagues found a mean of 3.8 µmol/100 g/min (standard deviation [SD] 1.8) for the low-grade gliomas and 6.6 µmol/100 g/min (SD 3.3) for the high-grade gliomas.[9] Expressing tumor or brain glucose metabolic rates in units of micromoles (or milligrams) per 100 mL per minute requires appreciation of the FDG mathematical model.

Di Chiro employed a tumoral-to-nontumoral metabolic ratio and obtained a median ratio of 1.4 with high-grade gliomas and < 1.4 with low-grade gliomas.[9] Of greater interest was the relationship of this ratio to survival rates, with patients with higher-grade gliomas having a median survival of 5 months and those with ratios < 1.4 having a median survival of 19 months. One group of investigators found a 78 percent 1-year survival rate with gliomas of low metabolic rate compared to a 29 percent 1-year survival rate with tumors of a higher metabolic rate.[22] Delbeke and colleagues employed tumor-white matter (T/WM) and tumor-cortex (T/C) ratios[23] after a review of 58 tumors, 32 of which were high-grade gliomas and 26 of which were low-grade gliomas. They achieved a 94 percent sensitivity and a 77 percent specificity, with a T/WM ratio cutoff of 1.5 for the low-grade tumors with high-grade tumors having higher ratios (Figure 6–1).

The term "tumoral greed" has been used by Di Chiro to describe the suppressed cortical uptake of FDG seen in patients with cerebral tumors.[9] This suppressed uptake is seen in areas surrounding the neoplasm as well as in areas remote from the neoplasm. Crossed cerebellar diaschisis (decreased FDG uptake in the cerebellar hemisphere contralateral to the tumor) has also been observed. Deafferentation is the apparent mechanism of this effect.

Positron emission tomography FDG studies have also been used to address the question of the malignant degeneration of low-grade gliomas. In 1977, Muller and colleagues studied the biologic progression of 137 low-grade gliomas and found that 56 percent of grade I tumors evolved to a grade II variety and that 31 percent progressed to glioblastoma multiforme.[24] Francavilla and colleagues studied 12 patients with known low-grade gliomas that subsequently underwent malignant degeneration.[25] There was increased FDG accumulation, when compared to the baseline studies, in those tumors proven to have undergone malignant degeneration.

Hypoxia of cerebral gliomas has been found to have an impact on the response to therapy, and cerebral perfusion studies as well as PET scans with F-18 fluoromisonidazole may find more widespread use in this type of a scenario.[26] Tumor hypoxia leads to what is termed "hypoxic radioresistance" and may require the modification of radiotherapy with hyperbaric-oxygen therapy or chemical radiosensitizing drugs. Valk and colleagues demonstrated the feasibility of assessing tumor hypoxia in three patients using a combination of Rb-82 and F-18 fluoromisonidazole.

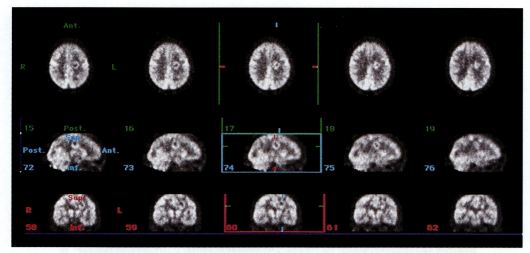

Figure 6–1. Glioblastoma recurrence in a 66-year-old male. The row of positron emission tomography fluorodeoxyglucose images shows intense uptake in a circumferential pattern within a recurrent glioma in a 66-year-old male. He was treated with radiation initially. A follow-up magnetic resonance imaging (MRI) scan showed a peripherally enhancing lesion in the left cerebral hemisphere at the site of the previously treated tumor.

Carbon-11 methionine has been used successfully for the definition of gliomas and can be combined with FDG studies to differentiate tumor necrosis from viable tumor. Using these two tracers and stereotactic biopsies in 14 patients, Goldman and colleagues found that C-11 methionine was able to accurately identify viable tumor tissue in treated cerebral gliomas. Ogawa and colleagues used both C-11 methionine and PET FDG imaging for evaluation of the grade and extent of cerebral tumors in 10 patients. They concluded that whereas FDG had the more definite role in depicting tumor grade, C-11 methionine was better at defining the anatomic extent of the tumors.[27] Both tracers were able to demonstrate the metabolic heterogeneity of human gliomas.

Tumor response to therapy is another area where PET FDG imaging has been found to help. Decreased FDG uptake compared to pretherapy scans was found to be indicative of a favorable outcome, and the tumors regressed completely. On the other hand, very little or no change from the baseline uptake was observed in those patients who did poorly despite treatment.

One of the first clinical applications of PET imaging was in the differentiation of tumor necrosis from recurrence. Contrast-enhanced CT and MRI can depict a treated tumor as a peripherally enhancing mass within the brain parenchyma, giving rise to the diagnostic dilemma of tumor recurrence versus post-treatment changes. Positron emission tomography FDG imaging is able to differentiate the two more clearly for FDG shows very little or no uptake within an area of tumor necrosis and more significant uptake in an area of true recurrence (Figure 6–2). Positron emission tomography FDG imaging is now an established and recognized modality for this application and is being increasingly used in many centers.[28]

ROLE OF POSITRON EMISSION TOMOGRAPHY IN THE MANAGEMENT OF MENINGIOMAS

Meningiomas are usually considered to be benign. However, a few meningiomas show aggressive behavior by invading the adjacent brain matter or other structures, leading to a poor outcome. Some meningiomas recur after successful surgical removal. To predict the possibility of a recurrence, a number of parameters have been used, including the type of surgery and histologic and cytologic features. In 1987, Di Chiro and colleagues investigated intracranial meningiomas with PET FDG imaging in 17 patients and correlated the glucose metabolism of the meningiomas with the histopathology and the clinical outcome. In this study, nonrecurrent meningiomas were found to have a lower glucose utilization rate (1.9 mg/100 mL/min, SD 1.0), with no recurrence

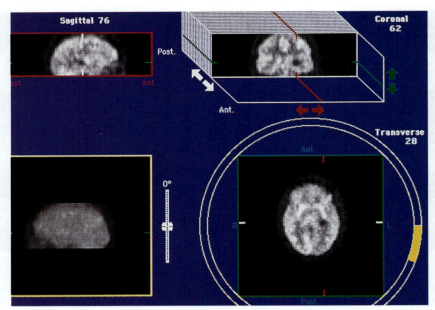

Figure 6–2. Radiation necrosis. A set of transaxial tomographic images from a positron emission tomography fluorodeoxyglucose (FDG) brain scan of a 30-year-old female with treated glioblastoma. A follow-up magnetic resonance imaging scan showed gadolinium enhancement in the left parietal region (scan not shown). There is no uptake of FDG in the region of the treated glioblastoma, suggesting radiation necrosis.

reported for 3 to 4 years following surgery. On the other hand, the metabolic rate was significantly higher (in the order of 4.5 mg/100 mL/min, SD 1.9) in 11 patients who had tumor recurrence. The metabolic rates also correlated well with the rate of tumor enlargement as demonstrated by follow-up CT examinations. In their histopathologic correlation, these investigators found that the syncytial or atypical type of meningioma had the highest metabolic rate, followed by the papillary and angioblastic varieties.[29] In their study on a small series of different brain tumors, including gliomas and meningiomas, Heiss and colleagues were not able to distinguish the histologic type of tumor by virtue of the FDG uptake values.[30] On the other hand, they noted considerable heterogeneity of regional FDG uptake within individual tumors, including the three meningiomas.

IMAGING OF MISCELLANEOUS CEREBRAL TUMORS

Pituitary adenomas constitute about 4 percent of intracranial primary tumors. The tumors can arise from any of the six different cells that constitute the gland, and about 70 percent are usually associated with a high hormone secretion. The type of hormone and the resulting syndrome are dependent on the cell of origin. Prolactinomas are the most common of the pituitary adenomas. In 1987, Bergstrom and colleagues studied the uptake of C-11–labeled L- and D-methionines in four patients with normal pituitary glands and made the interesting discovery that methionine uptake in the pituitary gland is quite chemically stereospecific.[31] Positron emission tomography imaging with C-11 methionine by the same investigators was found to be very useful for the follow-up of prolactinomas after treatment with bromocriptine. So marked was this response that the decrease in C-11 methionine could be observed in a matter of a few hours following the intramuscular administration of bromocriptine.[32,33] Amino acid metabolism decreased by 40 percent in the first few hours after bromocriptine administration, and a re-examination by PET at 7 to 9 days showed a further decrease. This was followed by significant tumor shrinkage, which was confirmed by anatomic studies.

Pinealomas constitute only 1 percent of all intracranial tumors although they constitute 3 to 8 percent of all intracranial tumors in the pediatric age group. Histologically, they tend to be most commonly either germinomas (33 to 50%) or gliomas (25%). Pinealomas can also show fairly intense uptake of FDG, as is demonstrated in Figure 6–3.

Metastatic disease to the brain has also been found to be FDG avid on PET imaging. Colorectal cancer (Figure 6–4), lung cancer (Figure 6–5), breast cancer, and lymphoma (Figure 6–6) are but a few examples of cancers shown to metastasize to the brain and to be detected on PET scans. Both primary and secondary central nervous system (CNS) lymphomas are FDG avid, and PET FDG imaging serves as a very useful diagnostic test, especially in patients with acquired immunodeficiency syndrome (AIDS)–associated lymphoma, for whom CNS toxoplasmosis is an important differential diagnosis. In a series of 11 patients with AIDS and CNS lesions that were suspicious for lymphoma or toxoplasmosis, Hoffman and colleagues were able to diagnose lymphoma successfully in 5 patients, using a visual and semiquantitative analysis with PET FDG scans[34–36] (Figures 6–7 and 6–8). Hiesiger and colleagues compared the utility of C-11–labeled putrescine and C-11–labeled 2-deoxy-D-glucose in eight patients with primary and metastatic brain tumors and found that PET images with the C-11–labeled putrescine were better at identifying tumors that had a lower glucose metabolic rate than were the images obtained with C-11–labeled deoxyglucose.[37] Recently, neurocytoma (a tumor seen in young adults) has been classified by the new World Health Organization as a neuronal tumor. This same tumor was previously classified as an oligodendroglioma, owing to its histologic appearance. It is derived from the subependymal plates of the lateral ventricle and can proliferate within the ventricle. Mineura and colleagues studied four patients with this tumor and assessed the perfusion parameters with O-15–labeled tracers and the metabolic rate with FDG. The study showed that CBF and CBV were higher than in the contralateral gray matter in three of the four patients whereas the tumor cerebral metabolic rate of glucose uptake (CMRGl) was lower than that of the gray matter.[38]

Despite the advances made in PET imaging and its validation as an extremely useful diagnostic tool, MRI and CT remain the chief modalities for the initial diagnosis of cerebral tumors, including gliomas, in most neurologic practices. Several investigators have compared gadolinium-enhanced T1-weighted MR images with PET FDG scans of brain tumors. Davis and colleagues studied 36 lesions and found a 93 percent concordance between enhancement of brain tumors with gadolinium and FDG uptake on PET imaging. They also concluded that some anaplastic astrocytomas can be non-enhancing with

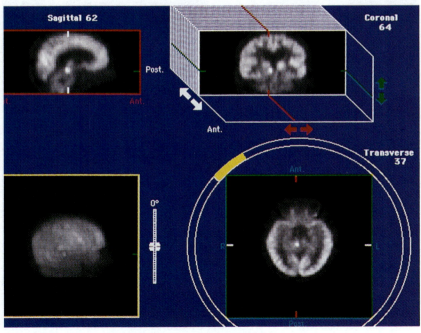

Figure 6–3. Fluorodeoxyglucose uptake in a pinealoma.

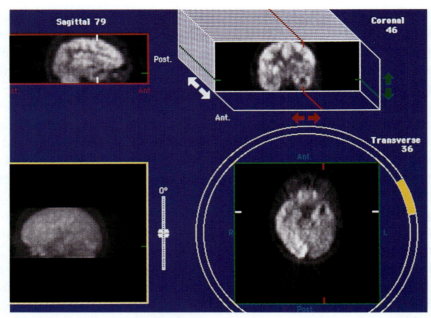

Figure 6–4. Positron emission tomography fluorodeoxyglucose scan in a 60-year-old patient with metastatic colon cancer. There is evidence of at least two hyperintense foci (one in the left temporal lobe and the other in the right occipital lobe) indicative of mutiple metastases.

gadolinium and that others may be hypometabolic. It is in cases such as this that both modalities may complement each other and that co-registered images may offer optimal targets for biopsy.[39] In recent years, MRS has helped elucidate the nature of biochemical changes occurring within cerebral

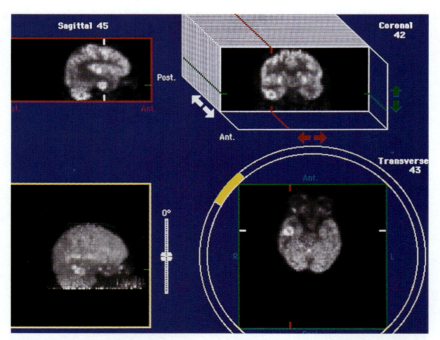

Figure 6–5. A male patient with lung cancer. Contrast-enhanced anatomic studies showed a single enhancing lesion in the right temporal region. The positron emission tomography fluorodeoxyglucose (FDG) scan showed intense FDG uptake in the same region, suggesting a metastatic focus.

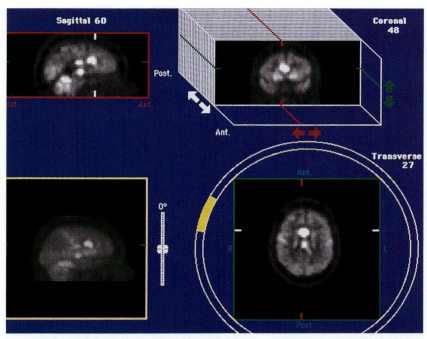

Figure 6–6. Positron emission tomography scans of a 67-year-old woman who had high-dose methotrexate therapy for central nervous system lymphoma. There is avid fluorodeoxyglucose uptake in several foci within the brain, including the corpus callosum and cerebellum (seen on the sagittal scan).

tumors. Magnetic resonance spectroscopy measures the by-products of tumor metabolism whereas PET imaging measures the substrates used for metabolism. Studies with MRS have largely been carried out on cerebral gliomas and meningiomas. Magnetic resonance spectroscopy has demonstrated normal spectra of phosphorus-31 in low-grade gliomas and has demonstrated decreased and split phosphodiester peaks and an alkaline pH in the higher-grade tumors. One correlative study of PET and MRS of gliomas demonstrated decreased N-acetylaspartate (NAA) and increased choline signal intensities within tumor spectra. Both the hypo- and hypermetabolic tumors by PET showed lactate signal intensities on MRS. Meningiomas that showed a variable FDG uptake showed very low phosphocreatine levels. Thus, the information obtained by MRS can complement that obtained by PET studies. Positron emission tomography and MRI/MRS co-registration is being increasingly used to better localize abnormal regions seen on PET FDG imaging. One of the reasons the metabolic imaging is superimposed on the anatomic imaging is the better spatial resolution of lesions obtained on the CT/MRI images. Most co-registration methods applied to brain imaging with PET and MRI use surface-matching or volume-matching algorithms. Serial MR and PET images are aligned, and an anatomic and functional image is generated that allows for better localization of the functional abnormality seen on the PET scans. This is especially valuable for increasing the accuracy of interpretation of tumor recurrence or radiation necrosis. Likewise, such a combination of modalities can aid in the proper sampling of tissue for biopsies.[39–42]

PEDIATRIC IMAGING

In the pediatric population, brain tumors account for a large proportion of deaths from cancer. One-half of pediatric brain tumors arise in the posterior fossa and consist of astrocytomas, medulloblastomas, ependymomas, and brainstem gliomas. The atypical teratoid/rhabdoid tumor is a special type of tumor that has been recently described.[43]

A considerable body of experience has accrued in the field of pediatric imaging with PET over the past few years. The CNS applications of PET have included studies on epilepsy, intraventricular hemorrhage, neonatal asphyxia, tumors, and the effects of radiation and chemotherapy on the brain.[44–47]

One of the practical difficulties faced by the physician imaging the pediatric patient is that of sedation. As certain sedatives can affect the blood flow or

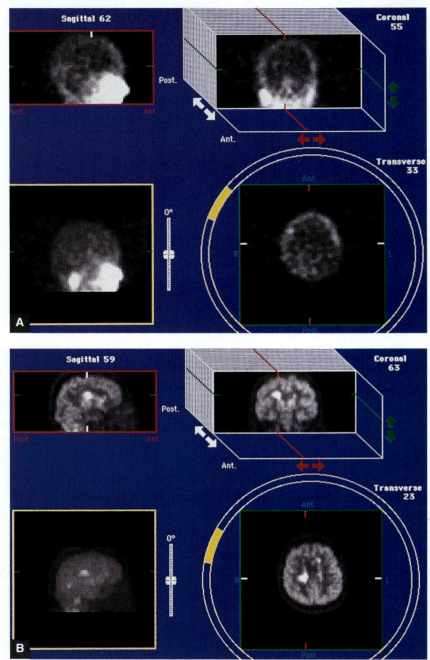

Figure 6–7. Central nervous system (CNS) lymphoma in a human immunodeficiency virus–positive patient. A young male patient who had acquired immunodeficiency syndrome presented with neurologic symptoms. Computed tomography scans of the brain showed multiple masses in both hemispheres, enhancing with contrast. *A,* At an outside facility, he had a thallium scan that did not reveal any uptake of the isotope within the masses. *B,* He was then referred for a positron emission tomography fluorodeoxyglucose (FDG) scan, which clearly demonstrated intense FDG uptake in all the cerebral masses, suggesting CNS lymphoma rather than toxoplasmosis (which had been considered the most likely diagnosis).

metabolism of the CNS, sedation is commonly advised. This sedation is usually carried out at 30 minutes post injection. Tumor blood flow and metabolism have not been shown to be affected significantly by sedatives.[44] In 1992, Hoffman and colleagues published their results of PET FDG studies conducted on 17 children in the age range of 3 to 16 years with posterior fossa tumors. Some of the children had PET imaging before and after radiation and chemotherapy. These investigators used the FDG uptake in the white and gray matter as a reference and graded the tumor uptake on a scale of 1 to 5. Highly malignant tumors such as medulloblastomas had the highest uptake of FDG whereas uptake was less in the pilocytic astrocytomas and lowest in the gliomas. It was observed that the clinical outcome in the case of posterior fossa tumors was not necessarily predictable by the degree of FDG uptake. This was especially true in the case of brainstem gliomas, in which involvement of the vital structures in the brain stem by the tumor can act as an important factor influencing survival, quite independently of the histologic grade of the tumor. The constraints of the study did not allow the investigators to determine whether PET FDG scanning would allow accurate differentiation of tumor from necrosis within the posterior fossa.[45] In 1993, Holthoff and colleagues reported their findings on 15 children and young adults with posterior fossa tumors and primitive neuroectodermal tumors who had repeated PET studies during the course of their treatment. They reported a good correlation between the metabolic rates of the tumors as measured by FDG avidity and by clinical response.[46]

One other area of concern in the pediatric population has been the long-term effects on the brain of chemotherapy and radiation treatment in children with systemic cancers such as leukemia. In acute lymphocytic leukemia, prophylaxis against leukemic infiltration of the CNS has included therapeutic irradiation of the brain or chemotherapy and has helped reduce the incidence of CNS relapses considerably. Phillips and colleagues evaluated 12 long-term survivors of childhood leukemia by PET FDG imaging and documented that the glucose metabolism of cerebral white matter was reduced in all of their patients who had had a combination of radiation therapy and chemotherapy but not in the patients who had received chemotherapy alone. The other pertinent findings by these authors were a decreased glucose metabolism in the thalamus and heterogeneity of the pattern of glucose metabolism within the cortical and subcortical gray matter in all of their patients.[47] As in the case of adult tumor imaging, image alignment, registration, and fusion play the same role in pediatric brain tumor management and follow-up.[48]

FUTURE DIRECTIONS

Future applications of PET brain tumor imaging will focus on radiopharmaceutical development (new tracers) as well as on newer PET systems with improved resolution.

Research into the expression of peripheral benzodiazepine receptors (pBDZRs) is also under way. These receptors are expressed on the surface of glial cells and have been located on the outer membrane of cell mitochondria and nuclei, thus indicating a probable role in the metabolism of oxygen. Using ^{3}H-labeled pBDZR/ligand PK 11195, Black and colleagues found an increased level of pBDZR in rat and human gliomas in vitro. The higher-grade gliomas had a higher specific ligand-binding rate than the lower-grade gliomas and a fivefold increase compared to normal glial cells.[11] Other receptors under investigation are muscarinic cholinergic receptors (mAChRs), which are found in various tumors, including gliomas. By synthesizing and employing different benzilate stereoisomers, Lang and colleagues found that the various isomers had different selectivities for the mAChRs. An extension of the same study demonstrated a clearance that was proportional to the muscarinic receptor concentration.[49–51] Areas still under investigation are the application of PET imaging with radiopharmaceuticals such as iodine-124–labeled iododeoxyuridine to study the DNA burden of tumoral tissues.[11,12,48] Multidrug resistance has been measured in animals using substrates to P glycoprotein labeled with carbon-14 (^{14}C) and ^{3}H.

Technical advances in PET, in addition to new radiopharmaceuticals, will also focus on higher-resolution PET systems using detector materials such as cerium-doped lutetium orthosilicate (LSO),[52] in addition to image registration approaches that will make routine the incorporation of PET biochemical and anatomic (MRI, CT) fusion imaging into clinical studies.

REFERENCES

1. Saha GB, MacIntyre WJ, Go RT. Radiopharmaceuticals for brain imaging. Semin Nucl Med 1994;24:324–49.
2. Ericson K, Bergstrom M, Eriksson L, et al. Positron emission tomography with ^{68}Ga-EDTA compared with transmission computed tomography in the evaluation of brain infarcts. Acta Radiol 1981;22:385–98.
3. Hawkins RA, Phelps ME, Huang S-C, et al. A kinetic evaluation of blood-brain barrier permeability in human brain tumors with [^{68}Ga] EDTA and positron computed tomography. J Cereb Blood Flow Metab 1984;4:507–15.
4. Jarden JO, Dhawan V, Poltorak A, et al. Positron emission tomographic measurement of blood-to-brain and blood-to-tumor transport of ^{82}Rb: the effect of dexamethasone and whole-brain radiation therapy. Ann Neurol 1985;18:636–46.
5. Pardridge WM. CNS drug design based on principles of blood-brain barrier transport. J Neurochem 1998;70:1781–92.
6. Aronen HJ, Gazit IE, Louis DN, et al. Cerebral blood volume maps of gliomas: comparison with tumor grade and histologic findings. Radiology 1994;191:41–51.
7. Siegal T, Rubinstein R, Tzuk-Shina T, Gomori JM. Utility of relative cerebral blood volume mapping derived from perfusion magnetic resonance imaging in the routine follow up of brain tumors. J Neurosurg 1997;86:22–7.
8. Leenders KL. PET: blood flow and oxygen consumption in brain tumors. J Neurooncol 1994;22:269–73.
9. Di Chiro G. Positron emission tomography using [F] fluorodeoxyglucose in brain tumors—a powerful diagnostic and prognostic tool. Invest Radiol 1986;22:360–71.
10. Blasberg RG. Prediction of brain tumor therapy response by PET. J Neurooncol 1994;22:281–6.
11. Black KL, Ikezaki K, Santori E, et al. Specific high-affinity binding of peripheral benzodiazepine receptor ligands to brain tumors in rat and man. Cancer 1990;65:93–7.
12. de Wolde H, Pruim J, Mastik MF, et al. Proliferative activity in human brain tumors: comparison of histopathology and L-[1-C^{11}] tyrosine PET. J Nucl Med 1997;38:1369–74.
13. Goldman S, Levivier M, Pirotte B, et al. Regional methionine and glucose uptake in high-grade gliomas: a comparative study on PET-guided stereotactic biopsy. J Nucl Med 1997;38:1459–62.
14. Alger JR, Frank JA, Bizzi A, et al. Metabolism of human gliomas: assessment with H-1 MR spectroscopy and F-18 fluorodeoxyglucose PET. Radiology 1990;177:633–41.
15. Hara T, Kosaka N, Shinoura N, Kondo T. PET imaging of brain tumor with [methyl – ^{11}C] choline. J Nucl Med 1997;38:842–7.
16. Heiss W-D, Wienhard K, Wagner R, et al. F-Dopa as an amino acid tracer to detect brain tumors. J Nucl Med 1996;37:1180–2.
17. Roelcke U. PET: brain tumor biochemistry. J Neurooncol 1994;22:275–9.
18. Mineura K, Sasajima T, Kowada M, et al. Perfusion and metabolism in predicting the survival of patients with cerebral gliomas. Cancer 1994;73:2386–94.
19. Leenders KL, Beaney RP, Brooks DJ, et al. Dexamethasone treatment of brain tumor patients: effects on regional cerebral blood flow, blood volume and oxygen utilization. Neurology 1985;35:1610–6.
20. Sasajima T, Mineura K, Sasaki J, et al. Positron emission tomographic assessment of cerebral hemocirculation and glucose metabolism in malignant glioma following treatment with intracarotid recombinant human tumor necrosis factor-α. J Neurooncol 1995;23:67–73.
21. Lammertsma AA, Wise RJS, Cox TCS, et al. Measurement of blood flow, oxygen utilisation, oxygen extraction ratio, and fractional blood volume in human brain tumors and surrounding oedematous tissue. Br J Radiol 1985;58:725–34.
22. Alavi JB, Alavi A, Chawluk J, et al. Positron emission tomography in patients with glioma. Cancer 1988;62:1074–8.
23. Delbeke D, Meyerowitz C, Lapidus RL, et al. Optimal cutoff levels of F-18 fluorodeoxyglucose uptake in the differentiation of low-grade from high-grade brain tumors with PET. Radiology 1995;195:47–52.
24. Muller W, Afra D, Schroder R. Supratentorial recurrences of gliomas: morphological studies in relation to time intervals with astrocytomas. Acta Neurochir (Wien) 1977;37:75–91.
25. Francavilla TL, Miletich RS, Di Chiro G, et al. PET in the detection of malignant degeneration of low-grade gliomas. Neurosurgery 1989;24:1–5.
26. Valk PE, Mathis CA, Prados MD, et al. Hypoxia in human gliomas: demonstration by PET with fluorine-18-fluoromisonidazole. J Nucl Med 1992;33:2133–7.
27. Ogawa T, Inugami A, Hatazawa J, et al. Clinical positron emission tomography for brain tumors: comparison of fluorodeoxyglucose F 18 and L-methyl-11-C methionine. AJNR Am J Neuroradiol 1996;17:345–53.
28. Di Chiro G, Oldfield E, Wright DC, et al. Cerebral necrosis after radiotherapy and/or intraarterial chemotherapy for brain tumors. AJR Am J Roentgenol 1988;150:189–97.
29. Di Chiro G, Hatazawa J, Katz DA, et al. Glucose utilization by intracranial meningiomas as an index of tumor aggressivity and probability of recurrence: a PET study. Radiology 1987;164:521–6.
30. Heiss WD, Heindel W, Herholz K, et al. Positron emission tomography of fluorine-18-deoxyglucose and image guided phosphorus-31 magnetic resonance spectroscopy in brain tumors. J Nucl Med 1990;31:302–10.
31. Bergstrom M, Muhr C, Ericson K, et al. The normal pituitary examined with PET and (methyl-^{11}C)-L-methionine and (methyl-^{11}C)-D-methionine. Neuroradiology 1987;29:221–5.
32. Bergstrom M, Muhr C, Lundberg PO, et al. Amino acid distribution and metabolism in pituitary adenomas using PET with D-[^{11}C] methionine and L-[^{11}C] methionine. J Comput Assist Tomogr 1987;11:384–9.
33. Bergstrom M, Muhr C, Lundberg PO, et al. Rapid decrease in amino acid metabolism in prolactin secreting pituitary adenomas after bromocriptine treatment: a PET study. J Comp Assist Tomogr 1987;11:815–9.
34. Rosenfeld SS, Hoffman JM, Coleman RE, et al. Studies of

primary central nervous system lymphoma with F-18-fluorodeoxyglucose positron emission tomography. J Nucl Med 1992;33:532–6.
35. Ogawa T, Kanno I, Hatazawa J, et al. Methionine PET for follow-up of radiation therapy of primary lymphoma of the brain. Radiographics 1994;14:101–10.
36. Hoffman JM, Waskin HA, Schifter T, et al. FDG-PET in differentiating lymphoma from nonmalignant CNS lesions in patients with AIDS. J Nucl Med 1993;34:567–75.
37. Hiesiger E, Fowler JS, Wolf AP, et al. Serial PET studies of human cerebral malignancy with [1-^{11}C] putrescine and [1-^{11}C] 2-deoxy-D-glucose. J Nucl Med 1987;28:1251–61.
38. Mineura K, Sasajima T, Itoh Y, et al. Blood flow and metabolism of central neurocytoma. Cancer 1995;76:1224–32.
39. Davis WK, Boyko OB, Hoffman JM, et al. F-18–2-deoxyglucose PET correlation of gadolinium enhanced MR imaging of CNS neoplasia. AJNR Am J Neuroradiol 1993;14:515–23.
40. Hanson MW, Glantz MJ, Hoffman JM, et al. FDG-PET in the selection of brain lesions for biopsy. J Comput Assist Tomogr 1991;15:796–801.
41. Scott AM, Macapinlac H, Zhang JJ, et al. Clinical applications of fusion imaging in oncology. Nucl Med Biol 1994;21:775–84.
42. Nelson SJ, Day MR, Buffone PJ, et al. Alignment of volume MRI and high resolution F-18 fluoro-deoxyglucose PET images for the evaluation of patients with brain tumors. J Comput Assist Tomogr 1997;21:183–91.
43. Vezina LG. Diagnostic imaging in neuro-oncology. Pediatr Clin North Am 1997;44:701–19.
44. Shulkin BL. PET applications in pediatrics. Q J Nucl Med 1997;41:281–91.
45. Hoffman JM, Hanson MW, Friedman HS, et al. FDG-PET in pediatric posterior fossa brain tumors. J Comput Assist Tomogr 1992;16:62–8.
46. Holthoff VA, Herholz K, Berthold F, et al. In vivo metabolism of childhood posterior fossa tumors and primitive neuroectodermal tumors before and after treatment. Cancer 1993;72:1394–403.
47. Phillips PC, Moellar JR, Sidtis JJ, et al. Abnormal cerebral glucose metabolism in long term survivors of childhood acute lymphocytic leukemia. Ann Neurol 1991;29:263–71.
48. Treves ST, Mitchell KD, Habboush IH. Three dimensional image alignment, registration and fusion. Q J Nucl Med 1998;42:83–92.
49. Lang L, Aloj L, Kiesewetter DO, et al. A review of new oncotropic tracers for PET imaging. Nucl Med Biol 1996;23:669–72.
50. Gurwitz D, Razon N, Sokolovsky M, Soreq H. Expression of muscarinin binding sites in primary human brain tumors. Dev Brain Res 1984;14:61–70.
51. Brunetti A, Alfano B, Soricelli A, et al. Functional characterization of brain tumors: an overview of the potential clinical value. Nucl Med Biol 1996;23:699–715.
52. Brennan KM, Moses WW, Derenzo SE. Advances in positron tomography for oncology. Nucl Med Biol 1996;23:659–67.

7

External Beam Radiotherapy

GLENN BAUMAN, MD, FRCP(C)
DAVID A. LARSON, PHD, MD

The efficacy of radiation for central nervous system (CNS) tumors is predicated on the delivery of an adequate dose of radiation to a target of interest within the brain. The safety of radiotherapy is maximized by reducing the effective dose to uninvolved brain tissue and other critical structures (optic chiasm, eyes, spinal cord, and brain stem) surrounding this target. Modern innovations in treatment delivery, such as accurate patient immobilization, imaging-based target definition within a reference coordinate (stereotactic) space, and conformally shaped beams and with dynamic intensity modulation, allow the dose of radiation delivered to be better confined or "conformed" to a target of interest. Stereotactic radiosurgery and stereotactically guided brachytherapy arose as subsets of this general principle, largely due to the earlier availability of technology to implement these simpler versions of conformal radiotherapy. Advances in external beam radiation treatment planning and delivery systems have now brought us to the point where fractionated stereotactic conformal external beam radiotherapy is in routine clinical use (Figures 7–1 and 7–2).[1] We would define modern "conventional radiotherapy" for CNS tumors as linear accelerator–based fractionated external beam megavoltage radiotherapy using stereotactic conformal (and, increasingly, intensity modulation) technologies. The full benefit of the newer technology will be determined by clinical trials but holds potential for both increasing tumor control (by allowing the safe escalation of radiation dose) and decreasing the risk of late radia-

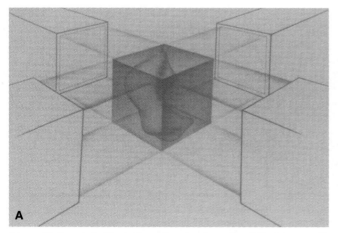
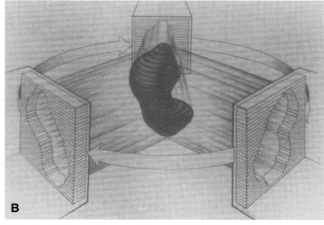

Figure 7–1. *A,* An illustration of nonconformal radiation therapy. Use of a few simply shaped rectangular radiation fields produce a treatment volume that is cuboidal and includes a considerable amount of normal tissue. *B,* An illustration of conformal radiation therapy. Multileaf collimation of multiple or moving radiation beams produces a shape that conforms closely to the "beam's-eye view" configuration of the tumor. Intensity modulation can alter radiation fluency within the beam's-eye view field shape to increase conformality even further. (Reproduced with permission from Lichter AS, Fraass BA, McShan DL, et al. Recent advances in radiotherapy treatment planning. Oncology 1998;2:43–57.)

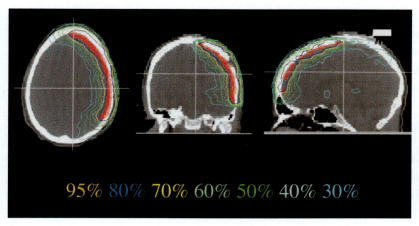

Figure 7–2. Dose distribution of an intensity-modulated treatment for a patient with a malignant meningioma. Tumor studding over the dural convexity was treated while minimizing irradiation of the underlying brain. Dose prescribed was 59.4 Gy delivered to the 80% isodose surface. Delivery of this treatment requires accurate patient immobilization, three-dimensional volume reconstruction of the tumor from MRI and CT fusion, inverse treatment planning to generate the intensity profile of the beam, and a dynamic beam intensity modulation. This technology is rapidly becoming widely available.

tion toxicity (by minimizing the volume of brain receiving high-radiation doses). Until these clinical trials have matured, one has to look to the past (using older radiotherapy techniques) for the clinical benefit of radiation treatments and understand that modern innovations may improve on these results. In the meantime, our treatment philosophy is to use the best modern treatment tools to minimize toxicity and maximize tumor control.

PATIENT ASSESSMENT

The radiation oncologist is a physician with postgraduate training in the use of radiation for the treatment of neoplastic disease. A complete patient assessment by the radiation oncologist is essential prior to radiation treatment and should include a history and physical, with special attention paid to specific neurologic signs and symptoms and the overall performance status and general health of the patient. Coexisting illnesses such as collagen vascular disease, uncontrolled hypertension, diabetes, or multiple sclerosis may be associated with a higher risk or late radiation effects and should be considered when deciding on the use of radiation as well as technique and dose. A review of all surgical procedures, pathology reports, and diagnostic imaging should be undertaken, ideally in a multidisciplinary team setting with neurosurgical, neuropathologic, neuro-oncologic, neuroradiologic, and radiation oncologic input.

For many patients with primary brain tumors, factors exclusive of treatment such as age, performance status, and tumor histology are the strongest prognostic factors for outcome. Careful considera-

tion of these pretreatment factors will assist in determining the appropriate role of radiation treatment and in counseling the patient regarding the expected benefit of the treatment.

Empiric radiation treatment of patients on the basis of imaging alone should be discouraged. In most cases, at minimum, a stereotactic biopsy is associated with a low risk of morbidity and will confirm the diagnosis of malignancy for patients with intracranial lesions. Radiation without biopsy should be restricted to several well-defined scenarios in which the risk of misdiagnosis is minimized. Examples might include a child with a typical imaging and clinical picture of a diffusely infiltrating pontine glioma, a cancer patient with a typical imaging picture of multiple CNS metastases, or a human immunodeficiency virus (HIV)-positive patient not responding to empiric toxoplasmosis therapy with a typical picture of a CNS lymphoma.

IMMOBILIZATION

Modern, stereotactic conformal radiotherapy requires the reproducible, accurate immobilization of the patient for both treatment planning and radiation delivery. Use of custom immobilization devices (eg, masks, relocatable stereotactic frames) combined with fiducial markers allows the precise alignment of patients on a daily basis on the linear accelerator for treatment. Current plastic mask–based systems can accomplish this task with a set-up accuracy of ± 2 to 3 mm (Figure 7–3).[2] Noninvasive, relocatable stereotactic frame systems can accomplish this task with an accuracy approaching the uncertainty of the diagnostic imaging (± 1 to 2 mm). Immobilization to the level of ± 2 to 5 mm is probably sufficient for most targets > 1 to 2 cm in size and is usually considerably less than the interphysician variability of target definition.

IMAGING AND SIMULATION

Once an immobilization device has been constructed, the patient is imaged in the treatment position. In the past, radiotherapy fields were designed with reference to bony anatomic landmarks using fluoroscopy and plain simulator radiographs. Following simulation, manual acquisition of patient contours and delineation of the target volumes for computerized dosimetry were necessary. This manual registration of tumor volumes derived from diagnostic imaging onto the simulator radiographs and contours was both tedious and of limited accuracy. For modern conventional radiation treatment planning, the acquisition of a set of axial planning computed-tomographic (CT) images through the brain volume of interest is required. This planning CT scan differs from diagnostic CT scans in that the planning CT images are acquired under the same conditions (on a flat couch with a custom immobilization device) used for treatment of the patient on the linear accelerator. Computed tomography contains the electron density information needed for radiation-dose calculations but may not be the ideal imaging for many brain tumors. Fusion of magnetic resonance imaging (MRI) (pre- and/or postoperative) and planning CT images may facilitate tumor volume definition.[4,5] Dedicated CT simulators are becoming available in many radiation oncology departments.[1] These CT simulators incorporate powerful imaging workstations for efficient target contouring[3] and image manipulation, such as image fusion between CT and other modalities such as MRI as well as "virtual" simulation of beam arrangements (Figure 7–4).

PLANNING TARGET VOLUME DEFINITION

Once planning CT images are in the treatment planning computer, the radiation oncologist will define the gross tumor volume (GTV) on the axial planning CT images, expanding this volume to include other areas at risk of tumor spread to generate the clinical target volume (CTV). Fusion of tumor volumes identified on MRI with the planning CT can assist in this process. The CTV is subsequently enlarged by a "safety margin" (usually 3 to 5 mm) to account for inaccuracies in imaging and patient set-up error to generate the planning target volume (PTV). Any critical structures such as the brain stem, optic chiasm, and spinal cord are also contoured.

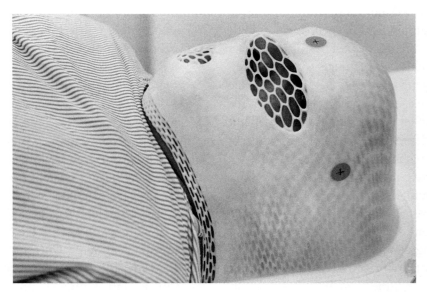

Figure 7–3. Immobilization mask for CNS irradiation. Fiducial markers on the shell allow accurate patient positioning day to day. The mask itself is fastened to the treatment couch during radiation to prevent patient movement.

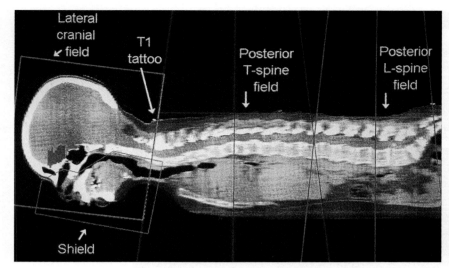

Figure 7–4. A sagittal, isocentric, multiplanar reformatted image of a 15-year-old male patient demonstrating virtual simulation of all fields and shielding. Accurate matching of the cranial and thoracic spine fields is achieved by interactive collimator rotation of the former directly on the workstation monitor. (Reproduced with permission from Mah K, Danjoux CE, Manship S, et al. Computed tomographic simulation of craniospinal fields in pediatric patients: improved treatment accracy and patient comfort. Int J Radiat Oncol Biol Phys 1998;41:997–1003.)

TREATMENT PLANNING

Once the GTV, CTV, PTV, and critical structures have been identified by the radiation oncologist on the planning CT images, the radiation dosimetrist will design a plan to deliver a uniform radiation dose (usually homogeneous within 5%) to the PTV while minimizing dose to any critical structures outside the PTV. In the past, due to limitations of imaging and computerized dosimetry, this task was usually accomplished using a limited number of simply shaped radiation beams of uniform intensity. The resulting dose distribution usually erred on the side of caution, irradiating large volumes of normal brain to minimize the chance of a "geographic miss" of the tumor (see Figure 7–1). Modern conformal radiotherapy seeks to minimize the high dose deposited outside the PTV by the use of multiple, nonoverlapping, radiation beams shaped to the configuration of the tumor in the beam's-eye view (see Figures 7–1, 7–5, and 7–6). Currently, most treatment planning is performed manually, through the iterative, "forward" optimization of two to six radiation beams with (relatively) conventional beam angles, beam's-eye view blocking, and beam modifiers (compensators, wedges). Dose-volume histograms provide a graphic summary of the dose received by the PTV and surrounding critical structures, and it may be used to compare rival treatment plans. In addition, using biologic models, the dose-volume histograms may be used to generate estimates of normal tissue complication probability (NTCP) and tumor control probability (TCP), which can also be used to rank rival proposed radiation plans.[1]

A recent innovation is the availability of "inverse treatment planning" software, whereby the radiation oncologist specifies the desired dose distribution (conforming to the PTV) and organs at risk to be avoided. Back calculation (analogous to the image-reconstruction algorithms used by CT scanners) then yields the appropriate beam-delivery parameters (angle, shape, intensity, profile) to produce the distribution desired in the patient.[1] The delivery of such "inversely planned" treatments may require the use of intensity modulation radiotherapy (IMRT) to dynamically alter the beam intensity across the beam profile. Such treatments may produce a conformal dose deposition with a reasonable dose homogeneity throughout the PTV and a rapid dose falloff outside of the PTV (see Figure 7–2).

TREATMENT DELIVERY

Fractionated radiation treatments for primary CNS tumors are typically performed using high-energy (4 MV or greater) photon (x-ray) beams generated by linear accelerators. Treatments are typically delivered on a daily basis, Monday to Friday, over 5 to 6 weeks (25 to 30 treatments). Individual fractions are typically 1.8 to 2.0 Gy, and total doses are in the range of 50 to 60 Gy. Currently, most tumors are treated with a limited number (2 to 6) of static fields, conformally

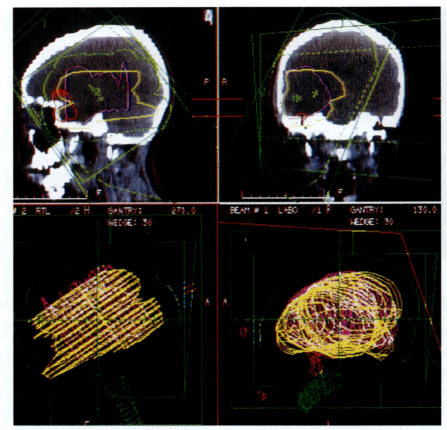

Figure 7–5. Example of a patient with a high-grade glioma (anaplastic astrocytoma) treated with conformal external beam radiation. The area of contrast enhancement plus a margin for tumor spread is included in the planning target volume.

shaped to the beam's-eye view of the tumor with custom-poured metal alloy (cerrobend) blocks or multileaf collimators. For most intracranial targets, such conformally shaped static fields will yield dose distributions equivalent to that produced by multiple-arc, single-isocenter radiosurgery-type treatments.[6] The

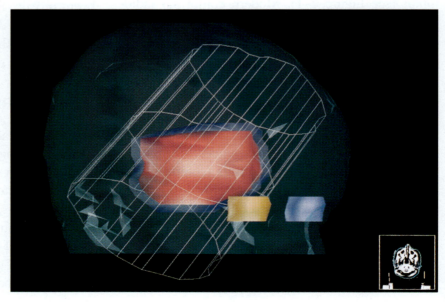

Figure 7–6. A 4-year-old boy with a subtotally excised pilocytic astrocytoma treated with conformal external beam radiotherapy. The well-circumscribed nature of this low-grade tumor allows very tightly conformal radiation fields, thus minimizing uninvolved brain irradiation and potential late cognitive toxicity. A three-field technique (right and left laterals, anterosuperior oblique) was used. Only the anterosuperior field is shown for clarity. Clinical and planning target volumes are indicated by red and blue surfaces and the radiation beam aperture by the wireframe.

intensity of the beam across the field is typically uniform, although simple beam modifiers ("wedges" or "compensators" that selectively attenuate portions of the radiation beam) may be placed in the field to ensure that the dose is homogeneously distributed throughout the PTV. By more sophisticated modulation of the beam intensity across the PTV, very conformal complex dose distributions may be produced, even for irregularly shaped tumors (see Figure 7–2). This intensity modulation may be accomplished by the alteration of field shape "on the fly" by dynamic movement of multileaf collimator leaves (dynamic MLC) or the dynamic modulation of the slit aperture of an arced radiotherapy beam. For now the technical expertise needed to plan and deliver (and verify the accuracy of) intensity-modulated radiotherapy restricts its use primarily to academic centers, but the technology is becoming widely available.

RADIATION FRACTIONATION

Radiation effects are manifest as cell attrition due to apoptosis or reproductive cell death as a result of radiation-induced deoxyribonucleic acid (DNA) damage. The brain is unique in that the normal parenchymal cell populations (neuronal, glial, vascular) are either static or slowly dividing, and, as a consequence, the clinical manifestation of radiation side effects within the normal brain usually do not appear until months or years after radiation is completed ("late" or "delayed" reaction). Like other late-reacting tissues, the normal CNS parenchyma is very sensitive to the size of individual doses (fractions) of radiation, reflecting a large capacity for radiation damage repair at lower doses per fraction. Tumor cells, for the most part, have less capacity for sublethal damage repair and are spared to a lesser degree by lower fraction size compared to normal tissue. Tumor cells will also reassort into more radiosensitive phases of the cell cycle between fractions as compared to the slowly cycling normal CNS cells. Fractionation also allows hypoxic cells to become reoxygenated between treatments, also increasing their sensitivity to radiation. Thus, differences in radiosensitivity between normal and tumor cells can be exploited by fractionation to improve the therapeutic ratio. In contrast, single-fraction radiation treatments (ie, radiosurgery) cannot exploit differences in repair, reassortment, and reoxygenation. This potential disadvantage can be overcome by the use of large single doses of radiation but can be done safely only if the normal brain can be excluded from the high-dose volume. Thus, radiosurgical techniques are most useful for treating small, well-circumscribed tumor volumes and are less appropriate for treating larger volumes of normal brain infiltrated by tumor. Most conventional radiation treatments are delivered with individual fractions of 1.8 to 2.0 Gy, daily (Monday to Friday). **Hyperfractionation** involves delivering multiple, usually smaller (< 1.1 to 1.2 Gy) fractions per day (2 to 3 times a day) over a similar time period (5 to 6 weeks) but to a higher total dose. The smaller doses per fraction allow more sublethal damage repair by the normal brain and permit modest dose escalations of 15 to 20 percent over conventionally fractionated treatments. **Accelerated hyperfractionation** involves delivering multiple fractions (2 to 3 times per day) of similar size to daily fractionation (usually 1.6 to 2.0 Gy) over a shorter period of time (3 to 4 weeks), with the intent of reducing tumor cell repopulation that may occur over a more protracted (5- to 6-week) course of radiation. Both approaches have been explored for malignant supratentorial and brainstem gliomas, but, to date, no dramatic clinical advantage over daily fractionation to conventional doses has been noted. The use of altered fractionation schemes in other primary brain tumors has not been extensively explored. **Accelerated hypofractionation** uses fewer, larger fraction sizes (typically 3 to 5 Gy/d) to a lower total dose (20 to 40 Gy) over 1 to 3 weeks. Such schemes may be used for the palliative treatment of patients with malignant or metastatic brain tumors; it minimizes the inconvenience of multiple treatments for very ill or poor prognosis patients.

CHEMICAL MODIFIERS OF RADIATION EFFECT

Hypoxic cells have been demonstrated in vitro to exhibit up to a threefold decrease in radiosensitivity and may represent a radioresistant cell population, especially in tumors that have areas of central necrosis. Hypoxic cell sensitizers, high concentrations of oxygen (hyperbaric oxygen, carbogen), and hemoglobin modifiers have been used to address this issue. Dose-limiting toxicity, poor drug delivery to tumor, and reoxygenation during standard fractionated treatment may account for the lack of therapeutic benefit observed in clinical trials to date. Halogenated pyrimidines are thymidine analogues that are incorporated into the DNA of actively cycling cells. Cells incorporating these analogues have been demonstrated to exhibit increased radiosensitivity. Actively cycling tumor cells theoretically may preferentially take up the analogue over slowly cycling normal brain parenchyma, resulting in differential cell sensitization. A large Radiation Therapy Oncology Group (RTOG) phase III trial examining the use of 5-bromodeoxyuridine (BUDR) for anaplastic astrocytoma failed to confirm a survival benefit for this agent. Chemotherapeutic agents have the potential to interact with radiation to increase tumor-cell kill either additively (independent toxicity, spatial cooperation) or synergistically (by radiosensitization). Cisplatin, topotecan, tirapazamine, and paclitaxel are chemotherapy agents that have shown synergistic effects against malignant glioma cells when combined with radiation in vitro. The clinical utility of these agents in malignant gliomas is being explored in phase I/II clinical trials by cooperative groups like the RTOG.

ACUTE TOXICITY OF RADIOTHERAPY

Occasionally a transient worsening of preradiation symptoms occurs early in the course of irradiation. This worsening has been attributed to a transient increase in vascular permeability leading to increased peritumoral edema and usually responds to a short-term increase in corticosteroid dose.[7] Persistent or refractory symptoms may also be due to tumor progression, and patients may require repeat imaging while on treatment if their clinical condition worsens despite steroid use. Concomitant medical problems (infection, thromboembolism, hyperglycemia) are also common in brain tumor patients and may contribute to clinical worsening; these should be ruled out. Nausea and vomiting independent of changes of intracranial pressure may be seen, particularly with posterior fossa/brainstem irradiation. Alopecia within the irradiated areas is experienced and may be permanent with higher total doses. Radiation dermatitis is usually mild but may be treated with topical hydrocortisone if necessary. Otitis externa can be seen if the ear is included in the irradiation fields, and serous otitis media can occur. Mucositis and esophagitis may be seen with craniospinal irradiation due to the exit of the spinal fields through the oropharynx and mediastinum. Fatigue may be seen on treatment, particularly with large-volume cerebral or craniospinal irradiation. Blood counts can drop while on treatment, again, particularly for those patients receiving craniospinal irradiation, and neutrophils and platelet counts should be checked weekly in these patients.

SUBACUTE TOXICITY OF RADIOTHERAPY

The acute side effects of radiation usually subside within 4 to 6 weeks after radiation. In the interval 6 to 12 weeks after irradiation, neurologic deterioration may occur as an "early-delayed" or subacute side effect.[7] This early-delayed effect has been attributed to changes in capillary permeability as well as transient demyelination secondary to damage to oligodendroglial cells. Symptoms usually respond to a course of steroid therapy and improve over several months. The main difficulty is in distinguishing such changes from tumor recurrence. Within the spinal cord, a subacute reaction (presumably) due to transient demyelination may be seen. This self-limited side effect, termed Lhermitte's sign, is experienced as transient tingling and paresthesia within the extremities, particularly on neck flexion.

DELAYED CENTRAL NERVOUS SYSTEM TOXICITY OF RADIOTHERAPY

Cranial irradiation can produce neuropsychological changes and focal brain injury.[7] In children, it is clear that large-volume irradiation of the brain, higher radiation doses, and younger age at irradiation (< 5 years old) are related to subsequent changes in intellect as measured by serial intelligence quotient (IQ) testing. In adults, decreases in new learning ability, recent memory, abstraction, and problem solving can be seen, particularly following cranial irradiation, and may be accompanied by parenchymal T2 changes on MRI (Figure 7–7A). A rare late effect of radiotherapy is CNS parenchymal necrosis with resulting mass effect and/or focal deficits (Figure 7–7B). Focal necrosis is more often a result of radiation alone, whereas a more diffuse leukoencephalopathy may be seen after combined treatment with chemotherapy, particularly methotrexate, and radiation. Necrosis may mimic tumor progression; metabolic imaging (single-photon emission computed tomography [SPECT], positron emission tomography [PET], MRI) may help distinguish recurrent tumor from necrosis. Symptomatic necrosis is usually treated with steroids and/or surgical debulking.[7–9]

ANAPLASTIC ASTROCYTOMA AND GLIOBLASTOMA MULTIFORME

Malignant gliomas grow in an infiltrative manner and have a propensity for spread among white matter tracts within and between hemispheres. Tumor infiltration is commonly associated with significant peritumoral edema, and biopsy of the edema (as delineated by CT or MRI) confirms the presence of infiltrating tumor cells. The major microscopic tumor burden, however, lies within several centimeters of the preoperative contrast-enhanced volumes on CT or MRI, and most patients fail within several centimeters of this region after surgery.[10] Careful review of the T2-weighted MRI in designing the radiation plan, particularly for those patients with evidence of bilateral extension across the corpus callosum, will minimize the chance of a geographic miss. In rare cases in which diffuse brain infiltration is evident (ie, gliomatosis cerebri), whole brain irradiation may still be necessary. Randomized trials of radiotherapy have demonstrated a clear survival benefit for radiotherapy added to surgery for patients with malignant gliomas.[10] Randomized trials by the British Medical Research Council and Scandinavian Brain Tumor Study group demonstrated superiority of 60 Gy over 45 Gy.[10] A randomized RTOG study comparing 70 Gy with 60 Gy did not, however, demonstrate superiority to the high-dose treatment using nonconformal radiotherapy techniques.[10] Dose escalation through hyperfractionation using nonconformal techniques to doses as high as 81.6 Gy was performed on a prospective RTOG trial. A potential survival advantage with a dose of 72 Gy (and decreased survival at higher doses) led to a randomized trial comparing 72 Gy (1.2 Gy bid) to 60 Gy (2.0 Gy once daily), with no benefit to hyperfractionation noted.[11] Several groups have reported dose escalation using stereotactic conformal external beam radiotherapy to doses of 80 Gy or more[12] but without dramatic

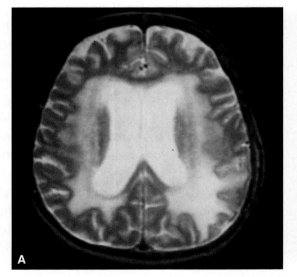
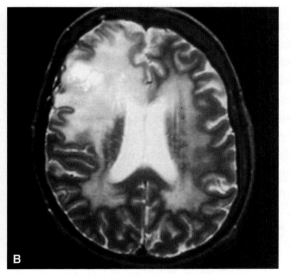

Figure 7–7. *A*, Post-treatment T2-weighted MRI demonstrating increased signal in previously treated brain parenchyma. Such MRI changes may be asymptomatic or associated with cognitive changes. *B*, Post-treatment, contrast-enhanced, T1-weighted MRI demonstrating enhancing changes due to radiation necrosis. Radiation necrosis may be difficult to differentiate from recurrent tumors on MRI. Symptomatic patients are treated with steroids and/or surgical debulking.

improvements in survival over conventional doses. Treatment of localized partial brain volumes encompassing either the preoperative contrast-enhanced tumor volume or the peritumoral edema with a 2- to 3-cm margin is recommended. Radiation Therapy Oncology Group trials for malignant glioma typically specify a "shrinking-field" technique, treating the preoperative edema with a 2-cm margin to 46 Gy with a subsequent boost to the preoperative contrast-enhancing tumor with a 2.5-cm margin to a total dose of 60 Gy.

In most patients, the maximum benefit of radiotherapy both clinically and radiologically is evident by 3 to 4 weeks postradiation. A good response as measured by a decrease in tumor size on CT or MRI in the setting of stable or reduced steroid requirements is a favorable prognostic indicator.[13] Approximately 20 percent of patients will exhibit clinical or radiographic evidence of tumor progression while on radiation. Median survival for patients with anaplastic astrocytomas is approximately 3 years, with a 20 percent 5-year survival rate. The outlook for patients with glioblastoma treated with radiation is considerably worse: median survivals of 12 to 18 months for the most favorable patients and few long-term survivors. Elderly or poor-performance-status patients with malignant gliomas may tolerate radiotherapy poorly, and the survival observed (6 to 8 months) is disproportionately short compared to the 6-week duration of a conventionally fractionated radiation schedule. Hypofractionated (larger dose per fraction) short radiation schedules (30 Gy/10 fractions to 40 Gy/15 fractions) may be associated with similar palliative benefits and are often better tolerated among these poor prognosis patients.[14] Re-treatment with conventionally fractionated radiation is rarely helpful for patients with recurrent malignant glioma after prior fractionated radiotherapy. Promising results for a hypofractionated re-treatment schedule using stereotactic conformal radiation techniques have recently been reported.[15]

LOW-GRADE ASTROCYTOMA AND OLIGODENDROGLIOMA

Like malignant gliomas, low-grade astrocytomas and oligodendrogliomas are characterized by infiltration of the surrounding parenchyma but with relatively less tumorigenic edema and mass effect than high-grade gliomas. Pilocytic tumors, in particular, may be well circumscribed and are often particularly amenable to complete surgical resections. Magnetic resonance imaging is more sensitive than CT scanning for target volume delineation as these tumors often appear as low-intensity, nonenhancing regions on T1-weighted scans and high-intensity on T2-weighted scans. Image fusion of the diagnostic MRI and planning CT can facilitate target volume delineation for these tumors.

As some low-grade gliomas may behave indolently, and radiation may be associated with late CNS toxicity, controversy exists as to the optimal timing of radiation for patients with these neoplasms. In general, postoperative radiotherapy is not recommended for most younger patients with total resection of a low-grade glioma. The benefit of immediate postoperative radiotherapy in patients with subtotally resected low-grade gliomas remains controversial. Retrospective reviews have suggested a benefit of radiation added to surgery, but this benefit is most pronounced in older series, less so in more modern series. Preliminary results of an European Organization for the Research and Treatment of Cancer (EORTC) trial (randomizing patients between immediate or deferred radiotherapy) suggest a progression-free but not overall survival advantage to immediate postoperative radiotherapy.[16] Pretreatment patient factors (age, performance status, tumor histology) are of prognostic value in patients with low-grade gliomas as they are in high-grade gliomas. Whether these prognostic factors can be used to select patients for immediate versus delayed radiation remains to be demonstrated. Patients receiving postoperative radiotherapy could be treated to doses of 45 to 54 Gy in 25 to 30 fractions. Randomized trials have not demonstrated an advantage to high-dose radiotherapy (60 to 65 Gy) over more modest doses of radiotherapy (45 to 54 Gy) for low-grade glioma.[17,18] Focal tailored radiation fields covering the preoperative tumor volume (as visualized on the T2-weighted MRI) with a 2- to 3-cm margin are appropriate (see Figure 7–6). Use of stereotactic conformal radiotherapy techniques can be expected to benefit these patients by minimizing the potential long-term toxicity in this patient population with a long (5- to 10-year) expected life span (see Figure 7–6). Anaplastic oligodendrogliomas have a more aggressive course than low-grade oligodendrogliomas. Maximal surgical resection followed by adjuvant radiotherapy (60 Gy/30 fractions) to the MRI T2-weighted preoperative tumor volume with a 2- to 3-cm margin is recommended. Ongoing trials are evaluating the benefit of chemotherapy combined with radiotherapy for these tumors. Survival is considerably longer than for patients with other malignant gliomas, however, with median survival of up to 5 to 7 years reported following surgery and radiation.

BRAINSTEM GLIOMA

Low-grade brainstem lesions typically grow in a focal fashion and may present with discrete neurologic deficits referable to the anatomic area of involvement. Higher-grade lesions tend to grow in an infiltrative manner and extend along the white matter tracts into the cerebellum or diencephalon, diffusely expand the brain stem, and present with mixed symptoms including cranial neuropathies, long-tract signs, and obstructive hydrocephalus.

Due to the morbidity of resection of most brainstem lesions, radiation therapy has been the mainstay of treatment for most patients with brainstem gliomas. In those patients with diffuse lesions, inclusion of the entire brain stem from the diencephalon to the C2 vertebral level is recommended. Any cerebellar extension must also be covered with an appropriate margin. More focal lesions may be treated with tighter fields (2- to 3-cm margins on the GTV). Design of the portals is greatly facilitated by correlation with the sagittal MRI contrast-enhanced T1- and T2-weighted images. Use of conformal treatment planning to avoid simple opposed lateral beam arrangements may spare the middle ear and auditory apparatus (as well as temporal lobes) from late side effects of radiation.

The finding that most brainstem tumors fail within the irradiated volume has led to attempts to dose escalate to improve local control. Hyperfractionation for brainstem gliomas has been extensively investigated in phase I/II trials. Total doses up to 78 Gy in 78 fractions delivered at 1 Gy bid have been delivered. Improved survivals with doses of 72 Gy (1 Gy bid) were noted among single institution series as well as phase I/II trials.[19] This dose escalation represents an approximately 20 percent increase in effective tumor dose for a 5 percent increase in effective normal tissue dose as compared to a conventional fractionation. A randomized comparison of conventional (54 Gy, 1.8 Gy OD) versus hyperfractionated radiotherapy (72 Gy, 1 Gy bid), both combined with concurrent cisplatin, failed to confirm a survival advantage for hyperfractionation.[19] Although the optimum dose-fractionation scheme has yet to be determined, conventionally fractionated (50 to 54 Gy in 25 to 30 fractions/5 to 6 weeks) or hyperfractionated (72 Gy, 1 Gy bid/7 wk) schedules are commonly used. Hyperfractionated radiotherapy to higher doses or combined with chemotherapy may be associated with higher risks of symptomatic brainstem injury.[20,21]

EPENDYMOMA

The majority of ependymomas present within the posterior fossa, within the region of the fourth ventricle; however, supratentorial and spinal ependymomas are also seen. Ependymomas have a well-documented capacity for cerebrospinal fluid (CSF) spread. Pooled patient data suggest an overall risk of CSF involvement of about 12 percent with a 5 percent incidence on presentation. In those patients with suspected or diagnosed ependymoma, neuraxis staging with contrast-enhanced MRI and CSF cytology is essential.

Like gliomas, these tumors may be locally invasive, and postoperative radiotherapy after a subtotal resection to reduce or delay local recurrence is usually recommended. In the past, the finding of a disproportionate number of high-grade and infratentorial tumors among those patients with CSF relapse led to the recommendation that patients presenting with these tumors be treated with craniospinal irradiation. More recent retrospective reviews have demonstrated that the overall incidence of isolated spinal relapses is low, even among the highest-risk patients, and the majority of spinal failures are associated with local recurrences. Given the potential morbidity of craniospinal irradiation, especially in young patients, a more selective use of this modality is appropriate.[22,23] Careful neuraxial staging of all patients is essential. Pathologic review by a pathologist familiar with these tumors is essential to rule out ependymoblastoma and medulloblastoma as these tumors have a much higher risk of neuraxial spread. Those patients with demonstrated neuraxial spread (positive MRI or positive CSF cytology) or high risk of CSF dissemination (ependymoblastoma) should receive craniospinal irradiation (36 to 40 Gy) with local boosts to the areas of gross disease and primary tumor (total dose 50 to 54 Gy). Patients in whom craniospinal radiotherapy is not indicated should be treated with generous local fields encompassing the preoperative tumor volume with margins of 2 to 3 cm to doses of 50 to 54 Gy. Ependymomas of the posterior fossa commonly can extend to the upper cervical cord, and this area should be included if there is evidence of extension on imaging. Anaplastic ependymomas are treated in a manner similar to low-grade ependymomas; however, the dose to the primary tumor is usually somewhat higher (54 to 60 Gy). Many clinicians (but not the current authors) would recommend craniospinal irradiation in the setting of high-grade posterior fossa tumors given perceived higher risk of spinal seeding for these patients. Spinal failure in the absence of local failure is rare in most series and may be seen in patients despite prophylactic spinal irradiation. A recent review of the literature suggests only a modest reduction in the incidence of spinal recurrence from 9.5 to 6.7 percent in high-grade tumors treated with prophylactic spinal irradiation.[22]

MEDULLOBLASTOMA AND PRIMITIVE NEUROECTODERMAL TUMOR

The radiation treatment of "small round blue cell" tumors (primitive neuroectodermal tumor [PNET]) of the CNS, medulloblastoma, ependymoblastoma, and pineoblastoma follow similar principles. Dissemination throughout the CSF is relatively common and complete neuraxis staging preradiation is essential. An attempt at complete resection preradiation is important as most series have demonstrated improved survival for those patients with tumor debulked to < 1.5 cm². Given the risk of CSF relapse, prophylactic treatment of the whole craniospinal axis to doses of 30 to 40 Gy is recommended (see Figure 7–4). Trials attempting to substitute chemotherapy for whole cranial or craniospinal radiation have been unsuccessful, with the majority of patients failing in the CSF when radiation to these areas is omitted. Single-institution trials have reported good results with a lower dose (18 to 25 Gy) of craniospinal irradiation in selected patients. However, in a randomized trial by the Children's Cancer Study Group/Pediatric Oncology Group, an excess of early CSF relapses (17/63 vs 5/63) was noted among the patients receiving low-dose irradiation and prompted early termination of the trial.[24] For patients with unfavorable-risk (bulky residual or positive CSF) medulloblastoma or PNET other than medulloblastoma, conventional-dose craniospinal irradiation, combined with chemotherapy, is indicated. For favorable-risk medulloblastoma patients (negative CSF, residual tumor < 1.5 cm²), addition of chemotherapy to low-dose craniospinal radiation (18 to 23 Gy) may reduce the risk of CFS failure that can occur with low-dose radiation alone.[25] The most common site of failure after radiation is the site of the original tumor, and most retrospective analyses suggest an improvement in survival rate with a radiation boost to this area to 50 to 54 Gy.[26] For patients with medulloblastoma, this boost is usually delivered to the whole posterior fossa. Conformally planned radiation to encompass the posterior fossa may spare the morbidity associated with full-dose radiation to the middle ear and temporal lobes. The use of hyperfractionation schedules or radiosurgery boosts in an attempt to dose escalate the boost dose beyond 50 to 54 Gy is the subject of current trials.

PINEAL REGION

Germinoma

Germinomas are radiosensitive tumors and cure rates with radiotherapy are high. Adequate surgical sampling and correlation with serum and CSF β-human chorionic gonadotropin and α-fetoprotein markers are essential to rule out the presence of nongerminomatous elements. Modern series with biopsy-proven germinomas and negative neuraxis staging treated to partial brain fields have demonstrated low rates of isolated spinal recurrence (< 10%); thus, routine craniospinal irradiation for all patients with germinoma is not recommended. Currently, craniospinal radiotherapy is reserved for those patients with demonstrated CSF spread (on MRI or CSF cytology) and possibly patients with multiple midline tumors. Doses of 30 to 36 Gy to the neuraxis with a local field boost to 50 to 55 Gy are recommended for those patients for whom craniospinal irradiation is indicated. Partial cranial fields including the whole ventricular system to a dose of 30 Gy followed by a local field boost to 50 to 54 Gy to the preradiation tumor volume with a 2- to 3-cm margin are suggested for patients without indications for neuraxis irradiation[27] (Figure 7–8).

Nongerminomatous Germ Cell Tumor

Nongerminomatous germ cell tumors (NGGCTs) are less radiosensitive than germinomas, and maximal safe resection is generally recommended for the majority of patients prior to radiation. Poor survival among NGGCT patients has led some clinicians to recommend routine craniospinal irradiation after surgery. More recently neoadjuvant and/or adjuvant platinum-based chemotherapy has been used in an attempt to improve survival.[23] Consolidative local field (for patients with a negative neuraxis) or craniospinal radiotherapy (for patients with CSF spread) should be added following chemotherapy using doses similar to that for germinomas.[27]

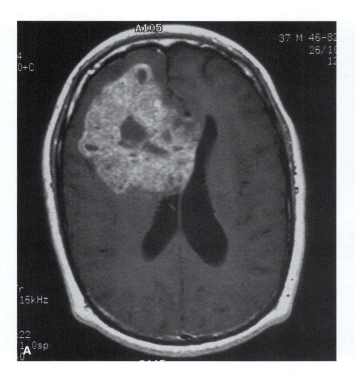
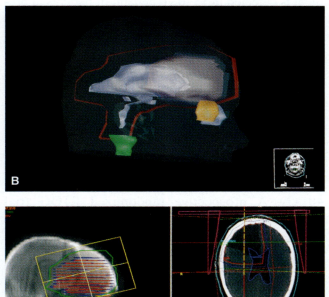
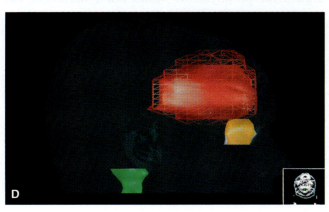

Figure 7–8. *A*, Patient with a large, frontal primary CNS germinoma. The tumor was grossly excised and craniospinal axis staging with MRI and cytology was negative. *B*, Initial phase of treatment included the whole ventricular system and tumor bed (pale red). Custom field shaping protected the eyes (orange, blue) and upper spinal cord (green). *C*, Tumor bed (solid red) was subsequently boosted by a three-field technique for a total dose of 50.4 Gy in 28 fractions. *D*, Prescription isosurface for boost is indicated by red wire mesh.

Pineocytoma and Pineoblastoma

Those patients with subtotal resections should receive postoperative radiotherapy using conformal techniques to treat the preoperative tumor volume with a 2- to 3-cm margin to a dose of 50 to 54 Gy. Patients with pineoblastomas are treated in a manner similar to those with unfavorable-risk medulloblastoma.

PRIMARY CENTRAL NERVOUS SYSTEM LYMPHOMA

Primary CNS lymphomas typically appear as solitary or multiple periventricular masses on CT scan or MRI and they frequently will seed the CSF space either at presentation or at relapse. Vitreous or retinal involvement is detected in 15 to 20 percent of patients at presentation. Primary intraocular lymphoma is associated with the subsequent development of CNS lymphoma in up to 80 percent of patients. For these reasons, preradiation ophthalmic assessment and neuraxis staging are recommended. For nonimmunosuppressed patients, whole brain radiotherapy (45 to 50 Gy/25 fractions/5 wk) is recommended. The posterior orbits should be included for all patients, and for those patients with demonstrated ocular involvement, the whole globe should be included to 30 to 40 Gy. A prospective randomized RTOG trial demonstrated no benefit from a local field boost of 20 Gy added to whole brain radiotherapy of 40 Gy compared to whole brain radiotherapy alone.[28] Treatment recommendations in patients with apparently isolated ocular lymphoma treatment are controversial. The frequent association of ocular lymphoma with synchronous or metachronous CNS involvement argues for prophylactic whole brain radiation, but irradiation to only the involved globe in the absence of demonstrable CNS disease is acceptable. If radiation to the globe only is undertaken, a technique that facilitates subsequent matching to whole cranial fields should be used. Craniospinal irradiation has been suggested for those patients with documented CSF involvement; however, intrathecal chemotherapy is more frequently used. Combined intrathecal and intravenous chemotherapy and cranial radiation is associated with improved survival over radiation alone in prospective phase I/II studies.[29]

MENINGIOMA

The current treatment of choice for benign meningiomas is complete surgical resection. Complete resection, without significant morbidity, may be difficult for patients with base of skull, cerebellopontine angle, or cavernous sinus meningiomas. For these patients, a conservative subtotal resection followed by postoperative radiation gives local control rates similar to that of a gross total excision with potentially decreased morbidity (Figure 7–9).[30] Postoperative radiation to doses of 50 to 54 Gy in 25 to 30 fractions to the preoperative tumor volume with a 1- to 2-cm margin is recommended. Special attention should be paid to the region of the infratemporal fossa for base of skull/sphenoid wing meningiomas as extracranial extension through cranial nerve foramen is not uncommon.

Meningiomas with evidence of adverse pathologic features (anaplasia, high mitotic rate, atypia), adverse histologic subtypes (papillary, angioblastic, hemangiopericytoma), and those with evidence of brain, skull, or scalp invasion should be considered as aggressive or malignant tumors. In the setting of malignant or aggressive meningioma, postoperative radiation is recommended even if gross total resection has been performed as a high rate of local recurrence is noted with surgery alone.[31] Postoperative radiotherapy (50 to 60 Gy/25 to 30 fractions) to the preoperative tumor volume with a 2- to 3-cm margin has been associated with longer intervals to recurrence and higher rates of local control compared to surgery alone for malignant meningioma.[32]

BRAIN METASTASES

Brain metastases are a common neuro-oncologic problem seen by the radiation oncologist. Traditionally, patients with brain metastasis have been treated with short, palliative courses of whole brain radiation, 30 Gy in 10 fractions (3 Gy/fraction) or 20 Gy in 5 fractions (4 Gy/fraction). Randomized trials of higher doses using conventional or hyperfractionated schedules have not demonstrated a benefit over short schedules. A recursive partitioning analysis of patients treated with whole brain radiation on a series of RTOG protocols defined three distinct groups of

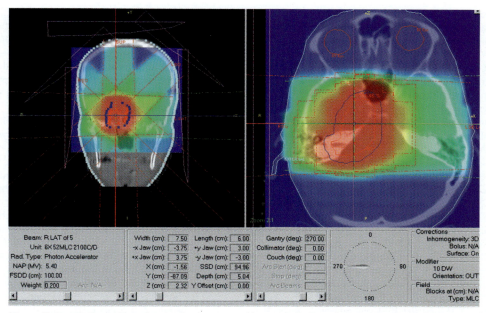

Figure 7–9. Patient with an incompletely resected base-of-skull meningioma involving the right cavernous sinus and sphenoid wing. A five-field conformal radiotherapy plan allows for treatment of the residual tumor while sparing the surrounding brain and eyes.

patients. The most favorable subset of patients (controlled systemic disease, good performance status, age < 65) had a median survival of approximately 6 months, and the most unfavorable (poor performance status) only 3 months when treated with whole brain radiotherapy alone.[33] Randomized trials and single-institution series have suggested a survival benefit to surgical resection or radiosurgical boost combined with whole brain radiotherapy for patients with solitary brain metastasis, especially those with otherwise favorable prognostic factors.[34] A randomized trial of surgical resection for solitary metastases with or without whole brain radiotherapy confirmed the importance of postoperative cranial irradiation in preventing subsequent intracranial metastases.[35] Patients with "radiosensitive" tumors (ie, metastatic germ cell tumors) might benefit from higher-dose (45 to 50 Gy/25 fractions) whole brain radiotherapy, especially in the setting of an isolated intracranial failure.

SPINAL CANAL

Meningiomas and neurofibromas are usually amenable to complete surgical resection with excellent local control. By analogy to intracranial tumors, postoperative radiotherapy (45 to 50 Gy/ 25 fractions) encompassing the preoperative tumor volume plus a 2- to 3-cm margin usually is added for incompletely excised tumors with high rates of local control (> 80%) expected.[36] Patients with ependymomas and spinal cord gliomas should have complete staging of the neuraxis prior to radiotherapy to rule out CSF dissemination and/or an occult intracranial primary presenting with CSF spread. Subtotally resected low-grade lesions should receive postoperative radiotherapy (45 to 50 Gy/25 fractions) as should all high-grade lesions (50 to 54 Gy/25 to 30 fractions). The preoperative tumor volume (including any syrinx, if enhancing) should be treated with a 2- to 3-cm margin. Irradiation of the whole craniospinal axis (using doses similar to that for medulloblastoma) is occasionally necessary for those patients with documented leptomeningeal spread.[36]

REFERENCES

1. Purdy JA. Advances in three-dimensional treatment planning and conformal dose delivery. Semin Oncol 1997;26:655–72.
2. Verhey LJ. Immobilizing and positioning patients for radiotherapy. Semin Radiat Oncol 1995;5:100–14.
3. Mah K, Danjoux CE, Manship S, et al. Computed tomographic simulation of craniospinal fields in pediatric patients: improved treatment accuracy and patient comfort. Int J Radiat Oncol Biol Phys 1998;41:997–1003.

4. Khoo VS, Dearnaley DP, Finnigan DJ, et al. Magnetic resonance imaging (MRI): considerations and applications in radiotherapy treatment planning. Radiother Oncol 1997;42:1–15.
5. Hamilton RJ, Sweeney PJ, Pelizzari CA, et al. Functional imaging in treatment planning of brain lesions. Int J Radiat Oncol Biol Phys 1997;37:181–8.
6. Laing RW, Bentley RE, Nahum AE, et al. Stereotactic radiotherapy of irregular targets: a comparison between static conformal beams and non-coplanar arcs. Radiat Oncol 1993;28:241–6.
7. Schultheiss TE, Kun LE, Ang KK, Stephens LC. Radiation response of the central nervous system. Int J Radiat Oncol Biol Phys 1995;31:1093–112.
8. Mulhern RK, Ochs J, Kun LE. Changes in intellect associated with cranial radiation therapy. In: Gutin PH, Leibel SA, Sheline GE, editors. Radiation injury to the nervous system. New York: Raven Press; 1991. p. 325–40.
9. Valk PE, Dillon WP. Diagnostic imaging of the central nervous system radiation injury. In: Gutin PH, Leibel SA, Sheline GE, editors. Radiation injury to the nervous system. New York: Raven Press; 1991. p. 211–38.
10. Leibel SA, Scott CB, Loeffler JS. Contemporary approaches to the treatment of malignant gliomas with radiation therapy. Semin Oncol 1994;21:198–219.
11. Scott CB, Curran W, Yung W, et al. Long term results for RTOG 9006: a randomized trial of hyperfractionated radiotherapy (RT) to 72 Gy and carmustine vs standard RT and carmustine for malignant glioma patients with emphasis on anaplastic astrocytoma (AA) patients [abstract]. Proc Am Soc Clin Oncol 1998;17:348a.
12. Sandler HM, Radany EH, Greenberg HS, et al. Dose escalation using 3D conformal radiotherapy for high grade astrocytomas. Am Soc Ther Radiol Oncol 1994;30:214.
13. Barker FG, Prados MD, Chang SM, et al. Radiation response and survival time in patients with glioblastoma multiforme. J Neurosurg 1996;84:442–8.
14. Bauman GS, Gaspar LE, Fisher BJ, et al. A prospective study of short-course radiotherapy in poor prognosis glioblastoma multiforme. Int J Radiat Oncol Biol Phys 1994;29:835–9.
15. Shepherd SF, Laing RWW, Cosgrove VP, et al. Hypofractionated stereotactic radiotherapy in the management of recurrent glioma. Int J Radiat Oncol Biol Phys 1997;37:393–8.
16. Karim ABMF, Cornu P, Bleehen N, et al. Immediate postoperative radiotherapy in low grade glioma improves progression free survival but not overall survival: preliminary results of an EORTC/MRC randomized phase III study. Proc Am Soc Clin Oncol 1998;17:400a.
17. Karim ABMF, Hatlevoll R, Menten J, et al. A randomized trial on dose-response in radiation therapy of low-grade cerebral glioma: European Organization for Research and Treatment of Cancer (EORTC) study 22844. Int J Radiat Oncol Biol Phys 1996;36:549–56.
18. Shaw E, Arusell R, Scheithauer B, et al. A prospective randomized trial of low- versus high-dose radiation therapy in adults with supratentorial low-grade glioma: initial report of a NCCTG-RTOG-ECOG study. Proc Am Soc Clin Oncol 1998;17:401a
19. Freeman CR, Farmer JP. Pediatric brainstem gliomas: a review. Int J Radiat Oncol Biol Phys 1998;40:265–71.
20. Packer RJ, Zimmerman RA, Albright AL, et al. Outcome of children with brainstem gliomas after treatment with 7800 cGy of hyperfractionated radiotherapy. A CCG phase I/II trial. Cancer 1994;74:1827–34.
21. Freeman CR, Kepner J, Kun LE, et al. A detrimental effect of a combined chemotherapy-radiotherapy approach in children with diffuse intrinsic brain stem glioma? Int Radiat Oncol Biol Phys 2000;47:561–64.
22. Vanuytsel LJ, Brada M. The role of prophylactic spinal irradiation in localized intracranial ependymoma. Int J Radiat Oncol Biol Phys 1991;21:825–9.
23. Vanuytsel LJ, Bessell EM, Ashley SE, et al. Intracranial ependymoma: long-term results of a policy of surgery and radiotherapy. Int J Radiat Oncol Biol Phys 1992;23:313–9.
24. Deutsch M, Thomas PRM, Krischer J, et al. Results of a prospective randomized trial comparing standard dose neuraxis irradiation (3600 cGy/20) with reduced neuraxis irradiation (2340/13) in patients with low-stage medulloblastoma. Pediatr Neurosurg 1996;24:167–77.
25. Goldwein JW, Radcliffe J, Johnson J, et al. Updated results of a pilot study of low dose craniospinal irradiation plus chemotherapy for children under five with cerebellar primitive neuroectodermal tumors (medulloblastoma). Int J Radiat Oncol Biol Phys 1996;34:899–904.
26. Halperin EC. Impact of radiation technique upon the outcome of treatment for medulloblastoma. Int J Radiat Oncol Biol Phys 1996;36:233–9.
27. Wolden SL, Wara WM, Larson DA, et al. Radiation therapy for primary intracranial germ-cell tumors. Int J Radiat Oncol Biol Phys 1995;32:943–9.
28. Nelson DF, Martz KL, Bonner H, et al. Non-Hodgkin's lymphoma of the brain: can high dose, large volume radiation therapy improve survival? Int J Radiat Oncol Biol Phys 1992;23:9–17.
29. DeAngelis LM. Current management of primary central nervous system lymphoma. Oncology 1995;9:63–78.
30. Lunsford LD. Contemporary management of meningiomas: radiation therapy as an adjuvant and radiosurgery as an alternative to surgical removal. J Neurosurg 1994;80:187–90.
31. Vanuytsel L, Brada M. The role of prophylactic spinal irradiation in localized intracranial ependymoma. Int J Radiat Oncol Biol Phys 1991;21:825–30.
32. Goldsmith BJ, Wara WM, Wilson CB, Larson DA. Postoperative irradiation for subtotally resected meningiomas. J Neurosurg 1994;80:195–201.
33. Gaspar L, Scott CB, Rotman M, et al. Recursive partitioning analysis of prognostic factors in three Radiation Therapy Oncology Group (RTOG) brain metastasis trials. Int J Radiat Oncol Biol Phys 1997;37:745–51.
34. Noordijk EM, Vecht CJ, Haaxma-Reiche H, et al. The choice of treatment of single brain metastasis should be based on extracranial tumor activity and age. Int J Radiat Oncol Biol Phys 1994;29:711–7.
35. Regine WF, Mohiuddin M, Tibbs PA, et al. A randomized prospective trial of the benefit of post-operative radiotherapy in the treatment of single metastases to the brain. Int J Radiat Oncol Biol Phys 1998;42:196.
36. Linstadt DE, Wara WM, Leibel SA, et al. Postoperative radiotherapy of primary spinal cord tumors. Int J Radiat Oncol Biol Phys 1988;16:1397–403.

8

Interstitial Brachytherapy

G. EVREN KELES, MD
PENNY K. SNEED, MD
DAVID A. LARSON, PhD, MD
MITCHEL S. BERGER, MD

Although conventional radiotherapy is accepted as a standard approach in the treatment of malignant gliomas, several therapeutic modalities involving high doses of radiation (eg, stereotactic radiosurgery, three-dimensional conformal proton and photon radiation therapies, and interstitial brachytherapy) are being evaluated as adjuncts to standard management strategies. The goal of these techniques is to deliver high doses of radiation to a limited area without causing radiation-induced damage in the surrounding normal brain tissue.

Interstitial brachytherapy, which consists of the intratumoral placement of encapsulated radioactive sources, has been studied extensively in regard to its role as an adjunct to conventional radiation therapy. It has been shown that the radiation dose to the tumor may be significantly increased while limiting the dose received by the surrounding tissues. As most glioma recurrences occur locally (ie, adjacent to the initial resection cavity), achieving a high dose in a relatively limited tumor field has the potential of increasing the time to progression for these tumors, which are known to exhibit a dose-dependent response to radiation.

RATIONALE

Despite multimodality treatment including surgery, radiotherapy, and chemotherapy, gliomas mostly recur at the site of the original disease.[1] It is also well known that a total radiation dose of 6,000 cGy delivered through conventional techniques has a positive prognostic effect on survival for patients with high-grade gliomas whereas radiation doses of 5,000 and 7,000 cGy fail to show a better survival advantage.[2,3] Interstitial brachytherapy has the theoretic advantage of increasing the radiation dose received by the tumor while preventing the radiation-related side effects that are observed with higher doses of conventional radiotherapy.

Delivery of a relatively high dose of radiation to tumor while minimizing the effect of radiation on surrounding normal tissues is achieved mainly by a rapid decrease of radiation dose as the distance from the radioactive sources increases.[4] But minimizing radiation effects in normal tissue is also related to dose rate. Brachytherapy is usually delivered at dose rates of 5 to 100 cGy/h as compared with conventional external beam radiotherapy, which is typically delivered at the significantly higher rates of 100 to 200 cGy/min. Lower dose rates provide increased time for the repair of sublethal radiation damage in normal cells.[4] However, lower dose rates also provide increased time for the repair of sublethal damage in tumor cells. One of the challenges of brachytherapy is to provide a dose rate that is high enough to damage tumor cells yet not high enough to damage normal cells.

The use of hyperthermia in conjunction with interstitial brachytherapy has been an area of extensive research. In addition to heat being cytotoxic as a single modality, cells in hypoxic and low-pH environments, as well as those cells in the S phase of the cell cycle, which are more resistant to irradiation, are known to be affected by the addition of heat to radiation. Heat also inhibits the repair of sublethal damage from irradiation. Some of the methods used to achieve hyperthermia include the use of radio frequency, interstitial microwave antennas, and magnetic-loop induction.[4,5]

TECHNIQUE

Patients with hemispheric unifocal disease < 4 to 5 cm in greatest diameter, without leptomeningeal spread or subependymal invasion and not involving the corpus callosum, and a Karnofsky performance score greater than 60 or 70 in most series are generally considered to be eligible for interstitial brachytherapy. Florell and colleagues[6] reviewed the impact of patient selection on survival in patients with newly diagnosed supratentorial malignant gliomas. The median survival rates for implant-eligible and ineligible patients with glioblastoma multiforme were 13.9 and 5.8 months, respectively. The authors concluded that eligible patients live longer than ineligible ones by virtue of their younger age, more extensive resections, and better performance status and that the longer survival period following interstitial brachytherapy is partly the consequence of patient selection.[6]

Commonly used isotopes for interstitial brachytherapy are iodine-125, iridium-192, phosphorus-32, rhenium-186, and yttrium-90. The first two, that is, iodine-125 and iridium-192, are gamma-emitting isotopes whereas the other three isotopes emit beta particles. Gamma rays (photons lacking mass and electrical charge) have the ability to travel farther in tissue than beta particles.[4] Due to these characteristics, iodine-125 and iridium-192 are preferred for the treatment of solid tumors. Beta rays, which are negatively charged electrons emitted from some isotopes, have a limited depth of penetration. Therefore, isotopes that emit beta rays have been used mainly for irradiating tumor cells lining the cystic components of craniopharyngiomas and gliomas.[7–9] Other isotopes (eg, cobalt-60 and gold-198) have also been used (to a lesser extent) for interstitial brachytherapy for brain tumors.

Currently, the most commonly used source for interstitial brachytherapy is temporary high-activity or permanent low-activity iodine-125. Unlike temporary implants, permanent low-activity sources do not require a second procedure after craniotomy and are placed either during the operation that the patient undergoes for initial diagnosis or at the time of progression (Figure 8–1). At the operation, following maximal resection, seeds are evenly spaced along the resection cavity wall; a typical separation between seed midpoints is 0.5 to 1 cm.[10] Iodine-125 seeds may be secured in place with tissue adhesive or by being embedded in adjacent brain parenchyma at the designated spacing. Protecting the surgical team from radiation exposure is critical until the bone flap is replaced. Final computerized dosimetry is obtained from postoperative scans (Figure 8–2). Patients are followed up with postoperative serial magnetic resonance imaging (MRI). As a thin region of contrast enhancement may develop adjacent to the seeds, such changes seen by MRI are not considered evidence of treatment failure unless there is significant size progression or unless metabolic imaging (magnetic resonance spectroscopy [MRS] and positron emission tomography [PET]) indicate hypermetabolism indicative of tumor and not radiation necrosis.

For temporary implants, computed tomography images are obtained following the application of a stereotactic frame under local anesthesia. Computerized planning is performed on a three-dimensional reconstruction of the tumor volume to obtain the optimal distribution of radiation (Figures 8–3, 8–4, and 8–5). Stereotactic coordinates for placement of the catheters are calculated from these data and outer catheters are stereotactically placed and fixed to the scalp (Figure 8–6). Subsequently, inner catheters containing the radioactive seeds with necessary spacing are loaded into the outer catheters. Postimplant images are obtained to determine seed locations and the final isodose distribution and to calculate the time frame necessary to deliver a predefined radiation dose to the area of interest.

CLINICAL EFFICACY

Recurrent Gliomas

Brachytherapy for malignant gliomas has been used most commonly at the time of recurrence.[5,10–24]

Despite the fact that only approximately 10 to 40 percent of patients were considered eligible for interstitial brachytherapy, an additional median survival ranging from 26 to 65 weeks from the time of implant was observed.[5,10,12–16,18–24] Major studies evaluating the effect of interstitial brachytherapy on the survival of patients with recurrent high-grade gliomas are outlined in Table 8–1. In one of the larger series (66 patients with recurrent glioblastoma multiforme), median survivals from the date of implant for recurrent glioblastoma and nonglioblastoma malignant glioma were 49 and 52 weeks, respectively.[23] In this series, 40 percent of patients with malignant glioma underwent reoperation at a median of 33 weeks following implantation. Although 95 percent of the patients had pathologic evidence of tumor at

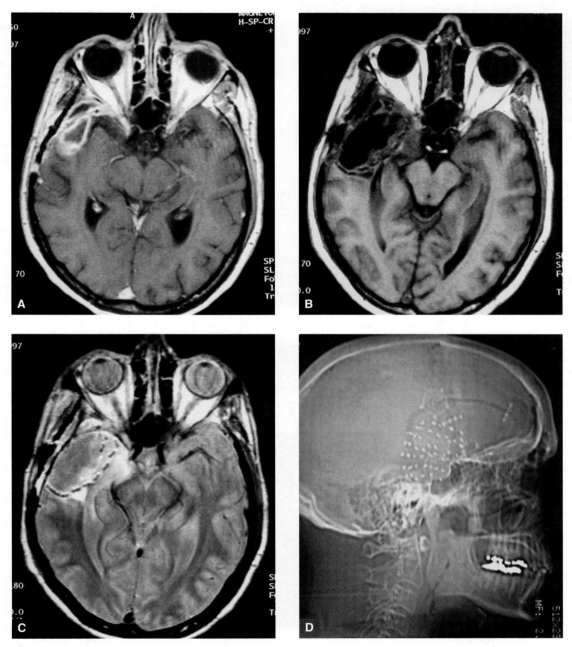

Figure 8–1. A 46-year-old male patient with a right temporal glioblastoma multiforme. *A*, Preresection contrast-enhanced T1-weighted axial magnetic resonance imaging (MRI) scan. *B* and *C*, Postoperative axial MRI scans depicting the resection cavity and radioactive implants. *D*, Postoperative lateral scout image showing the temporal craniotomy and radioactive seeds.

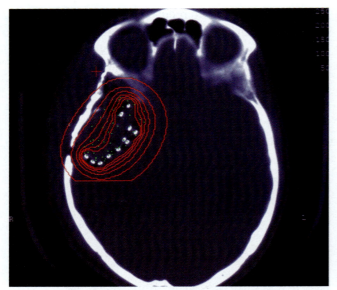

Figure 8–2. Isodose lines for the patient presented in Figure 8–1. The red lines represent isodose lines ranging from 300 Gy (*inner line*) to 50 Gy (*outer line*), in steps of 50 Gy.

reoperation, histologic findings did not affect survival. However, patients with glioblastoma multiforme who underwent reoperation had a statistically longer survival when compared with those who did not have a subsequent operation (medians of 90 and 37 weeks, respectively).[23] Similar findings regarding the prognostic effect of reoperation following interstitial brachytherapy were also reported in other series, including a study that compared stereotactic radiosurgery and brachytherapy for recurrent glioblastoma multiforme.[24] In that study, similar survival rates were reported for both treatment modalities.

Although temporary implants were used in the majority of the studies, there are also studies regarding the use of permanent seeds.[10–12] These studies report encouraging results, especially when implantation is preceded by maximal tumor resection. Halligan and colleagues[10] reported their experience with

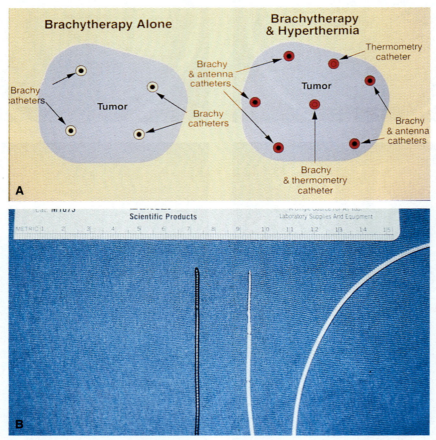

Figure 8–3. *A*, Schematic diagrams of end-on views of typical catheter arrangements for brachytherapy alone *(left)* and for brachytherapy with hyperthermia. For hyperthermia, catheters for housing heating antennas are placed closer to the tumor periphery, and additional catheters are required for thermometry. *B*, A helical-coil microwave antenna before *(right)* and after *(left)* placement of an electrically insulating coating.

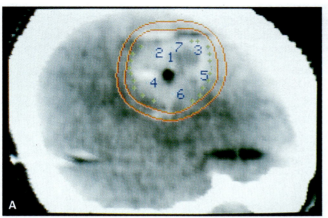 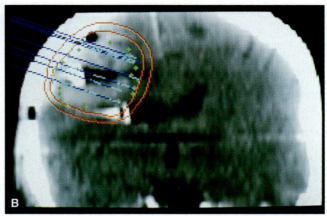

Figure 8–4. *A,* End-on view of a typical preplan for hyperthermia and brachytherapy, showing the catheter arrangement and 30- and 50-cGy/h isodose contours. *B,* Coronal view of the same preplan.

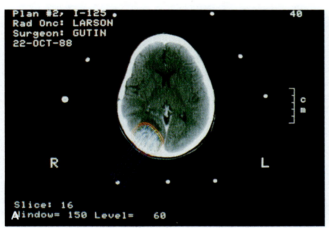 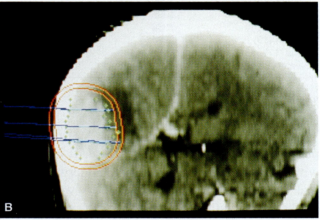

Figure 8–5. *A,* Axial view of a typical preplan for hyperthermia and brachytherapy showing the catheter and iodine-125 source arrangement and the 30- and 40-cGy/h isodose contours. *B,* Oblique view in the plane of the implant catheters for the same preplan.

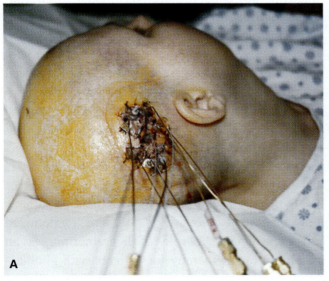 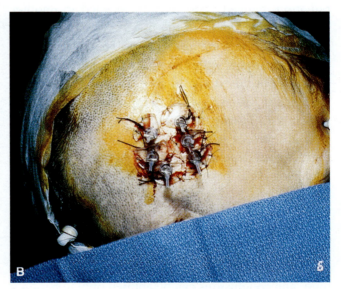

Figure 8–6. *A,* A patient with brain implant catheters. Heating antennas and thermometry probes are in place for brain hyperthermia treatment. *B,* A patient immediately after placement of brain brachytherapy catheters.

Table 8–1. SERIES EVALUATING THE PROGNOSTIC EFFECT OF BRACHYTHERAPY FOR PATIENTS WITH RECURRENT HIGH-GRADE GLIOMAS

Study (Reference No.)	Year	Implant	No. of Patients	Histology	Median Survival (mo)
Sneed (36)	1994	^{125}I / T	65	GBM	12
		^{125}I / T	45	GBM/AA	12
Bernstein (22)	1994	^{125}I / T	46	GBM/AA	10.6
Sneed (5)	1992	^{125}I / T*	25	GBM	11.8
		^{125}I / T*	16	AA	16
Halligan (10)	1996	^{125}I / P	18	GBM	16
		^{125}I / P	22	GBM/AA	16.3
Malkin (15)	1992	^{125}I / T	36	GBM/AA	10
Zamorano (12)	1992	^{125}I / T	23	GBM/AA	10
		^{125}I / P	11	GBM/AA	10
Larson (11)	1990	^{198}Au / P	13	GBM	9
		^{198}Au / P	20	AA	17
Schrieve (24)	1995	^{125}I / T	32	GBM/AA	11.5
Ryken (20)	1994	^{125}I / T	20	GBM/AA	5.5
Lucas (14)	1991	^{192}Ir / T	7	GBM	10.8
		^{192}Ir / T	13	AA	14.3
Loeffler (18)	1990	^{125}I / T	20	GBM	7
Chamberlain (21)	1995	^{125}I / T	16	GBM/AA	9.5
Kumar (13)	1988	^{60}Co / T	16	GBM	6.5
Kitchen (19)	1994	^{125}I / T	13	GBM/AA	6
Willis (17)	1988	^{125}I / T	12	GBM/AA	18
Stea (16)	1992	^{125}I / T*	6	GBM/AA	6

T = temporary; P = permanent; GBM = glioblastoma multiforme; AA = anaplastic astrocytoma.
*Patients also received hyperthermia.

permanent low-activity iodine-125 seeds in patients with high-grade astrocytomas who underwent maximal surgical resection. Median survival was 64 weeks from the time of implant for the subgroup of patients with glioblastoma multiforme. In this study, none of the patients required repeat craniotomy for radiation necrosis. Similarly, no reoperations for radiation-induced necrosis were needed in another series that incorporated the use of permanent gold-198 seeds following resection.[11] The median survival for patients with glioblastoma multiforme was 39 weeks in this study. In another series comparing permanent seeds with temporary iodine-125 implants following stereotactic biopsy, no significant differences in survival were observed.[12] However, steroid dependency after 6 months was 96 percent for the permanent low-dose-rate group, compared to 12.5 percent for those who received temporary high-dose-rate brachytherapy.

Although these results favor the use of interstitial brachytherapy for recurrent high-grade gliomas, it should be noted that the quality of evidence is not high, and conclusions can be applied only to patients who meet the inclusion criteria for each study.[25]

Newly Diagnosed Gliomas

Although early studies focused on patients with recurrent gliomas, the role of interstitial brachytherapy as a part of the initial management strategy for high-grade gliomas has also been evaluated. Several series have suggested a survival benefit for brachytherapy boost in selected patients. These studies are outlined in Table 8–2. Median survival from diagnosis ranges from 7 to 22 months for patients with primary glioblastoma multiforme treated with brachytherapy boost in conjunction with external beam radiotherapy.[12,26,27–32] The larger of these nonrandomized series reported similar median survival times of 18 and 19 months for patients with glioblastoma multiforme.[26,28]

In the literature, there are two randomized series that specifically addressed the prognostic effect of brachytherapy in the initial management of patients with malignant gliomas.[33,34] A third randomized series evaluated the role of hyperthermia as an adjunct to brachytherapy for patients with glioblastoma multiforme.[35] The prospective Brain Tumor Cooperative Group (BTCG) trial (BTCG study 87-

01), which randomized patients with primary malignant gliomas to brachytherapy using temporary high-dose-rate iodine-125 implants or to no brachytherapy prior to conventional external beam radiotherapy, showed a survival advantage ($p < .05$) for the implanted group.[33] Patients with a Karnofsky performance score of > 50 were included, and all 299 patients in this study received external radiotherapy (6,020 cGy to the tumor, plus a 3-cm border) and carmustine (BCNU) chemotherapy.[33]

The second study included 140 patients with a Karnofsky performance score of > 70, and patients were randomized to external beam radiation therapy (5,000 cGy) or external radiation plus temporary stereotactic iodine-125 implants.[34] This study did not show any survival benefit associated with the use of brachytherapy in newly diagnosed patients. Median survival for patients randomized to brachytherapy was 13.8 months versus 13.2 months for those who did not receive implants. Factors associated with improved survival in univariate analysis were younger age, better performance status, reoperation, and the use of chemotherapy at the time of recurrence. Multivariate analysis showed that treatment at recurrence (ie, reoperation or chemotherapy) and the patient's performance status are the most influential prognostic factors for this patient population.[34]

The third randomized study was conducted to determine if adjuvant interstitial hyperthermia improves the survival of patients with glioblastoma multiforme who are undergoing brachytherapy boost after conventional radiotherapy.[35] Time to tumor progression and survival were significantly longer for the group of patients who received hyperthermia than for the "no heat" group (median survival for the hyperthermia group was 85 weeks vs 76 weeks for the nonhyperthermia group; the 2-year survival rate for the hyperthermia group was 31 percent vs 15 percent for the nonhyperthermia group). The authors of this study concluded that adjuvant interstitial brain hyperthermia (given before and after brachytherapy boost) after conventional radiotherapy significantly improves the survival of patients with focal glioblastoma multiforme, with acceptable toxicity.[35]

Regarding anaplastic astrocytomas, the University of California, San Francisco, studies (which are the largest published series that evaluate the role of brachytherapy for patients with grade 3 astrocytomas) failed to show any benefit of brachytherapy in terms of survival.[23,36] The median survival time from diagnosis was 157 weeks and was not better than the survival times achieved with radiotherapy and adjuvant chemotherapy. Although there was no survival advantage with the use of brachytherapy boost, improved survival was observed with brachytherapy at the time of progression.[37]

Various radioactivity sources have been tried for the brachytherapy of low-grade gliomas, and there has been increasing use of temporary iodine-125 seeds during the last two decades. In one of the larger series (including 97 patients with pilocytic astrocytomas and 250 patients with grade 2 astrocytomas), 5- and 10-year survival rates were 85 percent and 83 percent for pilocytic astrocytomas and 61 percent and 51 percent for grade 2 astrocytomas.[38] Younger age, better performance status, and lower histologic

Table 8–2. NONRANDOMIZED SERIES EVALUATING THE PROGNOSTIC EFFECT OF INTERSTITIAL BRACHYTHERAPY IN PATIENTS WITH NEWLY DIAGNOSED HIGH-GRADE GLIOMAS

Study (Reference No.)	Year	Implant	No. of Patients	Histology	Median Survival (mo)
Sneed (28)	1995	^{125}I / T	159	GBM	19
		^{125}I / T	52	AA	36
Wen (26)	1994	^{125}I / T	56	GBM	18
Patchell (31)	1988	^{252}Cf / T	56	GBM/AA	10
Kumar (30)	1989	^{60}Co / T	30	GBM	7
Chun (32)	1989	^{192}Ir / T	20	GBM	14.5
		^{192}Ir / T	9	AA	15.5
Zamorano (12)	1992	^{125}I / T	25	GBM/AA	14
Malkin (29)	1994	^{125}I / T	20	GBM	22
Lucas (27)	1991	^{192}Ir / T	6	GBM	10
		^{192}Ir / T	7	AA	23

T = temporary; GBM = glioblastoma multiforme; AA = anaplastic astrocytoma.

grade were associated with better overall outcome. In this study, symptomatic radiation necrosis was observed in 2.6 percent of the patients, with permanent implants and larger tumor diameter being statistically significant risk factors for this complication.[38] The same group reported their updated results in 515 patients with low-grade gliomas with 5-year survival rates of 85 percent, 59 percent, and 37 percent for the age groups of < 19, 20 to 49, and > 49 years, respectively.[39] Reviewing their data on 247 patients with permanent iodine-125 implants and 268 patients with temporary iodine-125 implants, the authors concluded that radiation injury outside the treatment volume may be better avoided with temporary implants in the case of rapid tumor shrinkage in response to radiation.[39] However, the lack of class 1 evidence and the fact that these results were obtained in a highly selected patient population with smaller tumors and good performance status make the data difficult to generalize for patients with newly diagnosed low-grade gliomas.

COMPLICATIONS

Complications associated with the surgical technique are not specific to brachytherapy and include problems that may be encountered following any stereotactic approach or craniotomy. These include infection, hemorrhage, increased mass effect and intracranial pressure, and seizures, as well as systemic problems such as pneumonia, deep venous thrombosis, and pulmonary emboli.

Although uncommon, one side effect related to brachytherapy is increased mass effect and neurologic deterioration in the early postoperative period due to increased cell death and necrosis and resulting in increased swelling. This problem is more often encountered in tumors that are deeply located and larger. An acute complication rate of 11 to 12 percent was reported in two series, with no fatal complications.[22,26] In a larger series of 307 consecutive brachytherapy procedures, severe acute complications were observed in approximately 8 percent of the patients.[23]

The main radiation-related complication following interstitial brachytherapy is delayed radiation necrosis. With temporary high-activity implants, a certain degree of necrosis due to the high dose of radiation delivered through the implants occurs in the majority of patients. The reported incidence of symptomatic necrosis requiring reoperation varies from approximately 25 to 55 percent.[22–24,26,40] As the decision for reoperation is based on several factors, these figures do not represent the exact incidence of radiation necrosis. On neuroimaging studies, radiation necrosis is usually characterized by an enlarging mass with peripheral enhancement, similar to tumor progression. Both PET[41] and three-dimensional proton magnetic resonance spectroscopy (^{1}H-MRS)[42] have been evaluated, with promising results, for ability to distinguish between tumor progression and radiation-induced necrosis. Increased vasogenic edema due to radiation necrosis is initially managed with dexamethasone. In one series, the percentage of patients dependent on steroids was 97 percent at the time of brachytherapy, 67 percent at 1.5 years post-treatment, and 53 percent at 3 years post-treatment.[43] At the time of reoperation, histopathologic evaluation of the resected specimens revealed both tumor and radiation necrosis in the majority of cases.[23] Regardless of the histologic findings, patients who undergo reoperation have a better overall survival.[23,26] At the time of progression, however, most patients with higher-grade gliomas exhibit local tumor recurrence.[10,23,26,44,45]

A rare radiation-induced complication is the occlusion of a major artery, reported in patients with temporal lobe tumors where the high-dose volume included a major vessel.[46]

CONCLUSION

Within the last 30 years, advances in neuroimaging modalities and stereotactic techniques, together with better computerized treatment planning methods for dosimetry, have been helpful in achieving promising results with the use of interstitial brachytherapy for brain tumor patients. It should be noted, however, that most of the data are derived from single-arm uncontrolled studies and that only a fraction of the current literature is based on class 1 evidence. Nevertheless, interstitial brachytherapy appears to be a valid treatment option for patients with recurrent malignant gliomas and an adjunct to the initial management of patients with glioblastoma multiforme.

REFERENCES

1. Wallner KE, Galicich JH, Krol G, et al. Patterns of failure following treatment for glioblastoma multiforme and anaplastic astrocytoma. Int J Radiat Oncol Biol Phys 1989;16:1405–9.
2. Walker MD, Strike TA, Sheline GE. An analysis of dose effect relationship in the radiotherapy of malignant glioma. Int J Radiat Oncol Biol Phys 1979;5:1725–31.
3. Chang CH, Horton J, Schoenfeld D, et al. Comparison of postoperative radiotherapy and combined postoperative radiotherapy and chemotherapy in the multidisciplinary management of malignant gliomas. A joint Radiation Therapy Oncology Group and Eastern Cooperative Oncology Group study. Cancer 1983;52:997–1007.
4. Hall EJ. Radiobiology for the radiologist. 4th ed. Philadelphia: JB Lippincott; 1994.
5. Sneed PK, Gutin PH, Stauffer PR, et al. Thermoradiotherapy of recurrent malignant brain tumors. Int J Radiat Oncol Biol Phys 1992;23:854–61.
6. Florell RC, Macdonald DR, Irish WD, et al. Selection bias, survival, and brachytherapy for glioma. J Neurosurg 1992;76:179–83.
7. Hood TW, McKeever PE. Stereotactic management of cystic gliomas of the brain stem. Neurosurgery 1989;24:373–8.
8. Backlund EO. Colloidal radioisotopes as part of a multimodality treatment of craniopharyngiomas. J Neurosurg Sci 1989;33:95–7.
9. Pollack IF, Lunsford LD, Slamovits TL, et al. Stereotactic intracavitary irradiation for cystic craniopharyngiomas. J Neurosurg 1988;68:227–33.
10. Halligan JB, Stelzer KJ, Rostomily RC, et al. Operation and permanent low activity 125I brachytherapy for recurrent high-grade astrocytomas. Int J Radiat Oncol Biol Phys 1996;35:541–7.
11. Larson GL, Wilbanks JH, Dennis WS, et al. Interstitial radiogold for treatment of recurrent high grade gliomas. Cancer 1990;66:27–9.
12. Zamorano L, Yakar D, Dujovny M, et al. Permanent iodine-125 implant and external beam radiation therapy for the treatment of malignant brain tumors. Stereotact Funct Neurosurg 1992;59:183–92.
13. Kumar PP, Good RR, Jones EO, Leibrock LG. Intraoperative cobalt-60 treatment of glioblastoma multiforme. Radiat Med 1988;6:219–28.
14. Lucas GL, Ixton G, Cohen D, et al. Treatment results of stereotactic interstitial brachytherapy for primary and metastatic brain tumors. Int J Radiat Oncol Biol Phys 1991;21:715–21.
15. Malkin MG. Interstitial irradiation of malignant glioma. Rev Neurol 1992;148:448–53.
16. Stea B, Kittelson J, Cassady JR, et al. Treatment of malignant gliomas with interstitial irradiation and hyperthermia. Int J Radiat Oncol Biol Phys 1992;24:657–67.
17. Willis BK, Heilbrun P, Sapozink MD, et al. Stereotactic interstitial brachytherapy of malignant astrocytomas with remarks on postimplantation computed tomographic appearance. Neurosurgery 1988;23:348–54.
18. Loeffler JS, Alexander E 3rd, Hochberg FH, et al. Clinical patterns of failure following stereotactic interstitial irradiation for malignant gliomas. Int J Radiat Oncol Biol Phys 1990;19:1455–62.
19. Kitchen ND, Hughes SW, Taub NA, et al. Survival following interstitial brachytherapy for recurrent malignant glioma. J Neurooncol 1994;18:33–9.
20. Ryken TC, Hitchon PW, VanGilder JC, et al. Interstitial brachytherapy versus cytoreductive surgery in recurrent malignant glioma. Stereotact Funct Neurosurg 1994;63:241–5.
21. Chamberlain MC, Barba D, Kormanik P, et al. Concurrent cisplatin therapy and iodine-125 brachytherapy for recurrent malignant brain tumors. Arch Neurol 1995;52:162–7.
22. Bernstein M, Laperriere N, Glen J, et al. Brachytherapy for recurrent malignant astrocytoma. Int J Radiat Oncol Biol Phys 1994;30:1213–7.
23. Scharfen CO, Sneed PK, Wara WM, et al. High activity iodine-125 interstitial implant for gliomas. Int J Radiat Oncol Biol Phys 1992;24:583–91.
24. Shrieve DC, Alexander E 3rd, Wen PY, et al. Comparison of stereotactic radiosurgery and brachytherapy in the treatment of recurrent glioblastoma multiforme. Neurosurgery 1995;36:275–84.
25. Huncharek M, Muscat J. Treatment of recurrent high grade astrocytoma; results of a systematic review of 1415 patients. Anticancer Res 1998;18:1303–12.
26. Wen PY, Alexander EA 3rd, Black PM, et al. Long term results of stereotactic brachytherapy used in the initial treatment of patients with glioblastomas. Cancer 1994;73:3029–36.
27. Lucas GL, Luxton G, Cohen D, et al. Treatment results of stereotactic interstitial brachytherapy for primary and metastatic brain tumors. Int J Radiat Oncol Biol Phys 1991;21:715–21.
28. Sneed PK, Prados MD, McDermott MW, et al. Large effect of age on survival of patients with glioblastoma treated with radiotherapy and brachytherapy boost. Neurosurgery 1995;36:898–904.
29. Malkin MG. Interstitial brachytherapy of malignant gliomas: the Memorial Sloan-Kettering Cancer Center experience. Recent results. Cancer Res 1994;135:117–25.
30. Kumar PP, Good RR, Jones EO, et al. Survival of patients with glioblastoma multiforme treated by intraoperative high-activity cobalt-60 endocurietherapy. Cancer 1989;64:1409–13.
31. Patchell RA, Maruyama Y, Tibbs PA, et al. Neutron interstitial brachytherapy for malignant gliomas: a pilot study. J Neurosurg 1988;68:67–72.
32. Chun M, McKeough P, Wu A, et al. Interstitial iridium-192 implantation for malignant brain tumors. Part 2: clinical experience. Br J Radiol 1989;62:158–62.
33. Selker RG, Shapiro WR, Green S, et al. A randomized trial of interstitial radiotherapy (IRT) boost for the treatment of newly diagnosed malignant glioma (glioblastoma multiforme, anaplastic astrocytoma, anaplastic oligodendroglioma, malignant mixed glioma): BTCG study 87-01 [abstract]. Proceedings of the Congress of Neurological Surgeons 45th Annual Meeting; 1995 Oct 14–19, San Francisco (CA). p. 94–5.
34. Laperriere NJ, Leung PMK, McKenzie S, et al. Randomized study of brachytherapy in the initial management of

patients with malignant astrocytoma. Int J Radiat Oncol Biol Phys 1998;41:1005–11.
35. Sneed PK, Stauffer PR, McDermott MW, et al. Survival benefit of hyperthermia in a prospective randomized trial of brachytherapy boost + hyperthermia for glioblastoma multiforme. Int J Radiat Oncol Biol Phys 1998;40:287–95.
36. Sneed PK, Larson DA, Gutin PH, et al. Brachytherapy and hyperthermia for malignant astrocytoma. Semin Oncol 1994;21:186–97.
37. Prados MD, Gutin PH, Phillips TL, et al. Highly anaplastic astrocytoma: a review of 357 patients treated between 1977 and 1989. Int J Radiat Oncol Biol Phys 1992;23:3–8.
38. Kreth FW, Faist M, Warnke PC, et al. Interstitial radiosurgery of low-grade gliomas. J Neurosurg 1995;82:418–29.
39. Kreth FW, Faist M, Rossner R, et al. The risk of interstitial radiotherapy of low-grade gliomas. Radiother Oncol 1997;43:253–60.
40. Schupak K, Malkin M, Anderson L, et al. The relationship between the technical accuracy of stereotactic interstitial implantation for high grade gliomas and the pattern of tumor recurrence. Int J Radiat Oncol Biol Phys 1995;32:1167–76.
41. Valk PE, Budinger TF, Levin VA, et al. PET of malignant cerebral tumors after interstitial brachytherapy. J Neurosurg 1988;69:830–8.
42. Wald LL, Nelson SJ, Day MR, et al. Serial proton magnetic resonance spectroscopy imaging of glioblastoma multiforme after brachytherapy. J Neurosurg 1997;87:525-34.
43. Leibel SA, Gutin PH, Wara WM, et al. Survival and quality of life after interstitial implantation of removable high-activity iodine-125 sources for the treatment of patients with recurrent malignant gliomas. Int J Radiat Oncol Biol Phys 1989;17:1129–39.
44. Sneed PK, Gutin PH, Larson DA, et al. Patterns of recurrence of glioblastoma multiforme after external irradiation followed by implant boost. Int J Radiat Oncol Biol Phys 1994;29:719–27.
45. Agbi CB, Bernstein M, Laperriere N, et al. Patterns of recurrence of malignant astrocytoma following stereotactic interstitial brachytherapy with iodine-125 implants. Int J Radiat Oncol Biol Phys 1992;23:321–6.
46. Bernstein M, Lumley M, Davidson G, et al. Intracranial arterial occlusion associated with high-activity iodine-125 brachytherapy for glioblastoma. J Neurooncol 1993;17:253–60.

9

Radiosurgery for Brain Tumors

MICHAEL W. McDERMOTT, MD, FRCSC
PENNY K. SNEED, MD
RANDA ZAKHARY, MD, PhD
DAVID A. LARSON, PhD, MD

The treatment of brain tumors, primary and secondary, requires a multidisciplinary approach, and each phase of treatment has become more technically complex over time. Increasing levels of subspecialization for nurses and physicians are much more common today than even 10 years ago. Radiosurgery is a specialized radiotherapy technique that has grown rapidly in the last 10 to 15 years, and long-term results are now being reported. As opposed to standard fractionated radiotherapy, radiosurgery is the administration of the therapeutic dose of radiation in a single treatment session. The delivery of radiosurgery can be accomplished with a number of devices, each with its pros and cons. In the case of the Leksell Gamma Knife®, the device is dedicated to the treatment of intracranial targets.

At the University of California San Francisco (UCSF), our initial experience in radiosurgery was with a linear accelerator (LINAC)–based system. Since September 1991, we have used the Leksell Gamma Knife in two of its iterations: the U model (from 1991 to 1996) and the B model (from 1996 to the present). Our experience with this device is the basis of much of this chapter in terms of performing radiosurgery whereas the results of radiosurgery, for the most part, are applicable to LINAC, gamma-knife, or proton beam radiosurgery. This review is not meant to be exhaustive: rather, it is meant to point out the highlights of the treatment of primary and secondary brain tumors to those not familiar on a firsthand basis with the technology.

For the purposes of this discussion, "radiosurgery" will refer to stereotactic radiotherapy, in which the therapeutic dose is delivered in one session. The Radiation Therapy Oncology Group (RTOG) has defined radiosurgery as having the following components:[1]

1. Treatment of small targets
2. Application of a stereotactic head frame for target localization and accurate placement of an isocenter within the target volume
3. Convergence of multiple beams on the isocenter, with a steep dose gradient
4. Use of a single fraction of irradiation

Radiosurgery is not to be confused with stereotactic fractionated radiotherapy, in which relocatable stereotactic frames or frameless systems such as the Cyberknife (Accuray Inc., Santa Clara, CA) are used to deliver the full dose in several fractions.[2] Likewise, intensity-modulated radiation therapy (IMRT) is a technique in which multiple mobile vanes projecting into the primary collimator aperture allow for intensity changes across the beam.[3] Fractionated schedules for this treatment require accurate relocalization of the patient relative to the accelerator, with either skull-based talons or reinforced thermoplastic face molds. Fractionated stereotactic radiotherapy using a LINAC system frequently employs noninvasive relocatable frames using occipital pads, straps, and dental bite blocks.[4]

DELIVERY SYSTEMS

The most widely available system for the delivery of radiosurgery is a modified LINAC, used daily to treat other body sites on a fractionated-dose scheme.[5] Dedicated LINAC units are now commercially available, and mini-multileaf collimator units have also been adapted to these LINAC units. The first LINAC systems for radiosurgery were in use by 1984, and several variations followed. Each linear accelerator employs an electron gun that injects electrons into an accelerator tube; by the end of this tube, the electrons are traveling at close to the speed of light. Each electron collides with the metal target at the end of the tube, producing a photon of 4 to 10 MeV (typically 6 MeV). Movable primary collimators within the treatment head of the LINAC collimate the photon beam, and fixed secondary collimators can be attached to the treatment head to further "shape" the beam. The gantry on which the treatment head sits can rotate about an arc with a focal length of approximately 100 cm. With a combination of gantry and patient-couch rotation, a series of non-coplanar converging arcs that intersect the target is created that allows for the rapid decline in dose outside the treatment isocenter. The patient is fixed to the couch with a stereotactic head frame, the same head frame in which stereotactic imaging has been done with a fiducial localizing system that allows for calculations of target position in three dimensions and which is vital for treatment planning and dose-volume calculations. Assurance of accurate target localization and isocentric gantry and couch rotation is crucial for each isocenter of treatment. Thus, if one isocenter requires five non-coplanar arcs, confirmation of each arc for each couch position is required, and multi-isocenter treatments can be both labor and time intensive for the medical physics and radiation oncology staffs. A new instrument that is receiving increased use is the Cyberknife, a robotically controlled arm that positions a small X-band compact LINAC for delivery of multiple beams from a variety of angles, unconstrained by gantry or couch settings.[2,4] The localization of the intracranial target is based on co-registration of computed tomography (CT) and plain x-ray bony details and assumes constant relationships of the target to the skeleton. Patients can be placed in relocatable frames or thermoplastic head immobilizers for fractionated treatments.

The second most common system for radiosurgery is the Leksell Gamma Knife, models U, B, and C. There are 53 such units operating in North America and 144 units worldwide. This system houses 201 cobalt-60 sources that spontaneously decay with the release of two photons with an average energy of 1.2 MeV.[6] The photon beams from the primary collimator unit can be modified by the interposition of secondary head collimator units (or "helmets") that reduce the diameter of a single isocenter of treatment. The secondary collimator units are 4, 8, 14, and 18 mm in diameter. Plugging patterns in the secondary collimators allow for the deletion of entry and exit dose so that dose profiles can be shaped close to critical structures. The cobalt-60 sources have an activity at loading of about 30 Ci; the total activity of the 201-source unit is about 6,000 Ci, and the initial dose rate is 4 Gy/min. Given that the radioisotope has a half-life of 5.27 years, many units need to be reloaded after this time as the efficiency of treatment drops. The mechanical accuracy of the system is high, and the target isocenter is fixed so that each isocenter treatment requires confirmation of the x, y, and z coordinates set by treating physicians.

In the United States, there are only two active proton treatment facilities, at Loma Linda University and Harvard University.[7] The Berkeley unit was closed down in 1994. Although the cost of delivering stereotactic radiosurgery with protons is considerably higher (35% more) than with x-rays, theoretic advantages of isodose distributions exist because of the Bragg peak phenomenon. Particles lose energy along their path by way of collisions with electrons of atoms or the nuclei of atoms. The amount of energy the charged particle loses per unit of tissue traversed is inversely proportional to its velocity or energy. As the particle slows, more energy is deposited over a shorter distance. At the end of the particle path, there is a terminal collision of the treating particle with the target species so that both are annihilated and so that there is no exit dose. The range of particles is thus finite and is defined by their initial energy. However, the diameter of the

Bragg peak from a beam of uniform energy is generally too narrow to irradiate all but the smallest targets, so that several beams of closely related energies are combined to create a region of uniform dose over the depth of the target (the so-called spread-out Bragg peaks). Compared to photon irradiation, proton beams also have a sharp lateral dose decrease, which further adds to the precision of treatment and decreases the high-dose treatment volume.

RADIOBIOLOGY

The targets within tumors during radiosurgery are the proliferating tissues and the vessels supplying those tumors. The desired effects of treatment are reproductive cell death and tumor vessel thrombosis, while limiting the radiation effects in surrounding normal tissues. Kondziolka and colleagues and Lunsford and colleagues described the histopathologic changes that occur following radiosurgery in rat and baboon brain for a series of doses delivered in a single treatment.[8,9] In the rat brain, no pathologic changes were observed after 90 days for doses of 30, 40, 50, or 60 Gy delivered with a 4-mm collimator. Above 150 Gy, all rats had marked capillary endothelial cell damage, and all developed necrosis. In three baboons treated with 150 Gy to the caudate nucleus, all showed magnetic resonance imaging (MRI) evidence of a lesion 45 to 60 days after irradiation, and pathologic examination at 24 weeks confirmed tissue necrosis.

Photon radiosurgery of a given dose has a much higher radiobiologic effect on tumor tissue than the same dose given over a number of treatment sessions (fractionation). In normal tissue immediately adjacent to solid tumor tissue, the radiobiologic effect is also greater, and only by virtue of the steep dose falloff outside the target is the complication rate controlled. For normal tissues infiltrated by tumor, fractionation increases the therapeutic effect by (1) exploiting known differences in the ability of normal and tumor tissue to repair deoxyribonucleic acid (DNA) damage caused by ionizing radiation, (2) allowing for reoxygenation of tumor cells between fractions that may increase the sensitivity of tumor cells to radiation, (3) allowing for redistribution of cells into more sensitive phases of the cell cycle that may result in more damage to tumor tissue, and (4) irradiating repopulating tumor cells within the tumor with the successive doses in a fractionated schedule. These benefits of fractionation must be weighed against the disadvantages of tumor proliferation between treatments and the total time taken to reach a higher total dose in the target volume.

Hall and Brenner set forth their arguments for why they thought radiosurgery was suboptimal treatment for malignant tumors and for why it had an increased risk of toxic late effects in normal tissues.[10] They noted that late-responding tissues are more sensitive to changes in fractionation and that fractionation spares normal tissue for a given level of tumor damage. In a countering viewpoint, Larson and colleagues reviewed the radiobiology of radiosurgery as it is practiced for different target types.[11] Category I targets were those with late-responding target embedded within late-responding normal tissue, such as an arteriovenous malformation. Using a simple formalism for calculating the biologically effective dose (BED) for tissues with a low α/β, Larson and colleagues showed that the target within the prescription line experiences a BED of 100 to 200 Gy of fractionated radiotherapy whereas the tissue within a narrow rim of a few millimeters experiences only 10 to 30 Gy of treatment (Table 9–1). Category II targets were those with late-responding target surrounded by late-responding normal tissue, such as meningioma or schwannoma. Interior to the target periphery, the radiosurgery dose rises 20 to 40 Gy whereas a few millimeters beyond the target periphery, the dose drops to 5 to 10 Gy, a dose unlikely to cause any permanent effects. Category III targets were those with early-responding target embedded within late-

TABLE 9–1. COMPARISON OF RADIOSURGERY AND FRACTIONATED RADIOTHERAPY*		
	Fractionated Dose (2 Gy/fraction)	
Dose (Gy)	Normal Tissue, Late Responding (no. of fractions)	Tumor Tissue, Early Responding (no. of fractions)
10	30 (15)	16.7 (8)
20	110 (55)	50.0 (25)
30	240 (120)	100.0 (50)

*By biologically equivalent doses for early- and late-responding tissues.
Adapted from Larson D, Flickinger J, Loeffler J. The radiobiology of radiosurgery. Int J Radiat Oncol Biol Phys 1993;25:557–61.

responding normal tissue, such as a low-grade astrocytoma. In this example, the target tissue has an α/β of 10 whereas the normal tissue has an α/β of 2. With radiosurgery, the tumor tissue experiences a BED of 50 to 100 Gy or more of fractionated radiotherapy whereas the normal tissue within the target experiences a BED of 100 to 200 Gy of fractionated radiotherapy. For these targets, one would expect a higher complication rate with radiosurgery than with fractionated radiotherapy, and (to our knowledge) no one is currently treating these tumors at diagnosis with radiosurgery. Category IV targets were those with early-responding tissue surrounded by late-responding normal tissue; examples of these would be glioblastoma or brain metastases. Again, the target tissue receives a much higher dose within the prescription line than the normal tissue does outside of the prescription line. Malignant tumor tissue with a high α/β of 10 experiences a radiobiologic effect of 50 to 100 Gy or more of fractionated radiotherapy whereas the normal tissue outside the prescription line receives a radiobiologic effect of only 10 to 30 Gy of fractionated radiotherapy. Of note, the blood vessels within the tumor ($\alpha/\beta = 2$) receive a radiobiologic effect of 100 to 200 Gy or more of fractionated radiotherapy, which might be expected to cause vessel thrombosis on a delayed basis. Hypoxic tissues within the central part of the tumor will receive the highest dose, so that some inherent radioresistance of the hypoxic environment might be overcome. To date, published experience with brain metastases shows an excellent local control rate, supporting the use of radiosurgery over fractionation for these well-circumscribed tumors.[12–17]

RADIOSURGICAL TREATMENT USING THE GAMMA KNIFE

Patients are selected for treatment at a weekly multidisciplinary conference attended by neurosurgeons, radiation oncologists, radiation physicists, neuroradiologists, a clinical nurse specialist, and an administrator for the program. Consensus on treatment is reached for tumors deemed appropriate, and scheduling of treatment time is carried out. Patients are seen in consultation preoperatively by both a neurosurgeon and a radiation oncologist, and informed consent is obtained. Patient instructional videos are provided, and a path to the program Web site is provided to patients and families (see video clip on accompanying CD-ROM).

The morning of the procedure, the patient is brought to the preoperative area and changed into a gown and pants, and intravenous access is established. Intravenous sedation with lorazepam is offered prior to frame application. Droperidol is added for those patients who are claustrophobic. The neurosurgeon then reviews imaging studies to determine the anatomic position of the tumor(s) so that the frame can be positioned by placing the tumor as close as possible to the center of the frame (Figure 9–1). For a tumor in the right temporal lobe, the frame is positioned toward the right, "off center." We avoid using ear bars, which allows us greater freedom for frame positioning with patient comfort, and use a Velcro strap over the top of the patient's head to maintain the vertical position of the frame (Figure 9–2). With this technique, the frame is positioned, and the skin is marked for pin sites. The frame is then removed, and the skin over the pin sites is sprayed with ethyl chloride solution, which rapidly cools the skin and numbs it for injection of local anesthetic. We use a combination of 1.0 percent lidocaine and 0.5 percent bupivacaine with 3 cc of sodium

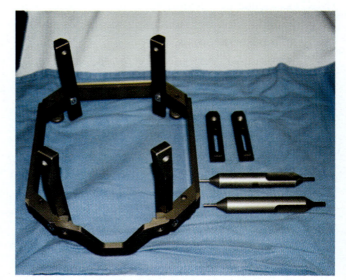

Figure 9–1. A Leksell stereotactic head frame used for gamma-knife radiosurgery, with front and long rear bars attached. Short rear bars and wrenches for securing bars are shown to the right. The frame is made of nonferromagnetic aluminum alloy, allowing it to be used for both magnetic resonance imaging and computed tomography.

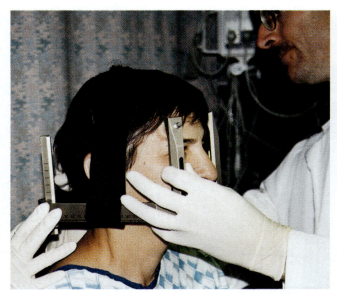

Figure 9–2. Positioning of a stereotactic frame, using a Velcro strap. For "off-center" positioning of the frame, pins of differing lengths are used at each corner. Here, placing the pins in diagonally opposed positions prevents the frame from slipping down.

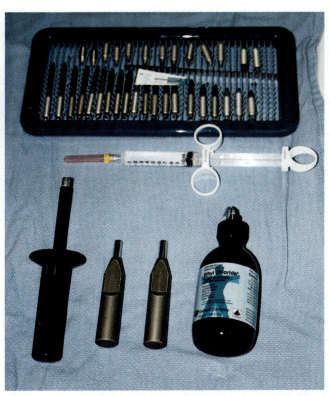

Figure 9–3. From top to bottom: tray containing a variety of pins of various lengths used to position a stereotactic head frame; local anesthetic solution (0.5% bupivacaine plus 1.0% lidocaine and sodium bicarbonate) in a syringe with a long 25-gauge needle; torque wrench (left), pin-tightening wrenches (middle), and ethyl chloride solution (right) for topical skin application.

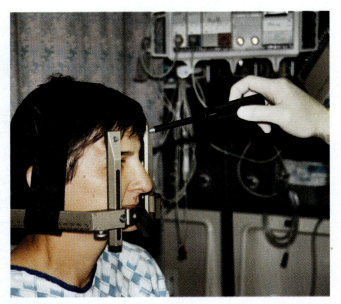

Figure 9–4. Final tightening of pins is done with a torque wrench for consistency and so that the frame is not overtightened, causing distortion of the frame base and an inability to match x values when the patient is in trunnions. We select a torque setting of 2 to 4-inch pounds for stereotactic frame application.

bicarbonate, injecting about 2 cc at each pin site (Figure 9–3). After injection, the frame is repositioned using the strap, and the pins are inserted at opposite corners to each other. The pins are tightened with thumb and index finger tension, and a torque wrench is then used to confirm a pressure of 2 to 4 inch-pounds of torque, which prevents the frame slipping from undertightening and prevents frame distortion from overtightening (Figure 9–4). Frame application using this technique has been successful under local anesthesia in all but a handful of 1,400 patients treated at our facility. Children under 14 years of age undergo frame application under general anesthesia.

Once the frame has been positioned, stereotactic imaging is done, using a fiducial localizing box attached to the stereotactic frame (Figure 9–5). The digital data file is sent to the Gamma Plan (Elekta Corp. Atlanta, GA) computer over the hospital ethernet, and images are scaled into stereotactic space. The neurosurgeon and radiation oncologist then outline the target volume(s), and the physicists derive the plan. For complex cases, targets are confirmed with the neuroradiologist prior to planning. The final plan is approved by both neurosurgeon and radiation oncologist, and a hard copy of the protocol is then printed out. The protocol defines the x, y, and z coordinates for each target isocenter; the gamma

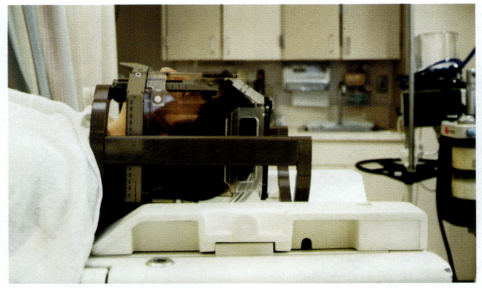

Figure 9–5. After frame application, stereotactic imaging is carried out with magnetic resonance (MR) imaging. A localizer box attaches to the frame base, and both are supported in a special cradle that fits into the patient table for the MR unit.

angle; the secondary head collimator size; and the irradiation time (Figure 9–6). For each target isocenter treatment or "shot," the treating physicians set the coordinates, have these checked, and then position the patient in the collimator unit by using trunnion bars that attach to "Z bars" on the base of the frame (see video on accompanying CD-ROM). For the U and B models of the Leksell Gamma Knife, each shot requires the re-entry of physicians into the treatment room for repositioning whereas with the C model, repositioning is done with computer-controlled electric motors for multiple shots with the same collimator (Figure 9–7).

At the end of the treatment time, the frame is removed, and patients under the age of 65 years and in good clinical condition are discharged after a 1-

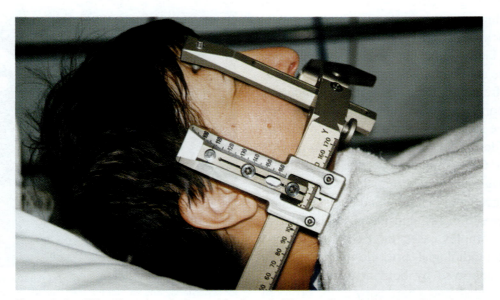

Figure 9–6. "Z bars" attach to the base of the frame holding a calibrated slider that allows the setting of z values in the vertical plane and y values in the horizontal plane. The x, y, and z values are calibrated in millimeters.

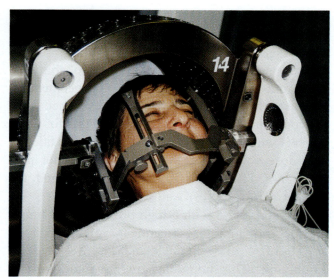

Figure 9–7. A patient positioned for treatment in a secondary head collimator unit. Horizontal trunnions attach to "Z bars" by a ball and pin set, and x value and gamma angle (axis of rotation through the center of the target) are set for treatment on a B model Gamma Knife.

hour period of observation. Those who are older than 65 years, who have limited motility, or who come for treatment from a distance are admitted overnight and discharged the next day. Those patients on steroids prior to treatment remain on the same dose for at least 5 days before a tapering of the dose is begun. Clinical follow-up is recommended at 3 weeks, 6 weeks, and 3 months. Repeat imaging is done at 2 to 3 months for malignant tumors (gliomas, metastases) and at 4 to 6 months for benign tumors (meningioma, schwannoma, pituitary adenoma). After the first year with no new lesions and with stabilization or response to treatment, the imaging interval is lengthened. After that time, the need for repeat studies at intervals of 6 to 12 months is determined on an individual basis.

CLINICAL RESULTS

Primary Tumors

Gliomas

To date, there have been no prospective studies showing a benefit for radiosurgery boost for primary malignant glioma following surgery and conventional fractionated external irradiation. The RTOG 93-05 trial is near the end of patient accrual, and results should be available soon. Reports from single- and multicenter reviews to date generally include patients with small tumors and in good neurologic condition. Most series since 1995 report median survivals that are 4 to 6 months longer than those of standard treatment; however, as in the case of brachytherapy, these patients were highly selected (Table 9–2).[18–23] Compared to high-activity brachytherapy implants, the early- and late-delayed toxicity of radiosurgery appears to be less. Immediate side effects from radiosurgery, such as nausea, dizziness, headaches, and seizures, are usually mild and self limited.[24] In a comparison of brachytherapy to radiosurgery using a linear accelerator for recurrent glioblastoma, Shrieve and colleagues noted that 22 percent of radiosurgery patients required reopera-

Table 9–2. RECENT RESULTS OF RADIOSURGERY FOR MALIGNANT GLIOMA*

Lead Author	No. of Patients	Original Pathology	Median Survival (mo)	Reference
Newly Diagnosed Gliomas				
Gannett	30	17 GM, 13 MG	12.9	18
Masciopinto†	31	31 GM	9.5	—
Sarkaria	115	96 GM, 19 AA	22.1	22
Larson	47	31 GM, 16 AA	14.5, 20.1	20
Kondziolka	107	64 GM, 43 AA	20.0, 56.0	19
Shrieve	78	78 GM	19.9	23
Recurrent Gliomas				
Hall	36	26 GM, 10 AA	7.0	26
Shrieve	86	72 GM, 4 AA, 10 A	10.2	25
Larson	132	66 grade IV, 27 grade III, 35 grade II, 4 grade I	9.2, 13.2, 12.2, NR	20
McDermott	79	37 grade IV, 19 grade III, 21 grade II, 2 grade I	9.4, 14.2, NR	27

A = astrocytoma; AA = anaplastic astrocytoma; GM = glioblastoma multiforme; MG = malignant glioma; NR = not reached.
*1995 to 2000.
†Data from Masciopinto JE, Levin AB, Mehta MP, Rhode BS. Stereotactic radiosurgery for glioblastoma: a final report of 31 patients. J Neurosurg 1995;82:530–5.

tion as compared to 44 percent of those treated with brachytherapy.[25] The same group reported their results in 1999 for 78 patients with newly diagnosed glioblastoma in whom radiosurgery was used to deliver a boost of irradiation after surgery and external irradiation.[23] In this study, the reoperation rate was 50 percent, and the median time to reoperation was 7.9 months, similar to prior figures with brachytherapy. Multivariate analysis revealed only age < 40 years as a significant predictor of outcome. When compared to the RTOG class outcomes for glioblastoma treated with standard irradiation, studies from Shrieve and colleagues and Kondziolka and colleagues noted improved survivals for classes III to V.[19,23] The 2-year survival rates for patients in classes III, IV, and V from these two radiosurgery series were 58 percent and 73 percent, 23 percent and 24 percent, and 23 percent and 26 percent, respectively. The corresponding 2-year figures for classes III, IV, and V from the RTOG standard-treatment groups were 35 percent, 15 percent, and 6 percent, respectively. Clearly, the results of the RTOG 93-05 trial (in which treatment with surgery, external radiation, and carmustine will be compared with the same treatment preceded by radiosurgery) are needed to clarify the impact of selection on outcome.

For recurrent gliomas, radiosurgery with or without chemotherapy is good salvage therapy for small localized enhancing tumors (Figure 9–8). In regard to recurrence, the results of radiosurgery are comparable to those of temporary or high-activity brachytherapy implants (see Table 9–2).[20,25–27] In one recent study, the influence of the probability of tumor outside the area of contrast enhancement on outcome was evaluated by magnetic resonance spectroscopy. Graves and colleagues found that for those patients with a low probability of tumor outside the high-dose volume, the median time to tumor progression (MTTP) was 8 to 10 months, and the median survival (MS) was 11 to 21 months.[28] By comparison, those with a high probability of tumor outside the high-dose treatment volume had an MTTP of 4 to 7 months and an MS of 9 to 13 months. This important finding indicates that functional metabolic imaging is an important tool for selecting patients for treatment, planning the target volume, and adding chemotherapy to the salvage regimen after radiosurgery (Figure 9–9). Lederman and colleagues reported on the results of "fractionated stereotactic radiosurgery" for 88 patients with recurrent glioblastomas for whom the MS was 7 months from treatment.[29] The authors found that MSs were longer for patients with tumors < 30 cc (9.4 months) than for those with tumors > 30 cc (5.7 months) ($p < .0001$). Stafford and colleagues reported the results of radiosurgery for recurrent ependymomas in 12 patients with 17 tumors.[30] With a follow-up of 2.5 to 60 months (median,

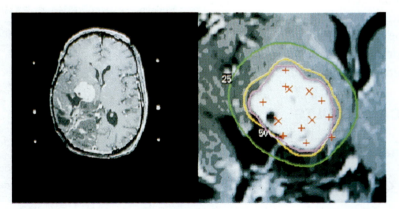

Figure 9–8. Recurrent right thalamic anaplastic astrocytoma. The astrocytoma was treated with Gamma Knife radiosurgery (11.0 Gy at 50 percent, 13 isocenters, 20.2 cc). The patient, a 39-year-old male, had been treated 16 years previously with radiotherapy (60 Gy) and 15 years previously with brachytherapy (111 Gy) and multiple surgeries for a right parietal glioblastoma. The enhancing volume was positron emission tomography positive. Note how the prescription isodose line (yellow) conforms closely to the shape of the contrast-enhancing tumor.

22.5 months), the overall MS was 3.4 years. Local control was very good for these recurrent tumors: 14 of 17 tumors were controlled, with an estimated 3-year control rate of 68 percent. There were 2 in-field failures and 1 marginal failure, and only 2 patients developed treatment-related complications. The authors felt that radiosurgery was a safe and effective way of providing local control in patients with recurrent ependymomas and that it deserved evaluation of its use in the management of high-risk patients after first operation.

Meningiomas

The standard treatment of meningiomas is surgical resection of the tumor and its dural attachment and associated hyperostotic bone. This resection is not always possible to achieve for meningiomas in a parasagittal, cavernous sinus, or skull base location. Arguments exist as to whether any residual tumor left after surgery should be treated. Donald Simpson's classic article from 1957 is still referred to for describing the natural history of risk of recurrence

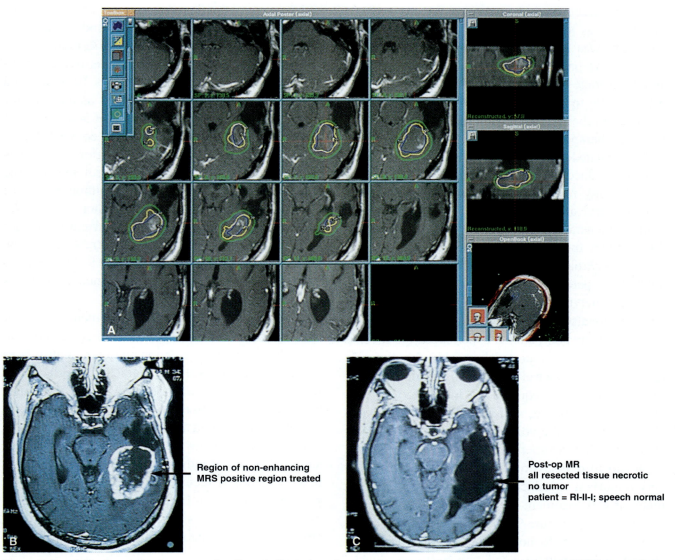

Figure 9–9. *A,* Treatment plan for recurrent malignant glioma, based on results of magnetic resonance spectroscopy (MRS) suggesting a high probability of tumor in non-enhancing tissue posterior and medial to the area of enhancement. *B,* Recurrent grade III. Two months after radiosurgery, a magnetic resonance (MR) image shows a large area of necrosis in an area of high-dose prescription (*arrow*). *C,* Recurrent grade III. Postoperative MR scan after reoperation for a necrotic tissue mass. Pathology is negative for tumor. The patient was alive, had normal speech, and was without further recurrence 12 months post radiosurgery but had right homonymous hemianopsia (RHH).

for meningiomas after varying degrees of surgical resection.[31] Recurrence rates of 9 percent (complete tumor and dural resection) to 40 percent (subtotal tumor resection) were reported for varying degrees of tumor and dural resection. In contrast, a recent review by Jung and colleagues found a very low recurrence rate among petroclival meningiomas after subtotal resection.[32] With modern imaging follow-up, the median progression-free survival was 66 months, and the 5-year progression-free survival rate was 60 percent. In the same article, the authors also reviewed 10 other series of these difficult tumors, beginning in 1980, and found that for the 400 combined cases (including their own), the average mortality was 4.5 percent (0 to 10%), the average morbidity was 23 percent (8 to 59%), the average cranial-nerve palsy rate was 48 percent (22 to 91%), and the average percentage of tumor resection was 63 percent (26 to 79%). A less aggressive surgical approach to these tumors, combined with postoperative radiotherapy or radiosurgery, is an option.

Fractionated external beam irradiation has been shown to reduce the likelihood of clinical recurrence for subtotally resected benign meningiomas and to prolong survival for patents with malignant meningiomas. Generally, doses of 5,400 cGy (in 180 to 200 cGy/day fractions, over 5.5 weeks) are administered by external techniques. Published control rates are 80 to 95 percent at 5 years and 70 to 85 percent at 10 years after treatment.[33–37] The complication rate with fractionated treatment is low, and only 3.6 percent of 140 treated patients experienced an adverse event in the series reported by Goldsmith and colleagues.[33] These control rates are the benchmarks for success that must be equaled by radiosurgery.

When appropriate, radiosurgery has the advantage of reducing the volume of normal brain irradiated during the treatment session and completing the treatment in one session. Targeting of the lesion is very important to reduce complications, and current imaging and treatment-planning software do much to achieve this (Figure 9–10). Those tumors with an en plaque shape do not lend themselves to radiosurgery and are better treated with fractionated techniques. For more spherically shaped meningiomas with a small dural attachment, it is not common to include the dural tail in the high-dose volume as this tail is felt to be consistent with hypervascular dura and not tumor. Hakim and colleagues reported the results of linear accelerator–based radiosurgery for intracranial meningiomas in 127 patients with 155 meningiomas.[38] The median follow-up was 31 months (range, 1.2 to 79.8 months), relatively short when compared to conventional irradiation treatment series. The median times of freedom from progression for benign, atypical, and malignant meningiomas were 20.9, 24.4, and 13.9 months, respectively. For benign meningiomas, the 3- and 5-year tumor control rates were both 89 percent. Permanent complications due to radiosurgery occurred in 4.7 percent of patients at a median of 10.3 months after radiosurgery. Kondziolka and colleagues reported the results of Gamma Knife radiosurgery for benign parasagittal meningiomas treated at 16 centers.[39] The median follow-up was 3.5 years, and 66 of 203 patients had radiosurgery as the primary form of treatment. In this group, the 5-year control rate was 93 percent ± 4 percent. In contrast, the 5-year control rate for those who had prior surgery was only 60 percent although the control rate for the treated volume was 85 percent and although most of the failures were due to distant tumor growth. We have also used radiosurgery for recurrent malignant meningiomas and have found the treatment to be effective and well tolerated (Figure 9–11). (Radiosurgery for recurrent malignant meningiomas is reviewed in a later chapter.)

The role of radiosurgery in the management of meningiomas will be further defined in coming years, but current information on tumor control rates and complications seems to indicate an established role. In one survey of patients 5 to 10 years after radiosurgery, 96 percent of patients felt that radiosurgery had provided a satisfactory outcome, and 93 percent of patients required no other tumor surgery.[40] Current indications for treatment include newly diagnosed, recurrent, or residual tumors after prior resection, with limitations on treatment being primarily based on size and proximity to critical structures such as the optic apparatus or brain stem.

Acoustic Neuromas

Acoustic neuroma, or schwannoma, is a benign tumor that occurs in the cerebellopontine angle (CPA) and

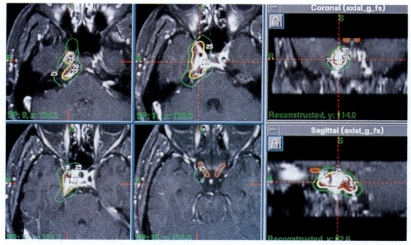

Figure 9–10. An example of a conformal treatment plan for cavernous sinus meningioma. The meningioma was treated to 16 Gy at 50 percent isodose line (IDL) to 5.5 cc (1.5 × 3.4 × 2.1 cm). The dose to the optic nerve/chiasm is limited to < 800 cGy.

that usually presents with a gradual onset of hearing loss, with or without associated tinnitus and dizziness. When the tumors become large, they can also cause symptoms related to compression and dysfunction of the fifth cranial nerve, with facial numbness; ipsilateral cerebellar dysmetria related to compression of the cerebellar peduncle; or symptoms referable to hydrocephalus due to kinking of the cerebral aqueduct or to the secretion of protein by the tumor, leading to a communicating form of hydrocephalus. Microsurgical resection has been the standard recommended treatment when the tumors are symptomatic. Lars Leksell, a Swedish neurosurgeon, began to use radiosurgery for the treatment of acoustic neuromas in the 1970s, and a number of clinical series have subsequently been reported. Three important series with more than 100 patients are summarized in Table 9–3.[40–42] Criticisms of radiosurgical treatment for this benign tumor are that the tumor is never removed completely and that there is still risk of radiation-induced injury to the brain stem and to the seventh, eighth, and fifth cranial nerves. There is a very low but theoretic chance of secondary tumor induction or malignancy generation following treatment, and this risk should be weighed against the risk of mortality with microsurgery and the risk of other unrelated tumors developing in another organ over the patient's lifetime. There is now evidence from patient questionnaires, surveys, and follow-up data after radiosurgery that the persistence of this benign intracranial

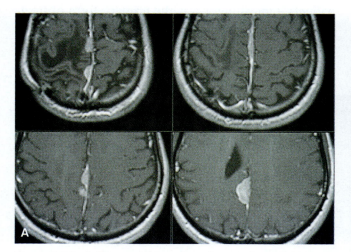
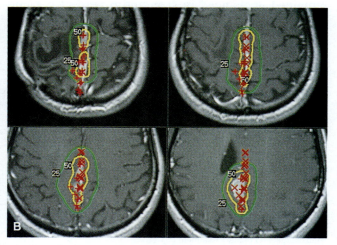

Figure 9–11. *A*, Recurrent falx malignant meningioma. *B*, Treatment plan for long, linear tumor recurrence in *A*.

tumor is not psychologically troublesome for patients and that their neurologic function can be well maintained.[43] The incidence of new cranial neuropathy following radiosurgery appears to be relatively low and acceptable from the patient's point of view. With modern imaging and beam shaping with collimator plugs, the dose to the adjacent brain stem can be limited to reduce the chance of complications (Figure 9–12).

Noren and colleagues reported the results from the Karolinska Institute in Sweden in 1993.[41] In the period of follow-up (12 to 120 months), 88 percent of tumors were either decreased in size or unchanged; 12 percent of tumors increased in size. The overall initial risk of facial weakness was 17 percent, but the risk decreased to 4 percent in long-term follow-up. Whereas 19 percent of patients experienced trigeminal neuropathy, there were no further cases after 1990, when the marginal doses were reduced. Using only pure-tone average as an assessment of useful hearing, Noren and colleagues reported a hearing preservation rate of 77 percent. Pure-tone average alone is generally regarded as a poor measure of useful hearing.

Kondziolka and colleagues reported long-term follow-up in 162 patients treated at the University of Pittsburgh between 1987 and 1992 in a survey between 5 and 10 years after the procedure.[43] Prior microsurgery had been performed in 26 percent of patients, and the average tumor margin dose was 16 Gy. Facial nerve function was normal in 76 percent of these patients before radiosurgery, and only 20 percent had useful hearing. After treatment, 62 percent of tumors became smaller, 33 percent remained unchanged in size, and 6 percent became slightly larger. Resection was performed in 4 patients (2%) within 4 years of radiosurgery. Normal facial nerve function was preserved in 85 percent of those who had normal facial function before radiosurgery. Eighty-four percent had normal trigeminal function after radiosurgery. Of the 32 patients who had useful hearing before radiosurgery, 47 percent maintained hearing within pretreatment levels. The authors identified treatment planning in the CT era as a significant predictor for worse hearing outcomes as compared to planning at later dates when MRI was used. The survey of patient satisfaction and outcomes was completed by 77 percent of surviving patients. When asked whether Gamma-Knife radiosurgery had met their initial expectations, 92 percent of patients said yes. Complications were described by 31 percent of patients and resolved in 56 percent of them. The most common complications described by patients after treatment were balance problems (6%) and facial twitching (5%). Radiosurgery was described as "successful" by all patients who had undergone previous microsurgery and by 95 percent of patients who had not undergone prior microsurgery. The authors concluded that this long-term follow-up 5 to 10 years after radiosurgery provided evidence that the treatment could provide long-term control of vestibular schwannomas while preserving neurologic function.

A recent article by Prasad and colleagues reviewed the experience at the University of Virginia, Charlottesville, as well as the preceding literature on the results of radiosurgery and microsurgery for acoustic neuroma.[42] Data from follow-ups of from 1 to 10 years were available on 153 patients treated with radiosurgery (mean, 4.27 years). In 96 percent of patients, radiosurgery was the primary form of treatment, and in 57 percent of patients, radiosurgery was used following microsurgery for treatment of recur-

Table 9–3. RESULTS OF RADIOSURGERY FOR ACOUSTIC NEUROMA*					
Lead Author	No. of Patients	Control Rate† (%)	Permanent Facial Neuropathy Rate (%)	Follow-Up	Reference
Noren	193	88	4	12–120 mo	41
Kondziolka	162	94	15	5–10 yr	43
Prasad	153	94‡ 89§	0	4–27 yr	42

*Gamma-Knife radiosurgery series with more than 100 patients.
†Tumor decreased in size or unchanged, not larger.
‡Radiosurgery as primary treatment (n = 96).
§Radiosurgery following microsurgery (n = 57).

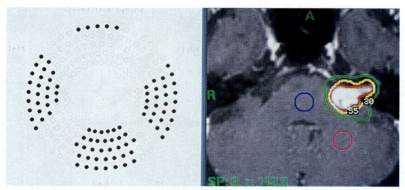

Figure 9–12. Example of a treatment plan for a left vestibular schwannoma, in which a plugging pattern is used to decrease the dose medially to the brain stem. The acoustic neuroma was treated to 13 Gy at 55 percent isodose line (IDL) to 2.6 cc (2.2 × 1.5 × 1.4 cm).

rence. The control rates in these two groups of patients were 94 percent and 89 percent, respectively. The authors reported a transient facial weakness incidence of 2.3 percent, and no patient had new permanent facial weakness. The transient incidence of trigeminal neuropathy was 4 percent and the permanent incidence was 1.6 percent. In 58 percent of the patients who had useful hearing before radiosurgery, hearing was preserved at the same level at a mean follow-up of 4.27 years. In contrast, 62.5 percent of all patients believed that their hearing was worse at follow-up than it had been before radiosurgery. The authors also summarized major microsurgical series of acoustic neuroma between 1984 and 1989. In those series with 190 to 1,000 patients, new facial neuropathy rates ranged between 1 and 19 percent, anatomic preservation of the seventh nerve was seen in 93 to 97.5 percent of patients, and hearing preservation was seen in 15 to 39 percent. Notably, there were other morbidities associated with open operation that were not seen with radiosurgery (eg, wound infection, cerebrospinal fluid leak), and there was a case mortality rate of between 0 and 2 percent. The authors concluded that microsurgery should be performed whenever surgical removal carried a risk-benefit ratio superior to that in their current study and that radiosurgery can be used to treat recurrent tumors after prior microsurgery as well as tumors in patients with medical conditions that preclude surgical treatment.

Clearly, some of the issues of outcome for radiosurgery, and microsurgery require further long-term follow-up. It is also clear that tumors associated with type 2 neurofibromatosis are more difficult to control with radiosurgery (Figure 9–13). It is doubtful that a randomized trial of microsurgery versus radiosurgery will ever be conducted. For the time being, it appears that the treatment is highly effective in inhibiting further tumor growth in more than 90 percent of patients in long-term follow-up (Figure 9–14).

Pituitary Adenomas

The standard treatment for pituitary adenomas is transsphenoidal microsurgical removal. Residual or recurrent tumors are often managed with postoperative irradiation using modern three-dimensional treatment-planning systems. Tumor control rates of from 76 to 97 percent have been achieved with fractionated external beam irradiation, but there is a risk of hypopituitarism related to the inclusion of the entire hypothalamic-pituitary axis in the field of irradiation.[44–46] Radiosurgery is now a well-accepted form of treatment for residual or recurrent tumors, especially when the tumors are localized to the sella or cavernous sinus. Suprasellar extension of tumor bringing it within 5 mm of the optic chiasm or nerves makes single-fraction treatment risky because of the late-delayed effects, with decline in vision or blindness. The single-fraction dose limit for the optic nerve and chiasm is approximately 800 cGy in current practice and must be lowered still in those who have had prior external irradiation.

Patients are selected for treatment on the basis of the failure of prior treatment where the pathologic

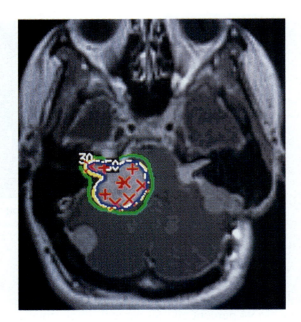

Figure 9–13. A patient with neurofibromatosis (NF) 2 and a large recurrent right-sided vestibular schwannoma, requiring a multi-isocenter treatment plan. The acoustic neuroma was treated to 12 Gy at 50 percent isodose line (IDL) to 11 cc (3.1 × 2.4 × 2.9 cm).

diagnosis has been established. Both functional and nonfunctional adenomas can be treated with the understanding that it takes months to years before hormone hypersecretion can be suppressed. This is not surprising given the fact that pituitary adenomas are slow-growing tumors and that DNA damage to cells will only be manifest when the cells attempt to divide. There is a component of tumor shrinkage and control that also relates to the effects on the tumor microvasculature, but again, this is a delayed effect (months to years). Landolt presented some intriguing data to suggest that the use of agents such as somatostatin and octreotide may actually offer some protection from the effects of irradiation for growth hormone (GH)–secreting and adrenocorticotropic hormone (ACTH)–secreting adenomas.[47] He recommends that patients be off medications for a period of time prior to radiosurgery.

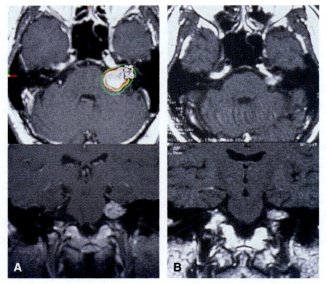

Figure 9–14. *A,* Images from the day of radiosurgery (RS) for a left-sided vestibular schwannoma. The acoustic neuroma was treated to 14 Gy at 50 percent isodose line (IDL) to 3.7 cc (2.4 × 1.9 × 1.7 cm). *B,* Fifteen-month follow-up images.

Kondziolka and colleagues have recently published the results of radiosurgery in 103 patients with pituitary adenomas over an 11-year period.[48] Seventy-four percent of patients had endocrine-active tumors, 32 percent had ACTH-secreting tumors, 22 percent had GH-secreting tumors, 16 percent had prolactin (PRL)-secreting tumors, and 4 percent had mixed GH- and PRL-secreting tumors. Radiation therapy had been administered to 17 percent of patients prior to radiosurgery. Over a mean follow-up of 40 months in 85 patients, tumor control was achieved in 95 percent of the patients. In 49 percent of these, the tumor volume was decreased; in 51 percent, it was unchanged. In the ACTH-producing tumors, normalization of cortisol levels occurred in 52 percent of patients at a mean of 16 months after treatment (Figure 9–15). For the GH-secreting tumors, normalization of GH-levels was achieved in 75 percent of patients and occurred at a mean of 29 months. This is in contrast to the University of Virginia experience, in which only 25 percent of GH-secreting tumors experienced remission at a mean of 20 months after treatment.[49] The results reported for Gamma Knife radiosurgery at the 10th International Leksell Society meeting in April 2000 are recorded in Table 9–4.[50–56]

Proton beam stereotactic radiotherapy, LINAC accelerator radiosurgery (SRS), and LINAC stereotactic radiotherapy (SRT) have also been used to treat pituitary adenomas. Yoon and colleagues reported an 80 percent imaging response/stabilization rate at a mean of 49.2 months after LINAC radiosurgery.[57] Seventy-nine percent of patients had an improvement in visual fields, and treatment-related complications were similar to those the same authors experienced with conventional radiation, with a 29 percent incidence of endocrine insufficiency. There were no visual or cranial neuropathy complications. Mitsumori and colleagues compared the results of SRS (n = 18) with those of SRT (n = 30).[58] The distribution of pathology was similar in the two groups, but in the SRS group, there were 4 patients who had received prior radiation, as opposed to none in the SRT group. The median tumor volume was also larger in the SRT group (5.73 cc versus 1.9 cc). The 3-year tumor control rates were 100 percent for SRS and 85.3 percent for SRT. Normalization of hormonal abnormalities was achieved in 33 percent of SRS patients at a mean of 8.5 months after treatment and in 54 percent of SRT patients at a mean of 18 months after treatment. Although the incidence of new endocrinopathy was similar in the two groups, 3 patients in the SRS group developed ring-enhancing lesions in the temporal lobe. None of the 48 patients developed neurocognitive or visual disorders attributable to treatment.

In summary, the treatment of residual or recurrent pituitary adenomas with radiosurgery is effective, both in terms of radiographic control of tumor and (to a lesser degree) with respect to normalization of hormone production. Preliminary data on the protective effects of receptor antagonists used for functional adenomas require further investigation and follow-up. Side effects from treatment appear

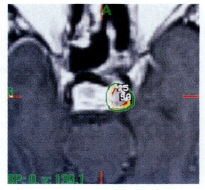 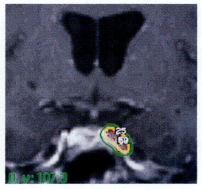

Figure 9–15. Treatment plan for a recurrent adrenocorticotropic hormone (ACTH)–secreting adenoma in the anterior superior left cavernous sinus. Residual ACTH-secreting pituitary adenoma was treated 1 month after transsphenoidal surgery (TSS) to 20 Gy at 50 percent isodose line (IDL) to 0.3 cc.

Table 9–4. RECENT RESULTS OF RADIOSURGERY FOR PITUITARY ADENOMAS*

Lead Author	No. of Cases	Control Rate (%)	Hormone Normalization Rate (%)	Complication Rate (%)	Reference
Baardsen	54	100	65.7 GH 100 (ACTH)	7.4 PI	50
Izawa	70	92	78 NS	2.8 V / RN	51
Leung	20	90	NFA	0	52
Mingione	68	98	NFA	0	53
Peker	14	100	100 GH/ACTH 83 PRL	0	54
Shin	16	100	67 GH 40 ACTH	6.2 PI	55
Vladyka	163	100	43 GH 85 ACTH 61 PRL	3.7 PI 0.6 V	56

ACTH = adrenocorticotropic hormone; GH = growth hormone; PRL = prolactin; PI = pituitary insufficiency; V = visual impairment; RN = radiation necrosis; NS = not stated; NFA = non-functional adenoma.
*As reported in the Proceedings of the 10th International Leksell Society Meeting; 2000 Apr. p.117–25.

similar to those previously reported from external irradiation, with a lower incidence of pituitary insufficiency. The key factors in avoiding problems appear to be (a) selection of appropriate patients (ie, tumor > 5 mm from optic apparatus) and (b) dose planning to limit the radiation dose to the optic chiasm and nerves (Figure 9–16).

Hemangioblastomas

Hemangioblastomas selected for radiosurgical treatment are usually those associated with von Hippel-Lindau syndrome, a neurocutaneous syndrome characterized by retinal and cerebellar hemangioblastomas. The cerebellar tumors are discovered more often now when they are small with current imaging techniques, and only the small tumors without an associated cyst are appropriate for treatment (Figure 9–17). When tumors that have a small associated cyst are treated, it is necessary to treat only the solid tumor and not the cyst wall. It is our experience that cysts may continue to grow in spite of radiosurgery, so if there is mass effect from the cyst more than from the tumor, the problem is better handled by open operation for cyst drainage and tumor removal.

A summary of recent clinical series using radiosurgery for hemangioblastomas is presented in Table 9–5. A multi-institutional report (by Patrice and colleagues in 1996) of the results of radiosurgery for 38 hemangioblastomas included patients treated on both linear accelerator and Gamma Knife units.[59] There were 18 primary tumors, and 20 were recurrent after failure of prior surgery. Eight patients were treated for multifocal tumors (total of 24). With a median follow-up time of 24.5 months (range, 6 to 77 months), the 2-year actuarial freedom from progression was 86 ± 12%. Smaller tumors (0.05 to 12.0 cc) were controlled better than larger tumors (32.0 to 10.53 cc), and tumors that received a median prescription dose of 14 Gy were more likely to fail than those that received a minimum dose of 16 Gy ($p = .0239$). In this study, 78 percent of surviving patients remained stable or clinically improved, and there were no permanent radiation complications. Niemela and colleagues reported that the median time to tumor response after treatment was 30 months.[60] Chang and colleagues observed radiographic response rates of complete response in 22 percent, shrinkage in 43 percent, and stabilization in 35 percent of 23 tumors followed for more than 2 years.[61] The reports by Niemela and colleagues and Pan and colleagues[62] both confirm the difficulty in controlling tumor-associated cyst growth after radiosurgery. In the report by Niemela and colleagues, 3 of the 5 tumor-associated cysts and 1 de novo cyst required surgical drainage after radiosurgery. Both reports concluded that radiosurgery was not a reliable method of treatment for controlling tumor-associated cysts. Complication rates seem acceptable,

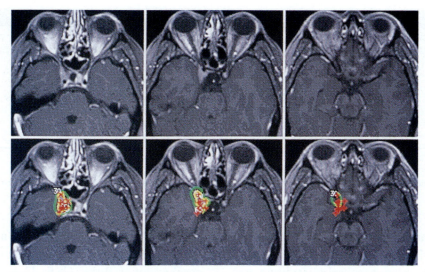

Figure 9–16. Treatment plan for a recurrent prolactin-secreting adenoma. Prolactinoma recurrent after transsphenoidal surgery 9 and 6 years earlier treated to 15 Gy at 60 percent isodose line (IDL) to 1.7 cc.

and Chang and colleagues, who reported radiation necrosis in 3 of 13 treated patients (23%), reduced their prescription dose to 20 to 25 Gy after the 2 patients treated with 35 Gy became symptomatic.

In summary, the current literature indicates that radiosurgery is an effective method for controlling hemangioblastomas, whether multiple or single, or primary or recurrent. The ideal tumors for treatment are small tumors (< 2 cm in diameter), tumors without associated cysts, and tumors that are several millimeters removed from the brain stem.

Malignant Skull Base Neoplasms

For the treating physicians, radiosurgery for malignant skull base neoplasms presents challenges related to tumor location, the aggressive nature of some histologies, and the high recurrence rate of the tumor in spite of treatment with surgery and fractionated radiation therapy techniques. Common neoplasms currently within the realm of accepted treatment for radiosurgery include nasopharyngeal carcinoma, adenoid cystic carcinoma, squamous

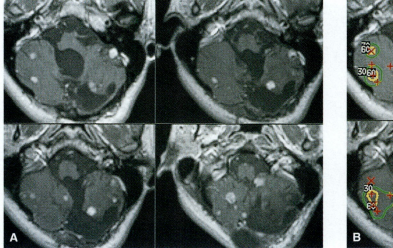
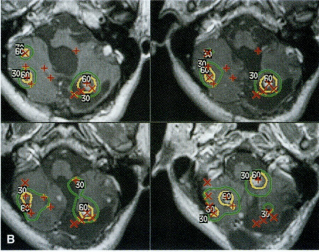

Figure 9–17. *A*, Pretreatment magnetic resonance images of a patient with von Hippel-Lindau syndrome and multiple small hemangioblastomas. *B*, Treatment plan, delivering 20 Gy to each lesion.

Table 9–5. RECENT RESULTS OF RADIOSURGERY FOR HEMANGIOBLASTOMAS					
Lead Author	No. of Patients	No. of Tumors	Control Rate (%)	Marginal Dose / Range	Complication Rate (%)	Reference
Niemela	10	11	91	25 Gy*/20–35 Gy	10.0	60
Patrice	22	38	86	15.5 Gy*/12–20 Gy	0	59
Pan	13	20	77	18 Gy/12–24 Gy	7.7	62
Chang	13	29	91	23.2 Gy/18–40 Gy	23.1	61
Jawahar†	27	29	84.5 (2 yr) 75.2 (5 yr)	16 Gy/11.7–20.0 Gy	NA	—

NA = not available.
*Mean dose.
†Data from Jawahar A, Kondziolka D, Garces YI, et al. Stereotactic radiosurgery for hemangioblastomas of the brain. Acta Neurochir (Wien) 2000;142:641–4.

cell carcinoma, chordoma, and chondrosarcoma (Figures 9–18 to 9–20).

Given the low incidence of primary bone neoplasms such as chordoma and chondrosarcoma, a large single-institution experience has yet to be presented. Muthukumar and colleagues reviewed 15 patients with malignant skull base tumors (9 with chordomas, 6 with chondrosarcomas) treated with Gamma Knife radiosurgery as an adjunct or alternative to microsurgical resection.[63] The mean tumor dose was 18 Gy (range, 12 to 20 Gy), and the mean tumor volume was 4.6 mL. Four of the treated patients died, 2 from progression of disease remote from the radiosurgery volume and 2 from unrelated disorders. Of the 11 surviving patients, 5 showed stabilization of disease, 5 showed a reduction in tumor size, and only 1 showed an increase in tumor volume (this patient went on to repeat microsurgical resection). During the mean interval follow-up of 4 years (range, 1 to 7 years), the authors felt that radiosurgery was a safe and effective treatment for small tumors. For larger skull base neoplasms, the advantage of fractionated particle beam radiotherapy is its ability to eliminate the exiting dose related to the Bragg peak effect, and it remains the benchmark treatment for these tumors. This is particularly true for tumors in close approximation to the brain stem or optic apparatus.

Complications of radiosurgery for these tumors are thankfully infrequent. In a review of 32 patients with newly diagnosed or recurrent skull base tumors, Miller and colleagues noted only one patient with radiation-induced optic neuropathy 12 months after radiosurgery.[64] Cmelak and colleagues noted major complications in 5 of 59 treatments of patients with skull-based malignancies and nasopharyngeal carcinoma.[65] This included 3 cranial nerve palsies, 1 cerebrospinal fluid (CSF) leak, and 1 case of trismus, for an overall rate of 8.4 percent. The authors found that complications were not correlated with radiosurgical volume, prior skull base irradiation, or radiosurgery dose > 20 Gy.

Nasopharyngeal carcinoma is a common malignancy in East Asia, and the persistence of local disease with later recurrence remains a problematic treatment issue. Tate and colleagues reported the results of stereotactic radiosurgery boost following radiotherapy in primary nasopharyngeal carcinoma.[66] Twenty-three patients received radiosurgery using a linear accelerator system following fractionated radiation therapy, and all had local control at a mean follow-up of 21 months (range, 2 to 64 months). External irradiation was combined with cisplatin chemotherapy in 15 of the 23 patients. Using a median radiosurgery boost dose of 12 Gy (range, 7 to 15 Gy) following fractionated doses between 64.8 and 70.0 Gy, the authors found no complications related to treatment by radiosurgery. However, 35 percent of patients (8 of 23) developed regional or distant metastases. The authors felt that radiosurgery provided excellent local control for advanced stages of nasopharyngeal cancer given the fact that 22 of 23 of their patients had stage IV disease.

Chua and colleagues reported their results of radiosurgery as a salvage therapy for locally persistent or recurrent nasopharyngeal carcinoma in 10 patients.[67] Tumor volumes ranged from 1.3 to 23.7 cc (median, 5.2 cc) and were treated with a median dose of 13.4 Gy. Median clinical follow-up was 10.5 months (range, 8 to 27 months), and the overall

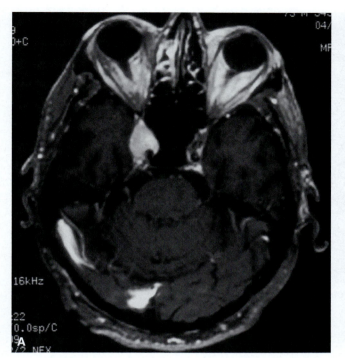 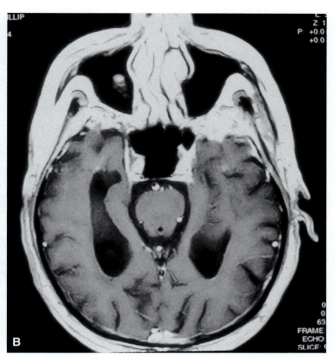

Figure 9–18. *A*, Right cavernous sinus adenoid cystic metastasis causing sixth-nerve palsy. *B*, Magnetic resonance image at 3-month follow-up, showing near-complete response with clinical improvement.

response to radiosurgery was 60 percent, with 10 percent of patients developing in-field progression. Only one patient developed a new cranial neuropathy in the absence of disease progression, suggesting that this was a form of radiosurgical toxicity. Lastly, Chang and colleagues recently described the use of radiosurgery for locally recurrent nasopharyngeal carcinoma in 15 of 186 patients with locally recurrent disease.[68] The addition of radiosurgery showed a trend toward improved 3-year survival ($p = 0.09$). The improved survival was related to tumor stage, a greater degree of improvement being noted for those with a higher stage of disease. In contrast, chemotherapy did not significantly affect survival.

Although the experience with radiosurgery for malignant skull base neoplasms is accumulating, there does appear to be a definite role for radiosurgery as a method of boosting local doses for tumors such as nasopharyngeal carcinoma and as primary treatment for small well-localized chordomas or chondrosarcomas that do not immediately abut the brain stem or optic apparatus. For recurrent malignant disease at the

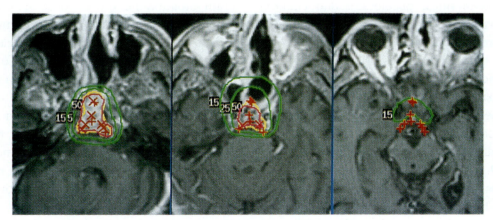

Figure 9–19. Treatment plan for a small upper clival and sellar chordoma.

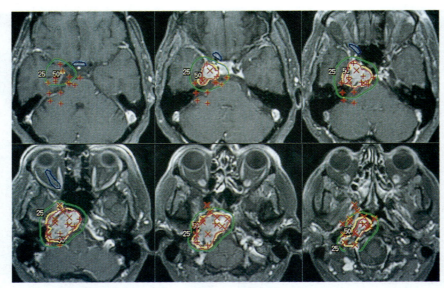

Figure 9–20. Multi-isocenter plan for a right petrous chondrosarcoma.

skull base, radiosurgery offers very reasonable palliation with good local control and few complications. Further experience and follow-up of treated patients will more accurately define the role of radiosurgery in this group of patients.

Brain Metastases

Brain metastases are a common oncologic problem, affecting up to 25 percent of cancer patients. Brain metastases account for nearly 40 percent of the patient load in the radiosurgery program at the UCSF. In the past, the majority of patients were managed with whole brain radiation therapy alone or with surgery plus whole brain radiation therapy, with reasonable survival and acceptable toxicity. Radiosurgery with linear accelerator and Gamma Knife units has demonstrated its effectiveness with respect to tumor control of treated lesions for patients with brain metastases. Radiosurgery has become an accepted method for palliation of patients with single metastases and small multiple brain metastases. A number of studies have revealed impressive local tumor control rates and survival rates, using radiosurgery alone equivalent to surgical series (Table 9–6).

One of the biggest issues is whether or not patients with brain metastases are best managed with radiosurgery alone or with the addition of whole brain radiation therapy. Whole brain radiation may cause diffuse white-matter damage and dementia in long-term survivors, and there is an interest in excluding whole brain radiation therapy in the initial management of patients with brain metastases.[12,15–17,69] The timing of the administration of these two forms of radiotherapy and their relative roles in the management of brain metastases are still not completely sorted out (Figure 9–21).

Kondziolka and colleagues reported the results of a prospective randomized trial of a whole brain radiation therapy with or without radiosurgery for patients with two to four brain metastases.[14] Selected patients had good performance status, with tumors < 2.5 cm in mean diameter and > 5 mm from the optic apparatus on MR imaging. Standard whole brain radiation therapy to a dose of 30 Gy in 12 fractions was administered, followed by radiosurgery to a dose of 16 Gy to the margin of each metastasis before, during, and within 1 month of whole brain radiation treatment. The study was to evaluate local control but was stopped early because of built-in interim analysis at 60 percent accrual. There was a highly significant difference in local control between the two arms; the median time to local failure was 6 months in the whole brain radiation therapy alone group versus 36 months for those receiving radiosurgery in addition. This study clearly demonstrated the superiority of combined therapy

Table 9–6. RECENT RESULTS OF RADIOSURGERY FOR BRAIN METASTASES

Author	Treatment Group	No. of Patients	No. of Mets	Median Local FFP	Median Brain FFP (mo)	Median Survival (mo)	Reference
Pirzkall (1998)	RS	158	1–3	89% at 1 yr	NS	~ 5.0	15
	RS + WBRT	78	1–3	92% at 1 yr	NS	~ 6.5	
Sneed (1999)	RS	62	1–6	21 mo	19.8*	11.3	17
	RS + WBRT	43	1–10	NR	18.1*	11.1	
Kondziolka (1999)	WBRT	14	2–4	6 mo	5.0	7.5	14
	WBRT + RS	13	2–4	36 mo	34.0	11.0	

FFP = freedom from progression; Mets = metastases; NS = not stated; NR = not reached; RS = radiosurgery; WBRT = whole brain radiotherapy.
*Allowing for successful salvage of a first failure.

for improving local control but was not designed to address whether improved local control produced a survival advantage. The median survival was 7.5 months for the group treated with whole brain radiation therapy alone versus 11 months for those who received combined treatment.

Two retrospective studies evaluating radiosurgery alone versus radiosurgery and whole brain radiation therapy for patients with brain metastases have been published. Pirzkall and colleagues evaluated 150 patients treated with radiosurgery alone and compared them to 78 patients treated with radiosurgery and whole brain radiation therapy.[15] Patients included in this review had one to three newly diagnosed brain metastases and Karnofsky performance scores of > 50. Patients were well balanced in terms of median age, performance status, and the presence or absence of extracranial disease. The actuarial local freedom-from-progression probabilities were 89 percent and 72 percent at 1 and 2 years, respectively, after radiosurgery alone versus 92 percent and 86 percent at 1 and 2 years, respectively, after radiosurgery plus whole brain radiation therapy ($p = .13$). The overall median survival times were not different between the two groups. When analyzed for those patients with no evidence of extracranial disease, the

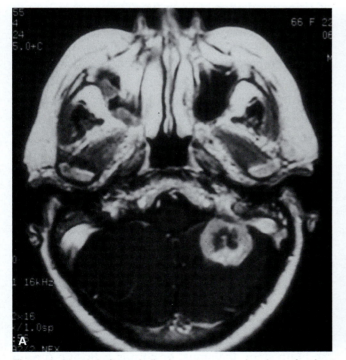 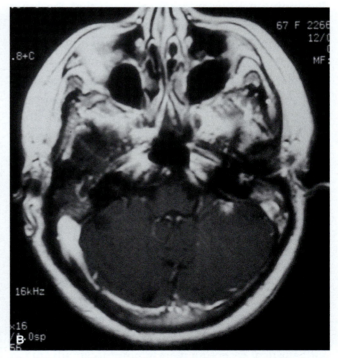

Figure 9–21. *A*, Left cerebellar breast metastasis prior to focal external irradiation and Gamma-Knife boost. *B*, Six-month follow-up image after completion of combined treatment.

median survival time for the group receiving radiosurgery alone was 8.3 months versus 15.4 months for the group treated with radiosurgery plus whole brain radiation therapy ($p = .08$).

Sneed and colleagues evaluated patients treated at UCSF between 1991 and 1997.[17] There were 62 patients who received radiosurgery alone while 42 patients received combined radiosurgery and whole brain radiation therapy. The two groups were balanced again for known prognostic factors, and the survival was identical for the two groups: 11.3 months for radiosurgery alone and 11.1 months for radiosurgery plus whole brain radiation therapy ($p = .80$). Analysis of patients without evidence of extracranial disease showed median survival times of 25.6 months for patients treated with radiosurgery alone versus 16.3 months for patients treated with radiosurgery plus whole brain radiation therapy. Importantly, freedom from progression of treated brain metastases was slightly but not significantly worse in the group receiving radiosurgery alone, with 1-year local freedom-from-progression probabilities of 71 percent for radiosurgery alone versus 79 percent for radiosurgery plus whole brain radiation therapy. In addition, the patients treated with radiosurgery alone had a twofold higher risk of developing new brain metastases, so that the brain freedom from progression was significantly worse in the group treated with radiosurgery alone. When an analysis was done allowing for a first salvage therapy for recurrence (salvage therapy consisting of radiosurgery, whole brain radiation therapy, surgery, or any combination of these), then the brain freedom-from-progression periods for the two groups were very similar: a median of 19.8 months for radiosurgery alone versus 18.1 months for radiosurgery plus whole brain radiation therapy ($p = .31$).

There is still a role for the surgical resection of brain metastases, particularly those metastases that are acutely symptomatic and related to increased intracranial pressure, causing focal neurologic dysfunction due to location, and metastases > 2.5 cm in diameter, with or without surrounding vasogenic edema. The results from prospective randomized trials of whole brain radiation therapy in combination with surgical resection clearly point to an advantage for combined treatments.

In summary, radiosurgery is an effective and appropriate form of therapy for patients with newly diagnosed or recurrent brain metastases. Combining radiosurgery and whole brain radiation therapy significantly improves local tumor control as compared to whole brain radiation therapy alone, but there is yet no evidence from a prospective study that indicates that this translates into a survival advantage. The two retrospective reviews of radiosurgery with or without whole brain radiation therapy cited above indicate that whole brain radiation therapy reduces the risk of new brain metastases but may not improve survival. A prospective randomized trial in patients with good performance status and limited extracranial disease is needed to evaluate radiosurgery plus up-front whole brain radiation therapy versus radiosurgery alone, and such a trial should include assessments of neurologic function, quality of life, and cost outcomes.

COMPLICATIONS

Complications after radiosurgery are usually divided by time intervals into acute (hours to days), early (weeks to months), and late-delayed (months to years) side effects. A variety of factors (including a history of prior irradiation, tumor type, tumor size, tumor location, and prescribed dose) determine how and when patients manifest the symptoms of toxicity. Flickinger proposed the integrated logistic formula for the prediction of permanent complications after radiosurgery alone or in combination with whole brain irradiation.[70,71] With this formula, a dose for a given volume can be selected that predicts a 3 percent risk of permanent complications. Subsequent studies, by the Pittsburgh group, of postradiosurgery imaging (PRI) changes after radiosurgery for arteriovenous malformations (AVMs) identified PRI changes in 30 percent of patients with AVMs, compared to 10 percent of meningioma and acoustic neuroma patients.[72] These studies also confirmed the fact that complications of treatment (and subsequent clinical symptoms) depend on the location of the treated lesion. After radiosurgery for AVMs, the risk of "postradiosurgery injury expression" was highest for lesions in the brain stem, thalamus, or corpus callosum (group 4) and declined, in order, for sites in the occipital lobe or basal ganglia (group 3); the cerebellum, temporal lobe, or parietal lobe (group 2); and the frontal lobe (group 1). Multivariate analysis found that the volume of brain receiving 12 Gy correlated significantly with the risk of radiation sequelae.

Recently, the RTOG published the final report of its prospective trial to define the maximum tolerated radiosurgical dose for recurrent malignant tumors after prior radiation.[16] The report analyzed 156 patients, 36 percent of whom had recurrent primary tumors and 64 percent of whom had recurrent metastases. Multivariate analysis revealed that tumor diameter, tumor dose, and Karnofsky performance score (KPS) were significant toxicity-associated variables. Tumors 21 to 40 mm in diameter (tumor margin dose, 15 to 18 Gy) were 7.3 to 16 times more likely to develop unacceptable toxicity compared to tumors < 20 mm. The incidence of unacceptable acute and chronic toxicities was 22% (35 in 156 patients). Fifteen were irreversible, 16 were life-threatening, and 4 were fatal (Table 9–7). Of the patients not on steroids at the time of treatment, 27 percent had to subsequently start them. Of the patients on steroids at the time of treatment, only 32 percent were able to discontinue them. Sixty-one percent of patients had an improved or stable KPS less than 3 months after treatment, and this percentage fell to 43 percent at 3 to 12 months. The actuarial risk of radionecrosis was 5 percent, 8 percent, 9 percent, and 11 percent at 6, 12, 18, and 24 months after radiosurgery, respectively.

To differentiate tumor recurrence from radiation necrosis after radiosurgery, a variety of functional imaging studies have been used, including single-photon emission computed tomography (SPECT), positron emission tomography (PET), and magnetic resonance spectroscopy (MRS). We have relied more than most centers on MRS because of the expertise of our neuroradiology research group.[28] A reduction in choline, choline/N-acetylaspartate (NAA) ratios, and ratios compared to normal brain can be seen in lesions that are radionecrotic.[73] Varying levels of creatine and lactate are expected, depending on the tumor type being imaged. In one study of 12 patients with glioblastoma treated with brachytherapy, MRS demonstrated spectral differences between residual tumor and contrast-enhanced radiation necrosis.[73] The study was also able to confirm the progression of tumor (in 9 patients) in previously normal areas outside the initial contrast-enhancing volume. The advantage of MRS technique is that it can be performed using standard 1.5-Tesla clinical MR units with software upgrades and special head coils. The volume of analysis in our research unit is now down to 0.13-cc voxels, making it sensitive and specific. Further developments will see increased use of MRS in combination with MRI to follow patients after radiosurgical treatment.

Table 9–7. COMPLICATION RATES AFTER RADIOSURGERY FOR RECURRENT MALIGNANT TUMORS*

Type of Complication	Incidence (%)	Median Time to Onset (mo)	Intervals to Onset (mo)
Irreversible edema requiring in-patient steroids	10	4.5	0.5–36.0
Radionecrosis requiring operation	10	5.0	4.0–27.0

*Includes malignant gliomas and metastases; final results of the Radiation Therapy Oncology Group (RTOG) 90-05 trial.

CONCLUSION

Radiosurgery is a powerful and effective form of radiotherapy delivered to intracranial targets in a single treatment session using stereotactic methods. The treatments are well tolerated and cause few complications in appropriately selected patients. There is a growing body of literature documenting responses for a variety of benign and malignant intracranial tumors. Further developments in treatment planning and delivery will shorten treatment times, thereby enhancing patient comfort and convenience. It is hoped that efforts to enhance the sensitivity of malignant tumors or to combine radiosurgery with other modalities of therapy will improve the already impressive local control rates achieved to date.

REFERENCES

1. Shaw E, Kline R, Gillin M, et al. Radiation Therapy Oncology Group: radiosurgery quality assurance guidelines. Int J Radiat Oncol Biol Phys 1993;27:1231–9.
2. Adler JR Jr, Chang SD, Murphy MJ, et al. The Cyberknife: a frameless robotic system for radiosurgery. Stereotact Funct Neurosurg 1997;69:124–8.
3. Barnett GH, Suh JH, Crownover RL. Recent advances in the

treatment of skull base tumors using radiation. Neurosurg Clin N Am 2000;11:587–96.
4. Shoshan Y, Suh JH, Barnett GH. Fractionated stereotactic radiosurgery. In: Germano IM, editor. LINAC and gamma knife radiosurgery. Park Ridge: American Association of Neurological Surgeons, 2000. p. 57–70.
5. Schultz CJ, Gillin M, Mueller WM. Modified linear accelerator radiosurgery: principles and techniques. In: Germano IM, editor. LINAC and gamma knife radiosurgery. Park Ridge: American Association of Neurological Surgeons, 2000. p. 19–30.
6. Yamamoto M. Gamma knife radiosurgery: technology, applications, and future directions. Neurosurg Clin N Am 1999;10:181–202.
7. Loeffler JS, Singer RJ, Chapman PH, Ogilvy CS. Proton-beam radiation therapy. In: Germano IM, editor. LINAC and gamma knife radiosurgery. Park Ridge: American Association of Neurological Surgeons, 2000; p. 71–4.
8. Kondziolka D, Lunsford LD, Claassen D, et al. Radiobiology of radiosurgery: part II. The rat C6 glioma model. Neurosurgery 1992;31:280–8.
9. Lunsford LD, Altschuler EM, Flickinger JC, et al. In vivo biological effects of stereotactic radiosurgery: a primate model. Neurosurgery 1990;27:373–82.
10. Hall EJ, Brenner DJ. The radiobiology of radiosurgery: rationale for different treatment regimes for AVMs and malignancies. Int J Radiat Oncol Biol Phys 1993;25:381–5.
11. Larson D, Flickinger J, Loeffler J. The radiobiology of radiosurgery. Int J Radiat Oncol Biol Phys 1993;25:557–61.
12. Chen JC, O'Day S, Morton D, et al. Stereotactic radiosurgery in the treatment of metastatic disease to the brain. Stereotact Funct Neurosurg 1999;73:60–3.
13. Chen JC, Petrovich Z, Giannotta SL, et al. Radiosurgical salvage therapy for patients presenting with recurrence of metastatic disease to the brain. Neurosurgery 2000;46:860–7.
14. Kondziolka D, Patel A, Lunsford LD, et al. Stereotactic radiosurgery plus whole brain radiotherapy versus radiotherapy alone for patients with multiple brain metastases. Int J Radiat Oncol Biol Phys 1999;45:427–34.
15. Pirzkall A, Debus J, Lohr F, et al. Radiosurgery alone or in combination with whole-brain radiotherapy for brain metastases. J Clin Oncol 1998;16:3563–9.
16. Shaw E, Scott C, Souhami L, et al. Single dose radiosurgical treatment of recurrent previously irradiated primary brain tumors and brain metastases: final report of RTOG protocol 90-05. Int J Radiat Oncol Biol Phys 2000;47:291–8.
17. Sneed PK, Lamborn KR, Forstner JM, et al. Radiosurgery for brain metastases: is whole brain radiotherapy necessary? Int J Radiat Oncol Biol Phys 1999;43:549–58.
18. Gannett D, Stea B, Lulu B, et al. Stereotactic radiosurgery as an adjunct to surgery and external beam radiotherapy in the treatment of patients with malignant gliomas. Int J Radiat Oncol Biol Phys 1995;33:461–8.
19. Kondziolka D, Flickinger JC, Bissonette DJ, et al. Survival benefit of stereotactic radiosurgery for patients with malignant glial neoplasms. Neurosurgery 1997;41:776–85.
20. Larson DA, Gutin PH, McDermott M, et al. Gamma knife for glioma: selection factors and survival. Int J Radiat Oncol Biol Phys 1996;36:1045–53.
21. Masciopinto JE, Levin AB, Mehta MP, Rhode BS. Stereotactic radiosurgery for glioblastoma multiforme. Stereotact Funct Neurosurg 1994;63:233–40.
22. Sarkaria JN, Mehta MP, Loeffler JS, et al. Radiosurgery in the initial management of malignant gliomas: survival comparison with the RTOG recursive partitioning analysis. Radiation Therapy Oncology Group. Int J Radiat Oncol Biol Phys 1995;32:931–41.
23. Shrieve DC, Alexander E 3rd, Black PM, et al. Treatment of patients with primary glioblastoma multiforme with standard postoperative radiotherapy and radiosurgical boost: prognostic factors and long-term outcome. J Neurosurg 1999;90:72–7.
24. Werner-Wasik M, Rudoler S, Preston PE, et al. Immediate side effects of stereotactic radiotherapy and radiosurgery. Int J Radiat Oncol Biol Phys 1999;43:299–304.
25. Shrieve DC, Alexander E 3rd, Wen PY, et al. Comparison of stereotactic radiosurgery and brachytherapy in the treatment of recurrent glioblastoma multiforme. Neurosurgery 1995;36:275–84.
26. Hall WA, Djalilian HR, Sperduto PW, et al. Stereotactic radiosurgery for recurrent malignant gliomas. J Clin Oncol 1995;13:1642–8.
27. McDermott M, Sneed P, Chang S, et al. Results of radiosurgery for recurrent gliomas. Radiosurgery 1996;1:102–12.
28. Graves EE, Nelson SJ, Vigneron DB, et al. A preliminary study of the prognostic value of proton magnetic resonance spectroscopic imaging in gamma knife radiosurgery of recurrent malignant gliomas. Neurosurgery 2000;46:319–28.
29. Lederman G, Wronski M, Arbit E, et al. Treatment of recurrent glioblastoma multiforme using fractionated stereotactic radiosurgery and concurrent paclitaxel. Am J Clin Oncol 2000;23:155–9.
30. Stafford SL, Pollock BE, Foote RL, et al. Stereotactic radiosurgery for recurrent ependymoma. Cancer 2000;88:870–5.
31. Simpson D. The recurrence of intracranial meningiomas after surgical treatment. J Neurol Neurosurg Psychiatry 1957;20:22–39.
32. Jung HW, Yoo H, Paek SH, Choi KS. Long-term outcome and growth rate of subtotally resected petroclival meningiomas: experience with 38 cases. Neurosurgery 2000;46:567–75.
33. Goldsmith BJ, Wara WM, Wilson CB, Larson DA. Postoperative irradiation for subtotally resected meningiomas: a retrospective analysis of 140 patients treated from 1967 to 1990. J Neurosurg 1994;80:195–201.
34. Hug EB, Devries A, Thornton AF, et al. Management of atypical and malignant meningiomas: role of high-dose, 3D-conformal radiation therapy. J Neurooncol 2000;48:151–60.
35. Maguire PD, Clough R, Friedman AH, Halperin EC. Fractionated external-beam radiation therapy for menin-

giomas of the cavernous sinus. Int J Radiat Oncol Biol Phys 1999;44:75–9.
36. Maire JP, Caudry M, Guerin J, et al. Fractionated radiation therapy in the treatment of intracranial meningiomas: local control, functional efficacy, and tolerance in 91 patients. Int J Radiat Oncol Biol Phys 1995;33:315–21.
37. Nutting C, Brada M, Brazil L, et al. Radiotherapy in the treatment of benign meningioma of the skull base. J Neurosurg 1999;90:823–7.
38. Hakim R, Alexander E 3rd, Loeffler JS, et al. Results of linear accelerator-based radiosurgery for intracranial meningiomas. Neurosurgery 1998;42:446–54.
39. Kondziolka D, Flickinger JC, Perez B. Judicious resection and/or radiosurgery for parasagittal meningiomas: outcomes from a multicenter review. Gamma Knife Meningioma Study Group. Neurosurgery 1998;43:405–14.
40. Kondziolka D, Levy EI, Niranjan A, et al. Long-term outcomes after meningioma radiosurgery: physician and patient perspectives. J Neurosurg 1999;91:44–50.
41. Noren G, Greitz D, Hirsch A, Lax I. Gamma knife surgery in acoustic tumours. Acta Neurochir Suppl (Wien) 1993;58:104–7.
42. Prasad D, Steiner M, Steiner L. Gamma surgery for vestibular schwannoma. J Neurosurg 2000;92:745–59.
43. Kondziolka D, Lunsford LD, McLaughlin MR, Flickinger JC. Long-term outcomes after radiosurgery for acoustic neuromas. N Engl J Med 1998;339:1426–33.
44. Flickinger JC, Nelson PB, Martinez AJ, et al. Radiotherapy of nonfunctional adenomas of the pituitary gland. Results with long-term follow-up. Cancer 1989;63:2409–14.
45. Rush S, Cooper PR. Symptom resolution, tumor control, and side effects following postoperative radiotherapy for pituitary macroadenomas. Int J Radiat Oncol Biol Phys 1997;37:1031–4.
46. Salinger DJ, Brady LW, Miyamoto CT. Radiation therapy in the treatment of pituitary adenomas. Am J Clin Oncol 1992;15:467–73.
47. Landolt A. Radiosurgery for functional pituitary adenomas. Proceedings of the 10th International Meeting of the Leksell Gamma Knife Society; 2000; April 14–20. Squaw Valley, CA.
48. Kondziolka D, Atteberry DS, Lunsford LD. Gamma knife radiosurgery for meningiomas, schwannomas, and pituitary tumors. In: Germano IM, editor. LINAC and Gamma Knife radiosurgery. Park Ridge: American Association of Neurological Surgeons; 1999. p. 207–19.
49. Laws ER, Vance ML. Radiosurgery for pituitary tumors and craniopharyngiomas. Neurosurg Clin N Am 1999;10:327–36.
50. Baardsen R, Pedersen P. Gamma knife radiosurgery for pituitary adenomas since 1989 in Norway. Proceedings of the 10th International Meeting of the Leksell Gamma Knife Society; 2000; Squaw Valley, CA. p. 117.
51. Izawa M, Hayashi M, Nakaya K, et al. Gamma knife radiosurgery for pituitary adenomas. J Neurosurg 2000;93 (Suppl 3):19–22.
52. Leung S, Yue C, Ho R. Minimally invasive approach for management of pituitary tumour. Proceedings of the 10th International Meeting of the Leksell Gamma Knife Society; 2000; Squaw Valley, CA.
53. Mingione V, Prasad D, Vance M, et al. Gamma surgery in nonfunctioning pituitary macroadenomas: a 10 year retrospective. Proceedings of the 10th International Meeting of the Leksell Gamma Knife Society; 2000; Squaw Valley, CA.
54. Peker S, Kilic T, Seker A, et al. Gamma knife radiosurgery for pituitary adenomas. Proceedings of the 10th International Meeting of the Leksell Gamma Knife Society; 2000; Squaw Valley, CA.
55. Shin M, Kurita H, Kawamoto S, et al. Stereotactic radiosurgery for pituitary adenoma invading the cavernous sinus. J Neurosurg 2000;93(Suppl 3):2–5.
56. Vladyka V, Subrt O, Lisak R, et al. Gamma knife radiosurgery for pituitary adenomas: evaluation of a series of 163 patients. Proceedings of the 10th International Meeting of the Leksell Gamma Knife Society; 2000; Squaw Valley, CA.
57. Yoon SC, Suh TS, Jang HS, et al. Clinical results of 24 pituitary macroadenomas with LINAC-based stereotactic radiosurgery. Int J Radiat Oncol Biol Phys 1998;41:849–53.
58. Mitsumori M, Shrieve DC, Alexander E 3rd, et al. Initial clinical results of LINAC-based stereotactic radiosurgery and stereotactic radiotherapy for pituitary adenomas. Int J Radiat Oncol Biol Phys 1998;42:573–80.
59. Patrice SJ, Sneed PK, Flickinger JC, et al. Radiosurgery for hemangioblastoma: results of a multiinstitutional experience. Int J Radiat Oncol Biol Phys 1996;35:493–9.
60. Niemela M, Lim YJ, Soderman M, et al. Gamma knife radiosurgery in 11 hemangioblastomas. J Neurosurg 1996;85:591–6.
61. Chang SD, Meisel JA, Hancock SL, et al. Treatment of hemangioblastomas in von Hippel-Lindau disease with linear accelerator-based radiosurgery. Neurosurgery 1998;43:28–35.
62. Pan L, Wang EM, Wang BJ, et al. Gamma knife radiosurgery for hemangioblastomas. Stereotact Funct Neurosurg 1998;70(Suppl 1):179–86.
63. Muthukumar N, Kondziolka D, Lunsford LD, Flickinger JC. Stereotactic radiosurgery for chordoma and chondrosarcoma: further experiences. Int J Radiat Oncol Biol Phys 1998;41:387–92.
64. Miller RC, Foote RL, Coffey RJ, et al. The role of stereotactic radiosurgery in the treatment of malignant skull base tumors. Int J Radiat Oncol Biol Phys 1997;39:977–81.
65. Cmelak AJ, Cox RS, Adler JR, et al. Radiosurgery for skull base malignancies and nasopharyngeal carcinoma. Int J Radiat Oncol Biol Phys 1997;37:997–1003.
66. Tate DJ, Adler JR Jr, Chang SD, et al. Stereotactic radiosurgical boost following radiotherapy in primary nasopharyngeal carcinoma: impact on local control. Int J Radiat Oncol Biol Phys 1999;45:915–21.
67. Chua DT, Sham JS, Hung KN, et al. Stereotactic radiosurgery as a salvage treatment for locally persistent and recurrent nasopharyngeal carcinoma. Head Neck 1999;21:620–6.

68. Chang JT, See LC, Liao CT, et al. Locally recurrent nasopharyngeal carcinoma. Radiother Oncol 2000;54:135–42.
69. Shaw E, Scott C, Souhami L, et al. Radiosurgery for the treatment of previously irradiated recurrent primary brain tumors and brain metastases: initial report of Radiation Therapy Oncology Group protocol (90-05). Int J Radiat Oncol Biol Phys 1996;34:647–54.
70. Flickinger JC. An integrated logistic formula for prediction of complications from radiosurgery. Int J Radiat Oncol Biol Phys 1989;17:879–85.
71. Flickinger JC, Schell MC, Larson DA. Estimation of complications for linear accelerator radiosurgery with the integrated logistic formula. Int J Radiat Oncol Biol Phys 1990;19:143–8.
72. Flickinger JC, Kondziolka D, Pollock BE, et al. Complications from arteriovenous malformation radiosurgery: multivariate analysis and risk modeling. Int J Radiat Oncol Biol Phys 1997;38:485–90.
73. Wald L, Nelson S, Day M, et al. Serial proton magnetic resonance spectroscopy imaging of glioblastoma multiforme after brachytherapy. J Neurosurg 1997;87:525–34.

10

Systemic Chemotherapy of Central Nervous System Tumors

KATHERINE E. WARREN, MD
HOWARD A. FINE, MD

Surgery and radiation are frontline treatments for patients with malignant primary brain tumors, but these modalities alone are rarely curative. Moreover, the major improvements in surgical and radiation techniques over the past 25 years have not translated into a substantially improved prognosis for the majority of patients with malignant brain tumors. The primary reason for treatment failure is the infiltrative nature of some tumors, particularly the malignant gliomas, which precludes performance of a true total resection. Cell-cycle kinetic studies have shown that the cells that migrate into the normal brain around the tumor are the most viable and have the highest capacity for proliferation.[1,2] For this reason, the tumors tend to recur after surgery or local radiation.[3,4]

Chemotherapy is a systemic treatment modality that can be used in attempts to eradicate the infiltrative tumor cells. It is used as adjuvant therapy with surgery and radiation in newly diagnosed patients and for recurrent disease, but its effectiveness in an adjuvant setting is difficult to ascertain. A modest improvement in median survival with the addition of single-agent or combination chemotherapy has been demonstrated in several trials.[5–7] In addition, a meta-analysis of 16 randomized clinical trials, which included more than 3,000 patients treated between 1975 and 1989, demonstrated a survival benefit for those patients with malignant gliomas treated with radiation and adjuvant chemotherapy compared to those treated with radiation therapy alone.[8] Overall median survival increased from 9.4 months for patients treated with radiation to 12 months for patients treated with radiation and adjuvant chemotherapy.[8] A separate retrospective analysis of 689 patients with glioblastoma multiforme diagnosed between 1975 and 1991 demonstrated that long-term survival was more likely in patients with a high performance status at diagnosis who received adjuvant chemotherapy compared to age, sex, and year-of-diagnosis controls who did not receive chemotherapy.[9] A study that reviewed data from two Brain Tumor Study Group protocols (including patients with glioblastoma multiforme or other types of anaplastic glioma) demonstrated an increased number of long-term survivors in the group of patients who received adjuvant chemotherapy with carmustine (BCNU) compared to the patients who were treated with radiation alone, regardless of prognostic factors.[10] Yet, because many trials are small, benefits in survival are modest at best, and confounding variables and prognostic factors have not been controlled for in many studies, the benefit of chemotherapy continues to be questioned, and its role in the treatment of these patients continues to be defined.

PRINCIPLES OF CENTRAL NERVOUS SYSTEM PHARMACOLOGY

A determinant of tumor response to a chemotherapeutic agent is the degree of exposure of the tumor cells to the active form of the drug. Exposure is determined by both the concentration of the drug at the tumor site and the length of time the tumor is exposed to the drug. The concentration of drug that reaches a tumor within the brain parenchyma is determined by numerous factors (Table 10–1). The central nervous system (CNS) is considered a pharmacologic sanctuary because drug delivery to the brain via systemic administration is often difficult and incomplete. Various methods have been attempted to increase drug delivery to the CNS, with the assumption that there is an increased likelihood of response if more drug reaches a tumor.

Drug Administration

Most chemotherapy drugs in current use are cytotoxic and kill cells when cells are actively dividing. Cytotoxic agents are generally classified as cell-cycle specific or cell-cycle nonspecific. Cell-cycle–specific agents act primarily during cell division and must be present in the tumor cells in effective concentrations at this critical point. In brain tumors, the actively dividing population is relatively small (10 to 30%);[11] therefore, continuous infusion (intravenous [IV] administration for ≥ 24 hours) would maximize the number of actively cycling cells exposed to sustained effective levels of drug.[12] Agents that are cell-cycle nonspecific can be administered as an IV bolus (IV administration in < 15 minutes). This achieves rapid peak plasma concentrations that then decline rapidly as the drug is distributed, metabolized, and excreted. Some chemotherapeutic agents (eg, temozolomide, lomustine (CCNU), procarbazine, and tamoxifen) may be administered orally. Although easier to administer, oral therapy is complicated by differences in bioavailability, which is affected by drug stability in gastric acid, absorption through gastric mucosa, inactivation by intestinal enzymes, hepatic metabolism, biliary excretion, and treatment-induced emesis.[13]

Blood-Brain Barrier

All systemically administered chemotherapeutic agents must cross the capillary endothelial cells of the cerebral vasculature to gain access to tumor cells in the brain. These capillary endothelial cells form a single layer of specialized vascular endothelial cells known as the blood-brain barrier (BBB). The BBB functions to maintain a precise neuronal environment by limiting the entry of toxins into the brain parenchyma. The endothelial cells comprising the BBB differ from other endothelial cells in that they have extended tight junctions, lack fenestrations and

Table 10–1. FACTORS AFFECTING DRUG LEVELS AT THE TUMOR SITE

Concentration of drug in the bloodstream
Degree of protein and tissue binding
Rate of blood flow to the tumor
Amount of drug able to cross the BBB
Diffusion of drug across the brain parenchyma
Amount of free, unbound drug crossing the tumor cell membrane

BBB = blood-brain barrier.

pinocytotic vesicles, and express specific transport mediators[14] (Figure 10–1). The passage of substances across the BBB depends on their size, lipid solubility, and ionization state.[15] Most hydrophilic substances and large lipophilic substances (which include many chemotherapeutic compounds) are restricted from entering the CNS. Smaller (< 180 MW [daltons]) lipophilic compounds are able to pass through the BBB, penetrating the lipid membranes by simple passive diffusion.

Drug Distribution

If a drug is able to cross the BBB, it is then distributed from the capillaries to the brain parenchyma, following the laws of diffusion. Diffusion of a lipid-soluble drug depends on its physicochemical properties, including the lipid/aqueous partition coefficients, molecular size, and charge.[16] Tissue characteristics including blood flow, cellularity, extracellular fluid composition, drug metabolism, and clearance will affect the tissue drug concentration. These tissue factors may differ in blood, tumor, and brain parenchyma.[17] Consequently, the final concentration of a drug in brain tissue or tumor is difficult to predict by its plasma pharmacokinetics.[18,19] Because it is not feasible to obtain tumor tissue biopsy specimens at multiple time points, the concentration of drug in the cerebrospinal fluid (CSF) is often used as a surrogate for the concentration of drug in the brain parenchyma. Although it is easier to obtain samples, it is unknown how predictive CSF drug levels are of drug levels in brain interstitium. The blood-CSF barrier differs from the BBB, and the distribution of drug in the CSF may be variable.[20] Microdialysis techniques for measuring the concentration of specific drugs in the extracellular fluid of

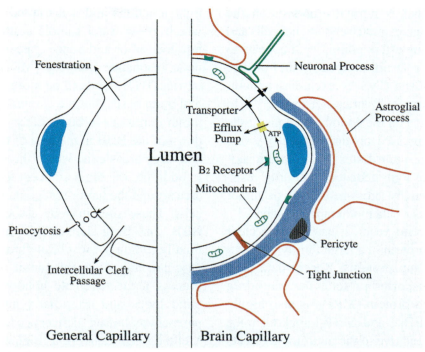

Figure 10–1. Schematic drawing comparing the typical endothelial cell to the endothelial cells of the blood-brain barrier (BBB). ATP = adenosine triphosphate. Reproduced with permission from Patel M, Blaney S, Balis F. A clinician's guide to chemotherapy. In: Grochow L, editor. Pharmacokinetics and pharmacodynamics. Baltimore: Lippincott, Williams & Wilkins; 1998. p. 68.)

the brain are currently being studied in a nonhuman primate model. The results are compared to CSF levels of drug to determine if CSF drug levels are indeed true surrogates for brain tissue levels of drug.[21]

PROBLEMS WITH CHEMOTHERAPY

Tumor Heterogeneity

Malignant primary brain tumors are heterogeneous. A variety of histologic subtypes may be observed within a single tumor,[22] and histologically similar tumors may not behave similarly. For example, astrocytic cells may be seen adjacent to oligodendroglial components of a single tumor. The regional cellular differences are reflected in differences in the chemosensitivity of the cells, with mixed cell populations from different regions of a tumor demonstrating different chemosensitivities.[23] This regional and clonal heterogeneity is thought to be at least partially responsible for the development of resistance to chemotherapeutic agents.[23] In addition to intratumor variations, behavior and chemosensitivity can differ markedly within a group of histologically similar tumors. Among the malignant gliomas, the median survival of patients with glioblastoma multiforme is 32 weeks, that of patients with anaplastic astrocytoma is 63 weeks, and that of patients with mixed anaplastic astrocytoma with an oligodendroglioma component is 278 weeks.[24,25] This variation makes it difficult to target therapy to a single disease. In addition, the number of available chemotherapeutic agents with which to treat the variety of CNS tumors is limited. Since the 1960s, only three drugs—temozolomide, BCNU, and CCNU—have been approved by the Food and Drug Administration (FDA) for specific use in brain tumor patients in the United States.

Drug Resistance

Drug resistance, either intrinsic or acquired, is frequently seen in tumors of the CNS, and many different mechanisms have been described. The best-characterized mechanism of drug resistance involves P glycoprotein. P glycoprotein (Pgp) is a 170-kDa transmembrane protein that is normally present on the luminal surface of brain capillary endothelial cells and that functions as a drug efflux pump.[26,27] It appears to play an important role in protecting the precise microenvironment of the CNS by excluding xenobiotics, including a variety of anticancer drugs.[28–30] In addition to its presence on the endothelial cells of the BBB, Pgp is overexpressed on the surface of some cancer cells, which contributes to a multidrug-resistance phenotype. Pgp-mediated multidrug resistance is characterized by cross-resistance of tumor cells to several classes of chemotherapeutic agents.[31]

Over the last several years, it has become clear that Pgp is just one protein in a large family of transmembrane efflux pump proteins. Recent data have shown that the transporter protein, the multidrug resistance–associated protein (MRP), is also highly expressed on the BBB,[32] and MRP knockout mice are extraordinarily sensitive to the neurotoxic effects of etoposide.[33] Thus, it is quite likely that other efflux pumps will prove to be important in brain tumor drug delivery and resistance.

Other mechanisms of drug resistance include the ability of a tumor cell to repair deoxyribonucleic acid (DNA) damage induced by cytotoxic agents or to make use of alternative pathways of metabolism.[34] O^6-alkylguanine-DNA-alkyltransferase (AGT) is a DNA repair protein that removes alkyl groups from the O^6 position of guanine. This is the site frequently alkylated (methylated) by alkylating agents, including BCNU and temozolomide. In a number of human tumor cell lines and animal models, in vitro cytotoxicity to nitrosoureas was inversely related to levels of AGT.[35–37] O^6-alkylguanine-DNA-alkyltransferase is expressed in many tumors and has been associated with tumor resistance and poor clinical response to methylating agents.

Several other mechanisms of drug resistance exist, including impaired drug transport or uptake, impaired intracellular metabolic activation, increased intracellular inactivation, and detoxification by nonspecific pathways.[38,39]

Blood-Tumor Barrier

The BBB is disrupted in many malignant brain tumors. Blood vessels in these tumors have abnormal tight junctions and a disrupted endothelial surface, which allow water-soluble contrast agents to cross into the tumor and hence appear enhancing on magnetic resonance imaging (MRI). This brain-tumor barrier (BTB) tends to be more permeable than normal brain tissue, but the amount of drug reaching the tumor continues to be severely restricted.[40,41] Breakdown of the BBB in the area of the tumor is variable, and large areas exist where the BBB remains intact. In addition, the brain adjacent to tumor (BAT) is the area around the tumor that contains infiltrating tumor cells. These sites may be associated with an intact BBB, and drug delivery to this area is difficult. Finally, although most brain tumors tend to be highly vascular, the aberrant tumor-induced angiogenic process tends to create abnormal vessels such as blind loops and arteriolar-venuole shunts, making parenchymal drug delivery even more inefficient. Methods for delivering higher concentrations of chemotherapeutic agents to the tumor and proximal brain tissue will need to be developed to affect the prognosis of patients with brain tumors.

Drug Interactions

Patients with tumors of the CNS are frequently prescribed medication to control signs and symptoms resulting from the tumor. These drugs include steroids, gastric acid inhibitors, and anticonvulsants. Each of these can have a prominent effect on the pharmacokinetics and delivery of chemotherapeutic agents. Dexamethasone is a glucocorticoid frequently administered to reduce cerebral edema and tumor-associated vascular permeability. Although it does improve symptoms in many patients, its mechanism of action is poorly understood, and doses vary widely. Recent studies in animal models have shown that dexamethasone can decrease the uptake of chemotherapeutic agents in the tumor and in the area around the tumor.[42,43] Clinical studies have also demonstrated pharmacokinetic effects on chemotherapeutic agents resulting from cytochrome P-450–inducing anticonvulsants. In a group of 59 patients with high-grade gliomas treated with 9-aminocamptothecin, higher-than-expected doses of the chemotherapeutic agent were required to reach a maximum tolerated dose (MTD).[44] In a phase I study of paclitaxel in patients with recurrent malignant glioma, the 27 patients on anticonvulsants reached an MTD that was 150 percent higher than that of patients not receiving anticonvulsants.[45] Some current phase I studies are stratifying patients by use of anticonvulsants.

APPROACHES TO OVERCOMING OBSTACLES TO CENTRAL NERVOUS SYSTEM CHEMOTHERAPY

Developing New Drugs

Drugs have been chemically modified and rationally synthesized to alter specific properties that may make them more amenable to CNS delivery. Spirohydantoin mustard is a rationally synthesized lipophilic alkylating agent. In phase I studies, neurotoxicity was frequent and dose limiting.[46] Despite its lipophilicity, the drug was highly protein bound, resulting in low CSF-plasma ratios.[46] Other methods of rational drug design for circumventing the BBB include complexing the drug to more lipophilic agents or coupling it to a molecule that has a specific transport system.[47]

Liposomes are drug carriers composed of synthetic phospholipid membranes organized as lamellar vesicles with aqueous compartments in which water-soluble drugs can be entrapped. Clinical studies have shown that liposomal doxorubicin decreases systemic side effects, including cardiac toxicity, while allowing higher doses.[48,49] One difficulty is that liposomes are preferentially taken up by fixed macrophages and therefore localize primarily in the liver, spleen, bone marrow, and lungs.[50] There is no evidence that incorporation of water-soluble agents into liposomes improves drug delivery to the CNS.

Overcoming Drug Resistance

P Glycoprotein/Multidrug-Resistance Reversal

A variety of drugs that inhibit Pgp have been investigated as modulators of multidrug resistance.[51,52] These include verapamil,[53] cyclosporine,[54] and cephalosporins,[55] which are thought to bind to Pgp and competitively inhibit the membrane pump, resulting in higher intracellular concentrations of the cytotoxic agents.[56] Although a handful of objective responses have been reported, particularly in lymphomas and myelomas,[57,58] Pgp modulation decreases the clearance of anticancer drugs that are Pgp substrates and enhances their toxicity. The enhanced toxicity presumably occurs because of inhibition of Pgp-dependent drug elimination pathways in the normal liver, which also expresses Pgp. In addition, the maximally tolerated dose of the Pgp modulators resulted in serum levels that were lower than the level needed to inhibit Pgp.[59] More potent modulators of Pgp, including the cyclosporin analogue PSC833, are currently undergoing clinical trials.

Inhibition of Repair Enzymes

Because the DNA repair protein AGT is a single-turnover DNA repair protein, the ability to repair the methylated site on the O^6 position of guanine is stoichiometrically related to the number of AGT molecules and the rate of protein resynthesis.[60,61] In a number of human tumor cell lines and animal models, inhibition of AGT activity markedly increased the sensitivity to nitrosoureas.[62,63] O^6-benzylguanine (O^6BG) is a potent inactivator of AGT.[60] It acts as an alternate and highly specific competitive AGT-binding substrate, irreversibly inactivating AGT.[64] Pretreatment with O^6BG has been shown to increase the cytotoxicity of temozolomide in vitro, in malignant glioma xenograft models,[65,66] and against a variety of human tumor xenografts grown in nude mice.[67,68] Adult and pediatric trials using O^6BG with cytotoxic agents are being conducted.

Improving Drug Delivery

Disruption of the Blood-Brain Barrier

Nonspecific osmotic disruption of the BBB has been clinically tested for the treatment of CNS malignancies. Neuwalt and colleagues demonstrated the feasibility of using hypertonic mannitol solutions to temporarily open the BBB to deliver higher doses of chemotherapeutic agents to the brain.[69] Although a modest number of responses have been seen,[70] (1) the procedure can be associated with considerable toxicity, (2) little additional chemotherapy is delivered to the bulk of the tumor, and (3) more chemotherapy is delivered to normal brain areas, which may potentiate the neurotoxicity of chemotherapeutic agents.[71–73]

Biomodulation of specific receptors on the BBB may be a means to achieve therapeutic drug concentrations in the tumor and in the brain around the tumor. Cereport (RMP-7, lobradamil) (Alkermes, Cambridge, MA) is a bradykinin analogue that interacts with the B2 (bradykinin)-receptor present on the BBB, resulting in selective permeabilization of the BBB at the blood-tumor interface and a small area around the tumor. The interaction of Cereport with the β_2-receptor results in the relaxation of tight junctions, allowing the entry of hydrophilic substances normally prohibited from entering the brain.[74] Studies performed in Wistar rats with implanted RG2 gliomas demonstrated that intracarotid infusion of Cereport increased the permeability for tracer molecules (ranging in molecular weight from 100 to 70,000 Da) within brain tumors.[75] The greatest increase in permeability was observed in the tumor area; less effect on permeability was noted as the distance from the tumor increased.[76] In preclinical studies using the rat RG2 glioma model, administration of intracarotid Cereport and carboplatin resulted in an increased delivery of carboplatin to the tumor and brain surrounding the tumor.[77] Animals that received both Cereport and carboplatin had an increased survival rate compared to animals that received carboplatin alone.[77] Clinical trials administering Cereport with carboplatin to adult and pediatric patients with malignant CNS tumors have recently been performed.[78,79]

High-Dose Chemotherapy

High-dose chemotherapy, followed by autologous bone marrow transplantation or peripheral stem cell transplantation, has been used with the rationale that increased delivery of chemotherapeutic agents across the BBB will occur secondary to higher serum levels. This may result in greater tumor cell kill, given the steep linear-log dose-response relationship of alkylating agents[80] and their non–cell-cycle–dependent cytotoxic properties.

High-dose chemotherapy has shown encouraging results, primarily for pediatric patients with relapsed medulloblastoma and intracranial germ cell tumors.[80] It has also been used in young children to avoid the toxic effects of craniospinal radiation.[80] High-dose chemotherapy with autologous stem cell rescue has been significantly less promising for adults with malignant glioma. In general, response rates and overall survival have not been impressive, and toxicity has been substantial.[81] Most high-grade astrocytomas have a relatively low proliferative index; therefore, a single pulse of high-dose chemotherapy may not achieve a high enough exposure to have an effect.

The major problem with high-dose chemotherapy is the increased systemic toxicity associated with higher doses. Although myelosuppression may be treated with infusion of stem cells, other toxicities are then unveiled, including neurotoxicity associated with high-dose thiotepa, renal and ototoxicity associated with carboplatin, cardiovascular toxicity associated with cyclophosphamide, mucositis associated with etoposide, and pulmonary and hepatic toxicities associated with the nitrosoureas.[80] The toxic mortality of high-dose chemotherapy for children with brain tumors ranges from 5 to 20 percent.[80]

Intra-arterial Therapy

Infusion of chemotherapeutic agents directly into the arterial supply of a tumor can provide a pharmacokinetic advantage by enhancing drug delivery to the tumor without increasing systemic drug exposure.[82,83] Intra-arterial administration augments local plasma peak drug concentrations and local exposure (as measured by the area under the concentration x time curve) compared to an equivalent intravenous dose, while decreasing systemic toxicity. This method may be more beneficial with drugs that undergo a large first-pass effect when given systemically and with drugs that have a high total body clearance.[84] A study by Levin and colleagues, using radiolabeled BCNU, demonstrated a fourfold increase in BCNU concentration in the brain following intracarotid administration compared to intravenous administration.[85] In a study involving 12 adult patients with recurrent glioblastoma, intra-arterial BCNU infusion resulted in a median survival time of 54 weeks following recurrence (92 weeks after diagnosis), but no major improvement in survival was demonstrated in a group of 43 patients treated adjuvantly post-irradiation.[86] It was hypothesized that the group receiving adjuvant intra-arterial BCNU had radiation changes that limited drug penetration into tissue,[86] although the effects of radiation on drug delivery across the BBB have been controversial.

Nitrosoureas, cisplatin, and carboplatin have been given by the intra-arterial approach and have led to a number of clinical responses.[87–89] However, the responses are modest, and the technique is associated with significant toxicity. In a study combining both intra-arterial and systemic chemotherapy, response rates of up to 54 percent in patients with grades II to IV gliomas were demonstrated, but 31 percent of patients developed neurotoxicity, and 12 percent developed serious permanent local toxicity.[90] A large phase III trial comparing intra-arterial BCNU to intravenous BCNU in newly resected malignant glioma adult patients demonstrated that the intra-arterial BCNU group actually had a lower survival rate than patients treated with intravenous BCNU. The reason for the decreased survival rate was unclear, but serious toxicity, including irreversible encephalopathy and blindness, was observed in the intra-arterial group.[91] No large randomized trial has yet demonstrated that intracarotid administration of chemotherapy is more advantageous than systemic administration.[91,92]

One difficulty with intra-arterial administration is that nonuniform drug distribution within the brain or brain tumor after intracarotid infusion may occur due to poor mixing or streaming of the drug solution within the artery.[93] Tissue regions that receive high concentrations of drug are at risk for toxicity whereas low drug concentrations in other tissue regions may be subtherapeutic.[94] In addition to increasing drug levels in the tumor with this technique, drug levels in the area of normal brain supplied by the artery are also increased, leading to an associated increase in neurotoxicity. Intracarotid administration of BCNU has also been associated with ocular toxicity, strokes, and an encephalitic picture.[95]

In adults, the majority of brain tumors are supratentorial and are supplied by the carotid arteries, but more than 50 percent of childhood brain tumors are infratentorial.[96] Infratentorial tumors are supplied by the vertebrobasilar arterial system, which is unique because of the convergence of the two vertebral arteries into the basilar artery. The effect of this arterial convergence on the distribution of drugs administered via the vertebral arteries is currently being studied.

Interstitial/Intratumoral Drug Delivery

Because most CNS tumors recur in or near the original tumor site,[97] improved local control may translate into improved survival. Interstitial therapy circumvents the BBB by administering drug directly into or adjacent to the brain tumor. The theoretic advantages are increased local drug concentrations; decreased systemic exposure; and high, prolonged levels of a chemotherapeutic agent. Different strategies for intratumoral drug delivery include topical applications, indwelling catheters, implantable drug delivery systems, and biodegradable polymers (wafers).

Biodegradable polymer matrices are molded wafers impregnated with a chemotherapeutic agent that is released in an active form for sustained periods in the area of the tumor. This technique increases a drug's therapeutic efficacy by producing high local-tissue concentrations over an extended period, with minimal systemic exposure.[98] Given BCNU's short plasma half-life and significant systemic toxicity,[99] BCNU-impregnated biodegradable wafers have been studied. These wafers, containing 3.8 percent BCNU, allow sustained-release delivery and higher local concentrations for extended periods of time. Preclinical studies demonstrated that BCNU could be released from polymer discs for up to 21 days in rat and rabbit brain.[100,101] Rats with implanted 9L gliomas that received BCNU-implanted polymers demonstrated improved survival compared to controls with empty polymers.[102]

In a phase I trial of BCNU loaded in the poly [bis] (p-carboxyphenoxy) propane-sebacic acid polymer in patients with recurrent glioma, the overall median survival was 46 weeks after implantation (87 weeks after initial diagnosis), with 86 percent of patients alive more than 1 year after diagnosis.[103] No significant systemic toxicities were observed during this study. One major complication was the later development of neurologic deterioration in a significant number (47%) of patients, thought to be due to the development of necrosis around the wafer. In a phase III trial randomizing patients with recurrent glioma to 3.85 percent BCNU polymer or empty polymer, there was a minimal although statistically significant improvement in median survival in the BCNU-treated group compared to the control group (31 weeks vs 23 weeks).[104] Significant complications due to necrosis did not occur in this study.[105]

Although polymer-mediated diffusion of cytotoxic agents continues to be an area of active research, there is a growing interest in enhanced convection delivery (ie, microperfusion), given its ability to homogeneously deliver molecules over a larger area of brain than can simple diffusion.

Intrathecal therapy

The most obvious method of circumventing the BBB in drug delivery is direct administration of chemotherapeutic agents into the CSF. Drugs can be injected intrathecally via the lumbar route or intraventricularly. For intraventricular administration, Ommaya reservoirs are frequently used. Ommaya reservoirs are subcutaneously implanted devices that have a catheter outlet in the CNS, usually within the ventricles or tumor bed. Chemotherapeutic agents can be administered percutaneously into the reservoir, which is then manually compressed to deliver the drug to the catheter tip in the tumor. Although convenient, the method does not allow continuous drug delivery to the tumor bed. Intrathecal administration of chemotherapeutic agents is associated with several advantages and disadvantages. One major advantage is that a significant concentration of drug can be achieved within the CSF with smaller doses of drug, decreasing systemic toxicity. Disadvantages include nonuniform distribution of drug throughout the subarachnoid space, variable diffusion and transport of the drug across the CSF-brain barrier,[20] neurotoxicity, and the lack of effective penetration of intrathecally administered drugs into the brain parenchyma.[106–108] For these reasons, intrathecal chemotherapy is currently used for meningeal disease. It is not useful for bulky parenchymal disease.

PHARMACOLOGY OF SPECIFIC AGENTS

Alkylating Agents

Nitrosoureas

The nitrosoureas, including BCNU and lomustine (CCNU), are cell-cycle–nonspecific alkylating agents. They spontaneously decompose into two active intermediates: an isocyanate group and a chloroethyldiazohydroxide group.[109] The chloroethyldiazohydroxide alkylates DNA, which leads to the cross-linking of DNA and resultant cellular instability. The isocyanate group produces carbamoylation of amino groups and depletion of glutathione, which inhibits DNA repair and interferes with ribonucleic acid (RNA) synthesis.

Because they are small, nonionized, and highly lipid soluble molecules, the nitrosoureas readily cross the BBB.[109] Lomustine is given orally; after systemic administration, CCNU concentration in the brain is equivalent to that in plasma.[84] Carmustine is given intravenously or intra-arterially; after systemic administration, BCNU concentration in the brain is 15 to 70 percent of that in plasma.[84]

Administration of nitrosoureas is the primary single-agent therapy used to treat gliomas. Several studies suggest that adjuvant therapy with nitrosoureas modestly improves survival for patients with malignant primary brain tumors[5,110–112] although a number of other trials have failed to demonstrate any survival advantage. Whether this discrepancy reflects the lack of statistical power to detect minimal antitumor activity in smaller clinical trials or whether it truly reflects a lack of antitumor activity remains unclear. Prior randomized trials have also failed to control for variables known to be extremely important in the prognosis of patients with glioma (ie, age, performance status, histology); therefore, the various trial outcomes may be biased by nonuniform distribution of these variables between treatment groups. A recent meta-analysis suggests that nitrosourea-based adjuvant chemotherapy has a modest benefit for patients with anaplastic gliomas but only a minimal benefit for those with glioblastoma. These benefits are probably restricted to the small group of patients with the best prognostic factors (ie, youth, minimal residual tumor after surgery, good performance status). Lomustine, as part of a multiagent chemotherapy regimen, has some benefit for patients with high-risk medulloblastoma.[113,114] In patients with high-risk medulloblastoma, prolonged survival was noted when CCNU and vincristine were added after surgery and radiation.[113,115]

The true activity of nitrosoureas for patients with recurrent or progressive malignant gliomas remains uncertain. Although the literature reports single-agent response rates of 40 to 50 percent, this is seldom seen in clinical practice. Most clinical trials in the literature were performed over 20 years ago, prior to the era of computed tomography (CT) and MRI. Thus, "response" was variably defined, usually using clinical or nuclear medicine ("brain scans") criteria. The true objective response rate of nitrosoureas therefore remains unknown although many believe it may be less than 10 percent for glioblastoma.

The major toxicities associated with nitrosoureas are nausea, emesis, myelosuppression, pulmonary fibrosis, and renal toxicity. The myelosuppression is cumulative (ie, it worsens with subsequent doses) and is typically delayed, occurring 3 to 5 weeks after treatment.[116,84]

Procarbazine

Procarbazine is an oral prodrug that is rapidly absorbed and that requires hepatic activation to its active form. It is metabolized to an azo-procarbazine and then converted by the cytochrome P-450 system into two active derivatives.[84] These active derivatives alkylate DNA at the O^6 position of guanine. Procarbazine can also induce DNA strand breakage and inhibit DNA, RNA, and protein synthesis. Procarbazine and its metabolites cross the BBB, with rapid equilibrium between plasma and CSF.[84]

Procarbazine can be used as a single agent or in multiagent regimens to treat malignant primary brain tumors. As a single agent, procarbazine has been compared to IV BCNU, methylprednisolone, and IV BCNU with methylprednisolone in patients with malignant glioma. The overall median survival was similar for the procarbazine and BCNU groups, but long-term survival at up to 24 months was superior in the procarbazine group.[5] Procarbazine in combination with CCNU and vincristine (PCV) was compared to single-agent BCNU as postradiation therapy in a randomized trial.[117] There was no significant difference in overall survival or time-to-tumor progression for the group as a whole. However, in the subset of patients with anaplastic gliomas (rather than glioblastoma), there was a significant difference in time-to-tumor progression and survival for the group receiving PCV. It is important to realize that this survival advantage was demonstrated only in the subset analysis of a very small group of patients. A recent retrospective analysis of the Radiation Therapy Oncology Group (RTOG) database, including more than 400 patients with anaplastic gliomas, revealed no survival advantage for patients treated with postradiation PCV versus BCNU.[118] Also, some investigators have reported procarbazine to be beneficial for patients with malignant gliomas that recur after radiation and nitrosourea therapy[119] whereas others suggest that procarbazine is significantly less active in patients previously exposed to nitrosoureas.[120]

Procarbazine is easy to administer and is generally well tolerated. The primary side effects are myelosuppression, nausea and vomiting, fatigue, rash, and neurotoxicity.[119] The dose-limiting toxicities are neutropenia and thrombocytopenia.[84] Procarbazine also inhibits monoamine oxidase and has a disulfiram-like effect. Patients must be cautioned to avoid sympathomimetic drugs, antihistamines, tricyclic antidepressants, and foods high in tyramine (wine, beer, cheese, chocolate, bananas, and yogurt) as the combination of these substances and procarbazine can cause acute hypertension or other interactions.[109,121] In addition, procarbazine can be associated with an acute hypersensitivity reaction resulting in life-threatening interstitial pneumonitis, particularly in patients allergic to the drug.[122]

Platinums

The platinum compounds cisplatin and carboplatin are cell-cycle–nonspecific bifunctional alkylating agents with demonstrated efficacy in the treatment of adult and childhood primary brain tumors.[3,123,124] Their cytotoxicity depends on the free, or unbound, fraction of drug. The platinum compounds alkylate the N7 position of guanine, producing inter- and intrastrand cross-links. Both agents are water soluble and penetrate the BBB poorly.[84]

Cisplatin has demonstrated variable activity against a wide range of tumors, including anaplastic astrocytoma, glioblastoma multiforme, medulloblastoma/primitive neuroectodermal tumor (PNET), CNS lymphoma, and germ cell tumors.[3,109,123,125] It can be given as a single agent or in combination with other drugs. In the pediatric population, cisplatin as a single agent is efficacious for recurrent medulloblastoma/PNET and for ependymoma.[126,127] Objective responses of primary and recurrent CNS germinomas have been documented, with cisplatin as a single agent.[128] In combination with CCNU or cyclophosphamide plus vincristine, cisplatin also is effective against high-risk and recurrent medulloblastomas.[129] Cisplatin has considerable side effects, which include severe nausea and vomiting (acute or delayed), nephrotoxicity, ototoxicity, myelosuppression, and peripheral neuropathy. Side effects are common, and frequent dose reductions are necessary.

Carboplatin is a cisplatin analogue with a similar activity profile and comparable cytotoxicity in vitro. It is more myelosuppressive than cisplatin but causes less ototoxicity, nephrotoxicity, nausea, emesis, and peripheral neuropathy.[84] It also has a higher unbound (ie, active) fraction in the plasma and greater CSF exposure than cisplatin.[130] As a single agent, carboplatin has demonstrated efficacy in pediatric patients for both low-grade gliomas and recurrent malignant primary brain tumors.[131,132] In adults, single-agent carboplatin has shown minimal activity for the treatment of recurrent malignant gliomas.[133]

Nitrogen Mustards

Several nitrogen mustards (including melphalan, chlorambucil, mechlorethamine, cyclophosphamide, and ifosfamide) have been used in the treatment of primary brain tumors. Their mechanism of cytotoxicity involves the formation of reactive carbonium ions that then interact with electrophilic regions of susceptible molecules, including DNA. Although cyclophosphamide has shown activity as a salvage treatment in adults and children with recurrent primary brain tumors,[109,134–137] the activity of nitrogen mustards against primary brain tumors is minimal at best.[109,138] Side effects are frequent and include myelosuppression, nausea and emesis, interstitial pneumonitis and pulmonary fibrosis, teratogenesis, and secondary malignancies.[139] In addition, cyclophosphamide and ifosfamide are associated with hemorrhagic cystitis.

Temozolomide

Temozolomide is an oral prodrug that is rapidly absorbed and that undergoes spontaneous hydrolysis to form the active metabolite 3-methyl- (triazen-1-yl) imidazole-4-carboxamide (MTIC).[140,141] Its mechanism of cytotoxicity is methylation of DNA, primarily at the O^6 position of guanine.[142,143]

In phase II testing of patients with recurrent anaplastic astrocytoma, a combined response and stabilization rate of 60 percent was demonstrated, with a progression-free survival rate of 48 percent at 6 months.[144] In phase II testing of patients with recurrent anaplastic astrocytoma or anaplastic oligoastrocytoma, 35 percent of patients demonstrated an objective response, and 26 percent had disease stabilization.[145] Single-agent activity for recurrent glioblastoma appears to be significantly lower.

Temozolomide is fairly well tolerated. The side effects include nausea, vomiting, constipation, diarrhea, thrombocytopenia, neutropenia, and anemia.[145]

Vincristine

Vincristine is a plant alkaloid that acts as a cell-cycle–specific agent. It enters cells via an energy-dependent carrier-mediated transport system and binds to tubulin during the S phase of the cell cycle, preventing polymerization and inducing metaphase arrest.[146] It undergoes extensive metabolism in the liver and is excreted primarily in the bile.[84] Vincristine is water soluble and penetrates the BBB poorly.[147]

Despite its limited CNS penetration, VCR is said to show activity as part of multiagent regimens against low-grade gliomas, medulloblastomas, oligodendrogliomas, and anaplastic astrocytomas.[113,148,149] It is important to note, however, that vincristine has never been rigorously evaluated as a single agent for primary brain tumors. Its primary side effects are neuropathy, constipation, and syndrome of inappropriate antidiuretic hormone (SIADH).[146]

Antibiotics: Anthracyclines

The anthracyclines are cell-cycle–nonspecific DNA-intercalating agents that interfere with DNA and RNA synthesis.[109] They include doxorubicin, dactinomycin, bleomycin, and plicamycin. In general, anthracyclines show minimal activity against brain tumors. They do not penetrate the BBB well and are also among the classes of drugs exhibiting multidrug-resistance phenotypes. Doxorubicin in combination with dacarbazine may have some activity for malignant meningiomas.[84] Bleomycin in combination with vinblastine and cisplatin may be active in patients with primary intracranial germ cell tumors.[84]

The primary side effects are bone marrow suppression, mucositis, extravasation injury, and cardiotoxicity. The cardiac toxicity is both acute and chronic. The acute cardiac toxicity is idiosyncratic and can occur at low doses. The chronic cardiac toxicity is related to cumulative dose and method of administration, with bolus dosing resulting in much more significant cardiac toxicity than does continuous infusion.

Antimetabolites

Methotrexate

Methotrexate is an S phase–specific folic acid analogue that reversibly binds to dihydrofolate reductase, blocking tetrahydrofolate production and reducing the intracellular pool of reduced folates. It has been used primarily for CNS lymphoma and leptomeningeal metastases and in multiagent regimens for the treatment of medulloblastoma and other high-grade pediatric malignant brain tumors.[3,125] High-dose single-agent methotrexate and combination chemotherapy regimens that include methotrexate have resulted in complete responses and long-term disease-free survival in patients with primary CNS lymphoma.[150–153]

The major side effects of high-dose methotrexate include myelosuppression, nephrotoxicity, nausea, emesis, diarrhea, mucositis, interstitial pneumonitis, and neurotoxicity. The neurotoxicity can present as acute encephalopathic syndrome, myelopathy, arachnoiditis, or progressive leukoencephalopathy.[154]

Cytarabine

Cytarabine is an S phase–specific pyrimidine analogue that is intracellularly phosphorylated to cytosine arabinoside triphosphate and incorporated into DNA, inhibiting DNA polymerase. Cytarabine can also slow DNA elongation and induce premature chain termination. It has little activity against malignant gliomas, but it may be efficacious in patients who have leptomeningeal metastasis from systemic malignancies.[84] It has also been used in multiagent regimens with methotrexate to treat primary CNS lymphoma.

Cytarabine can be administered intravenously or intrathecally. It does penetrate the BBB. Its major side effects include myelosuppression, nausea, emesis, and neurotoxicity, which can manifest as cerebellar syndrome, encephalopathy, seizures, or myelopathy.[155]

Topoisomerase Inhibitors

Etoposide

Etoposide (VP-16) is a semisynthetic derivative of the plant extract podophyllotoxin, an antimitotic agent that binds to tubulin. Etoposide causes single- and double-strand breaks in DNA through interactions with DNA topoisomerase II, inducing arrest in the G2 phase of the cell cycle. It also binds to tubulin and inhibits microtubule assembly. Etoposide is highly lipophilic but does not readily cross the BBB due to its large size.[84]

Etoposide has been used in a variety of schedules using different routes of administration, including oral, IV bolus, or continuous IV infusion over several days. When given orally, a higher dose is required because of decreased bioavailability.[146] Etoposide has been demonstrated to have minimal activity as a single oral agent in some patients with malignant gliomas[156,157] although it is not considered a particularly useful drug for this indication. Etoposide does have activity in several pediatric brain tumors, including PNETs and primary CNS germ cell tumors, and has been successfully used in combination with platinum compounds.

The major side effects are nausea, vomiting, neutropenia, and thrombocytopenia. A mild peripheral neuropathy may also occur.[146]

Camptothecin Analogues

The camptothecin analogues, including topotecan and irinotecan, have shown antitumor activity as single agents against a broad spectrum of tumor types. They cause stabilization of the covalent adduct between topoisomerase I and the 3'-phosphate group of the DNA backbone. Camptothecin analogues also inhibit the religation reaction catalyzed by topoisomerase I, which leads to multiple DNA single-strand breaks. They may also interfere with DNA repair processes and enhance cytotoxicity when combined with DNA-damaging agents.[158,159]

Topotecan is a water-soluble camptothecin analogue with excellent CNS penetration that binds directly to topoisomerase I without activation.[84] In xenograft studies, it demonstrated activity against ependymoma, high-grade gliomas, and medulloblastoma,[160] but activity in pediatric patients with low- and high-grade gliomas, medulloblastoma, and brainstem gliomas was not demonstrated in a phase II study.[161]

Irinotecan, also known as CPT-11, is a camptothecin derivative. It is a prodrug that requires de-esterification by carboxylesterases to yield its active metabolite, SN-38, which is 1,000 times more potent at inhibiting topoisomerase I.[84] Topoisomerase I plays a critical role in DNA replication and transcription. The enzyme normally functions in DNA to cause transient breaks in single-strand DNA, releasing the torsional strain caused by synthesis of a new strand of DNA or RNA around a double helix. Irinotecan stabilizes the topoisomerase I/DNA complex, inhibiting the reannealing of the parent DNA. When an advancing replication fork collides with the complex, double-strand DNA breaks occur, resulting in cell death.[162] In early trials of this agent, some responses were documented in patients with progressive, persistent, or recurrent malignant glioma.[163,164]

The primary side effects of camptothecin analogues are myelosuppression, nausea, emesis, and hypotension. Irinotecan is also associated with severe acute and delayed diarrhea.

Tamoxifen

Tamoxifen is a nonsteroidal antiestrogen with antiangiogenic properties that inhibits the activity of protein kinase C, a cytoplasmic enzyme involved in intracellular signaling pathways. Protein kinase C can induce cell proliferation and is strongly expressed in glioma cells. Tamoxifen has modest efficacy as a single agent in the treatment of patients with glioma[165] and recurrent anaplastic astrocytomas.[166] A few responses and disease stabilization have been reported in the pediatric population.[167,168]

Tamoxifen is given orally and is associated with a low incidence of toxicity.[165,169–171] The major side effect is nausea.

Paclitaxel

Paclitaxel is an agent that inhibits the disassembly of microtubules. It binds to the N-terminal amino acids of the β-tubulin subunit of microtubules and induces polymerization, resulting in cytotoxicity due to the disruption of normal microtubular function during cell division. As a single agent in phase I and II studies, paclitaxel demonstrated an overall stabilization rate of 35 percent in patients with recurrent gliomas although there were essentially no objective radiographic responses.[45,172] The primary side effects include myelosuppression, alopecia, nausea, peripheral neuropathy, and arthralgias. Of note, the pharmacokinetics of paclitaxel are altered by the concomitant use of anticonvulsants.[45]

Supportive Care Agents

A major component in the treatment of patients with tumors of the CNS is supportive care. Many patients have symptoms from the tumor, surrounding edema, or surgery; such symptoms include headaches, seizures, and increased intracranial pressure. It is important to note that the medications used to treat these symptoms may have an effect on the pharmacokinetics of cytotoxic agents, as previously described.

Corticosteroids

Steroids are used to control symptoms due to increased intracranial pressure. Glucocorticoids restore the integrity of the BBB through unclear mechanisms. Dexamethasone is a high-potency steroid most commonly used to treat symptoms associated with peritumoral edema. Its advantages over other synthetic glucocorticoids include a longer half-life, reduced mineralocorticoid effect, lower incidence of cognitive and behavioral complications, and decreased inhibition of leukocyte migration.[173]

Most patients with primary brain tumors require prolonged treatment with high doses of glucocorticoids to manage the cerebral edema associated with their tumor and treatment.[174] The side effects from the long-term use of steroids include hyperglycemia, infection, gastritis, osteopenia, peripheral edema, proximal myopathy, weight gain, and behavioral and personality changes.[175,176] Patients should therefore be maintained on the lowest possible dose of steroids that will control their symptoms. Glucocorticoids can also confound the evaluation of responses to therapy. Most brain scans use a water-soluble contrast agent to highlight the region with BBB disruption. Since steroids can partially restore the BBB, less contrast diffuses into the area and the tumor may appear smaller.[174] Therefore, responses to chemotherapy must be determined when a patient is on a stable or decreasing dose of steroids.

Anticonvulsants

Because anticonvulsants are associated with frequent side effects and may alter the pharmacokinetics of chemotherapeutic agents, the appropriate time to start a brain tumor patient on anticonvulsant therapy is controversial. Many agree that anticonvulsants should be started once the patient has a seizure. Benefit from the prophylactic use of anticonvulsants has not been determined.

Generalized seizures are usually treated with phenytoin or carbamazepine. Partial complex or focal motor seizures may be better controlled with carbamazepine or valproic acid. Plasma levels of anticonvulsants should be obtained after steady state has been achieved (usually after the fifth dose) and should be monitored on a regular basis once adequate levels have been obtained. Symptoms of toxicity from anticonvulsants are usually neurologic and include ataxia, nystagmus, slurred speech, confusion, and headaches, which can mimic tumor progression in some patients. In addition, many of the anticonvulsants affect plasma levels of other drugs.

FUTURE DIRECTIONS

Chemotherapy has improved the survival of some patients with CNS tumors to a modest extent, but the most effective choice of drug or drug regimens and method of delivery are unknown. New drugs are being developed as more is learned about the molecular biology of these tumors. The last decade has seen a change from the empiric development and testing of cytotoxic drugs to the development of drugs that affect specific molecular targets involved in signal-transduction pathways important for tumorigenesis.

Angiogenesis inhibitors, matrix metalloproteinases, and signal-transduction inhibitors are agents currently being developed and tested preclinically and clinically. Differentiating agents (such as the retinoids) and biologic response modifiers (such as interferon-β and monoclonal antibodies) are also being investigated. Gene therapy may enable the introduction of novel genetic material into tumor cells or the modification of cells for therapeutic benefit. It may be used to enhance sensitivity to chemotherapy, inhibit angiogenesis, or alter gene expression in the tumor cells. Pharmacologic advances in drug delivery, circumvention of drug resistance, definition of new molecular targets, and identification of chemosensitive tumors must be integrated to significantly improve the survival of these patients.

REFERENCES

1. Tannock I. The relation between cell proliferation and the vascular system in a transplanted mouse mammary tumor. Br J Cancer 1968;22:258–73.
2. Barendsen G, Broerse J. Experimental radiotherapy of a rat rhabdomyosarcoma with 15 MeV neurons and 300 kV x-rays. I. Effects of single exposure. Eur J Cancer 1969;5:373–91.
3. Kornblith P, Walker M. Chemotherapy for malignant gliomas. J Neurosurg 1988;68:1–17.
4. Muller H, Brock M, Ernst H. Long-term survival and recurrence-free interval in combined surgical, radio-and chemotherapy of malignant brain gliomas. Clin Neurol Neurosurg 1985;87:167–71.
5. Green S, Byar D, Walker M, et al. Comparisons of carmustine, procarbazine, and high-dose methylprednisolone as additions to surgery and radiotherapy for the treatment of malignant glioma. Cancer Treat Rep 1983;67:121–32.
6. Chang C, Horton J, Schoenfeld D, et al. Comparison of postoperative radiotherapy and combined postoperative radiotherapy and chemotherapy in the multidisciplinary management of malignant gliomas. Cancer 1983;52:997–1007.

7. Shapiro W. Therapy of adult malignant brain tumors: what have the clinical trials taught us. Semin Oncol 1986;13: 38–45.
8. Fine H, Dear K, Loeffler J, et al. Meta-analysis of radiation therapy with and without adjuvant chemotherapy for malignant gliomas in adults. Cancer 1993;71:2585–97.
9. Scott J, Rewcastle N, Brasher P, et al. Which glioblastoma multiforme patient will become a long-term survivor? A population-based study. Ann Neurol 1999;46:183–8.
10. DeAngelis L, Burger P, Green S, et al. Malignant glioma: who benefits from adjuvant chemotherapy? Ann Neurol 1998;44:691–5.
11. Levin V. A pharmacologic basis for brain tumor chemotherapy. Semin Oncol 1975;2:57–61.
12. Anderson N, Lokich J. Cancer chemotherapy and infusional scheduling. Oncology 1994;8:99–111.
13. DeMario M, Ratain M. Oral chemotherapy: rationale and future directions. J Clin Oncol 1998;16:2557–67.
14. Rapoport S, Robinson P. Tight-junctional modification as the basis of osmotic opening of the blood-brain barrier. Ann N Y Acad Sci 1986;481:250–67.
15. Fenstermacher J, Rall D, Patlak C, et al. Ventriculocisternal perfusion as a technique for analysis of brain capillary permeability and extracellular transport. Capillary Permeability, Proc Alfred Benzon Symp 1969;11:483–90.
16. Rall D, Zubrod C. Mechanisms of drug absorption and excretion: passage of drugs in and out of the central nervous system. Ann Rev Pharmacol 1962;2:109–28.
17. Stewart D. A critique of the role of the blood-brain barrier in the chemotherapy of human brain tumors. J Neurooncol 1994;20:121–39.
18. Collins J, Dedrick R. Distributed model for drug delivery to CSF and brain tissue. Am J Physiol 1983;245:R303.
19. Lippens R, Winograd B. Methotrexate concentration levels in the cerebrospinal fluid during high-dose methotrexate infusions: an unreliable prediction. Pediatr Hematol Oncol 1988;5:115.
20. Balis F, Blaney S, McCully C, et al. Methotrexate distribution within the subarachnoid space after intraventricular and intravenous administration. Cancer Chemother Pharmacol 2000;45:259–64.
21. Fox E, McCully C, Bacher J, et al. Comparison of in vitro and in vivo microdialysis calibration for tissue zidovidine concentrations in non-human primates. Proc Am Assoc Cancer Res 2000;41:721.
22. Burger P, Vogel S. The brain: tumors. In: Burger P, Vogel S, editors. Surgical pathology of the nervous system and its coverings. New York: John Wiley and Sons; 1976. p. 224–458.
23. Shapiro W, Shapiro J. Principles of brain tumor chemotherapy. Semin Oncol 1986;13:56–9.
24. Winger M, MacDonald D, Cairncross J. Supratentorial anaplastic gliomas in adults: the prognostic importance of extent of resection and prior low-grade glioma. J Neurosurg 1989;71:487–93.
25. Donahue B, Scott C, Nelson J, et al. Influence of an oligodendroglial component on the survival of patients with anaplastic astrocytomas. Int J Radiat Oncol Biol Phys 1997;38:911–4.
26. Thiebaut F, Tsuruo T, Hamada H, et al. Immunohistochemical localization in normal tissues of different epitopes in the multidrug transport protein P170: evidence for localization in brain capillaries and crossreactivity of one antibody with a muscle protein. J Histochem Cytochem 1989; 37:159–64.
27. Cordon-Cardo C, O'Brien J, Casals D, et al. Multidrug-resistance gene (P-glycoprotein) is expressed by endothelial cells at blood-brain barrier sites. Proc Natl Acad Sci U S A 1989;86:695–8.
28. Schinkel A, Mol C, Wagenaar E, et al. Multidrug resistance and the role of P-glycoprotein knockout mice. Eur J Cancer 1995;31A:1295–8.
29. Tatsuta T, Naito M, Oh-hara T, et al. Functional involvement of P-glycoprotein in blood-brain barrier. J Biol Chem 1992;267:20383–91.
30. Fojo A, Akiyama S, Gottesman M, et al. Reduced drug accumulation in multiple drug-resistant human KB carcinoma cell lines. Cancer Res 1985;45:3002–7.
31. Safa A. Multidrug resistance. In: Schilsky R, Milano G, Ratain M, editors. Principles of antineoplastic drug development and pharmacology. New York: Marcel Dekker; 1996. p. 457.
32. Huai-Yun H, Secrest D, Mark K, et al. Expression of multidrug resistance-associated protein (MRP) in brain microvessel endothelial cells. Biochem Biophys Res Commun 1998;243:816–20.
33. Lorico A, Rappa G, Finch R, et al. Disruption of the murine MRP (multidrug resistance protein) gene leads to increased sensitivity to etoposide (VP-16) and increased levels of glutathione. Cancer Res 1997;57:5238–42.
34. Levin V. Pharmacological principles of brain tumor chemotherapy. In: Thompson R, Green J, editors. Advances in neurology. New York: Raven Press; 1976. p. 315–25.
35. Catapano C, Broggini M, Erba E, et al. In vitro and in vivo methazolastone-induced DNA damage and repair in L1210 leukemia sensitive and resistant to chloroethylnitrosoureas. Cancer Res 1987;47:4884–9.
36. D'Atri S, Piccioni D, Castellano A, et al. Chemosensitivity to triazene compounds with O6-alkylguanine-DNA alkyltransferase levels: studies with blasts of leukemic patients. Ann Oncol 1995;6:389–93.
37. Gerson S, Berger N, Arce C, et al. Modulation of nitrosourea resistance in human colon cancer by O6-methylguanine. Biochem Pharmacol 1992;43:1101–7.
38. DeVita V. Principles of chemotherapy. In: DeVita V, Hellman S, Rosenberg S, editors. Principles and practice of oncology. Philadelphia: JB Lippincott; 1989. p. 276–93.
39. Seeber S. Cellular mechanisms of anticancer drug resistance. J Cancer Res Clin Oncol 1982;103:A51.
40. Groothius D, Fischer J, Lapin G, et al. Permeability of different experimental brain tumor models to horseradish peroxidase. J Neuropathol Exp Neurol 1982;41:164–85.
41. Neuwelt E, Barnett P, Bigner D, Frenkel EP. Effects of adrenal cortical steroids and osmotic blood-brain barrier opening on methotrexate delivery to gliomas in the rodent: the factor of the blood-brain barrier. Proc Natl Acad Sci U S A 1982;79:4420–3.
42. Straathof C, van den Bent M, Ma J, et al. The effect of dexamethasone on the uptake of cisplatin in 9L glioma and the area of brain around tumor. J Neurooncol 1998;37: 1–8.
43. Matsukado K, Nakano S, Bartus R, et al. Steroids decrease

uptake of carboplatin in rat gliomas–uptake improved by intracarotid infusion of bradykinin analog, RMP-7. Acta Neurochir Suppl (Wien) 1997;70:159–61.
44. Grossman S, Hochberg F, Fisher J, et al. Increased 9-aminocamptothecin dose requirements in patients on anticonvulsants. Cancer Chemother Pharmacol 1998;42:118–26.
45. Chang S, Kuhn J, Rizzo J, et al. Phase I study of paclitaxel in patients with recurrent malignant glioma: a North American Brain Tumor Consortium report. J Clin Oncol 1998;16:2188–94.
46. Heideman R, Kelley J, Packer R, et al. A pediatric phase I and pharmacokinetic study of spirohydantoin mustard. Cancer Res 1988;48:2292–5.
47. Langer R. New methods of drug delivery. Science 1990;249:1527–33.
48. Tardi P, Bowman N, Cullis P. Liposomal doxorubicin. J Drug Target 1996;4:129–40.
49. Cowens J, Creaven P, Greco W, et al. Initial clinical (phase I) trial of TLC D-99 (doxorubicin encapsulated in liposomes). Cancer Res 1993;53:2796–802.
50. Lopez-Berestein G, Kasi L, Rosenblum M, et al. Clinical pharmacology of 99m Tc-labeled liposomes in patients with cancer. Cancer Res 1984;44:375–8.
51. Gosland M, Lum B, Sikic B. Inhibition by modulators of drug resistance of 3H-vinblastine binding to plasma membranes of multidrug resistant and sensitive cells. Proc Am Assoc Cancer Res 1990;31:407.
52. Sikic B. Pharmacologic approaches to reversing multidrug resistance. Semin Hematol 1997;34:40–7.
53. Tsuruo T, Iida H, Tsukagoshi S, Sakurai Y. Overcoming of vincristine resistance in P388 leukemia in vivo and in vitro through enhanced cytotoxicity of vincristine and vinblastine by verapamil. Cancer Res 1981;41:1967–72.
54. Twentyman P, Fox N, White D. Cyclosporin A and its analogs as modifiers of Adriamycin and vincristine resistance in a multidrug resistant human lung cancer cell line. Br J Cancer 1987;56:55–7.
55. Goslan M, Lum B, Sikic B. Reversal by cefoperazone of resistance to etoposide, doxorubicin, and vinblastine in multidrug resistant human sarcoma cells. Cancer Res 1989;49:1901–5.
56. Kaye S. Reversal of multidrug resistance. Cancer Treat Rev 1990;17(Suppl A):37–43.
57. Miller T, Grogan T, Dalton W, et al. P-glycoprotein expression in malignant lymphoma and reversal of clinical drug resistance with chemotherapy plus high-dose verapamil. J Clin Oncol 1991;9:17–24.
58. Salmon S, Dalton W, Grogan R, et al. Multidrug resistant myeloma: laboratory and clinical effects of verapamil as a chemosensitizer. Blood 1991;78:44–50.
59. Fisher G, Sikic B. Clinical studies with modulators of multidrug resistance. Hematol Oncol Clin North Am 1995;9:363–82.
60. Gerson S, Liu L, Phillips W, et al. Drug resistance mediated by DNA repair: the paradigm of O6-alkylguanine DNA alkyltransferase. Proc Am Assoc Cancer Res 1994;35:699–700.
61. D'Incalci M, Citti L, Taverna P, et al. Importance of the DNA repair enzyme O6-alkylguanine alkyltransferase (AT) in cancer chemotherapy. Cancer Treat Rev 1988;15:279–92.
62. Bobola M, Blank A, Berger M, et al. Contribution of O6-methylguanine-DNA methyltransferase to monofunctional alkylating agent resistance in human tumor-derived cell lines. Mol Carcinog 1995;13:70–80.
63. Marathi U, Kroes R, Dolan M, et al. Prolonged depletion of O6-methylguanine DNA methyltransferase activity following exposure to O6-benzylguanine with or without streptozotocine enhances 1,3-bis(2-chloroethyl)-1-nitrosourea sensitivity in vitro. Cancer Res 1993;53:4281–6.
64. Pegg A, Boosalis M, Sampson L, et al. Mechanism of inactivation of human O6-alkylguanine-DNA alkyltransferase by O6-benzylguanine. Biochemistry 1993;32:11998–2006.
65. Friedman H, Dolan M, Pegg A, et al. Activity of temozolomide in the treatment of central nervous system tumor xenografts. Cancer Res 1995;55:2853–7.
66. Wedge S, Newlands E. O6-benzylguanine enhances the sensitivity of a glioma xenograft with low O6-alkylguanine-DNA alkyltransferase activity to temozolomide and BCNU. Br J Cancer 1996;73:1049–52.
67. Gerson S, Zborowska E, Norton K, et al. Synergistic efficacy of O6-benzylguanine and 1,3-bis(2-chloroethyl)-1-nitrosourea in a human colon cancer xenograft completely resistant to BCNU alone. Biochem Pharmacol 1993;45:483–91.
68. Dolan M, Pegg A, Biser N, et al. Effect of O6-benzylguanine on the response to 1,3-bis(2-chloroethyl)-1-nitrosoureas in the Dunning R3327G model of prostatic cancer. Cancer Chemother Pharmacol 1993;32:221–5.
69. Neuwelt E, Diehl J, Vu L, et al. Monitoring of methotrexate delivery in patients with malignant brain tumors after osmotic blood-brain barrier disruption. Ann Intern Med 1981;94:449–54.
70. Neuwelt E, Specht H, Howieson J, et al. Osmotic blood-brain barrier modification: clinical documentation by enhanced CT scanning and/or radionuclide brain scanning. AJNR Am J Neuroradiol 1983;4:907–13.
71. Nakagawa H, Groothius D, Blasberg R. The effect of graded hypertonic intracarotid infusions on drug delivery to experimental RG-2 gliomas. Neurology 1984;34:1571–81.
72. Rapoport S. Osmotic opening of the blood-brain barrier. Ann Neurol 1988;24:677–89.
73. Williams P, Henner W, Roman-Goldstein S, et al. Toxicity and efficacy of carboplatin and etoposide in conjunction with disruption of the blood-brain tumor barrier in the treatment of intracranial neoplasms. Neurosurgery 1995;37:17–28.
74. Sanovich E, Bartus R, Friden P, et al. Pathway across blood-brain barrier opened by the bradykinin agonist, RMP-7. Brain Res 1995;705:125–35.
75. Inamura T, Nomura T, Bartus R, et al. Intracarotid infusion of RMP-7, a bradykinin analog: a method for selective drug delivery to brain tumors. J Neurosurg 1994;81:752–8.
76. Elliott P, Hayward N, Dean R, et al. Intravenous RMP-7 selectively increases uptake of carboplatin into rat brain tumors. Cancer Res 1996;56:3998–4005.
77. Matsukado K, Inamura T, Nakano S, et al. Enhanced tumor uptake of carboplatin and survival in glioma-bearing rats by intracarotid infusion of bradykinin analog, RMP-7. Neurosurgery 1996;39:125–33.
78. Warren K, Patel M, Adamson P, et al. Phase I trial of RMP-7

and carboplatin in pediatric patients with brain tumors. Proc Am Soc Clin Oncol 1998;17:198a.
79. Cloughesy T, Black K, Gobin Y, et al. Intra-arterial Cereport (RMP-7) and carboplatin: a dose escalation study for recurrent malignant gliomas. Neurosurgery 1999;44:270–9.
80. Kalifa C, Valteau D, Pizer B, et al. High-dose chemotherapy in childhood brain tumors. Childs Nerv Syst 1999;15: 498–505.
81. Fine H, Antman K. High-dose chemotherapy with autologous bone marrow transplantation in the treatment of high grade astrocytomas in adults: therapeutic rationale and clinical experience. Bone Marrow Transplant 1992;10:315–21.
82. Collins J. Pharmacologic rationale for regional drug delivery. J Clin Oncol 1984;2:498–504.
83. Lutz R, Dedrick R, Boretos J, et al. Mixing studies during intracarotid artery infusions in an in vitro model. J Neurosurg 1986;64:277–83.
84. Newton H, Turowski R, Stroup T, et al. Clinical presentation, diagnosis, and pharmacotherapy of patients with primary brain tumors. Ann Pharmacother 1999;33:816–32.
85. Levin V, Kabra P, Freeman-Dove M. Pharmacokinetics of intracarotid artery 14C-BCNU in the squirrel monkey. J Neurosurg 1978;48:587–93.
86. Hochberg F, Pruitt A, Beck D, et al. The rationale and methodology for intra-arterial chemotherapy with BCNU as treatment for glioblastoma. J Neurosurg 1985;63:876–80.
87. Bashir R, Hochberg F, Lingwood R, et al. Pre-irradiation internal carotid artery BCNU in treatment of glioblastoma multiforme. J Neurosurg 1988;68:917.
88. Mahaley M, Hipp S, Dropcho E, et al. Intracarotid cisplatin chemotherapy for recurrent gliomas. J Neurosurg 1989; 70:371.
89. Newton H, Page M, Junck L, et al. Intra-arterial cisplatin for the treatment of malignant gliomas. J Neurooncol 1989; 7:39.
90. Stewart D, Grahovac Z, Hugenholtz H, et al. Combined intraarterial and systemic chemotherapy for intracerebral tumors. Neurosurgery 1987;21:207–14.
91. Shapiro W, Green S, Burger P, et al. A randomised comparison of intra-arterial versus intravenous BCNU, with or without intravenous 5-fluorouracil, for newly diagnosed patients with malignant glioma. J Neurosurg 1992;76: 772–81.
92. Cokgor I, Friedman H, Friedman A. Chemotherapy for adults with malignant glioma. Cancer Invest 1999;17:264–72.
93. Saris S, Blasberg R, Carson R, et al. Intravascular streaming during carotid artery infusions. J Neurosurg 1991;74: 763–72.
94. Saris S, Wright D, Oldfield E, Blasberg RG. Intravascular streaming and variable delivery to brain following carotid artery infusions in the Sprague-Dawley rat. J Cereb Blood Flow Metab 1988;8:116–20.
95. Rosenblum M, Delattre J, Shapiro W. Fatal necrotizing encephalopathy complicating treatment of malignant gliomas with intra-arterial BCNU and irradiation: a pathological study. J Neurooncol 1989;7:269–81.
96. Pollack I. Brain tumors in children. N Engl J Med 1994; 331:1500–7.
97. Hochberg F, Pruitt A. Assumptions in the radiotherapy of glioblastoma. Neurology 1980;30:907–11.
98. Brem H, Tamargo R, Olivi A, et al. Biodegradable polymers for controlled delivery of chemotherapy with and without radiation therapy in the monkey brain. J Neurosurg 1994; 80:283–90.
99. Loo T, Dion R, Dixon R, et al. The antitumor agent, 1,3-bis(chloroethyl)-1-nitrosourea. J Pharm Sci 1966;55:492–7.
100. Grossman S, Reinhard C, Colvin O, et al. The intracerebral distribution of BCNU delivered by surgically implanted biodegradable polymers. J Neurosurg 1992;76:640–7.
101. Yang M, Tamargo R, Brem H. Controlled delivery of 1,3-bis(2-chloroethyl)-1-nitrosourea from ethylene-vinyl acetate copolymer. Cancer Res 1989;49:5103–7.
102. Tamargo R, Myseros J, Epstein J, et al. Interstitial chemotherapy of the 9L gliosarcoma: controlled release polymers for drug delivery in the brain. Cancer Res 1993;53:329–33.
103. Brem H, Mahaley MJ, Vick N, et al. Interstitial chemotherapy with drug polymer implants for the treatment of recurrent gliomas. J Neurosurg 1991;74:441–6.
104. Brem H, Piantadosi S, Burger P, et al. Placebo-controlled trial of safety and efficacy of intraoperative controlled delivery by biodegradable polymers of chemotherapy for recurrent gliomas. Lancet 1995;345:1008–12.
105. Walter K, Tamargo R, Olivi A, et al. Intratumoral chemotherapy. Neurosurgery 1995;37:1129–45.
106. Fenstermacher J, Blasberg R, Patlak C. Methods for quantifying the transport of drugs across brain barrier systems. Pharmacol Ther 1981;14:217–48.
107. Blasberg R, Patlak C, Shapiro W. Distribution of methotrexate in the cerebrospinal fluid and brain after intraventricular administration. Cancer Treat Rep 1977;61:633–41.
108. Sipos E, Brem H. New delivery systems for brain tumor therapy. Neurol Clin 1995;13:813–25.
109. Gumerlock M, Neuwelt E. Principles of chemotherapy in brain neoplasia. In: Jellinger K, editor. Therapy of malignant brain tumors. New York: Springer-Verlag; 1987. p. 277–348.
110. Shapiro W, Green S, Burger P, et al. Randomized trial of three chemotherapy regimens and two radiotherapy regimens in postoperative treatment of malignant glioma. Brain Tumor Cooperative Group Trial 8001. J Neurosurg 1989; 71:1–9.
111. Walker M, Green S, Byar D, et al. Randomised comparisons of radiotherapy and nitrosoureas for the treatment of malignant glioma after surgery. N Engl J Med 1980;303: 1323–9.
112. Eyre H, Eltingham J, Gehan E, et al. Randomised comparisons of radiotherapy and carmustine versus procarbazine versus dacarbazine for the treatment of malignant gliomas following surgery: a Southwest Oncology Group Study. Cancer Treat 1986;70:1085.
113. Evans A, Jenkin R, Sposto R, et al. The treatment of medulloblastoma. Results of a prospective randomized trial of radiation therapy with and without CCNU, vincristine and prednisone. J Neurosurg 1990;72:572–82.
114. Packer R. Chemotherapy for medulloblastoma/primitive neuroectodermal tumors of the posterior fossa. Ann Neurol 1990;28:823–8.
115. Tait D, Thornton-Jones H, Bloom H, et al. Adjuvant chemotherapy for medulloblastoma: the first multi-center controlled trial of the International Society of Paediatric Oncology (SIOPI). Eur J Cancer 1990;26:464–9.

116. Wilson C, Boldrey E, Enot K. 1,3-bis (2-chloroethyl)-1-nitrosourea in the treatment of brain tumors. Cancer Chemother Rep 1970;54:273–81.
117. Levin V, Wara W, Davis R, et al. Phase III comparison of chemotherapy with BCNU and the combination of procarbazine, CCNU, and vincristine administered after radiation therapy with hydroxyurea to patients with malignant gliomas. J Neurosurg 1985;63:218–23.
118. Prados M, Scott C, Curran W, et al. Procarbazine, lomustine, and vincristine (PCV) chemotherapy for anaplastic astrocytoma: a retrospective review of Radiation Therapy Oncology Group protocols comparing survival with carmustine or PCV adjuvant chemotherapy. J Clin Oncol 1999;17:3389–95.
119. Newton H, Junck L, Bromberg J, et al. Procarbazine chemotherapy in the treatment of recurrent malignant astrocytomas after radiation and nitrosourea failure. Neurology 1990;40:1743–6.
120. Rodriguez L, Prados M, Silver P, et al. Reevaluation of procarbazine for the treatment of recurrent malignant central nervous system tumors. Cancer 1989;64:2420–3.
121. Maxwell M. Reexamining the dietary restrictions with procarbazine (an MAOI). Cancer Nurs 1980;451–7.
122. Coyle T, Bushunow P, Winfield J, et al. Hypersensitivity reactions to procarbazine with mechlorethamine, vincristine, and procarbazine chemotherapy in the treatment of glioma. Cancer 1992;69:2532–40.
123. Kyritsis A. Chemotherapy for malignant gliomas. Oncology 1993;7:93–100.
124. Pech I, Peterson K, Cairncross J. Chemotherapy for brain tumors. Oncology 1998;12:537–47.
125. Kim L, Hochberg F, Thornton A, et al. Procarbazine, lomustine, and vincristine (PCV) chemotherapy for grade III and grade IV oligoastrocytomas. J Neurosurg 1996;85:602–7.
126. Walker R, Allen J. Cisplatin in the treatment of recurrent childhood primary brain tumors. J Clin Oncol 1988;6:62–6.
127. Bertolone S, Baum E, Krivit W, et al. A phase II study of cisplatin therapy in recurrent childhood brain tumors. A report from the Children's Cancer Study Group. J Neurooncol 1989;7:5–11.
128. Allen J, Bosl G, Walker R. Chemotherapy trials in recurrent primary intracranial germ cell tumors. J Neurooncol 1985;3:147–52.
129. Packer R, Sutton L, Goldwein J, et al. Improved survival with the use of adjuvant chemotherapy in the treatment of medulloblastoma. J Neurosurg 1991;74:433–40.
130. Patel M, Godwin K, McCully C, et al. Plasma and cerebrospinal fluid pharmacokinetics of carboplatin and cisplatin [abstract 2753]. Proc Am Assoc Cancer Res 1996;37:403.
131. Allen J, Walker R, Luks E, et al. Carboplatin and recurrent childhood brain tumors. J Clin Oncol 1987;5:459–63.
132. Friedman H, Krischer J, Burger P, et al. Treatment of children with progressive or recurrent brain tumors with carboplatin or iproplatin: a Pediatric Oncology Group randomized phase II study. J Clin Oncol 1992;10:249–56.
133. Yung W, Mechtler L, Gleason M. Intravenous carboplatin for recurrent malignant glioma: a phase II study. J Clin Oncol 1991;9:860–4.
134. Longee D, Friedman H, Albright R, et al. Treatment of patients with recurrent gliomas with cyclophosphamide and vincristine. J Neurosurg 1990;72:583–8.
135. Allen J, Helson L. High-dose cyclophosphamide chemotherapy for recurrent CNS tumors in children. J Neurosurg 1981;55:749–56.
136. Friedman H, Mahaley M, Schold S, et al. Efficacy of vincristine and cyclophosphamide in the therapy of recurrent medulloblastoma. Neurosurgery 1986;18:335–40.
137. Carpenter P, White L, McCowage G, et al. A dose-intensive, cyclophosphamide-based regimen for the treatment of recurrent/progressive or advanced solid tumors of childhood. A report from the Australia and New Zealand Children's Cancer Study Group. Cancer 1997;80:489–96.
138. Coyle T, Baptista J, Winfield J, et al. Mechlorethamine, vincristine, and procarbazine chemotherapy for recurrent high grade gliomas in adults: a phase II study. J Clin Oncol 1990;8:2014–8.
139. Colvin M, Chabner B. Alkylating agents. In: Chabner B, Collins J, editors. Cancer chemotherapy principles and practice. Philadelphia: JB Lippincott; 1990. p. 276–313.
140. Newlands E, Blackledge G, Slack J, et al. Phase I trial of temozolomide (CCRG 81045:M&B 39831:NSC 362856). Br J Cancer 1992;65:287–91.
141. Brada M, Moore S, Judson I, et al. A Phase I study of SCH 52365 (temozolomide) in adult patients with advanced cancer. Proc Am Soc Clin Oncol 1995;14:470a.
142. Clark A, Deans B, Stevens M, et al. Antitumor imidazotetrazines: 32. Synthesis of novel imidazotetrazinones and related bicyclic heterocycles to probe the mode of action of the antitumor drug temozolomide. J Med Chem 1995;38:1493–1504.
143. Tisdale M. Role of guanine O6 alkylation in the mechanism of cytotoxicity of imidazotetrazines. Biochem Pharmacol 1987;36:457–62.
144. Levin V, Yung A, Prados M. A phase II study of Temodol in patients with anaplastic astrocytomas at first relapse [abstract]. Proc Am Soc Clin Oncol 1997;16:384.
145. Yung W, Prados M, Yaya-Tur R, et al. Multicenter phase II trial of temozolomide in patients with anaplastic astrocytoma or anaplastic oligoastrocytoma at first relapse. J Clin Oncol 1999;17:2762–71.
146. Chabner B, Myers C. Clinical pharmacology of cancer chemotherapy. In: DeVita V, Hellman S, Rosenberg S, editors. Cancer: principles and practice of oncology. Philadelphia: JB Lippincott; 1985. p. 308–9.
147. Jackson D, Sethi V, Spurr C, et al. Pharmacokinetics in the cerebrospinal fluid of humans. Cancer Res 1981;41:1466.
148. Levin V, Silver P, Hannigan J, et al. Superiority of postradiotherapy adjuvant chemotherapy with CCNU, procarbazine and vincristine (PCV) over BCNU for anaplastic gliomas: NCOG 6g61 final report. Int J Radiat Oncol Biol Phys 1990;18:321–4.
149. Glass J, Hochberg F, Gruber M, et al. The treatment of oligodendrogliomas and mixed oligodendroglioma-astrocytomas with PCV chemotherapy. J Neurosurg 1992;76:741–5.
150. Stewart D, Russell N, Atack E, et al. Cyclophosphamide, doxorubicin, vincristine, and dexamethasone in primary lymphoma of the brain: a case report. Cancer Treat Rep 1983;67:287–91.

151. McLaughlin O, Velasquez W, Redman J, et al. Chemotherapy with dexamethasone, high-dose cytarabine, and cisplatin for parenchymal brain lymphoma. J Natl Cancer Inst 1988;80:1408–12.
152. Chamberlain M, Levin V. Primary central nervous system lymphoma: a role for adjuvant chemotherapy. J Neurooncol 1992;14:271–5.
153. Brufman G, Halpern J, Sulkes A, et al. Procarbazine, CCNU and vincristine (PCV) combination chemotherapy for brain tumors. Oncology 1984;41:239–41.
154. Allegra C. Antifolates. In: Chabner B, Collins J, editors. Cancer chemotherapy principles and practice. Philadelphia: JB Lippincott; 1990. p. 110–53.
155. Baker W, Royer G, Weiss R. Cytarabine and neurologic toxicity. J Clin Oncol 1991;9:679–93.
156. Fulton D, Urtasun R, Forsyth P. Phase II study of prolonged oral therapy with etoposide (VP16) for patients with recurrent malignant gliomas. J Neurooncol 1996;27:149–55.
157. Chamberlain M. Recurrent supratentorial malignant gliomas in children. Long term salvage therapy with etoposide. Arch Neurol 1997;54:554–8.
158. Masumoto N, Nakano S, Esaki T, et al. Inhibition of cisdiaminedichloroplatinum (II)-induced DNA interstrand cross-link removal by 7-ethyl-10-hydroxy-camptothecin in HST-1 human squamous carcinoma cells. Int J Cancer 1995;62:70–5.
159. Rumbos H, Grosovsky A. Regulation of topoisomerase I activity following DNA damage: evidence for a topoisomerase I complex. Proc Am Assoc Cancer Res 1997;38:181.
160. Friedman H, Houghton P, Schold S, et al. Activity of 9-dimethylaminomethyl-10-hydroxycamptothecin against pediatric and adult central nervous system xenografts. Cancer Chemother Pharmacol 1994;34:171–4.
161. Blaney S, Phillips P, Packer R, et al. Phase II evaluation of topotecan for pediatric central nervous system tumors. Cancer 1996;78:527–31.
162. Burton E, Prados M. New chemotherapy options for the treatment of malignant gliomas. Curr Opin Oncol 1999;11:157–61.
163. Friedman H, Petros W, Friedman A, et al. Irinotecan therapy in adults with recurrent or progressive malignant glioma. J Clin Oncol 1999;17:1516–25.
164. Colvin O, Cokgar D, Ashley D, et al. Irinotecan treatment of adults with recurrent or progressive malignant glioma [abstract]. Proc Am Soc Clin Oncol 1998;17:1493.
165. Couldwell W, Weiss M, DeGiorgio C, et al. Clinical and radiographic response in a minority of patients with recurrent malignant gliomas treated with high-dose tamoxifen. Neurosurgery 1993;32:485–90.
166. Chamberlain M, Kormanik P. Salvage chemotherapy with tamoxifen for recurrent anaplastic astrocytoma. Arch Neurol 1999;56:703–8.
167. Pollack I, DaRosso R, Robertson P, et al. A phase I study of high-dose tamoxifen for the treatment of refractory malignant gliomas of childhood. Clin Cancer Res 1997;3:1109–15.
168. Ben Arush M, Postovsky S, Goldsher D, et al. Clinical and radiographic response in three children with recurrent malignant cerebral tumors with high-dose tamoxifen. Pediatr Hematol Oncol 1999;16:245–50.
169. Baltuch G, Shenouda G, Langleben A, et al. High-dose tamoxifen in the treatment of recurrent high grade glioma: a report of clinical stabilization and tumor regression. Can J Neurol Sci 1993;20:168–70.
170. Vertosick FT, Selker RG, Arena V. A dose escalation study of tamoxifen therapy in patients with recurrent glioblastoma multiforme. J Neurosurg 1994;80:385A.
171. Puchner M, Cristane L, Herrmann H. First results of a combined therapy (operation, tamoxifen [TAM], carboplatin [CP], radiotherapy [RT]) in patients with glioblastoma. J Neurooncol 1996;30:105.
172. Prados M, Schold S, Spence A, et al. Phase II study of paclitaxel in patients with recurrent malignant glioma. J Clin Oncol 1996;14:2316–21.
173. Mukwaya G. Immunosuppressive effects and infections associated with corticosteroid therapy. Pediatr Infect Dis J 1988;7:499–504.
174. Lesser G, Grossman S. The chemotherapy of adult primary brain tumors. Cancer Treat Rev 1993;19:261–81.
175. Weissman D, Dufer D, Vogel V, et al. Corticosteroid toxicity in neuro-oncology patients. J Neurooncol 1987;5:125–8.
176. Stiefel F, Breitbart W, Holland J. Corticosteroids in cancer: neuropsychiatric complications. Cancer Invest 1989;7:479–91.

Clinical Trials and Experimental Chemotherapy

SUSAN M. CHANG, MD

Neuro-oncologists face a great challenge in the management of patients with malignant glioma. After maximal safe resection and external beam radiation therapy, chemotherapeutic options are limited in their effectiveness. Despite clinical trials evaluating several agents over the past 20 years, the outcome of patients with malignant glioma remains poor.[1,2] Several principles have emerged regarding the successful design, conduct, and implementation of clinical trials specific to brain tumor patients.[3,4] Because the incidence of this disease is uncommon, accrual to clinical trials can be slow, and efforts are being made to enhance accrual rates. The formation of multi-institutional National Brain Tumor Consortia has been a major endeavor by the National Cancer Institute to support the development of new strategies in a cooperative and efficient way. This affords the opportunity for a number of motivated clinician-scientists to participate in a collaborative effort to improve the outcome of patients through clinical research.

Because of the limitations of chemotherapeutic agents for this disease, other strategies are needed. Intense research in the fields of cell biology, molecular cytogenetics, and immune modulation has added insight into the complex processes of oncogenesis, growth, and invasion of malignant glioma. New targets of cell proliferation, growth modulation, antiangiogenesis, anti-invasion, and immunotherapy are being explored in the clinical setting. Some of these strategies may be cytostatic rather than cytotoxic, and this needs to be considered when designing a trial and defining its end points. For example, one may theorize that anti-invasion measures as well as immunomodulatory strategies may be most successful at the time of minimal tumor burden, after maximal surgical resection and radiation therapy. The ability to detect the effect will be dependent on the timing of therapy evaluation. Also, if therapy is administered in the adjuvant setting, an important parameter of outcome will not be response rate but, rather, either progression-free survival or overall survival.

It has been demonstrated that there is great heterogeneity in outcome among patients with malignant glioma treated with equivalent modalities. Curran and colleagues[5] looked at the survival data in thousands of patients with malignant glioma treated on several Radiation Therapy Oncology Group (RTOG) protocols using a recursive partitioning analysis; they identified six classes of patients with median survivals ranging from a few months to years. The identification of important prognostic factors such as grade, histologic subtype, age, and performance status is an important first step when designing clinical trials in this disease. These prognostic factors must be considered so that the outcome of the experimental therapy is truly a reflection of the intervention and not patient selection.

Histologic confirmation of the diagnosis by central pathologic review has been shown to be important in the design and interpretation of clinical trials. The term "malignant glioma" is not specific to one histology but includes anaplastic astrocytoma, anaplastic oligodendroglioma, anaplastic mixed tumors, and glioblastoma multiforme. These histologies have different responses to radiation therapy and chemotherapy and also different survival expectations, and they represent a heterogeneous group of diseases. Although clinical trials in the past have included patients with malignant glioma, current trials study the different histologies independently. This enables the clinician to better interpret the results of trials and apply them to management of patients.

Despite similar histologic classification, there is still a range of outcomes both in terms of response to therapy and survival, even when other risk factors are similar. Recent information on the molecular genetics of tumors is giving us insight into more specific predictors of outcome. For example, in the pediatric tumor medulloblastoma, loss of genetic material from chromosome 17p appears to impact negatively in terms of prognosis. Cairncross and colleagues[6] also demonstrated the importance of allelic loss of 1p in anaplastic oligodendroglioma in predicting response to chemotherapy and better survival. In this study, all patients with this cytogenetic abnormality had an objective response to chemotherapy and a 95 percent 5-year survival rate, as opposed to only a 25 percent response and 25 percent 5-year survival rate in those who retained the allele. The role of other cytogenetic abnormalities in malignant glioma is being evaluated. Abnormalities of p53, a tumor suppressor gene important in the early transformation of glioma and that encodes the epidermal growth factor receptor (EGFR), may be important in predicting prognosis in the astrocytic tumors, but this is to be further evaluated along with other cytogenetic aberrations.[7] It is anticipated that future clinical trials may employ these molecular cytogenetic "diagnoses" as criteria for eligibility into studies.

Some of the outcome assessments chosen for the evaluation of therapy may be difficult to define or assess in this patient population. For phase I studies, even toxicity may be difficult to assess. Agents may have neurologic toxicity that may be difficult to distinguish from the neurologic effects of the tumor/cerebral edema and could interfere with the determination of the maximal tolerated dose. An example of the difficulty in interpreting adverse treatment effects is seen with the widely used National Cancer Institute Common Toxicity Criteria (CTC) used for grading side effects. Patients who develop a seizure on therapy would, by the CTC, be graded as having sustained a grade IV toxicity. However, seizures may have been present prior to the initiation of the experimental agent and may have occurred because of tumor progression or inadequate antiepileptic agents, rather than as a side effect of the medication. Similarly, any neurologic decline of increased weakness or sensory loss may be related to tumor progression, especially if there is localization consistent with the intracranial lesion. In such cases, the protocol should state how these side effects will be handled.

For some strategies, a typical dose-escalating phase I study may not determine the maximal tolerated dose (MTD). There may not be a dose-response curve and the biologically optimal dose may, in fact, not be at the MTD. Some of the newer agents not only are well tolerated at very high doses but are intended to be administered in a chronic dosing regimen. For these agents, continuous monitoring of toxicity is important. For phase I studies that evaluate new strategies using radiation, acute and chronic effects must be considered in the trial design.

Drug interactions with concomitant medications commonly used in this patient population, for example, anticonvulsants and corticosteroids, may alter the degree and type of toxicities and need to be considered when evaluating new agents. For example, an initial phase II study using doses of paclitaxel established for malignant glioma patients with solid tumors did not result in the expected level of toxicities; the paclitaxel was far better tolerated in the brain tumor patient population.[8] Because of the induction effect on the hepatic enzyme system, agents such as paclitaxel that are metabolized in the liver have accelerated clearance, and this results in lower serum drug concentrations. A phase I study stratifying patients by dose and use of anticonvulsants confirmed this finding. In addition, it was noted that the dose-limiting toxicity in patients on anticonvulsants was central neurotoxicity, not peripheral neuropathy.[9] Irinotecan is currently being evaluated in a phase I/II study that stratifies patients by the use of anticonvulsants.

Malignant gliomas are infiltrative in nature without clear borders on standard neuroimaging studies. The extent of the tumor can be difficult to define, especially in the presence of cerebral edema that can be hard to distinguish from tumor infiltration. Some studies use the change in the volume of contrast enhancement to assess response. Since objective responses are likely reflective of antitumor activity, many phase II studies use this as the measure of efficacy. However, a residual or progressive viable tumor is difficult to distinguish from the effects of surgery and radiation therapy, especially with focal radiation approaches such as radiosurgery and brachytherapy. Some of the newer investigational approaches involve the continuous infusion of agents via interstitially placed catheters or direct injection into the brain parenchyma after surgical excision. The interpretation of the subsequent magnetic resonance imaging (MRI) after these interventions will no doubt be difficult. Strict eligibility criteria to define a recurrent tumor need to be stated for protocols requiring progressive disease. Since treatment effects can mimic tumor progression on standard MRI scans, noninvasive studies such as positron emission tomography (PET) and MR spectroscopy are being used to differentiate these etiologies.[10,11] Patients who have necrosis as a result of therapy are managed differently and may have a different outcome from those with tumor progression. Clear definitions of measurable or evaluable disease as well as the criteria of "response" using clinical and radiographic criteria, including the consideration of steroid use, need to be stated. In a recurrent tumor that is rapidly progressive, stabilization of disease may be included in the response definition, and since the minority of patients with malignant glioma tend to exhibit a partial or complete response, this needs to be clearly indicated.[12]

Interpretation of the results of brain tumor studies can be difficult due to the use of different outcome measures in nonrandomized studies. Because of the lack of an appropriate historic control group and the problem of selection bias, efficacy of the treatment regimen is hard to determine. In the majority of phase II studies, response rate has been accepted as a measure of efficacy. For some studies, the median time to tumor progression may also be a study outcome. In the latter instance, the frequency of evaluating disease status needs to be stated since the end point is dependent on the time intervals at which progression will be assessed. The use of a set time at which the status of disease is assessed (eg, 6-month progression-free survival) also has been used. This has the advantage of not requiring the occurrence of a specific event and can allow for more timely completion of studies.

Recently, attention has been given to the important outcome of quality of life, which is assessed using validated patient questionnaires.[13] In patients with recurrent malignant glioma who have a median survival of 4 to 8 months, improvement in their quality of life is an important goal and needs to be incorporated into trials as an important objective. As an example, in a phase II randomized trial of temozolomide in patients with glioblastoma at first relapse, patients were randomized to procarbazine versus temozolomide and the primary end point was 6-month progression-free survival; one of the secondary objectives was to describe the health-related quality of life of patients on treatment.

CLINICAL TRIALS IN NEURO-ONCOLOGY

In the preceding section, some principles specific to the design and conduct of clinical trials in the brain tumor patient population have been emphasized. The importance of the basic principles of a specific question, clear objectives, defined outcome measures, specified patient selection, and statistical rigor in the design of a trial also cannot be overstated. In general, the types of clinical therapeutic trials can be described as phase I, II, or III. Phase I studies have the primary objective of determining the toxicities associated with a specified therapy. The determination of an MTD and, therefore, the defined phase II dose is another major objective. For some phase I studies, patient selection may be important. In some instances, patients who previously have been heavily pretreated with other agents may be excluded for fear of underestimating the MTD. Most phase I studies also have corollary pharmacokinetic and pharmacodynamic studies associated with them. For the brain tumor patient population, it has been important to characterize the pharmacologic interaction of the experimental agent with known agents that alter the hepatic metabolism of drugs. These agents include some anticonvulsants and corticosteroids. Because of hepatic enzyme induction by these agents, some chemotherapeutic agents may have accelerated metabolism, and, thereby, decreased toxicity may be noted at higher doses.

Although responses to therapy can be described in a phase I study, this is not the primary objective. In phase II studies, determination of efficacy is the main objective. These studies evaluate whether a therapy has sufficient antitumor activity to warrant further investigation in larger groups. These brain tumor trials typically accrue 40 to 50 patients, and a common end point may be the identification of at least a 20 percent response rate that is used to signify that the agent may be worthy of further clinical evaluation. Most phase II studies are open labeled and single arm in design; however, randomized phase II studies, although not comparative, provide the advantage of a concurrent "historic control," and, in some cases, if the difference between the two groups is large enough, this may reach statistical significance. Since the total number of patients treated with the therapy at the specified phase II dose tends to be limited in phase I studies, toxicity assessment is evaluated as a secondary objective in phase II studies.

Phase III studies aim to corroborate previous positive findings (confirmatory trials) or to modify an established regimen (explanatory trials). The evaluation of a new treatment is compared to a group of similar patients treated with a "control" therapy. A randomized trial design is usually implemented, and these studies tend to involve hundreds of patients. Primary and secondary outcome measures between the treatment groups should be predefined with a description of the statistical analyses that will be used to determine the significance of the findings. Phase III studies have many advantages and some limitations. One limitation is the large number of patients usually needed for these studies, which is difficult to achieve given the low incidence of this disease. This means that the time for accrual can be long, and these studies may only be possible through the cooperative effort of multi-institutions. Although brain tumor studies may be randomized, few can be double-blind, and for some end points such as progression-free survival, investigator bias cannot be eliminated. The obvious advantage of phase III studies given their randomized design is the minimization of bias and the ability to balance for the effect of unrecognized prognostic factors on outcome.

INITIAL THERAPY FOR MALIGNANT GLIOMA

Surgical Strategies

The main approaches to the treatment of patients with malignant glioma include maximal safe surgical resection, radiation therapy, and chemotherapy. Clinical trials are currently being conducted in an attempt to optimize the effect of surgery and radiation and to develop new strategies for chemotherapy. The development of surgically based clinical trials is a relatively new arena of research in this patient population. A phase I study of the use of gadolinium texaphyrin for MRI-guided resection of high-grade gliomas currently is being investigated. The objectives of this study are to determine the MTD of this agent as a tumor-retained contrast agent and to determine the intratumoral pharmacology and quantitative pharmacokinetics of this compound. Many of the newer therapies are administered interstitially, either via catheter placement with continuous infusion of the agent or via direct injection into the brain parenchyma after a surgical resection.

Radiation Strategies

Radiation therapy remains the mainstay of treatment for patients with cerebral glioma.[14] The main limitation of radiation therapy is the inherent resistance of tumor cells. This may be secondary to the ability of cells to repair the damage from ionizing radiation and the hypoxic environment of tumors as well as the relatively low growth fraction within primary brain tumors. Research strategies involve modification of the delivery of the radiation dose either by dividing the daily dose (hyperfractionated scheme) or by accelerated delivery. These strategies attempt to deliver a higher total dose, prevent tumor repopulation, and reduce the late effects on normal tissue. Since tissue hypoxia is one of the factors that influence the radioresistance of these tumors, attempts are being made to deliver higher concentrations of oxygen to the tumor in the hope that this may allow for more effective tumor cell kill. Agents can be used to preferentially sensitize tumor cells and not normal tissue, thereby improving the therapeutic efficacy. This strategy increases the radiochemical lesions within the deoxyribonucleic acid (DNA) and alters DNA repair mechanisms. Many agents are being evaluated.[15] Other strategies include increasing the number of cells at a more radiosensitive point in the cell cycle, thereby increasing the cytotoxic effect.

Focal radiation strategies allow for the delivery of higher doses of radiation to the tumor while sparing the normal tissue. A modification of the delivery of standard external beam radiation is using computer-assisted conformal radiation therapy. The RTOG is conducting a phase I/II study of conformal radiotherapy in patients with supratentorial glioblastoma multiforme. Other strategies include radiosurgery and brachytherapy (using either temporary or permanent radiation sources). The limitations for these strategies are the small percentage of patients who are eligible for this approach and the risk of radionecrosis as a consequence of delivering a high dose of radiation to the brain.

Cells are damaged by radiation as a function of time and temperature. Hyperthermia can inhibit the repair of DNA damage and increase radiosensitivity. Some experimental trials are investigating the use of hyperthermia in conjunction with radiation therapy. Boron neutron capture results in a highly localized generation of a high-linear energy transfer particle as a result of the interaction of a thermal neutron and a boron atom. The advantages of particle therapy include the higher and more localized delivered dose and an increased relative biologic effectiveness. The cellular damage also is less dependent on the degree of oxygenation of the tissue, an important factor in the radioresistance of high-grade tumors, especially glioblastoma multiforme. This approach is currently being investigated.

Current radiation-based studies for newly diagnosed malignant glioma are summarized in Table 11–1.

Using Chemotherapeutic Strategies

The treatment of brain tumor patients with chemotherapy poses a significant challenge for several reasons: (1) inherent and acquired mechanisms of drug resistance contribute to the poor responsiveness of gliomas; (2) the inability to deliver effective antineoplastic agents in sufficient concentrations to the tumor cells; (3) the blood-brain barrier is impermeable to most agents and restricts their entry into the brain parenchyma; (4) the systemic side effects of agents. Many different strategies using chemotherapy agents are being evaluated (Table 11–2).[16] These include the evaluation of new agents, combination chemotherapy, and the use of agents to reverse drug resistance. Increasing drug delivery is being explored via intra-arterial, intratumoral, or interstitial administration of drugs, as well as systemic high-dose standard agents using peripheral stem cell support or autologous bone marrow transplantation. The high-dose chemotherapy regimens are being evaluated primarily in the histologic subtype of pure

Table 11–1. RADIATION-BASED STUDIES FOR NEWLY DIAGNOSED MALIGNANT GLIOMA

Phase I	Phase II	Phase III
Drugs used during radiation		
Paclitaxel	RSR-13	XRT + DBD followed by
Cladribine	Interferon-β	DBD/BCNU vs XRT
Hydroxyurea + pentoxifylline	Intra-arterial CDDP + BCNU	BCNU vs BCNU/CDDP
Interferon-α + 13 CRA	BCNU/cisplatin/etoposide	(std vs accelerated XRT)
IUDR/accelerated XRT	Thalidomide	BCNU/CDDP x 3 + XRT
Gadolinium texaphyrin	Penicillamine and low copper diet	vs BCNU + XRT
Focal radiation		
Conformal radiotherapy	Brachytherapy + HT	Radiosurgery + XRT + BCNU
Stereotactic radiosurgery		vs XRT/BCNU
Particle therapy		
Boron neutron capture	Boron neutron capture	

13 CRA = 13-*cis* retinoic acid; IUDR = iododeoxyuridine; XRT = radiation; CDDP = cisplatin; BCNU = carmustine; DBD: = dibromodulcitol; HT = hyperthermia.

Table 11–2. CHEMOTHERAPY-BASED STUDIES FOR NEWLY DIAGNOSED MALIGNANT GLIOMA		
Phase I	Phase II	Phase III
BCNU/VP-16/thiotepa with peripheral blood stem cell support (pre-XRT) CI-980 (pre-XRT)	Temozolomide (pre-XRT) BCNU/temozolomide (pre-XRT) Aminocampthotecin (pre-XRT) High-dose CBDCA/thiotepa + stem cell or bone marrow support (pre-XRT) Intensive chemotherapy and autologous transplantation*	PCV ± DFMO (post-XRT) Intensive PCV + XRT vs XRT* XRT ± PCV *

*Eligible histology is anaplastic pure or mixed oligodendroglial tumors.
BCNU = carmustine; VP-16 = etoposide; XRT = radiation; CBDCA = carboplatin; PCV = procarbazaine, lomustine, vincristine; DFMO = difluoromethylornithine.

or mixed anaplastic oligodendroglioma. This tumor has shown chemosensitvity to standard doses of agents, and the hope is that more dose-intensive regimens would result in better long-term control and ultimately cure.

The side effects of radiation therapy can be debilitating and have an adverse effect on quality of life. Neoadjuvant strategies (prior to radiation therapy) also are being evaluated, especially in patients with anaplastic astrocytic and oligodendroglial tumors. If agents are found to be active and produce not only control but reduction of tumor size, it may delay or, ideally, obviate the use of radiation. A true assessment of the objective radiographic response to these agents is not confounded by the effects of prior radiation therapy using this paradigm.

Other Research Strategies

The intense laboratory research in the various fields of cell biology and molecular genetics that add insight into the complex process of oncogenesis has resulted in the development of exciting approaches. These include strategies of cell-growth modulation, tumor differentiation, anti-invasive agents, and antiangiogenic agents.[17–20] Several approaches using gene therapy are also being conducted. Murine cells engineered to produce a retroviral vector that carries a susceptibility gene (herpes simplex thymidine kinase) are placed within the tumor bed at the time of surgical debulking. The susceptibility gene is then incorporated into tumor cells that are actively dividing, and the antiretroviral drug ganciclovir is administered, thereby killing those tumor cells that have incorporated the gene.[21] Another gene therapy approach involves the replacement of genes known to be mutated or missing in malignant gliomas, for example, p53, which may be important in programmed cell death or apoptosis, and radio- or chemosensitivity.[22]

As more is being learned about the relationship of the effects of immune surveillance and the development of malignancies, strategies involving the modulation of the immune system are being explored in the treatment of patients with brain tumors.[23] Various approaches include the administration of cytokines (eg, interferon, interleukin-2), interstitial administration of radiolabeled antibodies, or recombinant proteins that consist of tumor antigen and conjugated toxins. Cellular adoptive immunotherapy approaches are also being explored.[24] Examples include the interstitial administration of lymphokine-activated killer cells and intravenous administration of T cells harvested from lymph nodes following vaccination with irradiated autologous tumor cells.

Yet another approach is photodynamic therapy in which photosensitizers are selectively taken up by tumor cells and are activated by the exposure to a particular wavelength of light. Evaluation of new photosensitizing agents is being conducted.

In this section, we have summarized some of the current experimental treatment protocols for adults with primary brain tumors (see Tables 11–1 and 11–2). These studies were published in the May/June edition of the listings of "*Current Clinical Trials: Oncology*" by the National Cancer Institute.

Other research strategies for newly diagnosed malignant glioma are summarized in Table 11–3.

INITIAL THERAPY FOR NEWLY DIAGNOSED GRADE II GLIOMA

After safe, maximal surgical removal of a glioma is performed, the strategies of radiation therapy and

Table 11–3. OTHER RESEARCH STRATEGIES FOR NEWLY DIAGNOSED MALIGNANT GLIOMA

Phase I	Phase II	Phase III
I-131-labeled antitenascin monoclonal Ab I-131-labeled monoclonal Ab fragment Me 1-14 F(ab)2 Adoptive immunotherapy Adeno- + HSV-TK gene therapy Astatine At 211 antitenascin monoclonal antibody 81C6 I-123 labelled antitenascin monoclonal antibody 81C6	Intracavitary IL-2 and LAK cell therapy	Photodynamic therapy using porfimer sodium

Ab = antibody; HSV-TK = herpes simplex virus thymidine kinase; IL = interleukin; LAK = lymphocyte activated killer.

Table 11–4. CHEMOTHERAPY-BASED PROTOCOLS FOR RECURRENT MALIGNANT GLIOMA

Phase I	Phase II	Phase III
BCNU wafers CI-980 Irinotecan Phenylbutyrate O_6-benzyl guanine/BCNU	Temozolomide DTIC Suramin Topotecan ISIS 3521 BCNU/temozolomide Interferon-α/BCNU ± tamoxifen Paclitaxel/topotecan/G-CSF Carboplatin/thymidine Paclitaxel/estramustine SU101	SU 101 vs procarbazine Procarbazine ± isoretinoin

BCNU = carmustine; DTIC = dacarbazine; G-CSF = granulocyte colony-stimulating factor.

chemotherapy may be considered. For patients who have had a gross-total resection of a grade II pure or mixed glioma, subsequent follow-up with surveillance scans is recommended. The role of radiation therapy subsequent to a subtotal resection or biopsy of a grade II glioma is still to be evaluated. The EORTC currently is conducting a phase III randomized comparison of early versus no or late radiotherapy for patients with low-grade gliomas. The role of adjuvant chemotherapy with CCNU (lomustine), procarbazine, and vincristine following radiation therapy is being evaluated by the RTOG in a randomized trial of patients with low-grade gliomas who are considered at high risk for recurrence. Patients greater than 40 years of age or those who have had either a biopsy or subtotal resection are eligible. For "low-risk" patients, a natural history study is being conducted.

TREATMENT FOR RECURRENT GLIOMA

There are several phase II studies evaluating single agents such as carboplatin, DTIC, temozolomide, antineoplastons A10 and AS2-1, and suramin as well as the combination of agents BCNU + interferon ± tamoxifen. Carmustine implant placement for recurrent low-grade tumors also is being evaluated in a phase II study. Chemotherapy-based protocols for recurrent malignant glioma are outlined in Table 11–4. Other research strategies for recurrent malignant glioma are summarized in Table 13–5.

SUMMARY

There continues to be an increasing number of clinical trials being conducted for patients with malignant glioma. A summary of these clinical trials involving

Table 11–5. OTHER RESEARCH STRATEGIES FOR RECURRENT MALIGNANT GLIOMA

Phase I	Phase II	Phase III
I-131-labeled antitenascin monoclonal Ab Recombinant chimeric protein composed of genetically altered IL-4 + *Pseudomonas* exotoxin Photodynamic therapy with porfimer sodium Astatine At 211 antitenascin monoclonal antibody 81C6 I-123 labelled antitenascin monoclonal antibody 81C6 Carmustine implant and irinotecan Adenovirus p53 gene therapy	Intracavitary IL-2 and LAK cell therapy Intracavitary IL-2 and allogeneic cytotoxic T lymphocytes Proxima GliaSite RTS	High- or low-dose photodynamic therapy using porfimer sodium

Ab = antibody; IL = interleukin; LAK = lymphocyte activated killer.

strategies of surgery, radiation therapy, and chemotherapy is presented here. Major advances in the understanding of the molecular biology and cytogenetics of malignant glioma will hopefully translate into effective therapeutic approaches.

REFERENCES

1. Lesser GJ, Grossman S. The chemotherapy of high-grade astrocytomas. Semin Oncol 1994;21:220–35.
2. Fine HA, Dear KB, Loeffler JS, et al. Meta-analysis of radiation therapy with and without adjuvant chemotherapy for malignant gliomas in adults. Cancer 1993;71:2585–97.
3. Perry JR, DeAngelis LM, Schold SC Jr, et al. Challenges in the design and conduct of phase III brain tumor trials. Neurology 1997;49:912–7.
4. Kaplan RS. Complexities, pitfalls, and strategies for evaluation of brain tumor therapies. Curr Opin Oncol 1998;10:175–8.
5. Curran WJ Jr, Scott CB, Horton J, et al. Recursive partitioning analysis in three Radiation Therapy Oncology Group malignant glioma trials. J Natl Cancer Inst 1993;26:704–10.
6. Cairncross JG, Ueki K, Zlastescu C, et al. Specific genetic predictors of chemotherapeutic response and survival in patients with anaplastic oligodendrogliomas. J Natl Cancer Inst 1998;90:1473–9.
7. Rainov NG, Dobberstein KU, Bahn H, et al. Prognostic factors in malignant glioma: influence of the overexpression of oncogene and tumor-suppressor gene products on survival. J Neurooncol 1997;35:13–28.
8. Prados MD, Schold SC, Spence AM, et al. Phase II study of paclitaxel in patients with recurrent malignant glioma. J Clin Oncol 1996;14:2316–21.
9. Chang SM, Kuhn JG, Rizzo J, et al. Phase I study of paclitaxel in patients with recurrent malignant glioma. J Clin Oncol 1998;16:2188–94.
10. Barker FG, Chang SM, Pounds TR, et al. 18-Fluorodeoxyglucose uptake and survival in patients with suspected recurrent malignant glioma. Cancer 1997;79:115–26.
11. Wald LL, Nelson SJ, Day MR, et al. Serial proton magnetic resonance spectroscopy imaging of glioblastoma multiforme after brachytherapy. J Neurosurg 1997;87:525–34.
12. MacDonald DR, Cascino T, Schold C Jr, et al. Response criteria for phase II studies of supratentorial malignant glioma. J Clin Oncol 1990;8:1277–80.
13. Weitzner M, Meyers C, Gelke C, et al. The Functional Assessment of Cancer Therapy (FACT) scale. Development of a brain subscale and revalidation of the general version (FACT-G) in patients with primary brain tumors. Cancer 1995;75:1151–61.
14. Laperriere NJ, Bernstein M. Radiotherapy for brain tumors. CA Cancer J Clin 1994;44:96–108.
15. Shenoy MA, Singh BB. Chemical radio-sensitizers in cancer therapy. Cancer Invest 1992;10:533–51.
16. Avgeropoulos NG, Batchelor TT. New treatment strategies for malignant gliomas. Oncologist 1994;4:209–24.
17. Feldkamp MM, Lau N, Guha A. Signal transduction pathways and their relevance in human astrocytomas. J Neurooncol 1997;35:223–48.
18. Lund EL, Spang-Thomsen M, Skovgaard-Poulsen H, et al. Tumor angiogenesis—a new therapeutic target in gliomas. Acta Neurol Scand 1998;97:52–62.
19. Giese A, Westphal M. Glioma invasion in the central nervous system. Neurosurgery 1996;39:235–52.
20. Cheson BD. The maturation of differentiation therapy. N Engl J Med 1992;327:422–3.
21. Ram Z, Culver KW, Oshiro EM, et al. Therapy of malignant brain tumors by intratumoral implantation of retroviral vector-producing cells. Nat Med 1997;3:1354–61.
22. Bischoff JR, Kirn DH, Williams A, et al. An adenovirus mutant that replicates selectively in p-53 deficient human tumor cells. Science 1996;274:373–6.
23. Jaeckle KA. Immunotherapy of malignant gliomas. Semin Oncol 1994;21:249–59.
24. Plautz GE, Barnett GH, Miller DW, et al. Systemic T cell adoptive immunotherapy of malignant gliomas. J Neurosurg 1998;89:42–51.

Gene Therapy Approaches

CANDELARIA GOMEZ-MANZANO, MD
JUAN FUEYO, MD
W.K. ALFRED YUNG, MD

The current therapies for glioblastoma multiforme are ineffective.[1] Therefore, it is urgently important to identify novel therapies that target specific differences between normal and malignant cells. Malignant gliomas are attractive targets for local gene therapy because of their absolute localization into the central nervous system (CNS) and absence of remote metastases. The development of new molecular techniques recently has yielded a battery of potential gene therapies for gliomas.[2,3] For the development of an efficient gene therapy strategy, accurate molecular targeting and proper delivery are critical. In this chapter, we review the most frequent molecular targets at each stage of the malignant progression of gliomas and the evolution of human adenoviruses as gene vehicles for cancer gene therapy strategies and as oncolytic tools.

CONCEPT OF GENE THERAPY

The initial goals of gene therapy were to cure relatively straightforward genetic disorders such as adenosine deaminase deficiency that are caused by a single defective gene.[4] These diseases could be cured by the transfer of a normal copy of the abnormal gene. However, cancer is now the target of the majority of gene transfer clinical trials in the United States. The development of retroviruses as gene vehicles to deliver genes inside cancer cells triggered the multiplication of gene therapy studies for gliomas. These vectors were very attractive because they are effective tools to transfer genes in vivo and are not able to complete their life cycle in postmitotic cells, which constitute the vast majority of normal brain cells. Many of the first gene therapy trials were done using retroviruses to transduce suicide genes into brain tumor cells. More recently, retroviruses are being replaced with replication-deficient adenoviruses (Figures 12–1 and 12–2), and other genes have been uncovered as potential targets.

The realization that any cancer results from defects in oncogenes and tumor-suppressor genes should propel the design of therapeutic strategies to target these fundamental molecular defects. The understanding of the critical role that cell-cycle and apoptosis regulation plays in the control of cancer should result in the development of strategies to inhibit tumor growth or kill cancer cells. Suitable molecular targets also have been found in such fields as angiogenesis or invasiveness, both characteristics of the most malignant forms of cancers. Other strategies are based (1) on the use of oncolytic viruses that replicate selectively in tumor cells or (2) on the expression of immunomodulators to trigger a selective immune response against the tumor.

The adaptation of gene therapy protocols to treat tumors has broadened the number of anticancer treatments. Within the past 10 years, a plethora of gene therapies against cancer have been developed that are proven to affect tumor growth in vivo. However, the field of gene therapy is still in its infancy. Improvements are needed at every level. At any rate, in the near future, understanding of the molecular mechanisms that regulate the origin, proliferation, and invasion of brain tumors will lead to more rational and less toxic therapies for cancer.

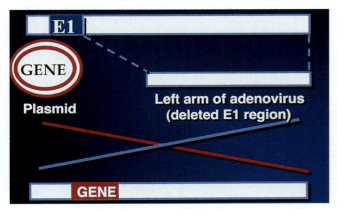

Figure 12–1. Genome of the adenovirus serotype 5. Structure of a recombinant replication-deficient adenoviral vector. The deletion of the E1 region from the genome of the adenovirus type 5 renders the adenovirus defective for replication. To construct the adenoviral vector, a shuttle vector carrying an expression cassette of the exogenous gene and part of the adenoviral sequence is cotransfected with another plasmid containing the adenoviral sequence (except the E1 region). The homologous recombination leads to the formation of a vector carrying the exogenous gene in the deleted E1 region.

manipulation in the laboratory of cancer-related genes is helping us to improve our understanding of the intricate molecular mechanisms that differentiate normal cells from cancer cells (Table 12–1).

One of the main problems of gene therapy is the so-called "vector gap." Despite the identification of genes that have a powerful anticancer effect, current vectors allow only an incomplete delivery of the therapeutic gene to every cancer cell in vivo. In addition, several strategies of gene therapy are based on the transfer or modification of a single gene. These single-gene strategies are not optimum to efficiently attack tumors, such as gliomas that are genetically heterogenic. Another obstacle to the development of gene therapy strategies is the incomplete understanding of the mechanisms regulating cancer growth (Table 12–2).

ADVANTAGES AND DISADVANTAGES OF GENE THERAPY

Gene therapy strategies are directed against the fundamental molecular defect of neoplastic cells. Therefore, gene therapy strategies may have a high therapeutic index based on specific gene target with low toxicity. Transfer of genes to cells in order to design therapies may have additional advantages. Thus, the functional

TARGETS IN GENE THERAPY FOR GLIOMAS

Among the most important targets for gene therapy strategies in brain tumors are tumor-suppressor genes, cell-cycle modulators, and growth factors.[5–9] These molecules are involved in inducing apoptosis (p53, E2F-1), blocking cell-cycle progression (p16, Rb), inducing proliferation (epithelial growth factor receptor [EGFR]), triggering angiogenesis (vascular

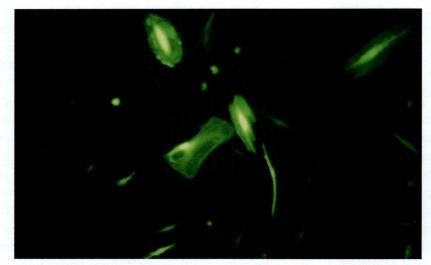

Figure 12–2. Examination of the infectivity of glioma cells. Shown are glioma cells infected with an adenovirus carrying the green fluorescence protein complementary deoxyribonucleic acid (cDNA). Infected cells acquire green fluorescence when observed through a fluorescence microscope (×200 original magnification). (Reproduced with permission from Fueyo J, Gomez-Manzano C, Alemany R, et al. Oncogene 2000;19:2–12.)

Table 12–1. ADVANTAGES OF GENE THERAPY
High therapeutic index: specificity with low toxicity
Based on the molecular defect of the neoplastic cells
Allows the examination of the fundamental mechanisms of cancer

endothelial growth factor [VEGF]), and favoring invasiveness (MMP2). In the development of gliomas and in their malignant progression, the gene abnormalities are thought to be additive, and, in this way, different mutations or amplifications can be observed in different stages of malignancy. Understanding the stepwise progression of these molecular defects may be critical for the development of more rational therapies for gliomas (Figure 12–3).

There is evidence that different genetic pathways may lead to the development of glioblastoma multiforme.[10] There are two major groups of human glioblastomas (primary and secondary); these are characterized by different molecular genetic defects.[10–12] Primary glioblastomas account for the vast majority of glioblastomas in older people (> 50 years) and have a short clinical history, usually less than 6 months.[10] In these tumors, there is no preclinical or histologic evidence of a preexisting, less malignant precursor lesion. In addition, the molecular abnormalities of primary glioblastomas are different from those observed in secondary glioblastomas. Thus, the EGFR amplification occurs significantly more often in elderly patients without loss of heterozygosity on chromosome 17p[13] or mutations in the *P53* gene.[14] In this group of glioblastomas, the amplification of MDM2, a molecule antagonistic of *P53*, is also observed;[15] this suggests that although *P53* is structurally intact, it might be functionally disabled. The presence of a mutant *P53* gene and abnormalities in chromosome 10 may be observed in a subset of primary glioblastomas such as the giant cell glioblastoma.[16] Secondary glioblastoma is characterized by the stepwise inactivation of genes in their formation. This type of glioblastoma often develops over months or years from low-grade or anaplastic astrocytomas and is mainly seen in young adults (< 50 years). Abnormalities of the Rb pathway are observed in both types of glioblastomas.[17] The classification of glioblastomas as primary and secondary has clinical and therapeutic implications: single-gene therapy strategies might apply for one type of glioblastoma only.

VECTORS AND DELIVERY

One of the most important areas of future research is vector design (see above, "Advantages and Disadvantages of Gene Therapy"). Improvement in the design and construction of delivery strategies is one of the most important factors responsible for the progress in the gene therapy field. Each delivery system has its own advantages,[18] suggesting that it may be more useful than others for specific cell types and tumors. Grossly, the delivery systems may be classified as viral and nonviral approaches (Table 12–3). The advantages of retroviruses include their integration into the genome and the requirement of cell division for transduction. Adenoviruses have high transduction efficiency and may infect many cell types, and the infection does not require cell division. Adeno-associated virus integrates into the

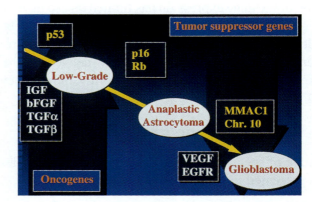

Figure 12–3. Genetic abnormalities in the malignant progression of gliomas. The stepwise inactivation of tumor-suppressor genes and overexpression/amplification of oncogenes is better defined in secondary gliomas. The inactivation of *P53* is one of the earliest events, the Rb pathway is abnormal in anaplastic astrocytomas, and abnormalities of the chromosome 10 (including inactivation of the MMAC1 gene) are observed in glioblastoma multiforme. The overexpression/amplification of epidermal growth factor receptor (EGFR) and vascular endothelial growth factor (VEGF) are other characteristics of this most malignant form of gliomas. IGF = insulin-like growth factor; bFGF = basic fibroblast growth factor; TGF = transforming growth factor. (Reproduced with permission from Gomez-Manzano C, Yung WK. Gene therapy for gliomas. BioMedicina 1999;2:242–44.)

Table 12–2. DISADVANTAGES OF GENE THERAPY
Incomplete delivery of the therapeutic gene to every cancer cell in vivo
Single-gene therapies: genetic heterogeneity of gliomas
Incomplete understanding of the mechanisms regulating proliferation, invasion, cell cycle, cell death

cell genome and does not express viral genes; the infection does not require cell division. Herpes simplex viruses have neuronal tropism and can carry a large insert (eg, 50 kb). Liposomes, mechanical administration, and protein–deoxyribonucleic acid (DNA) complexes can carry therapeutic nucleic acids with no limitations on the size or type.

Existing vectors, however, have limitations.[18] There is no current vector that is able to deliver the target gene to every cell of a tumor in vivo. For some viral vectors (eg, retroviruses) the achievable titers are low compared with what is needed for the treatment of large tumors. In addition, large-scale production may result in replication-competent viruses (eg, retroviruses, adenoviruses). Replication-deficient adenoviruses induce cellular toxicity and cell death. In addition, the virus may not be able to be administered to previously treated patients because of an immune response to viral antigens. The large-size genome of the herpes simplex virus has limited the possibility of its manipulation to decrease toxicity and to increase the ability to target tumor cells.

Nonviral vectors include liposomes, molecular conjugates, and naked DNA delivered by mechanical methods. These systems lack the ability to target specific cell types and mediate gene transduction mainly at the site of administration. In some cases, the duration of the gene expression has limited its use in vivo.

A universal gene delivery system has yet to be identified; however, the further improvement of present vectors as well as the use of new delivery strategies will likely expand the applicability and efficacy of gene therapy.

SPECIFIC STRATEGIES

A list of specific strategies and respective examples is presented in Table 12–4.

Table 12–3. GENE DELIVERY SYSTEM APPROACHES	
Viral	Nonviral
Adenovirus	Mechanical administration
Herpes simplex virus	Protein-DNA complexes
Adeno-associated virus	Liposomes
Retrovirus	
Vaccinia virus	
Avipoxvirus	
Baculovirus	

DNA = deoxyribonucleic acid.

Table 12–4. MOLECULAR TARGETS IN GLIOMAS	
Strategy	Example
Apoptosis inducers	p53, E2F-1
Cell-cycle modulators	Rb, p16
Signal transduction	MMAC
Control of angiogenesis	VEGF
Decrease of invasion	MMP-9, MMP-2
Induction of drug sensitivity	HSV-tk
Counteraction of oncogenes	EGFR
Oncolytic viruses	HSV
Anticancer immune response	IGF
Multiple-target strategies	

VEGF = vascular endothelial growth factor; HSV-tk = herpes simplex virus–thymidine kinase; EGFR = epidermal growth factor receptor; HSV = herpes simplex virus; IGF = insulin-like growth factor.

The p53 Paradigm

The *P53* gene is a prototype of a tumor-suppressor gene that is abnormal in gliomas (Table 12–5). Mutations causing loss of function of the *P53* gene are present in more than 30 percent of astrocytomas and constitute the earliest detectable genetic alteration in these tumors.[19,20] The wild-type p53 protein suppresses malignant transformation either by inducing apoptosis or by blocking cell-cycle progression (Figure 12–4). The p53 protein upregulates the expression of the p21 protein, a universal cyclin-dependent kinase inhibitor that regulates negatively the progression of the cell cycle. The p53 protein also transcriptionally activates the death gene bax that is related to the induction of apoptosis (Figure 12–5). Experimental transfer of p53 to glioma cells (Figure 12–6) first induces expression of the p21 protein and growth arrest and subsequently induces bax and apoptosis[21–23] (Figures 12–7 and 12–8). In addition to the direct effects of p53, other molecules

Table 12–5. TARGETING TUMOR-SUPPRESSOR GENES IN GLIOMAS		
Gene	% Abnormal	Studies
P53	50	In vitro
		In vivo
		Clinical trial
P16	60	In vitro
Rb	30	In vitro
		In vivo
E2F-1	—	In vitro
		In vivo
MMAC	50	In vitro
		In vivo

— = unknown.

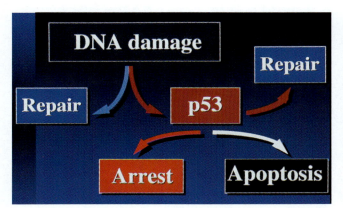

Figure 12–4. p53 functions (I): activation of p53 follows DNA damage. The functions of the p53 protein include DNA repair, arrest of cell-cycle progression, and apoptosis. These functions appear to be separable. DNA = deoxyribonucleic acid.

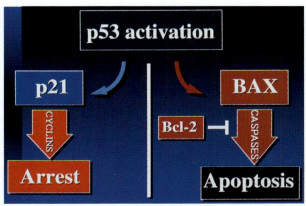

Figure 12–5. p53 functions (II): the p53 protein exerts its functions through transcriptional activation of other genes. Activation of p21, an inhibitor of the cyclin-dependent kinases, blocks the progression of the cell cycle. Bax is expressed during p53-mediated apoptosis. Bax-mediated apoptosis can be regulated by the expression of Bcl-2, an antiapoptotic molecule. (Reproduced with permission from Gomez-Manzano C, Yung WK. Gene therapy for gliomas. BioMedicina 1999;2:242–44.)

may enhance p53-apoptotic ability. It has been reported that coexpression of p16 and p53 induces apoptosis in p53-resistant cancer cells.[24] A possible rationale for this synergism is the downregulation of the Rb protein by the exogenous p16 protein.[24] In addition, p19ARF, which is the protein encoded by the alternate reading frame of the p16 locus, has recently been implicated in the activation of p53 by inhibiting the p53-antagonist MDM2 protein.[25]

The *P53* gene is a critical target to develop gene therapy strategies for cancer, and the toxicity and effect of the transfer of p53 to gliomas currently are being tested in the first clinical trial in gliomas using adenoviruses as transfer vectors. However, in gliomas, p53-transfer strategies may not have a wide-

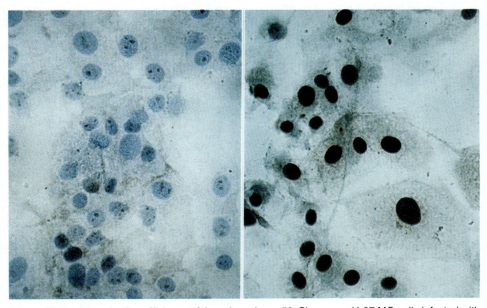

Figure 12-6. Transduction efficiency of the adenovirus-p53. Shown are U-87 MG cells infected with an adenovirus carrying the p53 complementary deoxyribonucleic acid. The overexpression of the exogenous protein is detected by immunohistochemistry using antibodies against the p53 protein. The exogenous p53 is mainly localized in the nucleus of the glioma cells (*right*). Parental U-87 MG cells express a very low level of endogenous wild-type p53 (*left*). DAB was used as chromogen. Sections were slightly counterstained with hematoxylin (×200 original magnification).

Figure 12–7. *A*, p53-mediated cell death. Examination of the viability of glioma cells treated with p53. Transfer of exogenous p53 complementary deoxyribonucleic acid to glioma cells induced cell death as assessed by growth curve assays using Trypan blue exclusion test. Transfer of p53 modified the morphology of the cells and produced a massive detachment of the treated cells from the culture dish by 5 days after the infection with the adenovirus-p53 (*B*) in comparison with the virus control-infected cells (*C*) (×100 original magnifcation). (Reproduced with permission from Gomez-Manzano C, Fueyo J, Kyritsis AP, et al. Adenovirus-mediated transfer of the p53 gene produces rapid and generalized death of human glioma cells via apoptosis. Cancer Res 1996;56:694–9.)

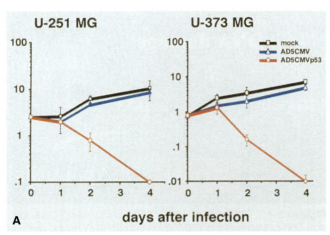

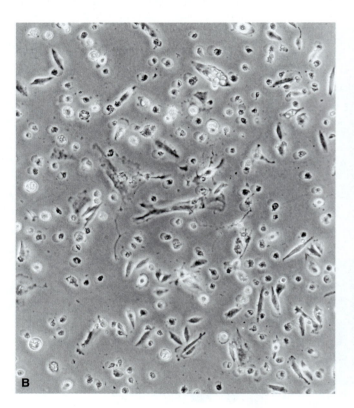

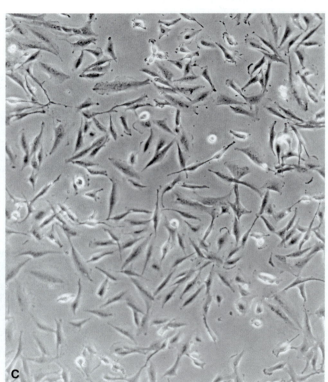

spread application because many gliomas express endogenous wild-type p53. In addition, the majority of mutant-p53 tumors harbor a subpopulation of cells that express wild-type p53 protein, and many gliomas overexpress p21 protein; expression of p21 is related to acquisition of an antiapoptotic phenotype.[22]

The Rb Pathway

Low-grade gliomas usually express wild-type Rb and p16 proteins. However, inactivation of these two proteins and amplification of cyclin D1 and cyclin-dependent kinase 4 (CDK4), which regulate the phosphorylation of the Rb protein (Figure 12–9), are among the most frequent abnormalities in anaplastic astrocytomas and glioblastomas.[26,27] Transfer of exogenous p16 or Rb to gliomas produces a cytostatic effect[28,29] and modifies the neoplastic phenotype of glioma cells, inhibiting their ability to form tumors in immunodeficient animals (Figure 12–10). The ultimate target of any alteration in the p16/Rb/E2F pathway is the deregulation of E2F

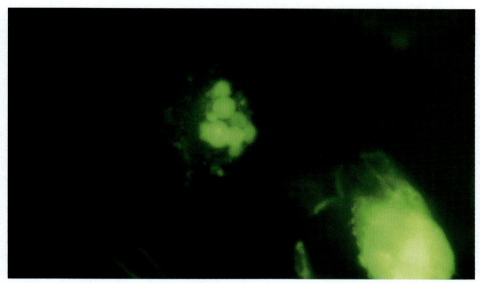

Figure 12–8. Features of p53-mediated apoptosis. Acridine orange staining of glioma cells infected with the p53 complementary deoxyribonucleic acid shows features of apoptosis. Shown are cells with nuclear condensation, nuclear fragmentation, and shrinkage of the cytoplasm (×400 original magnifcation). (Reproduced with permission from Gomez-Manzano C, Fueyo J, Kyritsis AP, et al. Adenovirus-mediated transfer of the p53 gene produces rapid and generalized death of human glioma cells via apoptosis. Cancer Res 1996;56:694–9.)

transcription factors. The E2F-1 protein transactivates several S-phase genes and drives cell-cycle progression through the G1 checkpoint. Furthermore, the E2F-1-mediated activation of proliferation is related to the acquisition of the neoplastic phenotype for ras-transformed fibroblasts. Thus, E2F-1 fulfills the criteria of an oncogene. However, the role of E2F-1, as in the case of the myc protein, appears to be dual since several lines of evidence indicate that the E2F-1 may also function as a tumor-suppressor gene.[30] In this regard, the E2F-1 protein has been shown to promote apoptosis in several systems, either alone or in association with p53. Furthermore, deletion of the E2F-1 gene results in spontaneous development of tumors in animals.[31,32]

In gliomas, the transfer of E2F-1 results in apoptosis[33] (Figures 12–11 and 12–12). This molecule is a potent anticancer tool, and preliminary studies suggest it may be more effective than p53 in eradicating glioma cells because it is able to induce apoptosis in p53-resistant cells.[23,33] Further, E2F-1 is able to override the growth arrest induced by p21 and p16, driving the cells to S phase and apoptosis. In glioma cells, E2F-1-mediated apoptosis has been shown to be independent of the status of the p53. The two main disadvantages of this apoptotic-inducer molecule are its potential toxicity and oncogenicity; transfer of the E2F-1 gene has been reported to induce apoptosis in normal fibroblasts.[34] However, the encouraging preliminary results obtained with the adenovirus-mediated transfer of

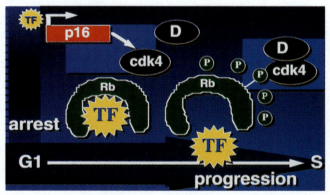

Figure 12–9. Regulatory loop: p16, Rb, E2F-1. Rb pathway. Cell-cycle control at the G1 checkpoint is exerted by the Rb protein. The Rb protein can bind and inactivate transcription factors (such as E2F-1), raising a block in the G1 phase of the cell cycle. The function of Rb is controlled by phosphorylation, which is mediated by cyclin D and cyclin-dependent kinases 4 and 6. Inhibition of the action of these molecules by the p16 protein induces activation of Rb and cell-cycle arrest. Deletion or mutation of Rb or p16 induces deregulated cell-cycle progression to S phase, multiplication of genetic defects, and eventually cancer. The Rb pathway is abnormal in the vast majority of the cancers including gliomas. TF = transcription factor; D = cyclin D; P = phosphorylation site.

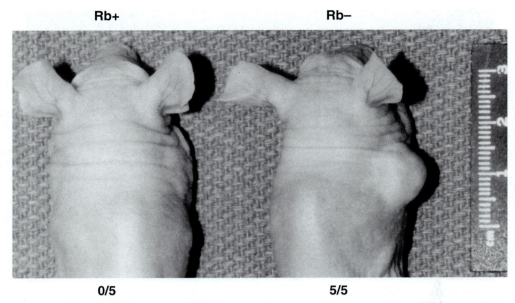

Figure 12–10. Transfer of tumor suppressor genes to gliomas. Rb transfer to gliomas: tumorigenicity. Rb inhibits tumorigenicity of glioma cells. Transfer of Rb to glioma cells results in the abolition of the glioma cells' ability to form tumors in nude mice. Rb-mediated inhibition of tumorigenicity is the strongest evidence of the tumor-suppressor role of Rb in gliomas. (Reproduced with permission from Fueyo J, Gomez-Manzano C, Yung WKA, et al. Suppression of human glioma growth by adenovirus-mediated Rb gene transfer. Neurology 1998;50:1307–15.)

Figure 12–11. E2F-1 mediated apoptosis. EsF-1 induces apoptosis in glioma cells. Transfer of E2F-1 to glioma cells induces apoptosis. During the E2F-1-mediated apoptosis, activation of the caspases is observed. One member of this enzymatic cascade is the protein PARP. *A,* Cleavage of PARP, resulting in the detection of fragments smaller than the full-length protein, is considered a biochemical marker of apoptosis. *B,* TdT analysis. Apoptosis can be quantitated by means of flow-cytometric analyses of deoxyribonucleic acid (DNA) breaks using the TUNEL assay. In this assay, apoptotic cells are situated in the superior window. This window is empty in the control cells. TdT = terminal deoxynucleotidyl nick end labeling.

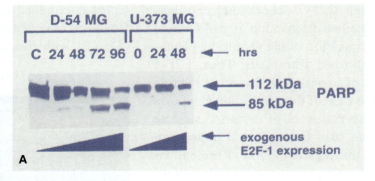

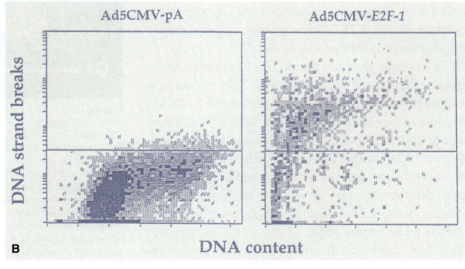

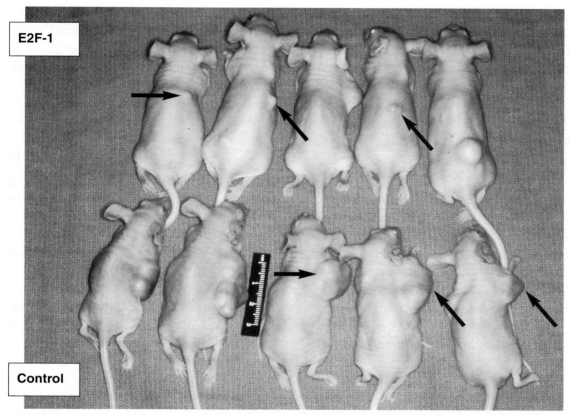

Figure 12–12. Transfer of tumor suppressor genes to gliomas. E2F-1 anticancer effect: in vivo studies. The antiglioma effect of E2F-1 is observed in vitro and in vivo. Transfer of E2F-1, using an adenoviral vector, to pre-established glioma tumors results in tumor inhibition ($p < .005$). (Reproduced with permission from Fueyo J, Gomez-Manzano C, Yung WKA, et al. Overexpression of E2F-1 in glioma triggers apoptosis and suppresses tumor growth in vitro and in vivo. Nat Med 1998;4:685-90.)

the E2F-1 gene into gliomas in vitro and in animal models should propel the development of clinical trials to assess the effectiveness of the transfer of E2F-1, alone or in combination with p53, in the treatment of gliomas.

In addition to the p16, Rb, and E2F-1 tumor-suppressor genes, the positive regulators of the cell cycle—cyclin D1, CDK4, and CDK6—are abnormally expressed in gliomas.[8,9] However, these alterations are not as frequent in these tumors as is the inactivation of tumor-suppressor genes. Theoretically, antisense strategies could be designed to counteract the oncogenic effect of these molecules in gliomas.

Antiangiogenesis: VEGF as a Target

Among the most suitable targets for new therapies of gliomas are the regulators of angiogenesis. These molecules are especially important in gliomas because hypervascularization is a major feature of these tumors. Indeed, the progression of an astrocytoma to anaplastic astrocytoma or glioblastoma multiforme is characterized by increased neovascularization.[35] Angiogenesis modulators are extraordinarily important in tumor growth, as is shown by the fact that neovascularization must occur for solid tumors to grow beyond a diameter of few millimeters.[36] One of these molecules is VEGF. This protein is efficiently secreted by tumor cells and promotes neovascularization. Messenger ribonucleic acid (mRNA) of VEGF has been shown to be overexpressed in the highly vascularized glioblastoma multiforme, indicating that VEGF plays a major role in the growth of gliomas. In addition, the transfection of VEGF complementary DNA (cDNA) to rat glioma cells results in hypervascularized tumors with abnormally large vessels, and the abrupt withdrawal of VEGF results in the regression of preformed tumor vessels.[37] Importantly, it has been shown that the transfection of antisense VEGF cDNA downregulates the endogenous VEGF and suppresses the ability of glioma cells to form tumors in mice.[38] In another study, ribozymes targeting VEGF downregulated VEGF in glioma cells in vitro.[39] In addition, it recently has been reported that adenovirus-mediated transfer of antisense VEGF to glioma cells in vivo inhibits tumor growth[40] (Figure 12–13).

Invasion: Metalloproteases

Glioma invasion involves cell adhesion and proteolytic modification of the extracellular matrix. The expression of numerous extracellular proteases has been documented in gliomas, but among the extracellular matrix–degrading proteinases, 72-kDa gelatinase-A (MMP-2) and the 92-kDa gelatinase-A (MMP-9) appear to be the principal MMPs that mediate the invasive phenotype in high-grade gliomas.[41] The control of the expression of MMP-2 and MMP-9 activity is still under intense examination, but it has been reported that MMP-2 activity is regulated both positively and negatively by growth factors and oncogenes. In gliomas, activation of MMPs is observed in the high grades (anaplastic astrocytoma and glioblastoma multiforme) but not in the low grades of malignancy or in normal tissue, suggesting that their activity contributes to the invasive capability of malignant gliomas. The suitability of MMPs as therapeutic targets in gliomas has been suggested by the fact that antibodies directed to either MMP-9 or its activator (urokinase/plasminogen) lead to a reduction in glioma invasion by approximately 70 percent.[41]

Genes that Activate Prodrugs

Another approach involves the conferring of drug sensitivity by transfixing tumor cells with a gene encoding an enzyme that can metabolize a nonprotoxic drug to its toxic form (suicide genes).

The thymidine kinase/ganciclovir approach takes advantage of the fact that the herpes virus thymidine kinase gene converts nontoxic nucleoside analogs such as ganciclovir into phosphorylated compounds that kill dividing cells. Thus, glioma cells genetically modified to express the herpes simplex virus–thymidine kinase (HSV-tk) gene can be killed by the administration of ganciclovir.[42] Preliminary studies in a rat glioma model showed that marked tumor regression occurred despite the fact that only a small fraction of cells were transduced by the exogenous gene. This cytotoxic effect of transduced on nontransduced cells is termed the "bystander effect." The thymidine kinase/ganciclovir approach currently is used in several clinical trials. Although the preliminary results of these studies are not completely satisfactory, it is expected that the substitu-

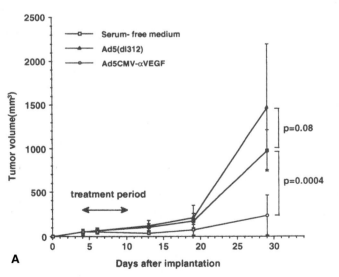
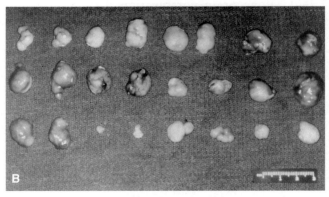

Figure 12–13. Antisense-VEGF therapy induces tumor inhibition. *A*, The growth rate of tumors in nude mice. Tumor volumes were measured by caliper and rendered as the mean ± standard deviation (mm³) for each group of mice. Treatment consisted of serum-free medium (mock infection) or either Ad5(dl312) (adenovirus control) or Ad5CMV-αVEGF. Intratumoral injections were given every other day for a total of four injections. *B*, The tumors removed from animals in the serum-free medium-treated group (*upper*), the Ad5(dl312)-treated group (*middle*), and Ad5CMV-αVEGF-treated group (*lower*). In these experiments, the transfer of antisense VEGF (αVEGF) induced a significant inhibition of the glioma growth. (Reproduced with permission from Im SA, Gomez-Manzano C, Fueyo J, et al. Antiangiogenesis treatment for gliomas: transfer of anti-sense vascular endothelial growth factor inhibits tumor growth in vivo. Cancer Res 1999;59:895–900.)

tion of retroviruses for adenoviruses as vehicles to transfer the herpex virus gene will improve the efficiency of this strategy.

The cytosine deaminase/5-fluorocytosine system is also popular among gene therapists.[43,44] In this system, the cytosine deaminase is used to convert 5-fluorocytosine to 5-fluorouracil in cancer cells.

The Antisense Strategy: Downregulation of Oncogenes

Several growth factors have been found amplified or overexpressed in low-grade gliomas (Table 12–6), including the basic fibroblast growth factor (bFGF), insulin-like growth factor (IGF), and the platelet-derived growth factor (PDGF) and its receptor PDGFR. These growth factors are involved in the unregulated cell proliferation and vascular neoformation. Another molecule overexpressed or amplified in glioblastoma multiforme is EGFR. The EGFR at 7p12 is the first gene found to be amplified in human glioblastomas and is the most commonly amplified gene in these tumors. The frequency of its amplification appears to correlate with increasing tumor grade, being present in 3 percent of low-grade astrocytomas, 7 percent of anaplastic astrocytomas, and nearly 40 percent of glioblastomas.[45,46] Several reports have addressed the role of EGFR in proliferation of and invasion by tumor cells. Although the oncogenic role of EGFR in gliomas is clear, there is no correlation between the amplification of EGFR and the prognosis of gliomas.

In addition to the wild-type phenotype, mutant forms of the EGFR have been identified in gliomas. At least one of these mutants confers enhanced tumorigenicity to human glioblastoma cells by increasing their proliferation and reducing apoptosis. Targeting of this mutant may induce apoptosis in gliomas expressing the mutant form of EGFR.[47]

In addition to EGFR, other mutated growth factor–related molecules have been found in high-grade gliomas. These include schwannoma-derived growth factor (SDGF, a member of the EGF family), VEGF, and the transforming growth factor (TGF)-α and -β families of proteins.[45,46] Although some gliomas overexpress growth factors, many gliomas coexpress growth factors and their receptors, suggesting that autocrine stimulation is the cause of the unregulated growth.[45,46]

Several antisense therapies designed against growth factors in gliomas have been examined.[46] For instance, transfer of the antisense sequence of the IGF-1 to C6 glioma cells has resulted in suppression of IGF-1 production, loss of in vivo tumorigenicity, and, most important, induction of a significant immunologic response that has caused the suppression of established C6 tumors without toxicity.[48] Similar studies performed with the IGF-1 receptor yielded similar results, including the trigger of anticancer immune response.[49] These results constituted the basis for a phase I clinical trial of this strategy. In another study, oligonucleotides complementary of the mRNA of the PDGF-B resulted in dose-dependent inhibition of the tumor growth.[50] Consistent with these results, transfection of glioma cells with a dominant negative form of PDGF has inhibited growth in vitro and suppressed tumorigenicity.[51] Other studies have demonstrated that antisense oligonucleotides[52–54] or complete antisense sequences[55] to bFGF, FGFR1, or TGF-α (see Table 12–6) also were able to suppress growth of glioma cell lines in cultures. In addition, treatment with oligonucleotides against TGF-β2 primer sequence enhanced lymphocytic proliferation and anticancer effect.[56] Importantly, subcutaneous implantation of glioma cells transfected to produce the antisense sequence of TGF-β2 resulted in the eradication of intracranial glioma tumors in rats.[57] These results prompted a phase I clinical study using this strategy.

Table 12–6. GROWTH FACTORS IN GLIOMAS	
Growth Factor	Effect
EGF/EGFR	Increase proliferation
PDGF/PDGFR	Glial transformation
bFGF/FGFR	Mitogenesis and angiogenesis
SDGF	Binds EGFR
	Mitogenesis
TGF-α	Binds EGFR
	Tumorigenesis
TGF-β	Local immunosuppression
IGF-1/IGF-1R	Glial tumorigenesis

EGFR = epidermal growth factor receptor; PDGFR = platelet-derived growth factor receptor; bFGF = basic fibroblast growth factor; FGFR = fibroblast growth factor receptor; SDGF = schwannoma-derived growth factor; TGF = transforming growth factor; IGF-1R = insulin-like growth factor 1 receptor.

Table 12–7. ONCOLYTIC VIRUSES			
Viruses	Targets	Advantages	Disadvantages
Herpes simplex virus	Cell division	Neurotropic Controllable (ganciclovir)	Toxicity
Adenovirus	p53 Rb	Tumor selective Cell cycle selective	Genetic heterogeneity Attacks normally dividing cells
Reovirus	Ras	Tumor selective	Few reports are available regarding its use

ONCOLYTIC VIRUSES

Details regarding oncolyte viruses are presented in Table 12–7.

Replication-Competent Adenoviruses

In cancer gene therapy, the failure to achieve enough tumor transduction to cause complete remission has led to the revival of replication-competent viruses (Figures 12–14 and 12–15). The lytic spread of virus throughout the tumor is an attractive solution. In gliomas, the work done with HSV-1 mutations provides a clear precedent of this strategy (see below, "Herpes Simplex Virus"). In comparison to HSV, adenoviruses theoretically are less toxic and easier to render tumor selective because they have a less complex genome. Thus far, the efforts have been aimed at improving the safety of replication-compe-

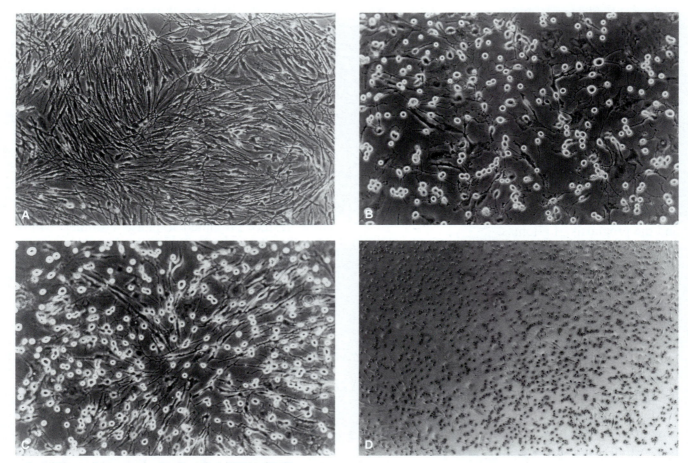

Figure 12–14. Infection of glioma cells with a mutant E1A oncolytic adenovirus. The infection of glioma cells with low doses of an oncolytic adenovirus resulted in a progressive cytopathic effect. Every dead cell released new progeny of oncolytic viruses that spread from cell to cell within the tumor. In gliomas, research performed with herpes simplex virus 1 mutants provides a clear example of the revival of replication-competent viruses. Time of infection: *A*, 0 hours; *B*, 2 days; *C*, 4 days; *D*, 6 days (×100 original magnification).

tent adenoviruses. Two strategies have been used to render adenoviral propagation selective for tumor cells: deletions and promoter regulation. As mentioned above, E1 proteins induce the cell cycle and inhibit apoptosis by binding to regulatory proteins such as p53 or Rb.[58] Therefore, in theory, mutant adenoviruses unable to inactivate p53 or Rb would propagate poorly in cells expressing p53 or Rb but more efficiently in tumor cells where p53 or Rb are already inactive. The specificity of a p53 nonbinding mutant for p53-defective cells is controversial.[59–62] Replication of p53 or Rb nonbinding mutants seems to correlate better with the capability of the infected cells to progress through the cell cycle than with the p53 or Rb status.[62,63] The strategy of controlling viral replication by substituting a viral promoter with a tumor-associated-antigen promoter has been attempted in prostate carcinoma, but the specificity of these promoters in the viral genome is a concern.[64,65] Despite potential problems of tumor specificity, both strategies have yielded promising preclinical results and have been translated into clinical trials (see below, "Results of Clinical Trials").

Herpes Simplex Virus

Herpes simplex virus type 1 mutants have been constructed for glioma therapy.[66–68] These mutants are attenuated for growth in nondividing cells but are replication competent within the tumor. An attenuated multimutated HSV-1 currently is being tested in a clinical trial. This double mutant, termed G207, has several properties favorable for treating gliomas:[67] (1) it is replication competent in dividing cells, including glioma cells; (2) it has attenuated virulence in normal cells; (3) it has been manipulated to be hypersensitive to ganciclovir treatment; and (4) it carries an easily detectable histochemical marker. Intratumoral treatment with the G207 virus decreased the growth of human glioma tumors implanted subcutaneously in nude mice and prolonged the survival of mice with intracerebral human glioma tumors. Toxicity studies showed that G207 is avirulent upon intracerebral inoculation of mice and HSV-sensitive nonhuman primates.

Another strategy consists of the use of HSV-1 to target tumor cells with upregulated mammalian ribonucleotide reductase, an enzyme whose expression is regulated by the Rb pathway.[69] In this strategy, the virus was modified to carry the transgene responsible for the bioactivation of the prodrugs cyclophosphamide and ifosfamide. The oncolytic effect, potentiated by the administration of the chemotherapeutics, was observed in vitro and in subcutaneous tumors established in immunodeficient animal models.

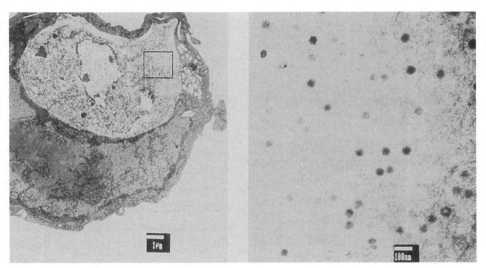

Figure 12–15. Electronic microscopy of a cancer cell infected with an oncolytic virus. Four days after infection with very low doses of an E1A-mutant replication-competent adenovirus, this cancer cell showed the production of numerous viral particles (*left*). The viral particles are observed clearly in a magnification of the marked area of the cell (*right*). (Reproduced with permission from Fueyo J, Gomez-Manzano C, Alemany R, et al. A mutant oncolytic adenovirus targeting the Rb pathway produces anti-glioma effect in vivo. Oncogene 2001;19:2–12.)

Reovirus

Human reovirus requires an activated ras-signaling pathway for infection of cultured cells. This property has been exploited for glioma therapy. Thus, a single intratumoral injection of viruses has resulted in regression of human U-87 MG glioblastoma tumors in immunodeficient mice models. In immunocompetent mice, a series of injections were required to obtain regression of the tumors.[70]

GENE IMMUNOTHERAPY

Gene immunotherapy is based on the use of recombinant DNA constructs to express cytokines and lymphokines. A major advantage of this approach is the potential to generate a systemic response against the tumor.[18] This strategy refers mainly to three different approaches: (1) presentation of tumor-rejection antigens by antigen-presenting cells; (2) vaccination with tumor cells that express cytokines; (3) expression of co-stimulatory molecules on the surface of tumor cells.

Presentation of Tumor-Rejection Antigens by Antigen-Presenting Cells

Autologous antigen-presenting cells can be harvested by mobilization from the blood of the patient or from biopsies of the brain tumor; they are then expanded in vitro with cytokines. To generate the antitumor immune response, antigen-presenting cells are transduced with the DNA or mRNA coding for the tumor antigen and then injected into the patient.

Vaccination with Cytokine-Expressing Tumor Cells

The second approach is based on the use of ex vivo vaccination with tumor cells that express cytokines. Disadvantages of this approach include the unavailability of tumor cells from every patient (inaccessible tumors) and the failure of the transduced cells to express the cytokine gene.

Expression of Co-stimulatory Molecules on the Surface of Tumor Cells

The transfer of co-stimulatory molecules (such as human leukocyte antigen [HLA]-type molecules) into tumor cells aims at generating T cell responses against the tumor. The identification of tumor-rejection antigens from brain tumors and of the critical components of afferent and efferent arms of the immune response are necessary to increase the efficiency of these systems.

RESULTS OF CLINICAL TRIALS

The results of the pioneer clinical trials have been published recently.[71–75] In the first clinical trial,[74] 15 patients (12 with recurrent malignant gliomas, 2 with metastatic melanomas, and 1 with metastatic breast carcinoma) were treated with stereotactic injections of murine fibroblast virus–producing cells that produce retroviruses carrying the HSV-tk gene. This pretreatment was followed by administration of ganciclovir. In spite of the low transduction efficiency (less than 0.17% of the tumor cells), this study showed a reduction of the tumor volume in 5 tumors. In addition, 3 patients showed a partial response and survived for more than 11 months. The adverse events of the treatment included meningeal inflammation, seizure, headache, and pancytopenia.

In another study,[75] 12 patients with recurrent glioblastoma were treated by direct injection of HSV-1-tk retroviral vector–producing cells into the surgical cavity margins after tumor debulking. Overall median survival was 206 days, with 25 percent of the patients surviving longer than 12 months; one of the patients was still free of detectable recurrence 2.8 years after treatment.

These preliminary trials show encouraging results that warrant further development. Future gene-based treatments (including regulation of the expression of molecules that are involved in cell-cycle control, apoptosis, cell migration, immune response, and angiogenesis) combined with other types of therapy could be more effective and less toxic (Table 12–8). Moreover, advances in vector design that increase both the efficiency of expression and the accuracy of the targeting should result in better response rates. In this regard, the substitution of retroviruses by adenoviruses as delivery vectors may result in a substantial improvement in the distribution of the therapeutic gene with subsequent enhancement of the clinical efficacy.

FUTURE DIRECTIONS

Multiple-Gene Strategies

Gliomas generally arise as the culmination of a multistep process that involves a variety of genetic abnormalities. Not every cell in the tumor has the same alterations. Combination of strategies that target proteins with different mechanisms of action (eg, apoptosis, antiangiogenesis) will probably be necessary for glioma treatment. The multiple-gene molecular approach may consist of a combination of proteins with different specific cytotoxicities: p53 triggers apoptosis; caspases are the executioner mechanism; p19 inactivates MDM2 and potentiates p53. In other strategies, one molecule may create the appropriate scenario for the action of a second one. Thus, antisense bcl-2 strategies can be combined with p53 to render resistant glioma cells sensitive to p53's apoptotic effect. Genes can cooperate to induce apoptosis (as with *P53* and E2F-1) or decrease invasiveness by targeting both MMAC1 and MMP-9. In addition, conventional chemotherapeutic agents and radiotherapy are able to augment the antitumoral effect of gene therapy strategies.

Improving Adenoviruses as Gene Therapy Tools

A strategy to improve efficacy of replicative adenoviruses is to convert the virus into a gene-carrying vector. This has been done with a p53 nonbinding mutant carrying the thymidine kinase gene.[76] Interleukin-12 is another candidate transgene to increase the oncolytic spread of replicative vectors because it can abrogate an antibody response against adenoviruses.[77] For gliomas, the molecular targets reviewed above that induce nonlytic therapeutic mechanisms are also rational candidates.

Other manipulations of the adenoviral vector could lead to increased tumor transduction; a promising strategy is the modification of the fiber to change the viral tropism.[78] A fiber with 20 carboxyterminal lysine residues confers an enhanced transduction of glioma cells.[79] Modified fibers are being incorporated in nonreplicative and replicative vectors.

Finally, to reach disseminated metastasis, a vector that could be delivered systemically is imperative. The major obstacle in this direction is the effective clearance of the adenoviral vectors by the macrophages of the liver and spleen.[80] As with stealth liposomes, adenoviral vectors have been sterically protected with polyethylene glycol to avoid interaction with these macrophages.[81] Although antibody neutralization was prevented, it remains to be explored whether approaches to change the surface of the virion will increase blood persistence, thus allowing systemic targeting.

In summary, different modifications of the adenovirus currently are still evolving to reduce the number of tumor cells that are not affected by the therapeutic effects of the delivered gene.

Specific and Inducible Promoters

An efficient control of gene expression at the transcriptional level is one of the most difficult goals to achieve. Active research is focused on identifying and developing gene regulatory elements that provide both cell-specific and stimulus-dependent expression to a delivered therapeutic transgene.[82,83]

Transgene expression may be restricted to a specific target population of cells or tissue by including the promoter region elements that bind tissue-specific positive or negative acting transcription factors. Promoters with high selectivity for glial cells include the glial fibrillary acidic protein, the myelin basic protein, and the JC virus promoter. Other promoters can be designed to be active in determined circumstances, such as during active cell division; E2F-1, cyclin, and CDK promoters may be active exclusively in dividing cells. In addition, some promoters may be more effective in cancer than in normal cells. Thus, the E2F-1 promoter may be active in glioma cells but not functional in nondividing glial cells.[84]

There is no question that a gene-delivery system would be more versatile in clinical applications if transgene expression was regulatable by administration of an effector. Early growth response gene-related promoter sequences that increase gene expression following exposure to radiation have been identified.[85] Using these structures, gene expression induced by irradiation resulted in a cell-specific anticancer effect. Other composite gene regulatory systems can be incorporated into gene

Table 12–8. HUMAN GENE TRANSFER PROTOCOLS FOR CANCER GENE THERAPY

Antisense
Chemoprotection
Immunotherapy/in vitro transduction
Immunotherapy/in vivo transduction
Prodrugs/ HSV-tk and ganciclovir
Tumor-suppressor gene
Single-chain antibody

HSV-tk = herpes simplex virus–thymidine kinase.
Adapted from National Institutes of Health office and reports of recombinant DNA activities.

delivery vectors to control the expression of the delivered gene with the administration of an effector molecule such as tetracycline.[86]

Discovery of New Targets

The two most frequent abnormalities in glioblastomas are monosomy of chromosome 10 and trisomies of chromosome 7.[87–91]

Chromosome 10: the PTEN/MMAC Gene

One of the most frequent abnormalities of glioblastomas are deletions of chromosome 10. MMAC1 (mutated in multiple advanced cancers) or PTEN (a phosphatase and tensin homologue deleted from chromosome 10) is a tumor-suppressor gene located on chromosome 10 that has been found mutated in malignant gliomas.[92,93] The MMAC1 protein apparently exerts its function by dephosphorylating a lipid of a key growth control pathway. Experiments with genetically modified mice have demonstrated that MMAC1 is essential for tumor suppression. Restoration of the MMAC1 activity to glioma cells has led to suppression of their neoplastic phenotype, providing evidence that MMAC1 is a tumor-suppressor gene in gliomas.[94] Although the function of the MMAC1 protein still is not completely understood, data from experiments in MMAC-null mice indicate that MMAC1 can suppress tumorigenesis through its ability to regulate cellular differentiation and anchorage-independent growth. Recent results indicate that at least part of PTEN's role is to regulate the activity of the serine/threonine kinase AKT/protein kinase B and, thus, influence cell survival signaling.[95] In addition, since MMAC1 is inactivated in the latest stages of the malignant progression of gliomas, it may play a role in angiogenesis or invasiveness. In this regard, the transfer of chromosome 10 to glioma cells induces thrombospandin-1 and inhibits angiogenesis.[96] In addition to PTEN/MMAC1, at least two other potential tumor-suppressor genes, DMBT1[97] (deleted in multiple malignant brain tumors) and H-neu[98] (a human homologue of the *Drosophila*-neuralized gene), have already been identified in chromosome 10. The functional role and frequency of their abnormalities in gliomas are still under investigation.

Chromosome 7

Findings collected by several authors indicate that abnormalities in the number and composition of chromosome 7 are frequent in glioblastomas.[87–91] Varying allelic imbalances of different loci along chromosome 7 (with a background of disomy, trisomy, tetrasomy, or polisomy) have been found by Liu and colleagues.[99] Interestingly, loci adjacent to EGFR are independently amplified, suggesting that a number of genes may be targeted for amplification in chromosome 7.

REFERENCES

1. Levin VA, Leivel S, Gutin PH. Neoplasms of the central nervous system. In: DeVita VT, Hellman SJ, Rosemberg SA, editors. Cancer. Principles and practice of oncology. Philadelphia: JB Lippincott; 1997. p. 2022–82.
2. Sasaki M, Plate KH. Gene therapy of malignant glioma: recent advances in experimental and clinical studies. Ann Oncol 1998;9:1155–66.
3. Spear MA. Gene therapy of gliomas: receptor and transcriptional targeting. Anticancer Res 1998;18:3223–31.
4. Friedmann T. A brief history of gene therapy. Nat Genet 1992;2:93–8.
5. Collins VP, James CD. Gene and chromosomal alterations associated with the development of human gliomas. FASEB J 1993;7:926–30.
6. Furnari FB, Huang HJ, Cavenee WK. Genetics and malignant progression of human brain tumours. Cancer Surv 1995;25:233–75.
7. Kleihues P, Ohgaki H. Genetics of glioma progression and the definition of primary and secondary glioblastoma. Brain Pathol 1997;7:1131–6.
8. Fueyo J, Gomez-Manzano C, Yung WKA, Kyritsis AP. The functional role of tumor suppressor genes in gliomas: clues for future therapeutic strategies. Neurology 1998; 51:1250–5.
9. Gomez-Manzano C, Fueyo J, Kyritsis AP, Yung WK. Tumor suppressor gene therapy for brain tumors. In: Chiocca AE, Breakefield X, editors. Gene transfer and therapy for neurological disorders. Totowa (NJ): Human Press Inc; 1998. p. 201–25.

10. Kleihues P, Burger PC, Plate KH, et al. Glioblastoma. In: Kleihues P, Cavanee WK, editors. Pathology and genetics of tumours of the nervous system. Lyon (France): International Agency for Research on Cancer; 1997. p. 16–24.
11. Watanabe K, Tachibana O, Sato K, et al. Incidence and timing of p53 mutations during astrocytoma progession in patients with multiple biopsies. Clin Cancer Res 1997; 3:523–30.
12. Reyes-Mugica M, Rieger-Christ K, Ohgaki H, et al. Loss of DCC expression and glioma progression. Cancer Res 1997;57:382–6.
13. von Deimling A, von Ammon K, Schoenfeld D, et al. Subsets of glioblastoma multiforme defined by molecular genetic analysis. Brain Pathol 1993;3:19–26.
14. Lang FF, Miller DC, Koslow M, Newcomb EW. Pathways leading to glioblastoma multiforme: a molecular analysis of genetic alterations in 65 astrocytic tumors. J Neurosurg 1994;81:427–36.
15. Biernat W, Kleihues P, Yonekawa Y, Ohgaki H. Amplification and overexpression of MDM2 in primary (de novo) glioblastomas. J Neuropathol Exp Neurol 1996;56:180–5.
16. Louis DN. The p53 gene and protein in human brain tumors. J Neuropathol Exp Neurol 1994;54:65–73.
17. Bigner SH, McLendon RE, Al-Dosari N, Rasheed A. Brain tumors. In: Vogelstein B, Kinzler KW, editors. The genetic basis of human cancer. New York: McGraw-Hill; 1998. p. 661–70.
18. Roth JA, Cristiano RJ. Gene therapy for cancer: what have we done and where are we going? J Natl Cancer Inst 1997; 89:21–39.
19. Nigro JM, Baker SJ, Preisinger AC. Mutations in the p53 gene occur in diverse human tumour types. Nature 1989;342:705–8.
20. Sidransky D, Mikkelsen T, Schwechheimer K, et al. Clonal expansion of p53 mutant cells is associated with brain tumour progression. Nature 1992;355:846–7.
21. Gomez-Manzano C, Fueyo J, Kyritsis AP, et al. Adenovirus-mediated transfer of the p53 gene produces rapid and generalized death of human glioma cells via apoptosis. Cancer Res 1996;56:694–9.
22. Gomez-Manzano C, Fueyo J, Kyritsis AP, et al. Characterization of p53 and p21 functional interactions in glioma cells en route to apoptosis. J Natl Cancer Inst 1997;14:1036–44.
23. Gomez-Manzano C, Fueyo J, Alameda F, et al. Gene therapy for gliomas: p53 and E2F-1 proteins and the target of apoptosis. Int J Mol Med 1999;3:81–5.
24. Sandig V, Brand K, Herwing S, et al. Adenovirally transferred p16INK4/CDKN2 and p53 genes cooperate to induce apoptotic tumor cell death. Nat Med 1997;3:313–9.
25. Evan G, Littlewood T. A matter of life and cell death. Science 1998;281:1317–22.
26. Ueki K, Ono Y, Henson JW, et al. CDKN2/p16 or RB alterations occur in the majority of glioblastomas and are inversely correlated. Cancer Res 1996;56:150–3.
27. Fueyo J, Gomez-Manzano C, Bruner JM, et al. Hypermethylation of the CpG island of p16/CDKN2 correlates with gene inactivation in gliomas. Oncogene 1996;13:1615–9.
28. Fueyo J, Gomez-Manzano C, Yung WKA, et al. Adenovirus-mediated p16/CDKN2 gene transfer induces growth arrest and modifies the transformed phenotype of glioma cells. Oncogene 1996;12:103–10.
29. Fueyo J, Gomez-Manzano C, Yung WKA, et al. Suppression of human glioma growth by adenovirus-mediated Rb gene transfer. Neurology 1998;50:1307–15.
30. Weinberg RA. E2F and cell proliferation: a world turned upside down. Cell 1996;85:457–9.
31. Field SJ, Tsay FY, Kuo F, et al. E2F-1 functions in mice to promote apoptosis and suppress proliferation. Cell 1996; 85:549–61.
32. Yamasaki L, Jacks T, Bronson R, et al. Tumor induction and tissue atrophy in mice lacking E2F-1. Cell 1996;85: 537–48.
33. Fueyo J, Gomez-Manzano C, Yung WKA, et al. Overexpression of E2F-1 in glioma triggers apoptosis and suppresses tumor growth in vitro and in vivo. Nat Med 1998;4: 685–90.
34. Kowalik TF, DeGregori J, Schwarz JK, Nevins JR. E2F1 overexpression in quiescent fibroblasts leads to induction of cellular DNA synthesis and apoptosis. J Virol 1995; 69:2491–500.
35. Plate KH, Breier G, Weich HA, Risau W. Vascular endothelial growth factor is a potential tumor angiogenesis factor in human gliomas in vivo. Nature 1992;359:845–8.
36. Folkman J. What is the evidence that tumors are angiogenesis dependent? J Natl Cancer Inst 1991;82:4–6.
37. Saleh M, Stacker SA, Wilks AF. Inhibition of growth of C6 glioma cells in vivo by expression of antisense VEGF sequence. Cancer Res 1996;56:393–400
38. Cheng SY, Huang HJS, Nagane M, et al. Suppression of glioblastoma angiogenicity and tumorigenicity by inhibition of endogenous expression of vascular endothelial growth factor. Proc Natl Acad Sci U S A 1996;93:8502–7.
39. Ke LD, Fueyo J, Cheng X, et al. A novel approach to glioma gene therapy: down-regulation of the vascular endothelial growth factor in glioma cells using ribozymes. Int J Oncol 1998;12:1391–6.
40. Im S-A, Gomez-Manzano C, Fueyo J, et al. Antiangiogenesis treatment for gliomas: transfer of antisense-VEGF inhibits tumor growth in vivo. Cancer Res 1999;59: 895–900.
41. Uhm JH, Dooley NP, Villemure JG, Yong VW. Mechanisms of glioma invasion: role of matrix-metalloproteinases. Can J Neurol Sci 1997;24:3–15.
42. Culver KW, Ram Z, Wallbridge S, et al. In vivo gene transfer with retroviral vector producing cells for treatment of experimental brain tumors. Science 1992;256:1550–2.
43. Aghi M, Kramm CM, Chou TC, et al. Synergistic anticancer effects of ganciclovir/thymidine kinase and 5-fluorocytosine/cytosine deaminase gene therapies. J Natl Cancer Inst 1998;90:370–80.
44. Rogulski KR, Kim JH, Kim SH, Freytag SO. Glioma cells transduced with an *Escherichia coli* CD/HSV-1 TK fusion gene exhibit enhanced metabolic suicide and radiosensitivity. Hum Gene Ther 1997;8:73–85.
45. Collis VP. Gene amplification in human gliomas. Glia 1995;15:289–96.
46. Campbell JW, Pollack F. Growth factors in gliomas: antisense and dominant negative mutant strategies. J Neurooncol 1997;35:275–85.
47. Nagane N, Coufal F, Lin H, et al. A common mutant epidermal growth factor receptor confers enhanced tumori-

genicity on human glioblastoma cells by increasing proliferation and reducing apoptosis. Cancer Res 1996;56:5079–86.
48. Trojan J, Johnson TR, Rudin SD, et al. Treatment and prevention of rat glioblastoma by immunogenic C6 cells expressing anti-sense insulin-like growth factor I RNA. Science 1993;259:94–6.
49. Resnikoff M, Sell C, Rubini M, et al. Rat glioblastoma cells expressing an antisense RNA to insulin-like growth factor-1 (IGF-1) are nontumorigenic and induce regression of wild-type tumors. Cancer Res 1994;54:2218–22.
50. Nitta T, Sato K. Specific inhibition of c-sis protein synthesis and cell proliferation with antisense oligodeoxynucleotides in human glioma cells. Neurosurgery 1994;34:309–15.
51. Shamah SM, Stiles CD, Guha A. Dominant-negative mutants of platelet-derived growth factor revert the transform phenotype of human astrocytoma cells. Mol Cell Biol 1993;13:7203–12.
52. Murphy PR, Sato Y, Knee RS. Phosphorothioate antisense oligonucleotides against basic fibroblast growth factor inhibit anchorage-dependent and anchorage-independent growth of a malignant glioblastoma cell line. Mol Endocrinol 1992;6:877–84.
53. Morrison RS. Suppression of basic fibroblast growth factor expression by antisense oligodeoxynucleotides inhibits the growth of transformed human astrocytes. J Biol Chem 1991;266:728–34.
54. Yung WK, Taylor S, Shi X, Steck PA. Modulation of transforming growth factor-alpha (TGF-α) autocrine growth regulation by antisense oligonucleotides in glioma cells. Proc Am Assoc Cancer Res 1993;34:524.
55. Redekop GJ, Nauss CC. Transfection with bFGF sense and antisense cDNA resulting in modification of malignant glioma growth. J Neurosurg 1995;82:83–90.
56. Jachmczak P, Bogdahn U, Schneider J, et al. The effect of transforming growth factor-$β_2$-specific phosphorothioate-antisense oligodeoxynucleotides in reversing cellular immunosuppression in malignant glioma. J Neurosurg 1993;78:944–51.
57. Fakhrai H, Dorigo O, Shawler DL, et al. Eradication of established intracranial rat gliomas by transforming growth factor β antisense gene therapy. Proc Natl Acad Sci U S A 1996;93:2909–14.
58. White E. Regulation of apoptosis by adenovirus E1A and E1B oncogenes. Semin Virol 1998;8:505–13.
59. Bischof JR, Kirn DH, Williams A, et al. An adenovirus that replicates selectively in p53-deficient human tumor cells. Science 1996;274:373–6.
60. Heise C, Sampson-Johanes A, Williams A, et al. Onyx-015, an E1B gene-attenuated adenovirus, causes tumor-specific cytolysis and antitumoral efficacy that can be augmented by standard chemotherapeutic agents. Nat Med 1997;3:639–45.
61. Rothmann T, Hernstermann A, Whitaker NJ, et al. Replication of ONYX-015, a potential anticancer adenovirus, is independent of p53 status in tumor cells. J Virol 1998;72:9470–8.
62. Goodrum F, Ornelles DA. p53 status does not determine outcome of E1B 55-kilodalton mutant adenovirus lytic infection. J Virol 1998;72:9479–90.
63. Fueyo J, Gomez-Manzano C, Alemany R, et al. A mutant oncolytic adenovirus targeting the Rb pathway produces anti-glioma effect in vivo. Oncogene 2000;19:2–12.
64. Rodriguez R, Schuur ER, Lim HY, et al. Prostate attenuated replication competent adenovirus (ARCA) CN706: a selective cytotoxic for prostate-specific antigen-positive prostate cancer cells. Cancer Res 1997;57:2559–63.
65. Shi Q, Wang Y, Worton R. Modulation of the specificity and activity of a cellular promoter in an adenoviral vector. Hum Gene Ther 1997;8:403–10.
66. Andreanski S, Soroceanu L, Flotte ER, et al. Evaluation of genetically engineered herpes simplex viruses as oncolytic agents for human malignant brain tumors. Cancer Res 1997;57:1502–9.
67. Mineta T, Rabkin SD, Yazaki T, et al. Attenuated multimutated herpes simplex virus-1 for the treatment of malignant gliomas. Nat Med 1995;1:938–43.
68. Mineta T, Rabkin SD, Martuza RL. Treatment of malignant gliomas using ganciclovir-hypersensitive, ribonucleotide reductase–deficient herpes simplex viral mutant. Cancer Res 1994;54:3963–6.
69. Chase M, Chung RY, Chiocca EA. An oncolytic viral mutant that delivers the CYP2B1 transgene and augments cyclophosphamide chemotherapy. Nat Biotechnol 1998;16:444–8.
70. Coffey MC, Strong JE, Forsyth PA, Lee PWK. Reovirus therapy of tumors with activated ras pathway. Science 1998;282:1332–4.
71. Recombinant DNA Advisory Committee. Regulatory issues. Hum Gene Ther 1995;6:1065–124.
72. Oldfield EH, Ram Z. Clinical protocol: intrathecal gene therapy for the treatment of leptomeningeal carcinomatosis (phase I–II study). Hum Gene Ther 1995;6:55–85.
73. Izquierdo M, Martin V, Felipe P, et al. Human malignant brain tumor response to herpes simplex thymidine kinase (HSV-TK)/ganciclovir gene therapy. Gene Ther 1996;3:491–5.
74. Ram Z, Culver KW, Oshiro EM, et al. Therapy of malignant brain tumors by intratumoral implantation of retroviral vector-producing cells. Nat Med 1997;3:1354–61.
75. Klatzmann D, Valery CA, Bensimon G, et al. A phase I/II study of herpes simplex virus type 1 thymidine kinase "suicide" gene therapy for recurrent glioblastoma. Study group on gene therapy for glioblastoma. Hum Gene Ther 1998;20:2595–604.
76. Freytag SO, Rogulski KR, Paielii DL, et al. A novel three-pronged approach to kill cancer cells selectively: concomitant viral, double suicide gene, and radiotherapy. Hum Gene Ther 1998;9:1323–33.
77. Yang Y, Trinchieri G, Wilson JM. Recombinant IL-12 prevents formation of blocking IgA antibodies to recombinant adenovirus and allows repeated gene therapy to mouse lung. Nat Med 1995;1:890–3.
78. Dmitriev I, Krasnykh V, Miller CR, et al. An adenovirus vector with genetically modified fibers demonstrates expanded tropism via utilization of a coxsackievirus and adenovirus receptor–independent cell entry mechanism. J Virol 1998;72:9706–13.
79. Yoshida Y, Sadata A, Zhang W, et al. Generation of fiber-mutant recombinant adenoviruses for gene therapy of malignant glioma. Hum Gene Ther 1998;9:2503–15.

80. Wolff G, Worgall S, van Rooijen N, et al. Enhancement of in vivo adenovirus-mediated gene transfer and expression by prior depletion of tissue macrophages in the target organ. J Virol 1997;71:624–9.
81. Chillon M, Lee JH, Fasbender A, Welsh MJ. Adenovirus complexed with polyethylene glycol and cationic lipid is shielded from neutralizing antibodies in vitro. Gene Ther 1998;5:995–1002.
82. Reeves SA. Retrovirus vectors and regulatable promoters. In: Chiocca AE, Breakefield X, editors. Gene transfer and therapy for neurological disorders. Totowa (NJ): Human Press; 1998. p. 7–38.
83. Henson WH. Promoters for expression of gene products within neurons and glia. In: Chiocca AE, Breakefield X, editors. Gene transfer and therapy for neurological disorders. Totowa (NJ): Human Press; 1998. p. 121–46.
84. Parr MJ, Manome Y, Tanaka T, et al. Tumor-selective transgene expression in vivo mediated by an E2F-responsive adenoviral vector. Nat Med 1997;3:1145–9.
85. Weichselbaum RR, Hallahan DE, Beckett MA, et al. Gene therapy targeted by radiation prefentially radiosensitizes tumor cells. Cancer Res 1994;54:4266–9.
86. Gossen M, Freundlieb S, Bender G, et al. Transcriptional activation by tetracyclines in mammalian cells. Science 1995;268:1766–9.
87. Rey JA, Bellow J, deCampos JM, et al. Chromosomal patterns in human malignant astrocytomas. Cancer Genet Cytogenet 1987;29:201–21.
88. Bigner SH, Mark J, Burger P, et al. Specific chromosomal abnormalities in malignant human gliomas. Cancer Res 1988;48:405–11.
89. Thiel G, Losanowa T, Kintzel D, et al. Karyotypes in 90 human gliomas. Cancer Genet Cytogenet 1992;58:109–20.
90. Hecht BK, Tuc-Carel C, Chatel M, et al. Cytogenetics of malignant gliomas: I. The autosomes with reference to rearrangements. Cancer Genet Cytogenet 1995;84:1–8.
91. Debiec-Rychter M, Alwasiak J, Liberski PP, et al. Accumulation of chromosomal changes in human glioma progression. Cancer Genet Cytogenet 1995;85:61–7.
92. Li J, Yen C, Liaw D, et al. PTEN, a putative protein tyrosine phosphatase gene mutated in human brain, breast and prostate cancer. Science 1997;275:1943–6.
93. Steck PA, Pershouse MA, Jasser SA, et al. Identification of a candidate tumor suppressor gene, MMAC1, at chromosome 10q23.3 that is mutated in multiple advanced cancers. Nat Genet 1997;15:356–62.
94. Cheney W, Johnson DE, Vaillancort M-T, et al. Suppression of tumorigenicity of glioblastoma cells by adenovirus-mediated MMAC1/PTEN gene transfer. Cancer Res 1998;58:2331–4.
95. Maehama T, Dixon JE. PTEN: a tumour suppressor that functions as a phospholipid phosphatase. Trends Cell Biol 1999;9:125–8.
96. Hsu SC, Volpert OV, Steck PA, et al. Inhibition of angiogenesis in human glioblastomas by chromosome 10 induction of thrombospondin-1. Cancer Res 1996;15:5684–91.
97. Mollenhauer J, Weimann S, Scheurlen W, et al. DBMT1, a new member of the SRCR superfamily, on chromosome 10q25.3–26.1 is deleted in malignant brain tumors. Nat Genet 1997;17:32–9.
98. Nakamura H, Yoshida M, Tsuiki H, et al. Identification of a human homologue of the *Drosophila* neuralized gene within the 10q25.1 malignant astrocytoma deletion region. Oncogene 1997;16:1009–19.
99. Liu L, Ichimura K, Pettersson EH, Collins VP. Chromosome 7 rearrangements in glioblastomas; loci adjacent to EGFR are independently amplified. J Neuropathol Exp Neurol 1998;57:1138–45.

Surgery for Brain Tumors

FRED G. BARKER II, MD
PETER SZTRAMSKI, RN

Surgery for brain tumors began in 1884, when Rickman Godlee performed an excision of a primary brain tumor in London, England. Although the operation provided a diagnosis, there was no lasting benefit for the patient, who died less than a month after surgery. More than a century of effort by the pioneer American neurosurgeon Harvey Cushing and his successors has provided a much brighter picture for today's patients who require surgery for brain tumors. In addition to providing a diagnosis, modern operations for brain tumors can often prolong life and improve its quality. Surgery can relieve symptoms due to mass effect, seizures, edema, and hydrocephalus. In addition, surgery can be used to achieve cytoreduction in brain tumors, to deliver adjuvant therapy with or without a preceding resection, and, in some cases, to provide a cure. This chapter describes some of the techniques that are used to achieve these goals in modern neurosurgical practice.[1]

DIAGNOSIS: STEREOTACTIC BIOPSY

When diagnosis of an intracranial mass lesion is the sole purpose of surgery, the most common operation performed is a stereotactic brain biopsy (Figures 13–1 and 13–2).[2,3] Although many proprietary devices are used to perform stereotactic biopsies, the basic principles are the same. After injection of a local anesthetic, a frame is fixed to the patient's head, using pins that pierce the skin and anchor the frame solidly to the outer table of the skull in the frontal and parietal regions. A fiducial device is affixed to the ring and an imaging study is obtained (usually computed tomography [CT] or magnetic resonance imaging [MRI]). A target is chosen on the images and target coordinates are generated that specify a point in three-dimensional space. The fiducial device is then exchanged for an arc that can guide a needle to the chosen target. After the entry point on the scalp surface is prepared and anesthetized, a short skin incision is made and a hole is created in the underlying skull and dura. Using the stereotactic arc, the biopsy needle is then advanced to the target point and a small piece of tissue is removed (about 10 mm × 1 mm × 1 mm). The tissue obtained is examined, usually with frozen-section pathology, and when a suitable specimen has been obtained, the incision is closed and the stereotactic frame removed.

The operative portion of this procedure takes about an hour and is generally well tolerated by the patient. Complication rates are low: about 1 percent of patients develop a postoperative infection, about 1 percent develop a hematoma large enough to cause a new neurologic deficit, and 3 percent suffer a postoperative seizure.[4,5] The procedure is usually followed by an overnight hospital stay, although some surgeons discharge the patient on the day of the procedure after an appropriate observation period.

The rate of achieving a diagnosis with a stereotactic brain biopsy is over 95 percent.[3] However, because many primary brain tumors are spatially heterogeneous, a small sample may not be representative of the entire tumor. For gliomas, this has two consequences. First, specimens obtained from resections of glial tumors are more likely to result in a higher grade diagnosis than stereotactic biopsies (Figure 13–3).[6] This is because the tumor is graded according to the most malignant area examined,

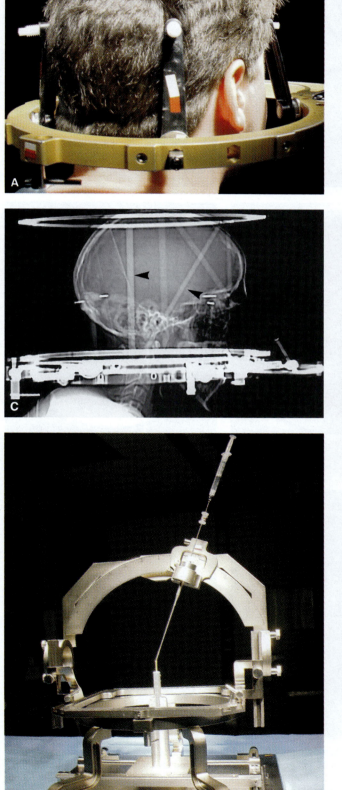
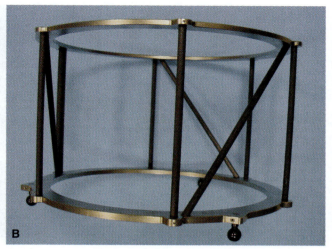
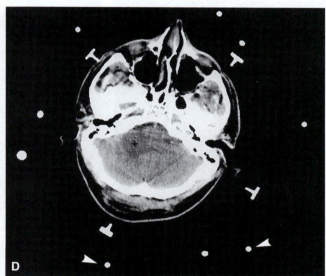
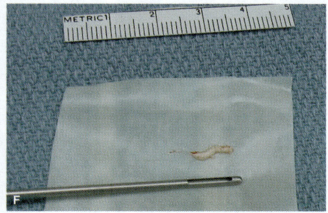

Figure 13–1. Stereotactic brain biopsy procedure. *A*, Stereotactic frame base ring attached to head using four percutaneous pins. *B, C*, Fiducial device attached to base ring for CT scan. *Arrows* indicate radiopaque fiducial bars. *D*, Contrast-enhanced axial CT image showing fiducial device (*arrows*) and target (*crosshair*). *E*, Stereotactic arc and needle assembled on targeting phantom to confirm targeting. *F*, Stereotactic biopsy needle and specimen.

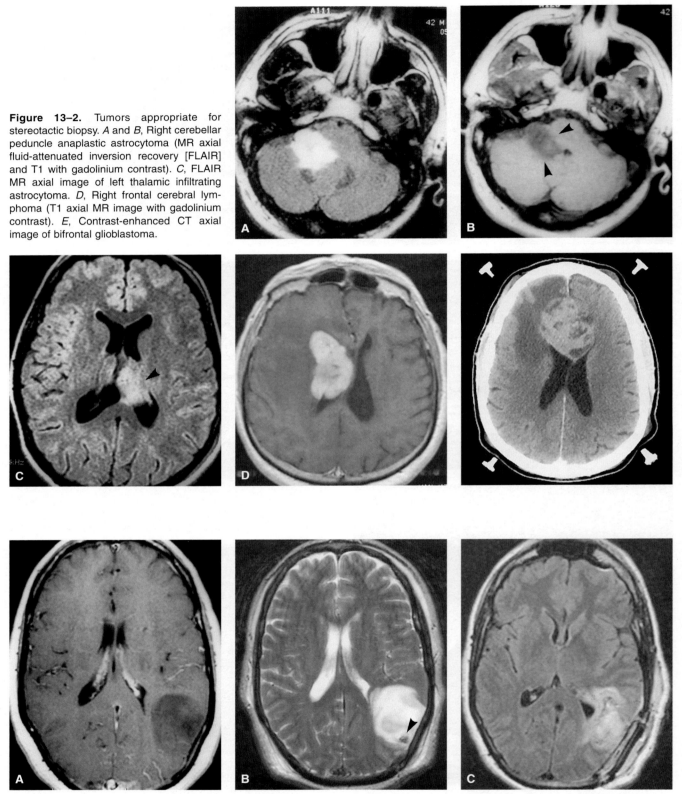

Figure 13–2. Tumors appropriate for stereotactic biopsy. *A* and *B*, Right cerebellar peduncle anaplastic astrocytoma (MR axial fluid-attenuated inversion recovery [FLAIR] and T1 with gadolinium contrast). *C*, FLAIR MR axial image of left thalamic infiltrating astrocytoma. *D*, Right frontal cerebral lymphoma (T1 axial MR image with gadolinium contrast). *E*, Contrast-enhanced CT axial image of bifrontal glioblastoma.

Figure 13–3. Because of heterogeneity within large gliomas, stereotactic biopsy of a large tumor can provide tissue that is not representative of the entire mass. *A* and *B*, Non-enhancing left parietal tumor in a 45-year-old man (T1 axial with gadolinium contrast and T2 axial MR images); (*arrow*), blood products in the biopsy site on the periphery of the tumor. Diagnosis from the biopsy was astrocytoma, grade 2. *C*, FLAIR MR axial image after resection of the mass. Final pathologic diagnosis was anaplastic astrocytoma (grade 3) because mitoses were found in the larger specimen.

even if the majority of the tumor is low grade. Second, resection specimens are more likely than stereotactic biopsy specimens to demonstrate areas of oligodendrocytic differentiation within the tumor.[7] This carries important prognostic information and may help in choosing postoperative therapy. When a tumor has a heterogeneous appearance on contrast-enhanced MR images, a target is typically chosen within the enhancing portion of the tumor, avoiding peripheral edema and central necrosis, to maximize the chance of providing viable tumor tissue of maximum biologic aggressiveness for diagnosis. When the tumor is non-enhancing or multiple areas of enhancing abnormality are present, an imaging modality that reflects tumor metabolism may help in selecting the portion of the tumor with the highest biopsy yield. Both 18-fluorodeoxyglucose positron emission tomography and magnetic resonance spectroscopy have been used for this purpose.

Stereotactic biopsy may be less safe or less effective in certain circumstances. Some tumors, such as pinealoblastoma and lymphoma, are intrinsically more likely to hemorrhage after a biopsy. Some locations within the brain are more risky targets. Tumors located in eloquent cortex or the brain stem may be associated with higher risks of postoperative neurologic deficits because of edema or hemorrhage. When the tumor is immediately adjacent to a major artery (such as the middle cerebral) or vein (as in the pineal region), vascular injury with a subsequent hematoma may be more likely.[5] Biopsy trajectories that avoid transgressing pial planes, such as Sylvian fissure, minimize the chances of injuring a major vessel. If all possible biopsy trajectories transgress a pial plane or cistern, as in the pineal region or cerebellopontine angle, an open or endoscopic biopsy may be a safer choice. Finally, very small targets (less than 5 mm in diameter) are difficult to take biopsy specimens from reliably because of the limitations on accuracy inherent in the equipment and imaging techniques that are used.[8]

A recent development in stereotactic biopsy technique is the use of intraoperative imaging with a handheld biopsy device.[9] This avoids the need for frame placement. Early results are promising, but whether the technique will match the success of frame-based biopsy is not yet clear.

Tumors for which stereotactic biopsy are ideal include those for which no further surgical therapy is planned. When a tumor appears to be a glioma or other intra-axial tumor that is resectable, most surgeons prefer to proceed directly with resection rather than perform a stereotactic biopsy as a separate, initial procedure.[10] Tumors for which biopsy is likely to be the only operation needed are those that are very responsive to radiation or chemotherapy (such as lymphomas) or those situated in locations for which the risk of excision is prohibitive (brain stem, thalamus, bifrontal gliomas) (Figure 13–2). When primary cerebral lymphoma is suspected, it is important not to administer corticosteroids preoperatively as these can cause rapid tumor cell lysis, resulting in the disappearance of the surgical target or a lack of identifiable lymphoma cells in the tissue specimen. Although germinomas are sufficiently responsive to radiation and chemotherapy that surgical excision is not indicated, they are often located in the pineal or suprasellar region, where an open or endoscopic biopsy may be safer than a stereotactic procedure.

Another situation in which stereotactic biopsy may be the only operation needed is when a mass has an appearance compatible with cerebral abscess or a demyelinating lesion. Stereotactic aspiration of a cerebral abscess can exclude the diagnosis of cystic tumor and provide a specimen for culture. Diffusion-weighted MRI scans can suggest the diagnosis of abscess preoperatively in most cases because the center of an abscess typically has a distinctive appearance of markedly restricted diffusion (Figure 13–4). Demyelinating lesions typically have a ring-enhancing appearance on gadolinium-enhanced MRI scans, often with a partial ring or crescent that is confined to the white matter, rather than a complete ring as is more typical in tumor or abscess (Figure 13–4).[11]

As already mentioned, endoscopic biopsy may sometimes offer a safer or more accurate alternative to stereotactic biopsy (Figures 13–5 and 13–6). Endoscopic biopsy is attractive when a fluid-filled space surrounds the biopsy target, such as a tumor within the lateral or third ventricles. Another difficult biopsy target is a thin-walled cyst because the window of the biopsy needle tends to be either within the cyst (providing only fluid) or within normal surrounding brain. An endoscope can be introduced into the cyst and a biopsy of the wall taken using grasping forceps. Finally, some tumors are surrounded by venous or arterial structures that make blind biopsy unsafe. Small masses in the pineal region may be more safely biopsied through the posterior third ventricle under endoscopic visual control, although experience in this area is still preliminary.

SURGICAL RESECTION

Most brain tumors are resectable with an acceptable degree of surgical risk. The indications for resecting a brain tumor, in addition to providing a diagnosis, are to relieve symptoms, to deliver adjuvant treatments, or to prolong life. Secondary goals may include providing tumor tissue for selection of adjuvant therapy (through in vitro chemosensitivity testing), for fabrication of adjuvant therapy (such as by making a tumor-based vaccine), or for research purposes.

Whatever the indication, the surgical procedure follows the same basic outline (see Figures 13–7 and 13–8 as well as video footage on CD-ROM). Preoperative prophylactic antibiotics are given, along with mannitol for osmotic diuresis (thereby reducing intracranial pressure and reducing the need for retraction), as well as corticosteroids, and an anticonvulsant if indicated. The skin and hair are sterilely prepped in

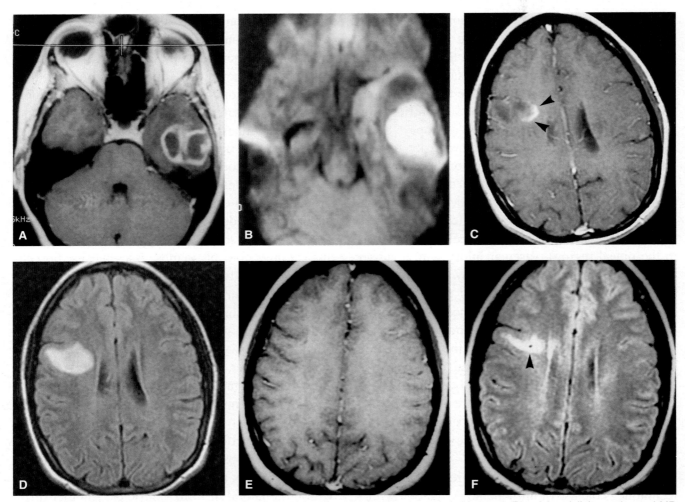

Figure 13–4. Non-neoplastic lesions that can be distinguished from tumors by stereotactic biopsy. *A*, T1 axial gadolinium-enhanced MR image of left temporal abscess (mixed anaerobic organisms). The image is also compatible with malignant glioma or metastases. *B*, Diffusion-weighted MR axial image. The bright signal on diffusion-weighted images is characteristic of abscess. *C*, *D*, *E* and *F*, Right frontal demyelinating plaque. *C* and *D*, Axial MR T1-weighted gadolinium-enhanced and FLAIR images. The characteristic partial ring of enhancement at the junction of the lesion with normal white matter of the centrum semiovale is seen (*arrows*). *E* and *F*, Axial MR T1-weighted gadolinium-enhanced and FLAIR images. After treatment, the lesion is smaller and has less enhancement. The biopsy site is seen (*arrow*).

the operative area. Most surgeons prefer to shave the hair-bearing scalp around the planned incision, although this is increasingly felt to be optional rather than required. A skin incision is made and the skin flap and any underlying muscle are reflected from the surface of the skull. Holes are made in the skull sur-

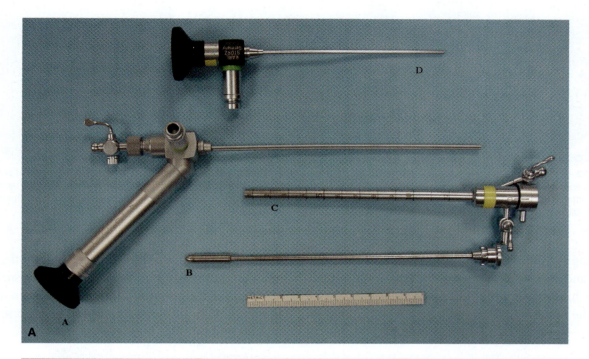

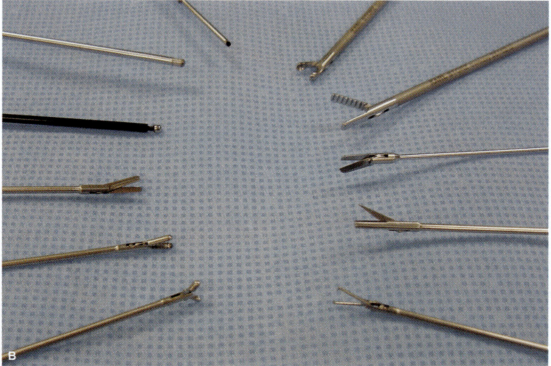

Figure 13–5. Endoscopic biopsy technique. *A,* Endoscopic biopsy equipment. A: angled endoscope with working channel; B and C: obturator and introducer sheath; D: straight endoscope without working channel. *B,* Endoscopic instruments. Clockwise from lower left: biopsy forceps, grasping forceps, scissors, monopolar and bipolar electrocautery wands, aspiration needle, cup and grasping forceps, scissors (three types).

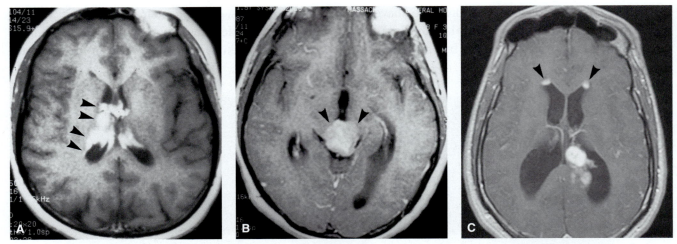

Figure 13–6. Tumors appropriate for endoscopic biopsy. Gadolinium-enhanced MR axial images. *A,* Intraventricular cerebral lymphoma involving ependymal lining and fornices, biopsy taken through right frontal horn. *B,* Pineocytoma—biopsy performed through third ventricle via lateral ventricle and foramen of Monro. *C,* Pilocytic astrocytoma in atrium of left lateral ventricle with drop metastases to both frontal horns (*arrows*). Biopsy performed through left lateral ventricle.

rounding the piece of bone to be removed (the "bone flap") and the circumference of the flap is cut, usually with a high-speed drill. The bone flap is separated from the underlying dura, to which it is adherent in varying degrees. The dura is incised and reflected to reveal the brain surface. A location on the surface is selected for the initial incision into the brain and the cortical surface is electrocauterized and incised. The

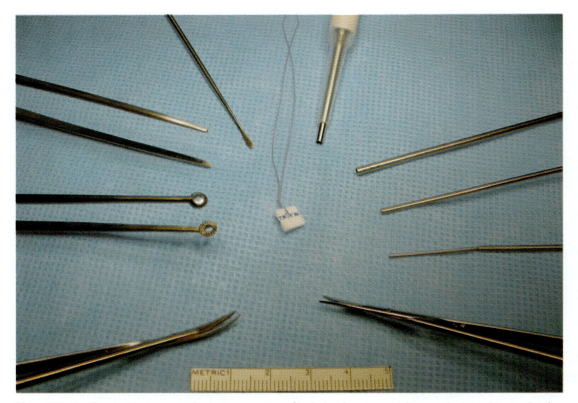

Figure 13–7. Surgical instruments for tumor resection. Clockwise from lower left: curved microscissors, ring forceps, bipolar electrocautery forceps, straight blunt dissector, ultrasonic aspirator, suction tubing (three sizes), straight microscissors. Center: quarter-inch cottonoid patty.

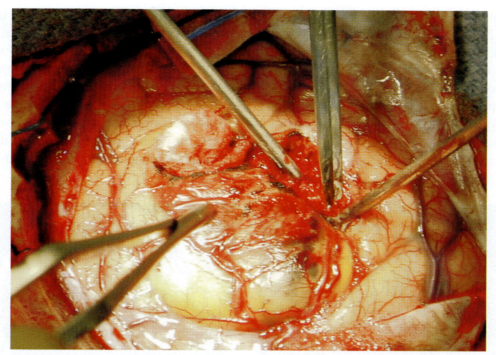

Figure 13–8. Dissection between tumor mass and surrounding cortex. The surgeon has just cauterized a surface vessel feeding the tumor using bipolar forceps (*upper right*). The vessel will be divided by the assistant using microscissors (*lower left*). Suction tubing, *upper left* and *lower right*. The tumor is a metastatic melanoma.

gray and white matter beneath are divided using bipolar electrocautery forceps and suction.

When the tumor is exposed, it can be removed in one of two ways: either by incising it and then debulking its mass from the center outward until its margins are reached or by first delineating the tumor's margins and then removing it en bloc or piecemeal. Hemostasis is then obtained in the walls of the resection cavity and the dura is closed, usually in a watertight fashion. The bone flap is replaced using circumferential wires or plates. If the bone flap cannot be replaced because of tumor involvement or because the bone was morcellated for removal, a cranioplasty can be fashioned to replace it. The muscle, muscle fascia, galea, and skin are then repaired in layers and a dressing is applied. Many variations on this basic sequence are used to address particular circumstances.[1,2]

Most brain tumor surgery can be performed under either local or general anesthesia. Local anesthesia facilitates earlier postoperative discharge from the hospital and permits constant monitoring of neurologic functioning during the operation.[12] By using propofol or other short-acting intravenous anesthetics, it is possible for patients to be asleep during the opening and closing portions of the operation (when discomfort is at a maximum) and awake only during the actual tumor resection. Most patients tolerate craniotomy under local anesthesia well, without significant discomfort.[12] Still, the majority of patients will select general anesthesia if given the choice. Tumors in the posterior fossa, in the skull base, or for which prolonged dissection or microsurgery will be required are essentially always removed under a general anesthetic. Resections that require intraoperative mapping of speech or sensory cortex must be performed under a local anesthetic, but cortical mapping of motor functions can be done under general anesthesia.

SURGERY TO RELIEVE SYMPTOMS

The primary means through which brain tumor removal relieves symptoms is by alleviating mass effect (Figure 13–9). Mass effect causes some symptoms that are location specific and others that are not.

Common location-specific symptoms include abulia or personality change (common in large anterior fossa meningiomas), motor or sensory deficits (caused by intra-axial or extra-axial tumors compressing primary motor or sensory cortex, or deeper pathways), aphasia (from compression of frontal, temporal, or parietal speech centers), visual deficit (compression of visual pathways anywhere between the optic nerve and primary visual cortex), or parietal lobe symptoms. General symptoms of mass effect include headache, nausea and vomiting, and lethargy. Any of these symptoms can potentially be relieved by removal of the causative mass, especially when the symptoms are of recent onset. (It is important to distinguish symptoms caused by mass effect from those caused by direct involvement of eloquent cortex, as when a malignant glioma infiltrates primary speech or motor centers.) The same rapid relief of symptoms can sometimes be

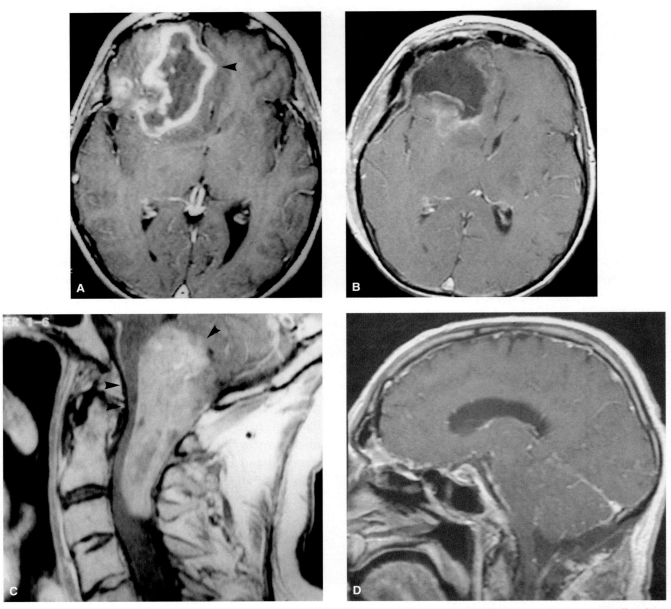

Figure 13–9. Surgery to relieve symptomatic mass effect. *A* and *B*, MR axial gadolinium-enhanced T1 images showing mass effect from right frontal glioblastoma causing headache and drowsiness. Note subfalcine herniation (*arrow*, *A*) and residual enhancing tumor posterior to resection cavity (*B*). *C* and *D*, MR sagittal gadolinium-enhanced images showing mass effect from compression of long tracts at craniocervical junction by fourth ventricular subependymoma. Symptoms were numbness below the neck, spastic gait, and tussive headache. *Arrows* show tumor and spinal cord compressed to a thin ribbon. Postoperatively, the symptoms were relieved (*D*).

seen after drainage of tumor cysts that cause mass effect (Figure 13–10).

A second type of symptoms that may be relieved by surgery are symptoms due to medically intractable seizures (Figure 13–11). The mechanism through which tumors cause seizures is ill-defined. The tumor itself can act as a seizure focus, and tumors can also induce seizure foci in the surrounding brain. Eventually, distant foci may be induced as well. Because the tumor itself is not necessarily the only seizure focus, or even the primary one, some surgeons recommend the use of techniques such as intraoperative electrocorticography to ensure that all important seizure foci are removed. Use of these adjuncts from the seizure surgery armamentarium has been reported to improve postoperative seizure control after some types of cerebral tumor removal, especially for low-grade tumors in the temporal lobes.[13]

Tumor removal often alleviates symptoms that are due to the edema within brain tissue adjacent to some intra-axial and extra-axial tumors (Figure 13–12). Small cerebral metastases are often surrounded by extensive cerebral edema, seemingly out of proportion to the size of the actual mass. When the symptoms are not relieved by corticosteroids, removal of the mass is the quickest means of palliation. Some small meningiomas (usually the secretory histologic subtype, most often based on the anterior cranial fossa floor) can cause a disproportionate amount of edema that is rapidly relieved by

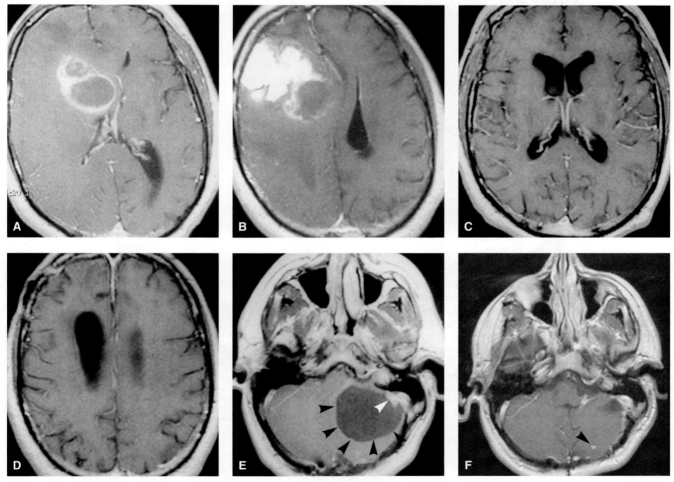

Figure 13–10. Surgery to relieve symptoms caused by tumor cysts. Gadolinium-enhanced MR axial images. *A, B, C* and *D*, Mass effect from right frontal anaplastic oligodendroglioma with cyst. Symptoms were headache, vomiting, and left hemiparesis. Postoperatively, symptoms were relieved (*C, D*). *E* and *F*, Cerebellar hemangioblastoma causing hydrocephalus, headache, vomiting, and imbalance due to large tumor cyst (*black arrows*). The tumor itself is less than 1 cm in diameter (*white arrow*). *F*, Cyst resolves after resection of tumor nodule. *Arrow* shows a smaller hemangioblastoma without associated cyst.

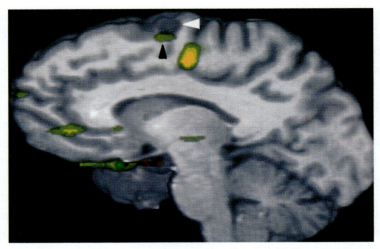

Figure 13–11. Surgery to relieve seizures. Functional MR sagittal image showing cavernous angioma (*white arrow*) in direct contact with supplementary motor area (*black arrow*). The mass caused medically intractable seizures that were relieved by resection.

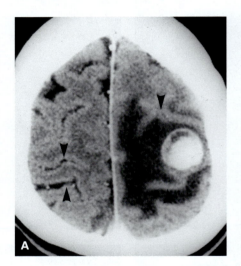
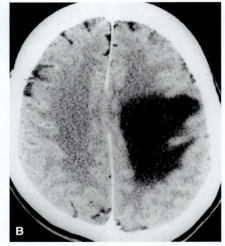

Figure 13–12. Surgery to relieve symptoms from tumor edema. Metastatic lung carcinoma to left precentral gyrus causing left hemiplegia from edema. *A*, contrast-enhanced CT axial image showing tumor in widened motor strip (*black arrows* show motor strip on each side). *B*, Axial CT image through a more inferior plane demonstrating severe edema distant from the mass. *C*, Photograph showing location of mass (indicated by forceps) within precentral gyrus just superior to hand motor centers, demonstrated using cortical mapping (number on gyral surface). Resection of the mass caused resolution of edema and return of normal right-sided strength, including handwriting, within 7 days.

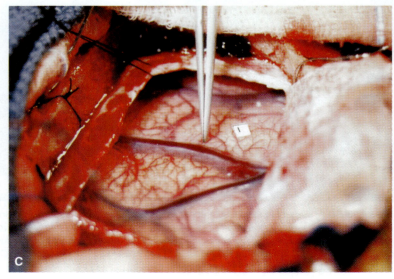

surgical removal. Radiation necrosis after intensive treatment of gliomas is another common source of intractable edema that can lead to steroid dependency and poor quality of life if the necrotic focus is not removed (Figure 13–13).[14]

SURGERY FOR CEREBROSPINAL FLUID ACCESS OR DRAINAGE

Brain tumors can obstruct the normal flow and absorption of cerebrospinal fluid (CSF) at several points. Cerebrospinal fluid is made by the choroid plexus in the lateral ventricles, passes through the foramina of Monro, the third ventricle, the aqueduct of Sylvius, and the fourth ventricle and its exiting foramina and finally passes over the cerebral hemispheres to its points of absorption near the superior sagittal sinus. The most common points of obstruction are the foramen of Monro and the aqueduct of Sylvius. Carcinomatous meningitis can cause hydrocephalus without a mass lesion by interfering with CSF passage through the basal cisterns or over the cerebral hemispheres. Treatment of hydrocephalus resulting from brain tumors usually requires placement of a ventriculoperitoneal shunt (Figure 13–14). Although seeding of the tumor to the peritoneum through the shunt has been reported, particularly in medulloblastoma, it is unusual.

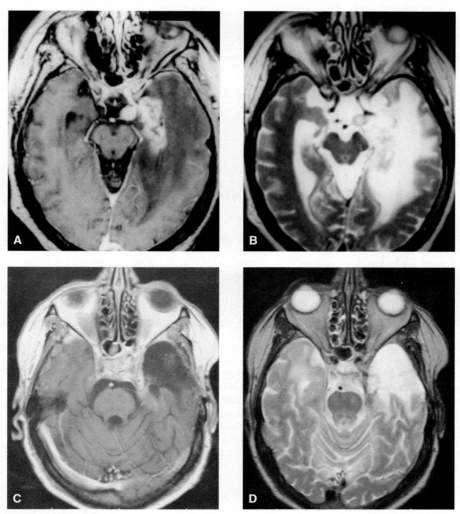

Figure 13–13. Surgery to remove radiation necrosis and relieve symptoms from surrounding edema. A and B, T1-weighted gadolinium-enhanced and T2-weighted MR axial images. Enhancing mass in medial left temporal lobe is radiation necrosis after radiation of a suprasellar meningioma. Edema extends far posteriorly (B). C, D, T1-weighted gadolinium-enhanced and T2-weighted MR axial images. After resection of the enhancing mass, edema is alleviated.

Hydrocephalus from obstruction of CSF flow in the aqueduct of Sylvius or fourth ventricle can be relieved by creating a third ventriculostomy, an opening in the floor of the third ventricle that permits CSF to pass directly into the basal cisterns (Figure 13–14). This is performed endoscopically and can sometimes be combined with an endoscopic biopsy of a posterior third-ventricular mass. Cerebrospinal fluid is

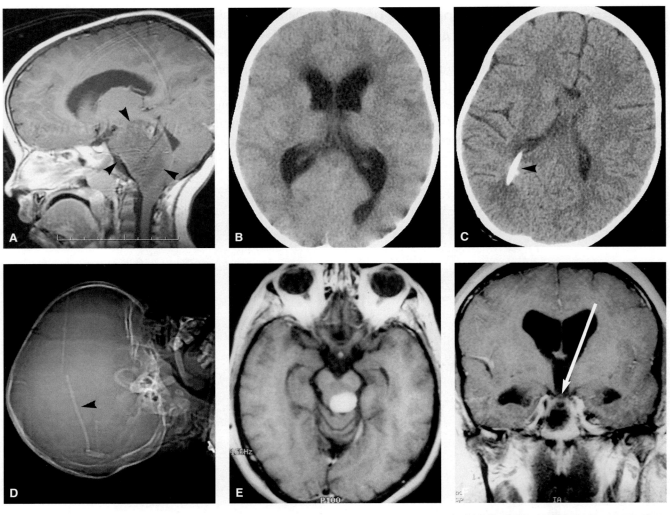

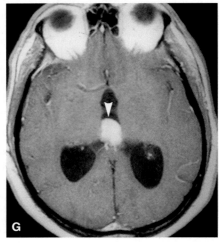

Figure 13–14. Surgery to relieve hydrocephalus. *A* and *B*, MR sagittal and axial gadolinium-enhanced images. Intrinsic malignant glioma of the pons in a child. Marked hydrocephalus from obstruction of the aqueduct of Sylvius. *C* and *D*, Axial CT image and lateral roentgenograph after shunt placement. The right occipital ventricular catheter is indicated by arrows. *E*, Obstruction of the aqueduct by metastasis from lung cancer. Treated with ventriculoperitoneal shunting and whole brain radiation therapy. *F* and *G*, Coronal and axial T1-weighted gadolinium-enhanced MR images. Pineocytoma with hydrocephalus. *F*, Coronal image demonstrating path for third ventriculostomy. *G*, Endoscopic biopsy of the portion of the mass presenting in the posterior third ventricle can be performed at the same procedure.

obtained directly from the lateral ventricles during the procedure for cytology and other studies. When hydrocephalus results from a fourth-ventricular mass, surgery to remove the tumor may relieve the hydrocephalus directly and only temporary CSF drainage into an external drainage system may be necessary.

Treatment of carcinomatous or lymphomatous meningitis may sometimes require long-term administration of intrathecal chemotherapy. Although this can be done using repeated lumbar punctures, implantation of a subcutaneous reservoir that is connected to an intraventricular catheter facilitates treatment (Figure 13–15). The catheter tip should be in one lateral ventricle (rather than the third ventricle) to allow dilution of medications by the larger volume of CSF contained in the lateral ventricle to prevent neurotoxicity. Such reservoirs can also be used to obtain CSF for cytology to follow treatment results.

SURGERY TO DELIVER ADJUVANT TREATMENTS

Some forms of adjuvant cancer treatment can only be delivered to brain tumors by surgical means. When the adjuvant treatment is available in liquid form, common means of delivery include injection through a stereotactic biopsy needle into non-resectable tumors and injection into the walls of a resection cavity after open surgical removal of a mass. These techniques are clearly most appropriate when an agent only needs to be delivered in a single dose. When multiple doses administered over time would be desirable, one of several techniques can be used to gain access. For short-term administration, a catheter may be left in a tumor resection cavity and is brought out through an opening in the skin, allowing repeated or continuous infusions over several days. For longer-

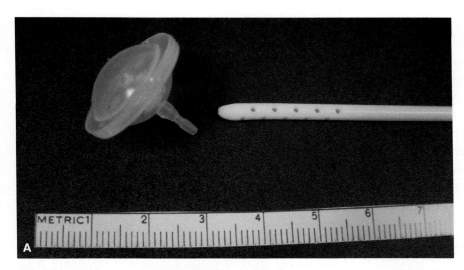
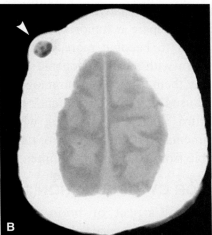
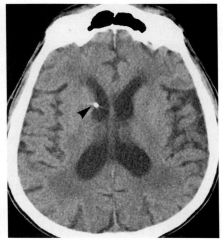

Figure 13–15. Surgery for long-term access to ventricular CSF. Ommaya reservoir placement for treatment of carcinomatous meningitis. *A,* Subcutaneous reservoir and ventricular catheter. *B,* Axial CT image showing subcutaneous reservoir. *C,* Axial CT image showing tip of ventricular catheter in frontal horn of right lateral ventricle.

term access, a catheter connected to a subcutaneous reservoir may be implanted for repeated administrations of a liquid agent over an arbitrary time period. When delivery over several days is possible using an implanted catheter, it is possible to take advantage of convection-based delivery.[15] In contrast to the diffusion-based distribution of therapeutic agents that occurs after a single dose is injected, convection-based delivery uses the mass action of slow fluid flow through interstitial fluid spaces to achieve a much wider volume of delivery over several days. The difference in distribution volume can be quite dramatic, convection-based methods can increase the volume of distribution by orders of magnitude when large molecules are being delivered.[15]

Adjuvant treatments available in liquid solutions or suspensions include genetically modified viruses intended to transduce tumor cells with a therapeutic gene (gene therapy), viruses modified so that they replicate selectively in tumor cells (viral therapy), and some chemotherapy agents. Agents commonly delivered directly into tumor cysts include those that work through local antineoplastic or irritant action (such as bleomycin) or radioisotopes that deliver ionizing radiation over a short path in tissue (such as phosphorus-32).

Other adjuvant treatments are only available as solids (Figure 13–16). These must be delivered by placement against the walls of a resection cavity. One such treatment is polymer wafers impregnated with carmustine (BCNU) (Gliadel®, Guilford Pharmaceuticals, Baltimore, MD). These have been shown to prolong median survival by 8 weeks after resection of recurrent malignant glioma.[16] Recently conducted trials have tested efficacy after initial resection of malignant glioma.[17] Wafers bearing higher concentrations of BCNU than the 3.85 percent used in Gliadel wafers have also been tested in the setting of recurrent glioma resections. To date, other types of wafers have not been tested in clinical trials.

Brachytherapy is the implantation of long-acting radiation sources into a tumor or surrounding tissue. The most common means of delivery into a glioma is to place catheters within or around the tumor. The catheters are then afterloaded with radioactive pellets of iodine-125 (I-125) or iridium-192, which are removed with the catheters after the calculated dose has been delivered. Randomized clinical trials have failed to show efficacy for tumor margin doses of 60 Gy delivered using I-125 implants over about 7 days.[18] Disadvantages of this treatment include the need for hospitalization during the treatment and a high rate of delayed radiation necrosis. Current testing focuses on small, permanently implanted seeds of I-125 that are placed against the wall of a resection cavity and deliver up to 160 Gy over a period of several months.[19]

Technology is also available for irradiating tumors intraoperatively by placing a probe into the tumor that emits radiation from its tip.[20] This results in a spherical dose distribution that resembles other forms of radiosurgery. Compared to standard radiosurgery, this form of interstitial irradiation may be useful when a specimen of the mass to be irradiated must be examined in order to establish a diagnosis (eg, single metastasis with no known primary) or when a tumor cyst can be stereotactically drained to reduce its size and then immediately treated with interstitial radiosurgery. Other forms of intraoperative irradiation are not often used for brain tumor treatment, although some applications have been reported, such as ex vivo high-dose irradiation of bone flaps that are infiltrated with tumor or irradiation of exposed dura that has been in contact with a malignant tumor using low-energy photons with very limited tissue penetrance.

Finally, there are some adjuvant therapies that are chosen on the basis of studies of resected tissue or that are actually made from resected tissue. For example, resected tissue from some tumors can be grown in tissue culture and used to test in vitro sensitivity to a panel of chemotherapeutic agents. The results are used to guide subsequent treatment with systemic chemotherapy.[21] Alternatively, the resected tissue can be used to prepare a tumor vaccine by modifying tumor cells to become more immunogenic, by mixing them with an immunogenic adjuvant, or by processing them to prepare immunogenic peptides that can be used to prime the patient's own dendritic cells in vitro.[22] These approaches, which are currently experimental, require amounts of tissue that are only available from a resection specimen.

SURGERY FOR CYTOREDUCTION

The most controversial aspect of brain tumor surgery is its role in prolonging survival. Most surgeons believe that surgery is effective in prolonging survival in malignant glioma and most other histologic brain tumor subtypes. (Exceptions are primary cerebral lymphoma, germinoma, and some malignant germ cell tumors, for which irradiation and/or chemotherapy are very effective.) Because there are no randomized trials that address this topic, all available evidence consists of studies linking more exten-

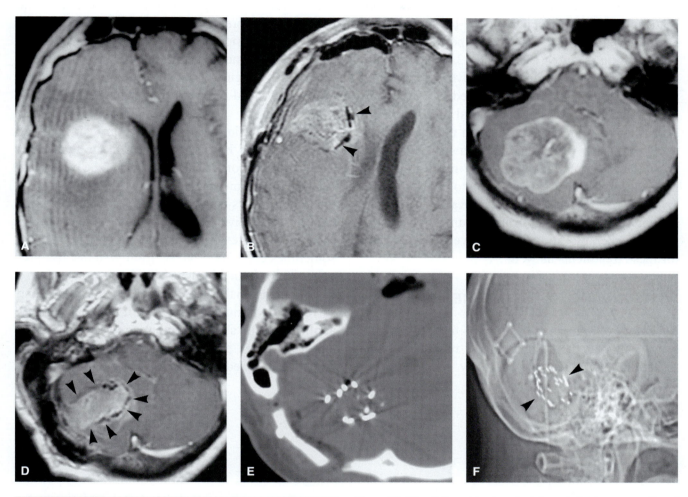

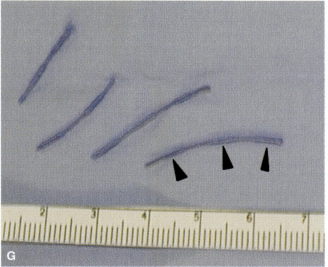

Figure 13–16. Adjuvant treatments delivered after tumor resection. *A and B*, MR axial gadolinium-enhanced T1-weighted images before and after resection of right frontoparietal recurrent malignant glioma. BCNU-impregnated wafers can be seen in the resection bed (*B, arrows*). *C* and *D*. T1-weighted axial gadolinium-enhanced MR images. Recurrent right cerebellar small cell lung carcinoma metastasis after whole brain radiation. *C*, Before resection. *D*, After resection with I-125 brachytherapy seeds permanently implanted in resection bed (*arrows*). *E* and *F*, Contrast-enhanced CT axial and lateral roentgenographic images. *Arrows* indicate brachytherapy seeds. *G*, Brachytherapy seeds before implantation. Individual radioisotope seeds are packaged as nodes (*arrows*) along a length of absorbable suture.

sive resection to longer subsequent survival. Most such studies have not adjusted for resectability, making it difficult to distinguish the benefit of surgery from the potential difference in natural history between resectable and unresectable tumors. However, the evidence that extensive resection of high-grade gliomas is associated with longer survival, even after adjustment for age and performance status, is strong (Figures 13–17 and 13–18).[23–27] Some studies suggest that more extensive resections of low-grade gliomas are also followed by longer survival.[28] Resection of single cerebral metastases has been shown to prolong survival in randomized trials.[29] Extensive resection is also a powerful prognostic factor in malignant gliomas in children[30] and in medulloblastomas.[31] In addition to improving survival per se, extensive tumor removals can improve patient tolerance of adjuvant treatments (such as radiation therapy) and may improve response rates for these treatments as well.[32,33]

IMPROVING EXTENT OF RESECTION

Recent developments in surgical technology and overall management have made more extensive resections more feasible in many specific situations. Preoperative embolization by interventional radiologists can facilitate resection of some skull-base tumors, such as meningiomas, and of hypervascular tumors such as choroid plexus carcinomas in children. Preoperative chemotherapy is rarely used to facilitate surgery but can be useful in some malignant tumors in children and in malignant primary pineal tumors to shrink the tumor away from surrounding structures and to reduce intraoperative blood loss (Figure 13–19). Radiation therapy is only rarely used on brain tumors in the pre-resection setting.

Technology in the operating room can facilitate tumor resection by distinguishing tissue that needs to be resected from tissue that needs to be preserved. Imaging-based methods primarily focus on showing the tumor and its boundaries, using images obtained either preoperatively or in real time in the operating room.[34] Frameless stereotactic guidance systems, sometimes called neuronavigation systems, use preoperatively obtained CT or MR images to generate a three-dimensional representation of the tumor and surrounding brain (Figure 13–20). Fiducial markers applied to the skin before imaging, or anatomic landmarks such as the tragus, lateral canthus, and glabella, are used to register the three-dimensional

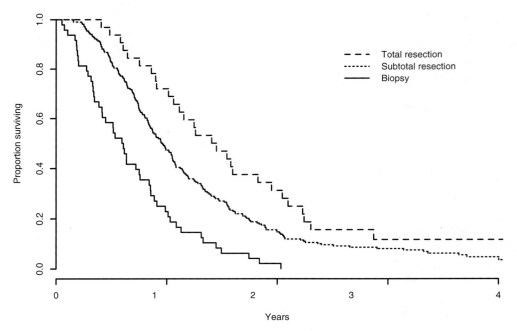

Figure 13–17. Kaplan-Meier curve showing survival in 301 patients with glioblastoma multiforme who underwent biopsy procedures or subtotal or total resections at diagnosis. The difference in survival was highly significant ($p < .001$).

imaging space to the patient's actual anatomy. Using a handheld probe, the surgeon can then indicate objects within the surgical field, while the guidance system shows the location of the probe in real time within the imaging space. Some systems can also highlight normal brain structures, such as the cerebral ventricles or pyramidal tract, on the images projected for view.

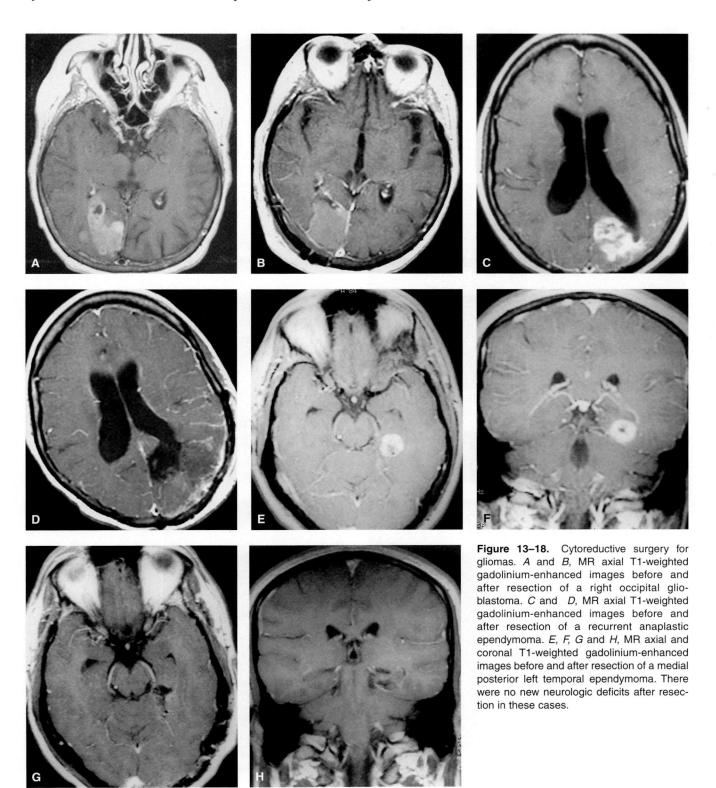

Figure 13–18. Cytoreductive surgery for gliomas. *A* and *B*, MR axial T1-weighted gadolinium-enhanced images before and after resection of a right occipital glioblastoma. *C* and *D*, MR axial T1-weighted gadolinium-enhanced images before and after resection of a recurrent anaplastic ependymoma. *E, F, G* and *H*, MR axial and coronal T1-weighted gadolinium-enhanced images before and after resection of a medial posterior left temporal ependymoma. There were no new neurologic deficits after resection in these cases.

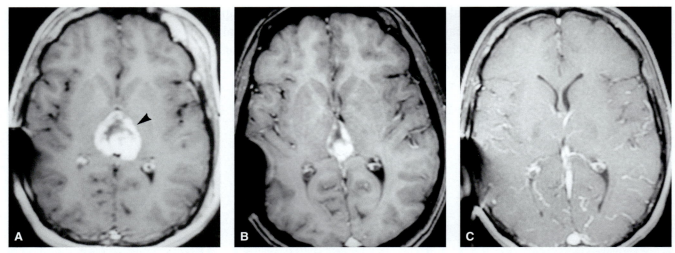

Figure 13-19. Neoadjuvant chemotherapy to facilitate resection of a malignant pineocytoma. MR axial T1-weighted gadolinium-enhanced images. *A*, At diagnosis. *B*, After neoadjuvant chemotherapy. *C*, After complete resection. At surgery, the tumor remnant was almost entirely necrotic.

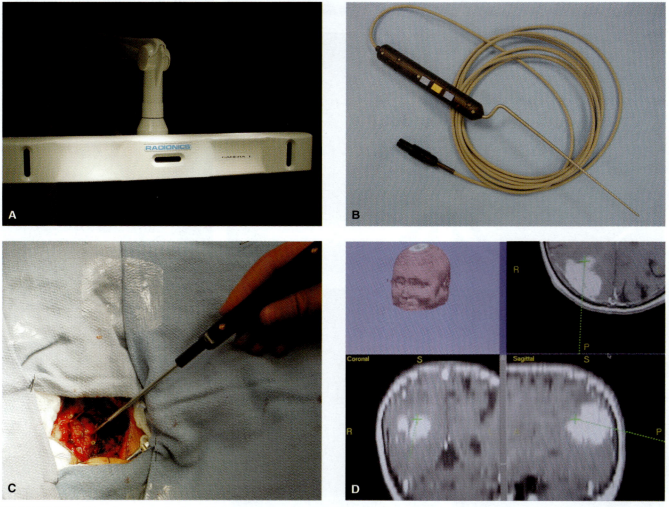

Figure 13-20. Frameless stereotactic guidance. *A*, Infrared camera; *B* and *C*, localization wands; *D*, device display screen during tumor resection.

Difficulties with neuronavigation systems include inaccuracies in registering imaging space to real space and, most importantly, the progressive shift in position of the tumor and surrounding brain that occurs during the operation. As the tumor is removed, surrounding brain will collapse inward to partially fill the resection cavity. As well, the entire brain usually shifts downward under the influence of gravity as CSF is progressively removed and as hyperosmolarity from mannitol administration shrinks the brain.[35] Despite these drawbacks, frameless stereotactic guidance systems can be useful for planning a small incision for lesions near the surface as well as for locating deep lesions. Frameless stereotactic guidance can be useful in resecting skull-base lesions as well as these do not shift during surgery.

Real-time intraoperative imaging modalities offer a solution to brain shift by allowing the operative area to be re-imaged at will. Ultrasonography, CT, and MRI are all available for intraoperative guidance. Intraoperative ultrasonography is widely available using non-dedicated ultrasound units. Ultrasonography allows location of deep lesions and can image residual tumor during a resection if the tumor tissue is hyperechoic, as is often the case. Disadvantages include low sensitivity for small areas of residual tumor and a requirement for a sufficiently large cranial opening to admit the imaging head. Intraoperative CT is ideal for real-time imaging during placement of catheters into difficult targets as currently available catheters are much better seen with CT than with MRI.[36] Intraoperative CT can also show small areas of residual enhancing tumor and allow remeasurement of cyst volumes after stereotactic drainage.

For most intraoperative imaging applications, MRI is the best available modality (Figure 13–21).[37,38] Intraoperative MRI suites require special surgical instrumentation that is not paramagnetic. Several scanner configurations are available: in some, the patient remains in the center of the magnet during the procedure, and in others the patient is moved in and out of the imaging area as needed. Most installations use a scanner that is dedicated to intraoperative use, but some installations permit use for imaging other patients when an operative procedure is not in progress.

With intraoperative MRI, as tumor resection progresses, repeated real-time MRI allows appreciation of residual tumor and its relationship to surrounding structures. The cycle of resection followed by imaging can be repeated until a satisfactory resection has been achieved. Intraoperative MRI can be combined with frameless stereotactic guidance, with the image set for the guidance system being updated periodically during the resection.[39] Inaccuracy due to intraoperative brain shift is thus less of a problem, although it is not entirely eliminated. Artifacts affecting intraoperative imaging include a very rapidly developing linear enhancement at the resection margin that can mimic residual tumor. Studies have shown an increase in the number of tumors for which imaging gross total resections can be achieved using intraoperative MRI, even after a resection using neuronavigation has been performed.[38,40,41]

Other methods for detecting residual tumor are not currently in wide clinical use. A variety of dyes that are administered intravenously can be used to give tumor tissue a different appearance from normal brain tissue, especially under ultraviolet light.[42] Reflectance spectroscopy is also under investigation as a means of distinguishing tumor tissue from normal brain tissue.

Functional methods are very useful for indicating parts of the brain that should not be resected because doing so would cause a neurologic deficit. Confident identification of functionally important brain structures can improve extent of resection by eliminating the requirement to leave residual tumor as a safety buffer.

Preoperatively, functional MRI can be used to demonstrate brain centers that show activation in response to motor or language tasks or sensory stimuli (Figure 13–22). Functional MRI uses the difference in signal characteristics between MR images obtained before and during an activity or stimulus to define the area of the brain that has increased oxygen extraction while the activity or stimulus is present. Areas of functional MRI-defined cortical activity correlate well with intraoperative cortical mapping, especially for primary motor and sensory cortices. Mapping of frontal speech areas is also reliably performed. Temporoparietal speech areas are more difficult to define clearly using functional

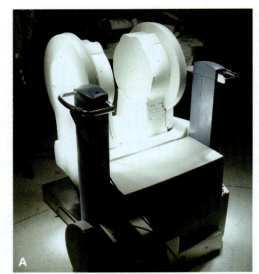

Figure 13–21. Intraoperative MRI. *A*, Portable intraoperative MRI unit. *B*, Patient in unit for preoperative MR scan. *C*, Intraoperative image of pituitary macroadenoma before resection.

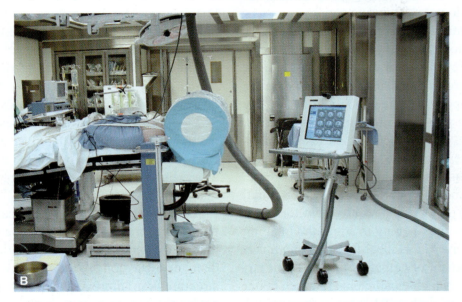

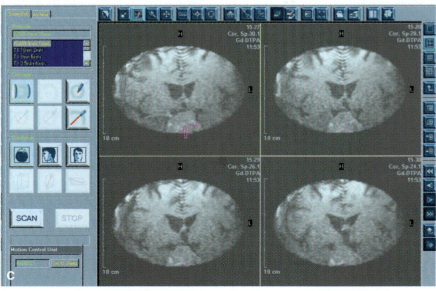

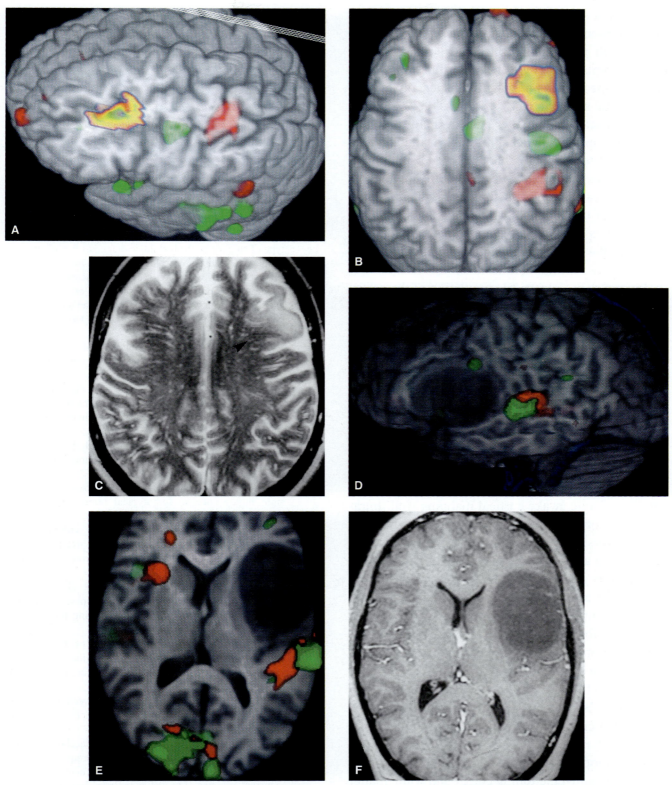

Figure 13–22. Functional MRI for preoperative definition of speech and motor centers. *A* and *B*, Left middle frontal gyrus oligodendroglioma. *A, B* (multicolor), and *C*, Functional MR image showing tumor, activation during language tasks (green) and right-hand motor tasks (red). *C*, Axial T2-weighted MR image. *D, E* and *F*, Left frontal astrocytoma. *D*, Functional MR image showing tumor (dark gray). Red and green areas represent brain activation during verb generation and semantic decision speech tasks, respectively. *F*, Axial T1-weighted gadolinium enhanced axial image. Resection of both tumors was possible without postoperative deficits.

MRI. When speech is at risk during a tumor resection, functional MRI can supplement awake craniotomy with intraoperative speech mapping, but it does not replace it. This is because functional MRI, although specific, is not sensitive, especially to temporoparietal speech areas.

Subcortical white-matter pathways are more difficult to map using MRI. Presently available functional MRI techniques cannot delineate subcortical white-matter pathways. Special diffusion tensor sequences can distinguish the predominant spatial direction of collections of axons within white matter, and this has some promise for future use in showing the relationship between critical white-matter pathways and mass lesions.[43]

Intraoperative electrical stimulation of the cortex (mapping) is the "gold standard" for identifying primary motor cortex, primary sensory cortex, and speech cortex.[44] Motor mapping can be performed under general anesthesia, but sensory and speech cortex mapping require an awake and cooperative patient. Patients with a significant preoperative aphasia are not good candidates for awake craniotomy because the operative team cannot communicate with them well enough to guarantee their cooperation during the procedure, and young children are poor candidates for the same reason. Most other patients tolerate awake cortical mapping well. Intraoperative cortical stimulation, combined with constant conversation with the patient as resection progresses, can allow resection of many tumors that are immediately adjacent to important speech centers. Sensory cortex can also be easily mapped in the awake patient. Motor mapping is the most common indication for intraoperative cortical stimulation. Because motor mapping is possible under general anesthesia, it is potentially applicable to all patients, including children. Extremity movements may sometimes be obtained with cortical stimulation even in patients who have no voluntary movement. Subcortical motor pathways can also be mapped using intraoperative stimulation. Because tumors can contain still-functioning cortex and white matter within their boundaries,[45] imaging techniques alone (such as intraoperative MRI) are not sufficient to guarantee safe resections when the tumor appears to abut eloquent brain areas.[46]

REFERENCES

1. Barker FG II, Gutin PH. Surgical techniques for gliomas. In: Berger MS, Wilson CB, editors. The gliomas. Philadelphia: WB Saunders; 1998. p. 349–60.
2. Apuzzo MLJ. Brain surgery. New York: Churchill Livingstone; 1993.
3. Krieger MD, Chandrasoma PT, Zee CS, Apuzzo ML. Role of stereotactic biopsy in the diagnosis and management of brain tumors. Semin Surg Oncol 1998;14:13–25.
4. Bernstein M, Parrent AG. Complications of CT-guided stereotactic biopsy of intra-axial brain lesions. J Neurosurg 1994;81:165–8.
5. Field M, Witham TF, Flickinger JC, et al. Comprehensive assessment of hemorrhage risks and outcomes after stereotactic biopsy. J Neurosurg 2001;94:545–51.
6. Glantz MJ, Burger PC, Herndon JE, et al. Influence of the type of surgery on the histologic diagnosis in patients with anaplastic gliomas. Neurology 1991;41:1741–4.
7. Donahue B, Scott CB, Nelson JS, et al. Influence of an oligodendroglial component on the survival of patients with anaplastic astrocytomas: a report of Radiation Therapy Oncology Group 83-02. Int J Radiat Oncol Biol Phys 1997;38:911–4.
8. Butler WE. Comparison of three methods of estimating confidence intervals for stereotactic error. Comput Aided Surg 1999;4:26–36.
9. Moriarty TM, Quinones-Hinojosa A, Larson PS, et al. Frameless stereotactic neurosurgery using intraoperative magnetic resonance imaging: stereotactic brain biopsy. Neurosurgery 2000;47:1138–45.
10. Jackson RJ, Fuller GN, Abi-Said D, et al. Limitations of stereotactic biopsy in the initial management of gliomas. Neurooncology 2001;3:193–200.
11. Masdeu JC, Quinto C, Olivera C, et al. Open ring imaging sign: highly specific for atypical brain demyelination. Neurology 2000;54:1427–33.
12. Taylor MD, Bernstein M. Awake craniotomy with brain mapping as the routine surgical approach to treating patients with supratentorial intraaxial tumors: a prospective trial of 200 cases. J Neurosurg 1999;90:35–41.
13. Berger MS, Ghatan S, Haglund MM, et al. Low-grade gliomas associated with intractable epilepsy: seizure outcome utilizing electrocorticography during tumor resection. J Neurosurg 1993;79:62–9.
14. Gutin PH. Treatment of radiation necrosis of the brain. In: Gutin PH, Leibel SA, Sheline GE, editors. Radiation injury to the nervous system. New York: Raven Press, 1991. p. 271–82.
15. Bobo RH, Laske DW, Akbasak A, et al. Convection-enhanced delivery of macromolecules in the brain. Proc Natl Acad Sci U S A 1994;91:2076–80.
16. Brem H, Piantadosi S, Burger PC, et al. Placebo-controlled trial of safety and efficacy of intraoperative controlled delivery by biodegradable polymers of chemotherapy for recurrent gliomas. The Polymer-Brain Tumor Treatment Group. Lancet 1995;345:1008–12.
17. Valtonen S, Timonen U, Toivanen P, et al. Interstitial chemotherapy with carmustine-loaded polymers for high-grade gliomas: a randomized double-blind study. Neurosurgery 1997;41:44–8 [discussion 48–9].

18. Laperriere NJ, Leung PM, McKenzie S, et al. Randomized study of brachytherapy in the initial management of patients with malignant astrocytoma. Int J Radiat Oncol Biol Phys 1998;41:1005–11.
19. Patel S, Breneman JC, Warnick RE, et al. Permanent iodine-125 interstitial implants for the treatment of recurrent glioblastoma multiforme. Neurosurgery 2000;46:1123–8.
20. Cosgrove GR, Hochberg FH, Zervas NT, et al. Interstitial irradiation of brain tumors, using a miniature radiosurgery device: initial experience. Neurosurgery 1997;40:518–23 [discussion 523–5].
21. Yung WKA. In vitro chemosensitivity testing and its clinical application in human gliomas. Neurosurg Rev 1989;12:197–203.
22. Pollack IF, Okada H, Chambers WH. Exploitation of immune mechanisms in the treatment of central nervous system cancer. Semin Pediatr Neurol 2000;7:131–43.
23. Barker FG, Prados MD, Chang SM, et al. Radiation response and survival time in patients with glioblastoma multiforme. J Neurosurg 1996;84:442–8.
24. Simpson JR, Horton J, Scott C, et al. Influence of location and extent of surgical resection on survival of patients with glioblastoma multiforme: results of three consecutive Radiation Therapy Oncology Group (RTOG) clinical trials. Int J Radiat Oncol Biol Phys 1993;26:239–44.
25. Keles GE, Anderson B, Berger MS. The effect of extent of resection on time to tumor progression and survival in patients with glioblastoma multiforme of the cerebral hemisphere. Surg Neurol 1999;52:371–9.
26. Scott JN, Rewcastle NB, Brasher PMA, et al. Which glioblastoma multiforme patient will become a long-term survivor? A population-based study. Ann Neurol 1999;46:183–8.
27. Lacroix M, Abi-Said D, Fourney DR, et al. A multivariate analysis of 416 patients with glioblastoma multiforme: prognosis, extent of resection, and survival. J Neurosurg 2001;95:190–8.
28. Berger MS, Deliganis AV, Dobbins J, Keles GE. The effect of extent of resection on recurrence in patients with low-grade cerebral hemisphere gliomas. Cancer 1994;74:1784–91.
29. Patchell RA, Tibbs PA, Walsh JW, et al. A randomized trial of surgery in the treatment of single metastases to the brain. N Engl J Med 1990;322:494–500.
30. Wisoff JH, Boyett JM, Berger MS, et al. Current neurosurgical management and the impact of the extent of resection in the treatment of malignant gliomas of childhood: a report of the Children's Cancer Group Trial No. CCG-945. J Neurosurg 1998;89:52–9.
31. Zeltzer PM, Boyett JM, Finlay JL, et al. Metastasis stage, adjuvant treatment, and residual tumor are prognostic factors for medulloblastoma in children: conclusions from the Children's Cancer Group 921 randomized phase III study. J Clin Oncol 1999;17:832–45.
32. Barker FG, Chang SM, Larson DA, et al. Age and radiation response in glioblastoma multiforme. Neurosurgery 2001. [In press]
33. Rostomily RC, Spence AM, Duong D, et al. Multimodality management of recurrent adult malignant gliomas: results of a phase II multiagent chemotherapy study and analysis of cytoreductive surgery. Neurosurgery 1994;35:378–88.
34. Zakhary R, Keles GE, Berger MS. Intraoperative imaging techniques in the treatment of brain tumors. Curr Opin Oncol 1999;11:152–6.
35. Nimsky C, Ganslandt O, Cerny S, et al. Quantification of, visualization of, and compensation for brain shift using intraoperative magnetic resonance imaging. Neurosurgery 2000;47:1070–9.
36. Butler WE, Piaggio CM, Constantinou C, et al. A mobile computed tomographic scanner with intraoperative and intensive care unit applications. Neurosurgery 1998;42:1304–10 [discussion 1310–1].
37. Barnett GH. The role of image-guided technology in the surgical planning and resection of gliomas. J Neurooncol 1999;42:247–58.
38. Wirtz CR, Knauth M, Staubert A, et al. Clinical evaluation and follow-up results for intraoperative magnetic resonance imaging in neurosurgery. Neurosurgery 2000;46:1112–22.
39. Nimsky C, Ganslandt O, Kober H, et al. Intraoperative magnetic resonance imaging combined with neuronavigation: a new concept. Neurosurgery 2001;48:1082–9.
40. Bohinski RJ, Kokkino AK, Warnick RE, et al. Glioma resection in a shared-resource magnetic resonance operating room after optimal image-guided frameless stereotactic resection. Neurosurgery 2001;48:731–42.
41. Knauth M, Wirtz CR, Tronnier VM, et al. Intraoperative MR imaging increases the extent of tumor resection in patients with high-grade gliomas. AJNR Am J Neuroradiol 1999;20:1642–6.
42. Haglund MM, Berger MS, Hochman DW. Enhanced optical imaging of human gliomas and tumor margins. Neurosurgery 1996;38:308–17.
43. Wieshmann UC, Symms MR, Parker GJ, et al. Diffusion tensor imaging demonstrates deviation of fibres in normal-appearing white matter adjacent to a brain tumour. J Neurol Neurosurg Psychiatry 2000;68:501–3.
44. Matz PG, Cobbs C, Berger MS. Intraoperative cortical mapping as a guide to the surgical resection of gliomas. J Neurooncol 1999;42:233–45.
45. Ojemann JG, Miller JW, Silbergeld DL. Preserved function in brain invaded by tumor. Neurosurgery 1996;39:253–8.
46. Skirboll SS, Ojemann GA, Berger MS, et al. Functional cortex and subcortical white matter located within gliomas. Neurosurgery 1996;38:678–84 [discussion 684–5].

14

Management of Primary Malignant Brain Tumors in Adults

ERIC BURTON, MD
MICHAEL PRADOS, MD

The malignant gliomas, which include anaplastic astrocytoma (AA), glioblastoma multiforme (GBM), anaplastic oligodendroglioma (AO), and anaplastic oligoastrocytoma (AOA), comprise the majority of the primary central nervous system (CNS) tumors diagnosed in the adult population. Understanding the management of patients with high-grade gliomas is important for the general oncologist who, at some point, will presumably be involved in their care. This chapter gives an overview of the care and treatment of patients with malignant gliomas from initial presentation through to the time terminal care is needed. Emphasis will be placed on recent advances in the different treatment modalities and current trends in management.

Despite improvements in surgical techniques, radiation therapy, and chemotherapy, the prognosis for high-grade gliomas remains poor. Median survival for GBMs is approximately 12 months and for anaplastic tumors 3 to 5 years. Survival at recurrence is generally in the order of several months for GBMs. Because of the poor survival associated with these tumors, novel treatment strategies are constantly being developed. One challenge is to introduce new therapies into settings where efficacy can be assessed and compared to standard therapies. This is best accomplished through clinical trials.

EPIDEMIOLOGY

Tumors of the CNS include a heterogeneous population of neoplasms. The American Cancer Society estimates there will be 17,200 new cases of brain and other nervous system cancers for 2001 in the United States (9,800 in males and 7,400 in females). The incidence rate of primary malignant brain tumors is 5.9 cases per 100,000 person years. In 2001, an estimated 13,100 deaths from primary malignant brain tumors are predicted. The most common of these is GBM, which is the cause of most deaths attributable to CNS tumors.[1]

CLASSIFICATION

Malignant gliomas arise from glial cells; glial cells include astrocytes, oligodendrocytes, and ependymal cells. Tumors of glial origin are classified as astrocytomas, oligodendrogliomas, mixed tumors (oligoastrocytomas), and ependymomas. The classification of malignant gliomas, as for most tumors, is based on the predominant cell type. Thus, astrocytomas typically demonstrate histologic features suggestive of astrocytes, whereas oligodendrogliomas have histologic features resembling oligodendrocytes, and mixed gliomas present histologic features of both types. Figure 14–1 shows the typical histologic appearance of a grade II, or low-grade, oligodendroglioma (Figure 14–1A) and a grade III, or anaplastic, oligodendroglioma (Figure 14–1B). However, in the case of mixed tumors such as oligoastrocytomas, it should be noted that the presence of both neoplastic cells occurs quite frequently, and this does not automatically imply a diagnosis of a mixed glioma. There is as yet no standard criterion that objectively defines how much of each tumor type is needed before a diagnosis of oligoastrocytoma can be given. Unfortunately, this allows interpretation that is highly subjective and at times results in discordant classification between pathologists.

In formulating the pathologic diagnosis of gliomas, the degree of differentiation and anaplasia within a tumor also must be established. Differentiation of a tumor is determined by how closely its neoplastic cells resemble normal cells. Anaplasia is a term that summarizes histopathologic features associated with malignant biologic behavior. This usually includes nuclear atypia, increased mitotic activity, atypical mitosis, cellular pleomorphism, cellular proliferation, vascular proliferation, and necrosis.[2] The significance of some of these features may vary considerably in different tumor types. For example, nuclear atypia and extensive endothelial proliferation indicate anaplasia and poor clinical prognosis in diffuse astrocytomas of the cerebral hemispheres, but they bear no such implications in a pilocytic astrocytoma.

The degree of anaplasia within a glioma is conveyed by assignment of a numerical "grade." The more anaplastic a tumor, the higher its grade and the poorer the prognosis. Grade III anaplastic astrocytomas and grade IV glioblastomas define the malig-

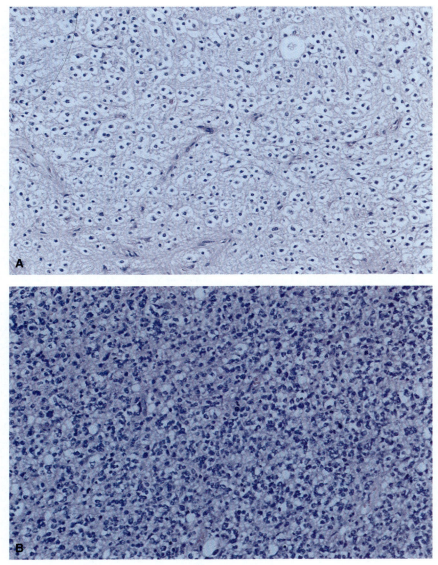

Figure 14–1. *A*, Grade II oligodendroglioma; *B*, grade III oligodendroglioma.

nant end of this spectrum according to the World Health Organization (WHO) criteria for tumor classification. In contrast, grade II astrocytomas have a low degree of anaplasia and a better survival outcome. Figure 14–2 shows the typical histologic appearance of astrocytoma grade II (Figure 14–2A), grade III (Figure 14–2B), and grade IV (Figure 14–2C) tumors.

The WHO has proposed one classification scheme for glial tumors. However, several other classification systems have been developed. Bailey and Cushing published the first of these in 1926. Examples of other classification systems are the Kernohan, Ringertz, Daumas-Duport/St. Anne-Mayo, and Duke schemes.[3] Depending on the particular schema, tumor grades may range from I to III or I to IV. Although all systems are based on the idea that glial tumors can be stratified by the degree of anaplastic features and, as such, malignant potential, the systems have differed in the relative weight given to histologic characteristics that determine grade. For example, by Duke criteria, a grade IV tumor must have necrosis, a feature common to GBMs. Alternatively, the WHO or Daumas-Duport/St. Anne Mayo systems do not necessarily require necrosis to classify a tumor as grade IV. Understandably, the variability in grading systems has led to discrepancies when comparing data from

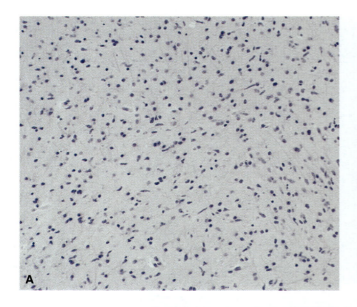
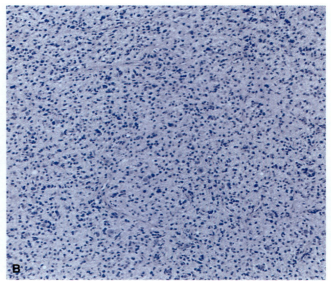
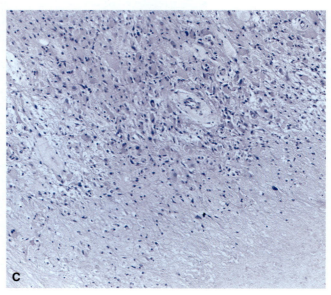

Figure 14–2. These astrocytic tumors show increasing degrees of anaplasia: *A*, grade II astrocytoma; *B*, grade III anaplastic astrocytoma; and *C*, grade IV glioblastoma multiforme.

different institutions. Recently, the trend has been toward using one of two systems for grading malignant gliomas: the WHO-II definition or the Daumas-Duport/St. Anne Mayo system. Still, even with standardized classification systems, in practice there continues to be a degree of subjectivity when pathologists evaluate tumors, and this can lead to differences in diagnoses and grading. Also, surgical sampling and previous radiation therapy (radiation may cause endothelial proliferation and necrosis) sometimes can make it difficult to grade newly diagnosed and previously treated tumors definitively.

CLINICAL PRESENTATION

The symptomatology produced by brain tumors is governed to a great extent by their rate of growth and location. For example, rapidly growing tumors and those located in eloquent cortex or along the ventricular system can manifest sooner than larger, slowly growing tumors in relatively silent areas. The change of neurologic function seen as a result of brain tumors can be divided into two categories: general signs and symptoms and focal signs and symptoms. There may be some overlap of these divisions. For instance, a headache may be indicative of generalized increased intracranial pressure (ICP) or it may be localized to the tumor location. Conversely, focal symptoms may result from generalized increased ICP that produces false localizing signs.

The general signs and symptoms usually are due to an increase in ICP, which may be caused by tumor mass, associated cerebral edema or vasogenic edema, obstruction of cerebrospinal fluid (CSF) flow, or obstruction of the venous system. The patient may present with headache, dizziness, nausea and vomiting, nuchal rigidity, or mental disturbances as a result of increased ICP.

Headache alone is the initial symptom in about 20 percent of patients with brain tumors. However, headaches occur at some time during the course of illness in approximately 70 percent of patients. Typically, they are not unusually severe and often are intermittent in nature. Classically, they are described as "morning headaches" that tend to improve as the day progresses. This type of headache is thought to be due to the relative hypoventilation that occurs during sleep. This in turn causes CNS arterial vasodilation and increased blood flow. This process reverses when the patient awakes and starts normal ventilation, lowering the blood CO_2. A physical finding associated with increased ICP is papilledema. Although not always present in patients with brain tumors, it may be the initial sign that prompts clinical investigation.

Headaches also may occur even when there is no evidence of increased ICP. Traction on pain-sensitive structures such as the major arteries, veins, and dural sinuses is the usual etiology. It should be noted that headaches are a common and nonspecific event during the lifetime of most people in the general population, and they rarely indicate the presence of a tumor.

Seizures represent the initial symptom in about 15 percent of patients with brain tumors. They may occur during the illness in approximately 30 percent of patients. Whether a tumor will produce seizures depends largely upon its location and growth characteristics. Seizures are more likely to occur with rapidly growing tumors that involve the cortex as opposed to slow-growing tumors located in the posterior fossa. The seizures may be focal in nature or generalized. Determining the nature of the seizure often is difficult since focal seizures may quickly generalize before a focal onset can be determined. As with headaches, seizures occur with much more frequency due to etiologies other than brain tumors. However, new-onset seizures in adults certainly should prompt an investigation to rule out focal lesions like tumors.

As opposed to generalized symptoms, focal signs and symptoms are due to interference with the local function of an area in the brain. Symptoms that result from tumors generally are gradual and progressive (subacute to chronic) as opposed to abrupt symptoms like those associated with strokes. The clinical symptoms depend on the anatomic location of the tumor.

Frontal lobe tumors can result in personality and cognitive changes. Generally, it is believed that bilateral involvement must be present to produce these symptoms. Patients may demonstrate symptoms of apathy, senseless joking, inappropriate playfulness, petulance, and irritability. There also may be signs of dementia with slowed reaction time, and, in more severe cases, there can be marked deterioration of thinking and behavior. Because of the mental disturbances seen in frontal lobe tumors, these patients sometimes are initially given primary psychiatric diagnosis and treated with antidepressants. Tumors located in the posterior area of the left frontal lobe may cause an expressive aphasia (if they involve Broca's area) with or without contralateral limb weakness. Right frontal lobe tumors also may cause contralateral weakness, but language involvement is less likely.

Tumors in the parietal lobe often cause disturbances of body perception when there is involvement of the sensory cortex or the associative areas. Involvement of the postcentral (sensory) gyrus produces defects in gnostic or discriminative types of sensation. Object perception may become impaired, and the patient may be unable to recognize familiar objects by their size, shape, or texture (astereognosis). Lesions of the parietal lobe, particularly in the nondominant hemisphere, can result in disturbances of body awareness such as unilateral neglect. These phenomena can occur in the left parietal lobe, but they may be obscured by language deficits that usually occur with left-sided parietal lesions.

Occipital lobe tumors can result in contralateral homonymous visual field deficits. Tumors in this area sometimes cause visual hallucinations, which consist of uniform flashes of light in different shapes. These are to be distinguished from the formed images observed by patients with temporal lobe lesions that cause seizures. The latter images usually are seen in the contralateral visual field, and they may occur as a solitary phenomenon or as the aura of a seizure.

Tumors of the dominant temporal lobe will produce disturbances in the comprehension of language. Tumors that extend posteriorly may be associated with anomia and alexia. Lesions in either temporal lobe may cause visual field deficits. Tumors that are anterior in location produce a contralateral superior homonymous quadrantanopsia. As the lesion extends posteriorly, the defect tends to become a hemianopsia. Of note, tumors in the anterior portion of the nondominant temporal lobe can be, in effect, asymptomatic. If seizures are caused by tumors in the temporal lobe they are usually complex partial in nature with auras of gastric upset, sensations of déjà vu, and olfactory or gustatory sensations.

Tumors located in the pituitary gland and hypothalamus often cause visual loss due to involvement of the optic nerve chiasm or optic tract. Tumors in this location can result in endocrinopathies such as diabetes insipidus or amenorrhea.

Tumors in the cerebellum can cause ataxia and possibly hydrocephalus due to compression of the fourth ventricle. Patients may present with weakness or cranial nerve findings with brainstem tumors. Tumors located in the brain stem and cerebellum often exhibit symptoms before the tumor is very large due to the close anatomic proximity of many critical areas.

DIAGNOSTIC NEUROIMAGING

Magnetic resonance imaging (MRI) of the brain is currently the standard imaging modality used in patients with, or suspected of having, brain tumors. It is more sensitive than computed tomography (CT) for detecting intracranial masses, and the multiplanar capability of MRI permits better assessment of the tumor and surrounding structures. This is especially helpful in surgical and radiation therapy planning and in assessing response to treatment. It was originally hypothesized that grading of primary gliomas could be accomplished based upon imaging characteristics. To an extent, this is true for gliomas; however, it is not uncommon for high-grade gliomas to have imaging characteristics of low-grade tumors approximately 30 percent of the time. This makes tumor biopsy or resection essential to determining a definitive pathologic diagnosis. Typical MRI findings for a malignant glioma usually demonstrate a single well-circumscribed lesion with heterogeneous signal changes seen within the tumor. This heterogeneous MRI signal seen in high-grade tumors usually represents areas of necrosis (which is dark or hypointense on the T1-weighted image) or varying degrees of cellular density and possibly hemorrhage. Vasogenic edema can also be associated with high-grade tumors. On MRI scan, this presents as a hypointense area surrounding the tumor bed. There can be varying degrees of associated mass effect. Intravenous gadolinium DTPA (pentetic acid) usually demonstrates enhancement of these tumors. Figure 14–3 shows the typical MRI appearance of a patient with GBM. The lesion enhances with contrast and has hypointense areas within the bulk of the lesion, in this case in the left frontal lobe area. The clinician must keep in mind that demyelinating lesions, vascular malformations, infection, and strokes all can mimic the MRI appearance of malignant gliomas. However, differing clinical presentations may assist in distinguishing between these other events.

An important challenge for imaging techniques in the CNS is to differentiate radiation injury and recurrent tumor. This radiographic dilemma most commonly arises if the patient has received additional radiation (beyond conventional external beam) with either radiosurgery or brachytherapy. Since both radiation injury and progressive tumor have similar imaging characteristics on conventional MRI, and the need to distinguish between the two is necessary for guiding future therapy, there is interest in using metabolic studies like positron emission tomography (PET) scanning and MR spectroscopy (MRS).

A PET scan, using ^{18}fluorine fluorodeoxyglucose, is used to determine the metabolic activity in the area of interest. Malignant gliomas show hypermetabolism of glucose, whereas radiation-injured or necrotic brain show reduced metabolism; this enables the radiologist to determine whether the suspicious areas are consistent with active tumor or dead tissue.[4] Figure 14–4 illustrates how PET imaging can help with differentiation of tumor from necrotic disease. Following initial therapy, it was not clear that the lesion depicted had responded to irradiation or if active disease was still present. Rather than consider a biopsy, a PET scan was done. Figure 14–4A is a noncontrast MRI of the lesion in the brain stem; Figure 14–4B reveals that this lesion enhances with contrast administration. Figure 14–4C shows the results of the glucose PET image, demonstrating increased uptake within the lesion. This lesion was clearly metabolically active with viable tumor rather than radiation injury.

Magnetic resonance spectroscopy, which is available with routine MRI equipment, can characterize areas consistent with radiation injury from normal brain or tumor by determining patterns of intracellular metabolites. The two metabolites of greatest interest when proton MRS is used are choline and N-acetylaspartate (NAA).[5] Tumors often show elevated levels of choline with reduced NAA metabolites, whereas necrotic brain has reduced levels of both. Specific ratios of these compounds are used to express the relative changes to normal brain and to determine tumor activity (Figure 14–5). Although MRS is still being studied, there are other potential advantages that MRS may have related to diagnosis and treatment planning. For example, the potential exists to distinguish neoplastic from non-neoplastic lesions or possibly to noninvasively classify tumors. It also may aid in defining targets for radiation therapy. More research into MRS image analysis is needed. New clinical trials often use MRS as one assessment, along with MRI, to follow disease activity.

PRINCIPLES OF THERAPY

The treatment of malignant gliomas typically involves the three modalities of surgery, irradiation, and chemotherapy. After the initial management of presenting symptoms (which may require anticonvulsants for seizures or steroids and possibly

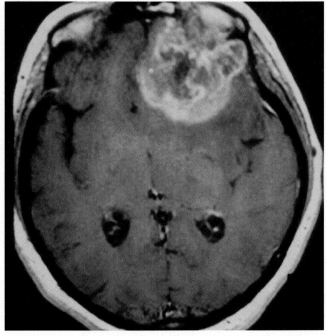

Figure 14–3. An axial T1-weighted MRI scan with gadolinium demonstrates a left frontal glioblastoma multiforme.

osmotic agents for tumor-associated edema with increased ICP), patients are usually referred for surgical evaluation. Surgery is needed to determine the histopathologic diagnosis (which will guide future therapy), to relieve symptoms due to mass effect, and to improve survival expectations. In virtually every large phase III study done in the setting of high-grade gliomas, the extent of surgical resection is associated with survival. Any degree of surgical resection larger than a biopsy will improve survival, and patients with extensive or gross-total tumor removal often will fare better than those with smaller partial resections. In almost all cases, surgery is followed by radiation therapy. In the case of grade III or IV malignant astrocytoma, irradiation following surgery is the most effective therapy for improving survival currently available. Chemotherapy may offer a modest survival benefit in patients with grade IV tumors, but it seems to be most beneficial in young patients and have little, if any, impact on survival in patients over the age of 60 years. Adjuvant chemotherapy following irradiation is a commonly accepted standard for patients with grade III tumors. Figure 14–6 is an algorithm describing typical treatment for the initial management of malignant gliomas.

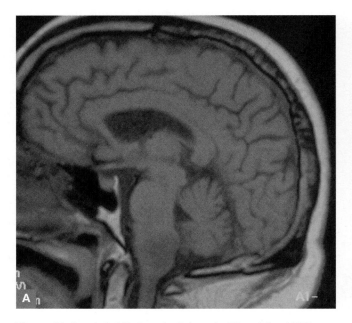
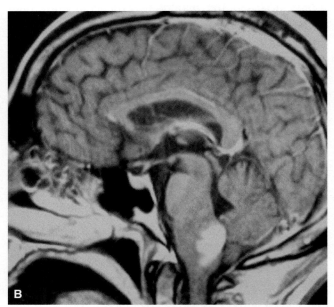
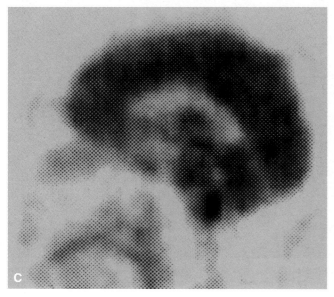

Figure 14–4. *A* and *B*, A sagittal view of a T1-weighted MRI: precontrast (*A*); postcontrast (*B*). *C*, Glucose PET scan demonstrating a metabolically active brainstem glioma centered in the medulla.

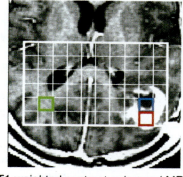
T1-weighted contrast enhanced MRI with PRESS region

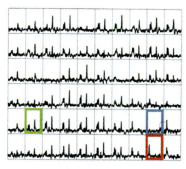
PRESS Excited region

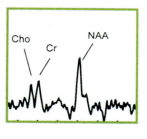
Normal Brain

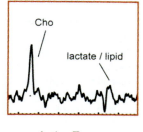
Active Tumor

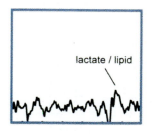
Necrosis

Point Resolved Spectroscopy (PRESS) is used to excite a region containing both the enhancing lesion and contralateral normal tissue. Individual voxels are then characterized by the size of the peaks corresponding to choline (Cho), creatine (Cr), N-acetylaspartate (NAA), and lactate/lipid. The typical patterns for normal white matter, tumor, and necrotic tissue are highlighted above.

Figure 14–5. Magnetic resonance spectroscopic image. (Illustration courtesy of Tracy McKnight, PhD.)

There are conditions other than the type of therapy given that influence survival. For example, age and performance status consistently are found to be independent factors that predict better survival outcomes for patients with malignant gliomas.[6] To illustrate this point, patients with GBMs who are less than 40 years of age and receive aggressive surgery with radiation and chemotherapy usually will survive longer than patients over 65 years who are treated in the same manner (median, 16 mo vs 9 mo, respectively).

Performance status, often measured on the Karnofsky Performance Scale (KPS), also has been shown to be an independent predictor of survival. Patients with lower KPS scores following surgery will have worse survival. Performance score often is an indirect measure of tumor burden, and, in many cases, the lower KPS score is due to a large tumor in an eloquent area of brain that is causing devastating neurologic deficits. Aggressive safe tumor resections frequently will increase the KPS of a patient dramatically.

Surgical Management

Surgery is a critical element in patient management. Aggressive surgical resection, although disputed by some oncologists, is felt to impact positively on the length and quality of survival in patients with malignant gliomas. Surgery is necessary to establish the diagnosis and concurrently relieve mass effect on adjacent structures. Aggressive resection also is the fastest method to reduce the total tumor burden, making the residual tumor more amenable to further ther-

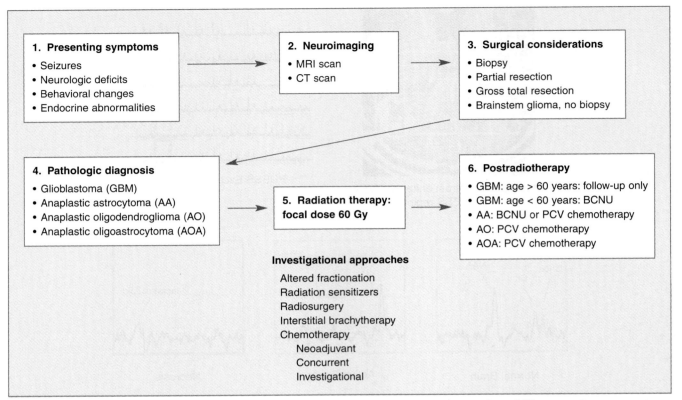

Figure 14–6. Management algorithm for the adult patient presenting with symptoms of a malignant glioma. MRI = magnetic resonance imaging; CT = computed tomography; BCNU = carmustine; PCV = procarbazine, CCNU (lomustine), and vincristine.

apies. Other benefits include better tissue sampling for histopathologic diagnosis and reduced dependence on steroids. Diffuse intrinsic lesions within the pons and medulla are the exception to the rule that surgery is needed to establish a diagnosis and reduce tumor burden. These lesions are so characteristic by radiologic imaging, with a uniform treatment outcome, that they usually are treated based on the radiographic diagnosis alone because of the significant risk of morbidity with surgery or biopsy.

The controversy surrounding extent of resection and outcome arises due to the mixed results from studies published over the past several years and design limitations of several studies that have demonstrated a benefit with aggressive resection. An example of one such study was published in 1993. The authors retrospectively compared resection versus biopsy in 152 patients with GBM at a single institution.[7] The analysis was adjusted for age and performance status. Patients undergoing resection followed by radiation survived longer than patients who received biopsy alone followed by radiation (median survival time, 50.6 wk and 33 wk, respectively). Other studies have demonstrated no benefit.[8] Many studies have been limited due to retrospective analysis or lack of control for independent prognostic factors that could bias outcomes. However, in terms of patient outcome, the weight of the evidence supports gross total resection's superiority to partial resection, and partial resection's superiority to biopsy.

Fortunately, two new surgical techniques have enabled neurosurgeons to perform aggressive resections while minimizing morbidity. One is an image-guided computer-assisted technique that allows real-time intraoperative guidance. The second is intraoperative cortical mapping. Cortical mapping localizes areas of eloquent cortex and subcortical white matter, making larger surgical extirpations possible without sacrificing safety. Image-guided (or surgical navigation systems) techniques link image data to the intended surgical region. There are several technologies that allow this, and each has advantages and disadvantages. The principal benefits of image guidance, as it relates to planning and operating on intracranial gliomas, are the abilities (1) to appropriately locate a minimal access craniotomy, (2) to define an optimal trajectory to the lesion with respect to functionally eloquent and vascular structures, and (3) to guide and gauge the extent of resection during surgery.[9]

Neurophysiologic techniques such as cortical mapping are adjuncts for safe resection in eloquent brain areas. Other techniques are somatosensory-evoked potentials, direct cortical stimulation, and awake-craniotomy. Methods such as these previously have been used in epilepsy surgery, and their adaptation in malignant glioma surgery has led to the ability to perform larger resections with an increased margin of safety when operating near eloquent cortex.[10]

Whereas image-guided systems and cortical mapping certainly allow more aggressive resections of brain tumors and minimize morbidity, it is important to keep in mind that due to the infiltrative nature of gliomas, tumor cells will extend beyond the areas seen on MRI. Therefore, even the most radical resection of a malignant glioma is not curative. As such, the optimal surgical goal is the most extensive resection possible that leaves the patient no worse off functionally. Figure 14–7 shows a series of MR images of a patient with a large GBM in the left frontal lobe prior to resection (Figure 14–7A) and following surgery (Figures 14–7B and 14–7C). This patient has less tumor burden and has been relieved of significant mass effect with improved neurologic function. From a prognostic standpoint, this patient typically would survive longer than a similar patient who had undergone only a small biopsy.

Patients with recurrent malignant gliomas should be evaluated for surgery in the same manner as newly diagnosed patients. Many patients with primary brain tumors can benefit from reoperation and enjoy a good functional status for months with GBM and years with AA. In a study published in 1998, 301 patients with GBM were assessed for survival and functional status after second resection.[11] This study detected a significant survival advantage in patients who underwent reoperation at the time of GBM recurrence over those who did not (median survival, 36 wk and 23 wk, respectively). Repeat resection also offers the opportunity to reduce mass effect and re-establish a pathologic diagnosis. Selection of patients for reoperation should be limited to those who have good preoperative KPS scores (> 60) and have additional treatment options available. Figure 14–8 is an algorithm depicting typical treatment of recurrent malignant glioma.

In summary, evidence supports aggressive resections as being beneficial to patients with high-grade gliomas at initial diagnosis and recurrence; the availability of intraoperative imaging and cortical mapping techniques has made it possible to do larger surgical resections without forgoing safety.

Radiotherapy

Conventional postoperative radiation generally follows surgery and has proven to be highly beneficial in the survival of patients with malignant gliomas. Radiation is given in most cases using three-dimensional treatment planning. This is done to limit exposure to the surrounding normal brain. Whole brain radiation is not used. The typical pattern of relapse is within 2 cm of the primary tumor site in 80 percent of cases, regardless of the extent of radiation.[12] Therefore, focal brain radiation is recommended to achieve local control and reduce toxicity. Radiation is usually targeted to the volume of the enhancing lesion seen on the MRI or CT scan with an additional 2- to 3-cm rim beyond that edge. Radiotherapy for gliomas is most commonly done with x-rays. The optimal dose of radiation for patients with high-grade gliomas is 60 Gy, and this is usually delivered in daily fractions of 180 to 200 cGy for approximately 6 weeks. Other fractionation schemes have been evaluated in the past and also are currently being tested in clinical trials. To date, none have demonstrated a survival benefit over that seen with single-dose fractions.

Resistance to irradiation and normal tissue tolerance limits the response of tumors to this modality. Doses above 60 Gy have an increased risk of severe radiation injury including necrosis to normal brain. Thus the dose is limited by this fact. In addition, several mechanisms of cellular resistance are known, including that of hypoxia. Chemical modifiers or radiation sensitizers have been used in an attempt to increase the therapeutic ratio of radiation therapy, but none has yet demonstrated any efficacy.[13]

Brachytherapy

Several methods of radiotherapy have been developed in the hope of increasing local disease control. The interest in focal therapy is fueled by the knowledge that the primary pattern of treatment failure is recurrence in or near the original tumor site in 80 to 90 percent of cases. Interstitial brachytherapy is one method used to increase the focal dose of radiation to the tumor. Brachytherapy has been performed using temporary high-activity sources and, more recently, with permanent low-activity iodine-125 sources. With temporary high-activity sources, stereotactic procedures are used to place the radiation sources precisely in the tumor bed at the time of surgical resection. The low- and high-activity seeds are used

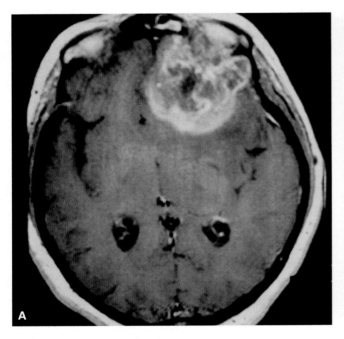
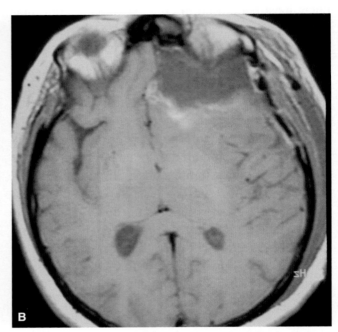
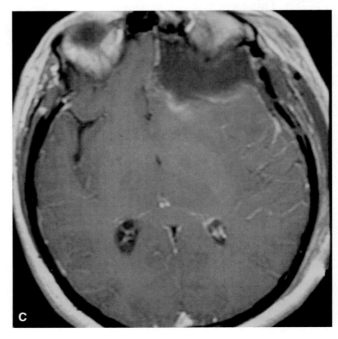

Figure 14–7. Axial T1-weighted MRI scan. *A*, Preoperative, left-frontal GBM; *B*, postoperative, noncontrast scan; *C*, postoperative, postcontrast scan.

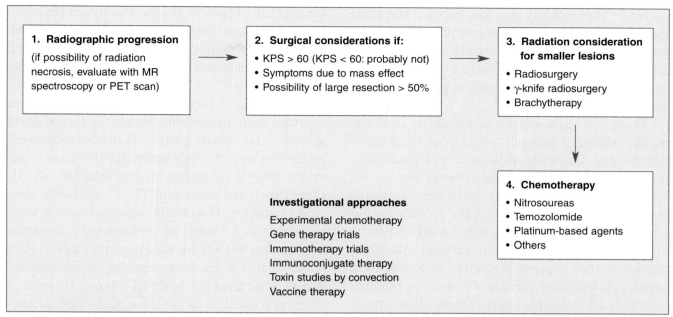

Figure 14–8. Management algorithm for patients with recurrent malignant gliomas. MR = magnetic resonance; PET = positron emission tomography; KPS = Karnofsky Performance Scale.

to deliver a total focal dose of additional radiation to 210 Gy and 50 Gy, respectively. Published phase II reports of temporary high-activity iodine-125 sources used as a "boost" after conventional radiation for stable disease and at tumor recurrence have reported encouraging results.[14–16] The median overall survival demonstrated in some studies was 19 months when brachytherapy was used as a boost after conventional radiation and approximately 13 months when used at tumor progression or recurrence. However, a more recent study reports less encouraging results. This trial randomized 140 patients with malignant astrocytomas to treatment with interstitial brachytherapy prior to conventional radiation. The control arm was treated with conventional radiation alone. No statistically significant improvement in survival for the patients treated with brachytherapy was noted (median survival, 13.8 mo vs 13.2 mo).[17] Because randomization and brachytherapy occurred prior to conventional irradiation, there may be selection factors that make it difficult to compare these results directly to studies using brachytherapy following irradiation. More work is needed to clarify the role of temporary implants in patients with newly diagnosed disease. Studies are ongoing to evaluate the role of permanent brachytherapy in both newly diagnosed and recurrent tumors. To date no prospective randomized trials have been done using brachytherapy at recurrence.

Stereotactic Radiosurgery

Another method used to deliver higher doses of radiation to focal areas is stereotactic radiosurgery. This technique delivers a large single fraction of radiation to a small tumor volume. The process typically involves placement on patients of a stereotactic frame that is used to direct multiple-source beams of radiation to the tumor target. There are several methods available, including linear accelerator-based radiosurgery, Gamma-Knife radiosurgery, and with heavy charged particle beams such as proton-beam radiosurgery. It appears that these techniques are comparable in their dose delivery and treatment outcome.

Like brachytherapy, radiosurgery has been used to treat patients with malignant gliomas after conventional radiation as a boost and at tumor recurrence. Single-institution studies suggest a survival benefit in both settings.[18] Typically, median survivals have been approximately 19 months when radiosurgery is used as a boost and 10 months when radiosurgery is used at recurrence. One retrospective, nonrandomized study compared radiosurgery and brachytherapy in the recurrent setting and found both to be equally efficacious.[19] Radiosurgery is a less invasive procedure and, as such, offers advantages over placement of permanent brachytherapy seeds, which requires a craniotomy. Some oncologists therefore advocate radiosurgery in place of brachytherapy in patients who are amenable to both therapies.[19]

There is a great degree of selectivity in determining whether a patient is eligible for focal radiation therapy. Generally, patients with a good functional status and small tumor volumes that do not involve critical areas of the brain are considered good candidates. The mere fact that patients are eligible for radiosurgery or brachytherapy implies a higher likelihood of better survival outcomes because of their superior prognostic factors as compared with ineligible patients. Prospective randomized trials are needed to confirm these observations. One phase III trial is ongoing in which patients with newly diagnosed GBMs are randomized to receive radiosurgery or not, before conventional radiation. Hopefully, this study will confirm the survival advantage radiosurgery has demonstrated in the nonrandomized single-arm studies.

Chemotherapy

At Initial Diagnosis

The role and benefit of chemotherapy in the treatment of patients with malignant gliomas are not as clearly defined as they are with surgery and radiation. The most commonly used agents are the nitrosoureas given as single agents or in combination with other drugs such as procarbazine and vincristine. The recommendations for these agents were based on studies conducted in the 1960s and early 1970s. A more recent meta-analysis of the larger studies in newly diagnosed malignant glioma patients demonstrated a proportionate increase in survival of patients treated with radiation and chemotherapy compared to those receiving only radiation.[20] However, analysis of the results with respect to histology demonstrated that only a subpopulation of patients with either AA or GBM had any benefit with chemotherapy. These were patients of good performance status, young age, and minimal residual disease after surgery. So the question remains whether chemotherapy is beneficial to the majority of patients, and similar studies suggest it may be better to avoid treating elderly patients with GBM with adjuvant chemotherapy due to the small likelihood of any survival benefit and the higher risk of drug toxicity.

Combination chemotherapy often is used as adjuvant chemotherapy for patients with malignant glioma. One small phase III trial randomized patients to receive single-agent BCNU (carmustine) or the drug combination of procarbazine, CCNU (lomustine), and vincristine (PCV) following standard irradiation. The results suggested that the combination was superior for patients with anaplastic astrocytoma but not for patients with GBM.[21] As a result of this study, some oncologists recommend that PCV be used for grade III tumors. However, a recent retrospective analysis was performed to determine whether any survival differences existed when a larger patient sample was available for comparison. In this analysis comparing patients with AA treated with either BCNU or PCV, no survival advantage for the three-drug regimen was found. These data would suggest that either BCNU or PCV might be appropriate as adjuvant chemotherapy in this patient population.[22] In the United States, patients with GBM are treated with surgery and irradiation, and some patients (typically younger and with good performance status) are treated with adjuvant BCNU chemotherapy. Patients with anaplastic gliomas other than GBM are treated with surgery, irradiation, and adjuvant chemotherapy (either BCNU or the combination of PCV).

For Recurrent Disease

Chemotherapy trials conducted in the setting of recurrent disease have demonstrated minimal and inconsistent effects. The most common agents used at recurrence are still the nitrosoureas, either BCNU or PCV. The next line of therapy usually involves platinum-based agents such as carboplatin or cisplatin. Other drugs used are high-dose tamoxifen, procarbazine, *cis*-retinoic acid, etoposide, or combinations of the above agents[23] (Table 14–1). Unfortunately, the reported response rates for chemotherapy used for patients with recurrent tumor is low and varies between 10 and 40 percent, with a progression-free interval of only several months. Newer alkylating agents and topoisomerase inhibitors also are being used with some success in the treatment of recurrent high-grade gliomas. Included in those groups are temozolomide and irinotecan. Fortunately, understanding some of the pathways of malignant transformation has made it possible to rationally test new therapies. Agents that inhibit signal-transduction pathways, cellular invasion, and new blood vessel formation (angiogenesis) are now being tested in clinical trials (Table 14–2). A brief discussion of these new agents is given in the next section.

Signal-Transduction Inhibitors

In some cases, tumor cells have amplification and/or overexpression of genes encoding for proteins that stimulate cell growth. This is known to be true for a family of growth factors and their protein-tyrosine kinase receptors that include platelet-derived growth factor (PDGF), vascular endothelial growth factor (VEGF), and epidermal growth factor receptor (EGFR). These proteins are overexpressed in a portion of malignant gliomas.[24,25] Several reports have noted constitutively active forms of these receptors and in some instances coexpression of the ligand and receptor. This suggests a possibility of autocrine and paracrine mechanisms for uncontrolled growth. In light of this finding, drugs that act to inhibit the signal pathways of these receptors are being evaluated.

Matrix-Metalloproteinase Inhibitors

Matrix metalloproteinases (MMPs) are a family of enzymes responsible for normal turnover and remodeling of the extracellular matrix; they are required for tumor angiogenesis and invasion. Elevated levels of MMPs are seen during tumor growth, and this observation has led to the development of MMP inhibitors as one strategy for treating patients with cancer.[26]

Angiogenesis Inhibitors

Several drugs are being studied because of their ability to inhibit angiogenesis. This interest has

Table 14–1. CHEMOTHERAPY AGENTS USED TO TREAT MALIGNANT GLIOMAS

Alkylating agents
  Nitrosoureas
    BCNU (carmustine)
    CCNU (lomustine)
  Nonclassic alkylating agents
    Procarbazine
    Temozolomide

Platinum analogues
  Carboplatin
  Cisplatin

Topoisomerase II inhibitors
  Etoposide (VP-16)

Topoisomerase I inhibitors
  Camptothecin analogues
    Irinotecan (CPT-11)
    Topotecan

Antimicrotubule agents
  Vinca alkaloids
    Vincristine
  Taxanes
    Paclitaxel

Protein kinase C inhibitor
  High-dose tamoxifen

Angiogenesis inhibitor
  Thalidomide

Table 14–2. CHEMOTHERAPY AGENTS CURRENTLY UNDER INVESTIGATION

Differentiation-related mechanisms
  Sodium phenylacetate
  Sodium phenylbutyrate
  Retinoids
    Cis-retinoic acid
    Fenretinide
    All-*trans* retinoic acid

Signal-transduction inhibitors
  Bryostatin
  SU-101
  UCN-01
  Hypericin
  Suramin

Matrix-metalloproteinase inhibitors
  Marimastat
  Bay 12-9566
  Ag 3340

Angiogenesis inhibitors
  TNP-470
  Angiostatin
  Endostatin
  Pentosan polysulfate
  Platelet factor 4
  SU-5416

sprung from the knowledge that tumors must develop new vasculature to grow and maintain vitality. Angiogenesis, which is normally a tightly regulated function, is upregulated in tumors. There are several incompletely understood mechanisms by which this may occur. One such mechanism may be overexpression of VEGF, which promotes neovascularization.[23] Thalidomide, a drug that inhibits angiogenesis, is thought to act by its negative effect on VEGF and is being evaluated for therapy. Many of the other drugs being evaluated as angiogenesis inhibitors have been isolated from the normal regulatory pathways (eg, angiostatin). Angiogenesis inhibition is an area of intense investigation.

Alternative Drug Delivery

Alternative delivery systems also are being investigated. Biodegradable polymer wafers that are impregnated with BCNU may be placed directly into the tumor bed at the time of surgery. Trials have demonstrated a slight survival benefit with this therapy at recurrence.[27] Agents that modify the blood-brain barrier, including bradykinin analogs, are being investigated as a way to increase drug delivery.

Chemosensitivity and Anaplastic Oligodendrogliomas

We now know that not all patients respond equally to chemotherapy. For instance, some patients with AO have shown exceptional chemosensitivity and frequently will show a complete response following chemotherapy using PCV. Molecular alterations seen in some AOs have been linked to chemotherapy response and survival. The allelic loss of chromosomes 1p and 19q is a molecular signature of these tumors and occurs in 50 to 70 percent of AOs. A link has been shown between this molecular marker and response to chemotherapy. In a recent study, 100 percent of the patients with either a loss of 1p or both 1p and 19q had an objective response to chemotherapy (24 of 24 and 22 of 22, respectively). In contrast, only 25 percent and 31 percent of the respective patients who retained these alleles had a response. The 5-year survival rate for patients with loss of heterozygosity at both 1p and 19q was 95 percent as opposed to a 25 percent 5-year survival rate in patients with AOs who retained these alleles.[28] The results of this study still must be confirmed by a larger series, but these findings do suggest that molecular markers may be used to identify chemosensitive tumors and assist in guiding treatment decisions.

In summary, chemotherapy will have a continued role in the treatment of patients with newly diagnosed and recurrent malignant gliomas, and, hopefully, an increasing knowledge of the molecular pathways involved in malignant transformation will enable researchers to develop more effective drug therapies.

TERMINAL CARE

Even with the advances made over the past several years, the majority of patients with malignant gliomas will have tumor recurrences and die from their disease. When further treatment no longer is given either because of patient and family wishes or because the medical risk of more therapy outweighs any potential benefit, efforts should be directed toward comfort care and avoiding prolonged suffering. Most patients and families at some point will want to know what the final months will be like. It is unlikely that the patient will be in any significant discomfort. If present, simple solutions exist that can help, including pain medications and steroids. Most patients will die after they become increasingly lethargic and finally lapse into coma. Patients and their families will need continued support from the treating physicians along with assistance in obtaining home health services and hospice care. Hospice care includes a team of physicians, nurses, and other support staff who can assist with "end-of-life" concerns. Most patients with brain tumors will die at home.

MOLECULAR PATHOGENESIS OF MALIGNANT GLIOMAS AND FUTURE DIRECTIONS

Great strides have been made over the past several years in understanding the cellular and molecular mechanisms involved in malignant transformation, and this currently is one of the most promising areas in the field of oncology. Although a full discussion is beyond the scope of this chapter, a few points will be made that demonstrate how understanding the molecular pathways involved in the evolution of high-grade gliomas has led to the development of new treatment strategies.

A tumor-suppressor gene frequently implicated in the pathogenesis of astrocytomas is p53. The p53 protein has been found to influence multiple cellular functions including progression through the cell cycle, deoxyribonucleic acid (DNA) repair after damage, genomic stability, and the tendency for cells to undergo apoptosis after treatment.[24] The p53 protein acts by modifying the transcription of multiple genes involved in these events, including p21, whose protein inhibits cell-cycle progression, and the BAX gene, which is involved in apoptosis.[29,30] Mutations of p53 have been reported in approximately 10 percent of primary GBMs (those that arise de novo without evidence of a low-grade precursor lesion) and 65 percent of secondary GBMs. Two points can be assumed from this: (1) there may be different genetic pathways that lead to the GBM phenotype, and (2) the p53 mutations may be an initiating event, at least in some tumors (those that arise from low-grade lesions). Several studies have demonstrated that introduction and overexpression of wild-type p53 in rodent and glioma cell lines result in growth arrest and induction of apoptosis in vitro and in vivo. Because of these laboratory observations, a rationale exists to test the hypothesis that p53 is an important factor in cell growth in patients with malignant glioma. A phase I clinical trial currently is ongoing in patients with recurrent malignant glioma. In this trial, a recombinant adenovirus vector is used to transduce the p53 gene into tumor cells of patients with recurrent tumors.

Other abnormalities of the cell-cycle regulatory pathway not necessarily associated with p53 have been demonstrated in malignant gliomas. One pathway that has been studied extensively involves the CDKN2 gene and its p16 protein product.[29,31] Other proteins involved in this regulatory system are cyclin-dependent kinases (CDK4), cyclins (cyclin D), and the retinoblastoma gene and protein (Rb). In the undisrupted pathway, the product of the CDKN2 gene (p16) binds to CDK4. This prevents its interaction with cyclin D. In turn, phosphorylation of Rb is inhibited, which prevents progression of the cell cycle from G1 to S. This last step is mediated by E2F, a transcription factor needed for cell-cycle progression. The most common alteration of this pathway seen in malignant gliomas is inactivation of the CDKN2 gene. This tumor-suppressor gene, located on chromosome 9p, is abnormal in approximately 33 percent of GBMs and 24 percent in AAs. However, loss of the ability to halt the cell cycle may result from altered expression of any of these genes, that is, loss of p16 expression, overexpression/amplification of CDKs, or loss of Rb function, and, in fact, all of these alterations have been associated to different degrees with malignant gliomas. It is believed that the loss of cell-cycle control may result in the introduction of mutations and improper reproduction of the genome (genomic instability) that has been implicated in the evolution of normal cells to cancer cells.

There have been encouraging preliminary results obtained with adenovirally mediated transfer of many of these genes in vitro and in animal models. This should propel the development of clinical trials based on the intratumoral transfer of these genes for treatment of malignant gliomas.

CONCLUSION

The principal management of malignant brain tumors remains surgery, radiation, and chemotherapy. The variations seen in these therapies, though not to be dismissed, have not significantly altered the survival of most patients with malignant brain tumors. What is encouraging is the heightened insight into the molecular basis of malignant transformation. The consequences will be the emergence of novel therapies and the use of molecular markers in tailoring treatment to specific genotypes. To give support to furthering these new developments, clinicians are urged to avoid the nihilistic attitude that is often an after-effect of caring for these patients and to allow for the possibility of enrollment into clinical trials when discussing treatment options with patients and their families.

REFERENCES

1. Greenlee RT, Hill-Harmon MB, Murray T, Thun M. Cancer statistics, 2001. CA Cancer J Clin 2001;57:15–36.
2. Kleihues P, Burger PC, Scheithauer BW. The new WHO classification of brain tumours. Brain Pathol 1993;3:255–68.

3. Daumas-Duport C, Scheithauer B, J OF, Kelly P. Grading of astrocytomas. A simple and reproducible method. Cancer 1988;62:2152–65.
4. Valk PE, Budinger TF, Levin VA, et al. PET of malignant cerebral tumors after interstitial brachytherapy. Demonstration of metabolic activity and correlation with clinical outcome. J Neurosurg 1988;69:830–8.
5. Taylor JS, Langston JW, Reddick WE, et al. Clinical value of proton magnetic resonance spectroscopy for differentiating recurrent or residual brain tumor from delayed cerebral necrosis. Int J Radiat Oncol Biol Phys 1996;36:1251–61.
6. Curran WJ Jr, Scott CB, Horton J, et al. Recursive partitioning analysis of prognostic factors in three Radiation Therapy Oncology Group malignant glioma trials [comments]. J Natl Cancer Inst 1993;85:704–10.
7. Devaux BC, JR OF, Kelly PJ. Resection, biopsy, and survival in malignant glial neoplasms. A retrospective study of clinical parameters, therapy, and outcome. J Neurosurg 1993;78:767–75.
8. Kowalczuk A, Macdonald RL, Amidei C, et al. Quantitative imaging study of extent of surgical resection and prognosis of malignant astrocytomas. Neurosurgery 1997;41:1028–38.
9. Barnett G. The role of image-guided technology in the surgical planning and resection of gliomas. J Neurooncol 1999; 42:247–58.
10. Matz P, Cobbs C, Berger M. Intraoperative cortical mapping as a guide to the surgical resection of gliomas. J Neurooncol 1999;42:233–45.
11. Barker FG II, Chang SM, Gutin PH, et al. Survival and functional status after resection of recurrent glioblastoma multiforme. Neurosurgery 1998;42:709–23.
12. Garden AS, Maor MH, Yung WK, et al. Outcome and patterns of failure following limited-volume irradiation for malignant astrocytomas. Radiother Oncol 1991;20:99–110.
13. Shafman TD, Loeffler JS. Novel radiation technologies for malignant gliomas. Curr Opin Oncol 1999;11:147–51.
14. Wen PY, Alexander E III, Black PM, et al. Long term results of stereotactic brachytherapy used in the initial treatment of patients with glioblastomas. Cancer 1994;73:3029–36.
15. Loeffler JS, Alexander E III, Wen PY, et al. Results of stereotactic brachytherapy used in the initial management of patients with glioblastoma. J Natl Cancer Inst 1990;82:1918–21.
16. McDermott MW, Sneed PK, Gutin PH. Interstitial brachytherapy for malignant brain tumors. Semin Surg Oncol 1998; 14:79–87.
17. Laperriere NJ, Leung PM, McKenzie S, et al. Randomized study of brachytherapy in the initial management of patients with malignant astrocytoma. Int J Radiat Oncol Biol Phys 1998;41:1005–11.
18. Shrieve DC, Alexander E III, Black PM, et al. Treatment of patients with primary glioblastoma multiforme with standard postoperative radiotherapy and radiosurgical boost: prognostic factors and long-term outcome. J Neurosurg 1999;90:72–7.
19. Shrieve DC, Alexander E III, Wen PY, et al. Comparison of stereotactic radiosurgery and brachytherapy in the treatment of recurrent glioblastoma multiforme. Neurosurgery 1995;36:275–84.
20. Fine HA, Dear KB, Loeffler JS, et al. Meta-analysis of radiation therapy with and without adjuvant chemotherapy for malignant gliomas in adults [comments]. Cancer 1993; 71:2585–97.
21. Levin V, Silver P, Hannigan J, et al. Superiority of post-radiotherapy adjuvant chemotherapy with CCNU, procarbazine and vincristine (PCV) over BCNU for anaplastic gliomas: NCOG 6G61 final report. Int J Radiat Oncol Biol Phys 1990;18:321–24.
22. Prados M, Scott C, Curran W, et al. PCV chemotherapy in anaplastic glioma: a retrospective review of Radiation Therapy Oncology Group (RTOG) protocols comparing survival with BCNU or PCV chemotherapy [abstract]. Neurooncology 1999;1:S47.
23. Burton E, Prados M. New chemotherapy options for the treatment of malignant gliomas. Curr Opin Oncol 1999;11: 157–61.
24. Cheng SY, Huang HJ, Nagane M, et al. Suppression of glioblastoma angiogenicity and tumorigenicity by inhibition of endogenous expression of vascular endothelial growth factor. Proc Natl Acad Sci U S A 1996;93:8502–7.
25. Rasheed BK, Wiltshire RN, Bigner SH, Bigner DD. Molecular pathogenesis of malignant gliomas. Curr Opin Oncol 1999;11:162–7.
26. Brown P. Matrix metalloproteinase inhibitors in the treatment of cancer. Med Oncol 1997;14:1–10.
27. Valtonen S, Timonen U, Toivanen P, et al. Interstitial chemotherapy with carmustine-loaded polymers for high-grade gliomas: a randomized double-blind study. Neurosurgery 1997;41:44–9.
28. Cairncross JG, Ueki K, Zlatescu MC, et al. Specific genetic predictors of chemotherapeutic response and survival in patients with anaplastic oligodendrogliomas. J Natl Cancer Inst 1998;90:1473–9.
29. Biernat W, Tohma Y, Yonekawa Y, et al. Alterations of cell cycle regulatory genes in primary (de novo) and secondary glioblastomas. Acta Neuropathol (Berl) 1997;94:303–9.
30. Nozaki M, Tada M, Kobayashi H, et al. Roles of the functional loss of p53 and other genes in astrocytoma tumorigenesis and progression. Neurooncology 1999;1:124–37.
31. Hill, JR, Kuriyama N, Kuriyama H, Israel MA. Molecular genetics of brain tumors. Arch Neurol 1999;56:439–41.

15

Management of Low-Grade Gliomas in Adults

EDWARD G. SHAW, MD

Low-grade gliomas are a pathologically and clinically diverse group of uncommon central nervous system (CNS) tumors that occur primarily in children and young adults. Prognosis is principally affected by age and pathologic type. Molecular genetic factors also may be prognostically significant. In general, more extensive surgical resection is associated with better prognosis. There is growing evidence that the timing of radiation, that is, whether it be early (postoperative) versus delayed (at the time of tumor progression), does not affect survival outcome. A definitive role for chemotherapy has yet to be defined.

EPIDEMIOLOGY AND ETIOLOGY

In 2001 in the United States, it is estimated that 17,200 CNS tumors will be diagnosed.[1] Of these, 15,000 will arise in the brain. Half of these would be gliomas, one-quarter of which would be low grade, resulting in approximately 1,900 new cases of low-grade gliomas per year.[2]

Etiologic factors for low-grade gliomas are largely unknown. The low-grade astrocytomas have been associated with von Recklinghausen's disease (type 1 neurofibromatosis) as well as type 2 neurofibromatosis.[3] Also, a direct association has been made between subependymal giant cell astrocytoma, an uncommon pathologic type of low-grade glioma, and tuberous sclerosis.[4]

PATHOLOGY

Grading Systems

The concept of dividing astrocytomas into separate grades associated with a distinct clinical prognosis dates back to the mid-1920s and early 1930s and the work of Bailey and Cushing, who recognized a subset of astrocytomas that had a more favorable outcome than glioblastoma.[5,6] There are four grading systems currently in use (Table 15–1).[7–12] All four of these grading systems share an assessment of the histologic features of nuclear abnormalities, mitoses, endothelial proliferation, and necrosis. At the present time, the four-tier grading scheme of the World Health Organization (WHO) is the most widely used and accepted.[7,12]

Classification

Historically, the low-grade gliomas have been thought of as a rather homogeneous group of brain neoplasms associated with a benign or favorable natural history. In fact, they are a diverse group of tumors found throughout the CNS whose outcome depends on a number of anatomic, pathologic, and treatment factors. Table 15–2 summarizes the current WHO classification of primary CNS tumors as it applies to the low-grade gliomas.[7,12] Astrocytic tumors can be classified broadly into three groups. The WHO grade II tumors, which are the most common, are the diffusely infiltrative low-grade astrocytomas. They include the fibrillary, protoplasmic, and gemistocytic types and represent 70 percent of low-grade cerebral astrocytomas.[13] Diffuse astrocytomas are usually poorly circumscribed and are capable of undergoing anaplastic transformation with an incidence as high as 79 percent.[14] The WHO grade I tumors are the pilocytic astrocytomas and comprise nearly all of the remainder of the cerebral astrocytomas. They tend to be better circumscribed and rarely transform to a more malignant phenotype.[15] Although pilocytic astrocy-

Grading Systems*	Grade I	Grade II	Grade III	Grade IV
Kernohan[8]	Cells: No anaplasia Cellularity: Mild Mitoses: None Vessels: Minimal endothelial or adventitial proliferation Transition zone to normal brain: Broad	Cells: Most appear normal, anaplasia in small numbers Cellularity: Mild Mitoses: None Vessels: As in grade I Transition zone: Less broad	Cells: Anaplasia in half of cells Cellularity: Increased Mitoses: Present Vessels: More frequent endothelial and adventitial proliferation Necrosis: Frequent, regional Transition zone: Narrowed	Cell: Extensive anaplasia, few "normal" appearing Cellularity: Marked Mitoses: Numerous Vessels: Marked proliferation Necrosis: Extensive Transitional zone: May be sharply demarcated
WHO[12]	Pilocytic astrocytoma	Astrocytoma: Tumor composed of astrocytes (fibrillary, protoplasmic, gemistocytic, giant cell, and combinations thereof); atypia evident, but no mitoses	Anaplastic astrocytoma: Astrocytoma showing mitotic activity; such tumors are not difficult to distinguish from glioblastoma	Glioblastoma: Anaplastic tumor, usually astrocytic, with high cellularity, endothelial proliferation, or necrosis with pseudo-palisading
St. Anne-Mayo[10]	None of the following four criteria: Nuclear abnormalities, mitoses endothelial proliferation, necrosis	One criterion	Two criteria	Three or four criteria
Ringertz[11]†	Astrocytoma: Tumor showing infiltrative growth pattern and mild to moderate hypercellularity; cytologic features resembling normal astrocytes with only mild nuclear abnormalities		Anaplastic astrocytoma: Cellular infiltrative astrocytomic tumor containing astrocytes with moderate pleomorphism; mitoses and moderate vascular proliferation may be seen but necrosis is absent	Glioblastoma multiforme: Markedly pleomorphic astrocytomic tumor with high cellularity and necrosis; may show limited infiltration

*The superscript references are the original references describing these grading systems; see also Kleihues et al[7] and Burger et al.[9]
†The Ringertz system of grading involves three grades only: astrocytoma is comparable to grades I and II in the other grading systems.

tomas occur more commonly in the cerebellum of children (juvenile pilocytic astrocytoma),[16] several series have described their behavior in the cerebral hemispheres.[17,18] Remaining are the uncommon low-grade glioma variants, including pleomorphic xanthoastrocytomas, subependymal giant cell astrocytomas, subependymomas, and several others, which will be discussed later in the chapter.

BIOLOGIC CHARACTERISTICS

In recent years, our understanding of the biology of low-grade astrocytomas has increased. This is due to studies of deoxyribonucleic acid (DNA) content, tumor proliferation, and both cytogenetics and molecular genetics.

Studies of Ploidy and Proliferation

In four separate series reporting the DNA content of 155 low-grade gliomas, the ratio of diploid to aneuploid tumors was approximately 2:1.[19-22] No consistent association between ploidy and survival has been noted in these series.

The assessment of tumor proliferation may offer greater insight into the malignant potential of the low-grade gliomas. Hoshino and colleagues observed a correlation between 5-bromodeoxyuridine (BUdR) labeling index and survival in 47 patients with low-grade astrocytomas. Of the 29 who had a labeling index of less than 1 percent, 26 remained alive without evidence of disease recurrence at the time of analysis, compared with only 9 of 18 patients who had a labeling index of 1 percent or more.[23] Coons and colleagues measured proliferation using a flow cytometric assessment of the percentage of cells in S phase. The median S phase fraction for a group of 27 low-grade astrocytomas was 4.3 percent. Survival was correlated significantly with the percent S phase fraction in multivariate analysis. Median survival was 49, 24, and 13 months, with S phase fractions of 0 to 2.9 percent, 3.0 to 5.9 percent, and 6.0 percent or more, respectively.[21]

Franzini and colleagues reviewed 70 patients with low-grade astrocytomas of the basal ganglia and thalamus, all of whom had a tritiated-thymidine labeling index performed on their biopsy specimens. The mean labeling index was 4.8 percent (range, 0.3 to 17.5%). Whereas the 3-year survival rate for the entire group was 57 percent, it was 0 percent when the labeling index was more than 5 percent, compared to 80 percent when the labeling index was less than 5 percent. The subset of patients who had a labeling index of less than 5 percent and who were less than 40 years old had a 100 percent 3-year survival rate.[24]

Studies of Molecular Genetics

The most common molecular genetic alteration in low-grade gliomas, which is present in 30 to 45 percent of low-grade astrocytomas, occurs on the p arm of chromosome 17, which is the location of the tumor-suppressor gene TP53. Its protein, p53, has multiple functions involved in the regulation of cell growth, apoptosis, transcription, and malignant transformation.[25]

Lang and colleagues detected TP53 mutations in 3 of 15 (20%) low-grade astrocytomas and mutant p53 protein accumulation in 5 of 8 (63%). Although they could not explain the aberrant expression of p53 protein in the absence of a TP53 gene mutation, they postulated that loss of p53 function in low-grade astrocytomas could be a predisposing factor for the accumulation of genetic damage leading to the progression of low-grade astrocytoma to glioblastoma.[26]

Chozick and colleagues theorized that the accumulation of mutant p53 protein, or the inactivation of wild-type p53 protein, might be a predictor of poor survival in patients with astrocytomas. They observed accumulation of abnormal p53 protein in 29 percent of 81 patients with grade II astrocytomas; the 4-year survival rate of these patients was 25 percent, compared with 87 percent for those who did not accumulate abnormal p53 protein. Other than age, p53 status was the most significant prognostic factor predictive of survival in multivariate analysis.[27] Ritland and colleagues observed allelic loss for chromosome 19 loci in 2 of 18 (11%) grade I, II, and III astrocytomas as compared with 21 of 54 (39%) grade IV astrocytomas. In most of these instances, the deletion was in the p arm of chromosome 19. These authors postulated that a tumor-suppressor gene important in the malignant transformation of low-grade to high-grade astrocytomas may reside on chromosome 19p.[28]

Growth factor expression may be prognostic for survival in low-grade astrocytomas. Abdulrauf and colleagues found a significant correlation in both uni- and multivariate analyses between vascular endothelial growth factor (VEGF) expression and survival in a series of 74 adults with supratentorial cerebral low-grade diffuse astrocytomas. Median survival time was 11.2 years in patients whose tumors expressed VEGF compared to 5.3 years in those whose tumors did not. Other growth factors, such as basic fibroblastic growth factor and epidermal growth factor, did not impact survival.[29]

Table 15–2. LOW-GRADE GLIOMAS* INCLUDED IN THE WHO CLASSIFICATION OF GLIOMAS

Type	WHO Grade
Astrocytic tumors	
Astrocytomas	II
Fibrillary	
Gemistocytic	
Protoplasmic	
Pilocytic astrocytomas	I
Pleomorphic xanthoastrocytomas	II
Subependymal giant cell astrocytomas	I
Subependymomas	I
Oligodendroglial tumors	
Oligodendrogliomas	II
Mixed glial tumors	
Mixed oligoastrocytomas	II
Neuronal and mixed glial-neuronal tumors	
Gangliogliomas	II
Central neurocytomas	II
Dysembryoplastic neuroepithelial tumors	I

*Exclusive of ependymal neoplasms.
Adapted from Kleihues et al[7] and Zulch.[12]

Immunohistochemical techniques also have been used to study the ontogeny of glial cells and have identified two lineages of astrocytes derived from distinct progenitor cells. Type II or fibrillary astrocytes are found in white matter and are derived from the O2A cell, a bipotential precursor that can differentiate toward astrocytes or oligodendrocytes. Type I or protoplasmic astrocytes reside in the cortex and are derived from a separate precursor cell. The type I and type II astrocytes express unique antigens that permit their characterization. Low-grade astrocytomas arising from the type I astrocyte lineage are associated with a more indolent clinical course, whereas those arising from the type II astrocyte lineage behave more aggressively.[30,31]

CLINICAL MANIFESTATIONS AND PATIENT EVALUATION

In this section, the clinical presentation and imaging of supratentorial low-grade gliomas will be reviewed based on information from collected series in the literature as recently reviewed by Shaw and colleagues.[32]

Clinical Presentation

The mean age at presentation is 37 years, with a mean age range of 10 to 66 years. Cases have been reported in patients as young as 7 months of age and as old as 78 years. Low-grade astrocytomas are more common in men than in women by a ratio of 1.4:1.

The most common symptom of a low-grade astrocytoma is seizure, which occurs in two-thirds of patients. Focal seizures are more common than generalized ones. Headache and weakness occur in approximately one-third of patients. Other symptoms are less common. The median duration from onset of symptoms to diagnosis is 6 to 17 months, with a range of 1 day to 17 years. The neurologic signs associated with low-grade astrocytomas have not been as thoroughly reported in the literature as have neurologic symptoms. About half of affected patients have a normal neurologic examination. The frequency of signs at presentation is as follows: sensory or motor deficit, 42 percent; altered mental status, 23 percent; papilledema, 22 percent; and aphasia, dysphasia, or decreased memory in 20 percent. Other signs are less common.[32]

The most powerful predictor of survival in patients with low-grade glioma is age. Children with low-grade astrocytoma have average 5- and 10-year survival rates of approximately 90 percent and 85 percent, respectively.[33–38] Adults who are under 40 years of age have a better survival than patients 40 years of age and older.[39–43] Piepmeier reported a mean survival time of 8.5 years in adults under 40 years versus 4.9 years for those 40 years of age and older.[42] In a more recent series, Leighton and colleagues observed a median survival time of 10.7 years compared to 8.1 years, for adults ≤ 40 versus > 40 years old, respectively.[43] Sex also appears to correlate with outcome, with females having a better survival rate than males.[33,44,45]

Of all the neurologic symptoms and signs associated with low-grade astrocytoma, seizures, particularly when preceding the diagnosis by 6 months or more and in the absence of other neurologic symptoms, are associated with a better prognosis.[33,39,46] In one series, the 5-year survival rate was 47 percent in patients presenting with seizures, 33 percent in those with headaches, 20 percent in those with altered mental status, and 0 percent when stupor was the presenting symptom.[47] In another series, the 5-year survival rate was 64 percent in low-grade glioma patients who had seizures, compared to 14 percent without.[48] Patients who present with a history of chronic epilepsy due to an underlying cerebral neoplasm frequently are found to have a low-grade astrocytoma. These patients are usually children or young adults whose seizure disorder and underlying tumor are often cured by complete resection.[49,50]

Imaging Characteristics

The computed tomographic (CT) and magnetic resonance imaging (MRI) characteristics of supratentorial low-grade astrocytomas have been described in multiple series in the literature as recently summarized.[32] The typical low-grade astrocytoma is lobar in location, involves the frontal or temporal lobes, measures greater than 5 cm in diameter, and is nonenhancing. Because of the infiltrative nature of low-grade astrocytomas, the CT appearance of a typical nonenhancing tumor is a poorly defined area of low attenuation (Figure 15–1A), whereas the T2-weighted MRI scan shows a more readily definable region of increased signal (Figure 15–1B), providing anatomic detail that is useful in defining the extent of the tumor and for both surgical and radiation therapy treatment planning.

Daumas-Duport and colleagues and Kelly and colleagues have performed imaging-histologic correlations of both CT and MRI scans in patients with astrocytic neoplasms of the brain undergoing stereotactic biopsies.[51,52] Three types of tumors can be identified (Figure 15–2), which correlate with the three morphologies of low-grade gliomas. The CT/MRI scan appearance of a type I tumor is that of a well-circumscribed area of contrast enhancement in the absence of surrounding low-attenuation change or edema (increased T2 signal). Pilocytic astrocytomas typically have this appearance (Figures 15–3A and 15–3B). The CT/MRI scan appearance of a type II tumor is that of a poorly defined area of low attenuation (increased T2 signal) that contains a focal area of contrast enhancement (Figures 15–4A and 15–4B). The type II tumors would be the 34 percent subset of low-grade astrocytomas that enhance. The CT/MRI scan appearance of a type III tumor, which characterizes two-thirds of low-grade gliomas, is that of a poorly defined area of low attenuation (increased T2 signal), as shown in Figures 15–1A and 15–1B.

Stereotactic biopsy–histologic correlations have helped to define the underlying pathologic makeup of type I, II, and III tumors. Type I tumors are comprised of solid tumor tissue embedded in surrounding normal brain parenchyma. The contrast-enhanced portion of type II tumors also contains solid tumor tissue, whereas the surrounding low-attenuation area on a CT scan or the area of increased signal on a T2-weighted MRI contains intact brain parenchyma infiltrated by tumor cells. Type III tumors are characterized by intact parenchyma infiltrated by tumor cells in the absence of any focal areas of solid tumor tissue. Generally, the MRI scan will define a larger area of increased signal on T2-weighted images for both type II and III tumors than will the CT scan. Also, microscopic

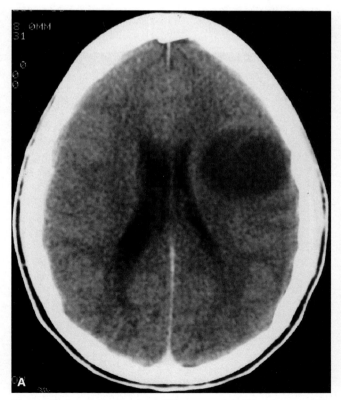
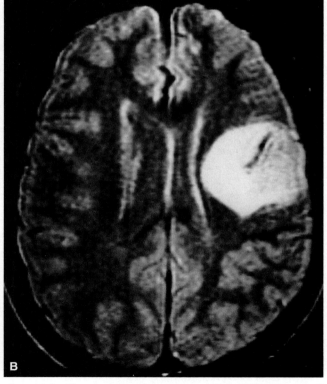

Figure 15–1. *A*, Postcontrast CT scan and, *B*, T1-weighted MRI scan of an adult with a nonenhancing posterior left frontal WHO grade II astrocytoma.

Spatial configuration	Solid tumor tissue	Isolated tumor cells*
Type I ●	+	0
Type II ✤	+	+
Type III ✤	0	+

Figure 15–2. Morphology of low-grade gliomas based on CT-histologic correlates (see text for explanation). *Within intact parenchyma. (Adapted from Daumas-Duport et al[51] and Kelly et al.[52])

tumor cells may extend up to several centimeters beyond the MRI-defined limits of the abnormalities seen in type II and III tumors.[52]

Understanding these imaging-based anatomic-pathologic relationships is important for both the neurosurgeon and radiation oncologist. Removal of the nonenhancing portion of a type II or III tumor in a patient whose tumor is located in a functionally intact area of brain may lead to significant neurologic deficits, whereas removal of the enhancing portion of a type I tumor even in deep locations such as the thalamus or basal ganglia should not result in deficits.[53] For the radiation oncologist treating a type II or III tumor, the initial treatment volume should include the MRI-based tumor extent, as defined by the T2-weighted MR images, with several centimeters of surrounding normal brain tissue as "margin," whereas a type I tumor could be irradiated with a minimal margin (≤ 1 cm) or conceivably by focal treatments such as stereotactic radiosurgery or brachytherapy.

The radiographic features of low-grade gliomas have been correlated with prognosis in a number of retrospective series. Although the presence of contrast enhancement on a CT scan in nonpilocytic low-grade gliomas would seemingly be associated with worse prognosis because of presumed higher-grade elements or malignant transformation, the data from multiple series are mixed, in that some associate contrast enhancement with a worse outcome,[39,42,45,47,54] whereas others have found no difference in survival rates.[55–58]

MANAGEMENT OPTIONS

Observation

The decision to observe a low-grade glioma following a radiographic or histologic diagnosis has been justified in the literature for several reasons, including the relatively favorable natural history of the dis-

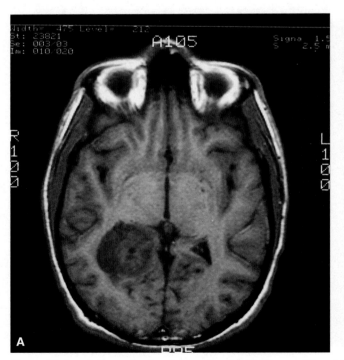 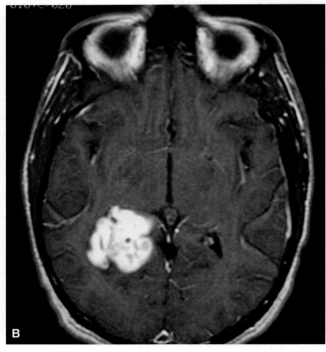

Figure 15–3. *A,* Precontrast and, *B,* postcontrast MRI scan (T1-weighted images) of an adult with a WHO grade I (pilocytic) astrocytoma of the right parietal lobe.

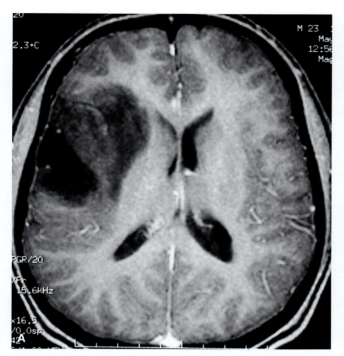 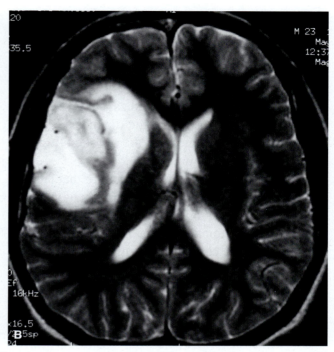

Figure 15–4. A, Postgadolinium T1-weighted and, B, T2-weighted MR images of a young adult with a WHO grade II astrocytoma of the right posterior frontal lobe.

ease (compared to malignant glioma), lack of proven benefit for early invasive interventions such as surgical resection or radiation therapy, and the potential morbidities of these treatments.[59–64]

Despite the favorable survival observed in certain subsets of low-grade glioma patients, the natural history of patients with any pathologic types of supratentorial low-grade gliomas, including the pilocytic astrocytomas (WHO grade I), diffuse astrocytomas, oligoastrocytomas, and oligodendrogliomas (WHO grade II), is significantly worse than that of an age- and sex-matched control population, for which the expected survival rate is greater than 95 percent (Table 15–3).[12,63] Based on this observation, it has been argued that all such patients should undergo aggressive surgical resection followed by radiation therapy; however, recent data from a prospective clinical trial have questioned the validity of this approach. The European Organization for the Research and Treatment of Cancer (EORTC) has conducted a phase III study in adults with supratentorial low-grade gliomas of all histologic types (excluding pilocytic astrocytomas) in which 311 patients were randomized either to observation (which could be considered a delayed radiation therapy approach) or to initial radiation therapy using 54 Gy to localized treatment fields. The 5-year progression-free survival rate was significantly better for the patients receiving initial radiation therapy (44% versus 37%), and two-thirds of the patients in the observation group ultimately required radiation. However, the overall 5-year survival rate was similar between the treatment groups (63% versus 66%).[65] These data suggest that observation is a reasonable strategy in an adult with a tissue-proven supratentorial low-grade glioma, although, ultimately, most patients will require radiation therapy.

Table 15–3. SURVIVAL OF SUPRATENTORIAL LOW-GRADE GLIOMAS*

Survival	Histologic Type			
	PA	DA	OA	O
Median (years)	NR	4.7	7.1	9.8
2 years (%)	88	80	89	93
5 years (%)	85	46	63	73
10 years (%)	79	17	33	49
15 years (%)	79	7	17	49

*WHO grades I–II. OA = oligoastrocytoma; O = oligodendroglioma; PA = pilocytic astrocytoma; DA = diffuse astrocytoma; NR = not reached. Adapted from the Mayo Clinic experience: Zulch[12] and Shaw.[63]

Surgery

The key surgical issues in the management of supratentorial low-grade gliomas are twofold. The first issue is whether to biopsy a patient whose clinical presentation and imaging studies suggest a low-grade glioma. Once a histologic diagnosis is established, the issue becomes whether to attempt gross-total resection of the tumor.

There are two series in the literature that suggest that as many as half of patients with an imaging diagnosis of low-grade diffuse astrocytoma (ie, WHO grade II astrocytoma) have a different pathologic diagnosis, most commonly a high-grade glioma. Wilden and Kelly reviewed their results in 34 patients who presented with a seizure disorder plus a nonenhancing tumor on CT scans. Stereotactic biopsy results revealed low-grade glioma (astrocytoma, oligoastrocytoma, or oligodendroglioma) in 26 patients (74%), high-grade glioma in 6 patients (17%), and ganglioglioma in 2 patients (6%). Three patients had subsequent surgical resection confirming their stereotactic biopsy result.[66] In another series with a similar outcome, Kondziolka reported the stereotactic biopsy results in 20 adults (17 of whom presented with a seizure) with CT scan evidence of a lobar, nonenhancing, low-attenuation lesion. Only half of the patients had a low-grade astrocytoma. Nine others (45%) had an anaplastic astrocytoma and 1 patient (5%) had encephalitis.[67]

Table 15–4 summarizes the outcome by extent of surgery in 10 "contemporary" (ie, patients who were operated on in or after 1970) supratentorial low-grade glioma series, with an emphasis on the diffuse astrocytomas and oligoastrocytomas.[33,41–43,47,55,68–71] Collectively, they show that about 60 percent of patients with supratentorial low-grade glioma undergo a gross-total or major subtotal resection, 30 percent a "less-than-major" subtotal resection, and 10 percent a biopsy. Nine of the series demonstrate

Table 15–4. OUTCOME BY EXTENT OF SURGICAL RESECTION IN CONTEMPORARY SUPRATENTORIAL LOW-GRADE GLIOMA SERIES*

Authors	Years of Study	Histologies	Surgical Data — Extent of Resection	N	Survival Rate — Median (yr)	5 Year (%)	10 Year (%)	p Value
Reichenthal et al[47]	1970–1982	A	STR+	45	NR	57	NR	NR
			STR–; Bx	11	NR	38	NR	
Janny et al[55]	1970–1989	A, OA	GTR; STR+	10	NR	88	68	.03
			STR–; Bx	22	NR	57	31	
North et al[33]	1975–1984	A, OA, PA	GTR	6	NR	85	NR	.002
			STR	62	NR	64	NR	
			Bx	9	NR	43	NR	
Piepmeier[42]	1975–1985	A, OA	GTR	19	8.5	NR	NR	.832
			STR	17	7.2	NR	NR	
			Bx	13	6.2	NR	NR	
Philippon et al[41]	1978–1987	A	GTR	45	NR	80	NR	< .001
			STR	95	NR	NR	NR	
			Bx	39	NR	45	NR	
Nicaloto et al[68]	1977–1989	A	GTR	17	NR	87	NR	.0001
			STR	59	NR	26	NR	
Piepmeier et al[69]	1982–1990	A	GTR	31	NR	NR	NR	.0013
			STR; Bx	24	12.0	NR	NR	
Bahary et al[70]	1974–1992	A, OA	GTR	14	NR	86	NR	.002
			STR	34	10.8	74	NR	
			Bx	15	4.2	38	NR	
Scerrati et al[71]	1978–1989	A, OA, O	GTR	76	NR	100	76	< .001
			STR+	31	NR	94	71	
			STR–	24	8.0	92	21	
Leighton et al[43]	1979–1995	A, OA	GTR; STR+	128	10.7	82	59	.006
			STR–	101	8.4	64	41	

A = astrocytoma; OA = oligoastrocytoma; PA = pilocytic astrocytoma; O = oligodendroglioma; GTR = gross-total resection; STR+ = more extensive subtotal resection; STR = extent of subtotal resection not reported; STR– = less extensive subtotal resection; Bx = biopsy; NR = not reported.
*Mostly diffuse astrocytoma and oligoastrocytoma.

a significant survival advantage for gross-total or major subtotal resection compared with minor subtotal resection or biopsy. In the more aggressively operated patients in these series, the average 5-year survival rate is 87 percent (range, 82 to 100%), whereas the comparable survival rate is 60 percent in the less aggressively resected patients (range, 24 to 64%). One series did not find a significant survival difference based on the extent of surgical resection.[42] The surgical data are similar for the low-grade oligodendrogliomas (Table 15–5). In the three reported series that date back to the 1950s, a significant survival benefit was seen in patients who underwent more aggressive surgery.[72–74]

Berger and colleagues use the pre- and postoperative tumor volume to predict the likelihood of recurrence in patients with supratentorial low-grade astrocytoma, oligoastrocytoma, and oligodendroglioma.[49] Using the preoperative tumor volume, no tumors recurred if the tumor volume was less than 10 cm^3, 14 percent recurred with a median time to recurrence of 58 months if the preoperative tumor volume was 10 to 30 cm^3, and 41 percent recurred with a median time to recurrence of 30 months if the preoperative tumor volume was greater than 30 cm^3. Similar results were observed based on the residual tumor volume. If it was less than 10 cm^3, 15 percent of tumors recurred with a median time to recurrence of 50 months, whereas those with more than 10 cm^3 of residual tumor had a 40 percent recurrence rate with a median time to recurrence of 30 months. Both pre- and postoperative tumor volumes were correlated with the likelihood of malignant transformation. If the residual tumor volume was less than 10 cm^3, half of the recurrences were high grade, whereas if the preoperative tumor volume was more than 30 cm^3, all recurrences were high grade.[75] In contrast, Lunsford and colleagues followed stereotactic biopsy of a supratentorial low-grade glioma with radiation therapy. The median survival time was 9.8 years for 35 consecutive patients treated between 1982 and 1992, only 3 of whom (9%) required subsequent cytoreductive surgery,[76] suggesting that extent of surgical resection in a "modern" treatment era may be less important.

Radiation Therapy

External Beam Radiation Therapy

The three key radiation therapy issues in the management of supratentorial low-grade gliomas include the timing of radiation (immediate or postoperative versus delayed or at recurrence), the proper treatment volume, and the appropriate dose.

Table 15–6 summarizes the outcome of surgery alone versus surgery plus radiation therapy in "contemporary" (ie, patients were treated in the megavoltage era of radiation, 1960 or later) supratentorial low-grade glioma series, with an emphasis on the diffuse astrocytomas and oligoastrocytomas.[41–43,55,57,68–70,77,78] Eight of the series did not identify a survival difference with postoperative radiation therapy, consistent with the findings of the EORTC prospective trial.[65] In these collected series, median survival times are in the range of 3.9 to 13 years (in two series, the median survival time was not reached[69,70]) with 5- and 10-year survival rates ranging from 29 to 84 percent and from

Table 15–5. OUTCOME BY EXTENT OF SURGICAL RESECTION IN CONTEMPORARY LOW-GRADE OLIGODENDROGLIOMA SERIES

Authors	Years of Study	Histologies	Extent of Resection	N	Median (yr)	5 Year (%)	10 Year (%)	p Value
Celli et al[72]	1953–1986	LG > HG	GTR; STR+	29	9.3	66	—	< .012
		O < OA	STR	71	4.8	48	—	
Mork et al[73]	1953–1977	LG > HG	GTR	177	3.8	—	—	.051
		O	STR		2.7	—	—	
Shaw et al[74]	1960–1982	LG < HG	GTR	19	12.6	74	59	.02
		O	STR	63	4.9	46	23	

LG = low grade; HG = high grade; O = oligodendroglioma; OA = oligoastrocytoma; GTR = gross-total resection; STR+ = more extensive subtotal resection; STR = extent of subtotal resection not reported; — = data not reported.

Table 15–6. RESULTS OF SURGERY ± RADIATION THERAPY FOR SUPRATENTORIAL LOW-GRADE GLIOMA SERIES*

Authors	Years of Study	Histologies	Surgical Data — Extent of Resection	N	Median (yr)	5 Year (%)	10 Year (%)	p Value
Bahary et al[70]	1974–1992	A, OA	Surgery	20	NR	66	—	NS
			S + RT	43	9.2	67	—	
Janny et al[55]	1970–1989	A, OA	Surgery	18	4.9	50	26	.8
			S + RT	15	3.9	45	27	
Leighton et al[43]	1979–1995	A, OA, O	Surgery	87	13.0	84	70	.003
			S + RT	80	8.0	62	35	
Nicolato et al[68]	1977–1989	A	Surgery	46	—	66	—	.12
			S + RT↓	9	—	44	—	
			S + RT↑	18	—	29	—	
Philippon et al[41]	1978–1987	A	Surgery	61	—	65	—	.43
			S + RT	118	—	55	—	
Piepmeier[42]	1975–1985	A, OA	Surgery	23	8.5	—	—	.174
			S + RT	26	6.5	—	—	
Piepmeier et al[69]	1982–1990	A	Surgery	45	NR	—	—	NS
			S + RT	10	9.0	—	—	
Shaw et al[77]	1960–1982	A, OA	Surgery	19	—	32	11	.034
			S + RT↓	72	5.0	49	21	
			S + RT↑	35	6.5	68	39	
Shibamoto et al[57]	1965–1989	A	Surgery	18	—	37	11	.048
			S + RT	101	—	60	41	
Westergaard et al[78]	1956–1991	A	Surgery	81	6.7	—	—	.35
			S + RT	82†	—	—	—	

A = astrocytoma; OA = oligoastrocytoma; O = oligodendroglioma; S = surgery; RT = radiation therapy; RT↓ = low-dose RT (< 53 Gy); RT↑ = high-dose RT (≥ 53 Gy); NR = not reached; NS = not significant; — = data not reported.
*Mainly astrocytoma and oligoastrocytoma.
†Only includes patients who received RT after 1969 when the minimum dose was 45 Gy.

11 percent to 70 percent, respectively, in both irradiated and nonirradiated patients.

Two series suggested a statistically significant benefit for postoperative radiation therapy.[57,77] In the Mayo Clinic series of Shaw and colleagues, the 5- and 10-year survival rates were 32 percent and 11 percent for patients who had surgery alone (most of whom were aggressively resected), compared with 47 percent and 21 percent in those receiving low-dose radiation (< 53 Gy) and 68 percent and 39 percent for those receiving high-dose radiation (≥ 53 Gy).[77] Shibamoto and colleagues reported similar results.[57]

When these various retrospective series are analyzed for the effect of radiation therapy as a function of age, there does appear to be a strong suggestion that radiation therapy improves survival in "older" patients. In the series by Philippon and colleagues, there was no survival benefit for postoperative radiation therapy when all patients were considered, regardless of age and extent of resection. However, in the subset greater than 50 years of age who had subtotal resection or biopsy of a grade I tumor, the 5-year survival rate was 70 percent with radiation versus 25 percent without; the 3-year survival rate was 50 percent with radiation versus 25 percent without in those with grade II tumors.[41] In the analysis of Shaw and colleagues, patients 35 years of age or older had a significantly poorer survival rate if postoperative radiation therapy was not given or if the dose of radiation was less than 53 Gy. Five- and 10-year survival rates were 37 percent and 5 percent in the "older" patients who had surgery alone or low-dose postoperative radiation, compared with 67 percent and 45 percent, respectively, when radiation was given with doses of 53 Gy or more.[77]

Table 15–7 summarizes the results of contemporary supratentorial low-grade oligodendroglioma series.[72,74,79–86] In six of them, a significant ($p \leq .05$)[72,81,83,85] or suggestive ($p < .10$)[74,86] survival advantage for patients receiving radiation therapy was seen. Median survival times are in the range of 2.2 to 5.6 years without radiation and 3.2 to 11.2 years with radiation. The 5-year survival rates ranged from 25 to 57 percent and 36 to 83 percent in the nonirradiated and radiated patients, respectively. Four oligodendroglioma series did not demonstrate a significant survival improvement in patients receiving radiation therapy,[79,80,82,84] although in three of the series, median survival times or 5-year rates were higher in the irradiated group.[79,80,84]

Radiation has several other effects besides the potential delay in recurrence or improvement in survival. In a small series of 5 patients with medically intractable epilepsy due to an underlying cerebral low-grade glioma, radiation therapy in doses of 54 to 61.2 Gy resulted in 1 patient becoming seizure free, 3 having more than a 90 percent decrease in seizure frequency, and 1 having a more than 75 percent but less than 90 percent reduction in seizure frequency.[87]

Radiation therapy also may decrease the likelihood of malignant transformation or at least delay its onset. Reichenthal and colleagues observed a 9 percent incidence of malignant transformation in the patients who received postoperative radiation therapy compared with 18 percent in those who had surgery alone.[47] Vertosick and colleagues reported a 56 percent likelihood of malignant transformation in their series and further observed that the median time to dedifferentiation was 5.4 years for patients who received radiation therapy compared with 3.7 years for those who had surgery alone.[88] The recent series of Leighton and colleagues reported an approximate 50 percent incidence of malignant transformation whether patients did or did not receive postoperative radiation therapy.[43] These data imply that radiation neither increases nor decreases the likelihood of malignant transformation, but, rather, this is a biologic phenomenon observed in low-grade gliomas independent of the treatment received.

External Beam Radiation Dose and Volume Considerations

For those patients who do receive radiation therapy, a decision must be made regarding the appropriate treatment field as well as the dose. Several series analyzing failure patterns in irradiated patients with low-grade hemispheric astrocytomas suggest that when progression occurs, it almost always is at the site of the primary tumor within the treatment volume,[33,48,56] implying that partial brain irradiation is appropriate. Since tumor cells have been identified

Table 15–7. RESULTS OF SURGERY ± RADIATION THERAPY FOR SUPRATENTORIAL OLIGODENDROGLIOMA SERIES*

Authors	Years of Study	Histologies	Surgical Data		Survival Rate			p Value
			Extent of Resection	N	Median (yr)	5 Year (%)	10 Year (%)	
Bullard et al[79]	1940–1983	LG + HG	S	34	4.5	48	16	.67
		O	S + RT	37	5.2	60	12	
Celli et al[72]	1953–1986	LG > HG	S	77	3.1	36	—	< .018
		O < OA	S + RT	28	6.3	57	—	
Chin et al[80]	1963–1977	LG + HG	S	11	NR	82	—	—
		O	S + RT	24	NR	100	—	
Gannett et al[81]	1956–1984	LG > HG	S	14	3.9	51	36	.032
		O > OA	S + RT	27	7.0	83	46	
Kros et al[82]	1972–1986	LG	S	10	2.0	20	0	> .05
		O	S + RT	23	3.8	40	0	
Lindegaard et al[83]	1953–1977	LG > HG	S	62	2.2	27	12	.039
		O	S + RT	108	3.2	36	8	
Reedy et al[84]	1950–1980	LG + HG	S	21	—	67	—	—
		O	S + RT	27	—	63	—	
Shaw et al[74]	1960–1982	LG < HG	S	8	2.0	25	25	.09
		O	S + RT↓	26	4.5	39	20	
			S + RT↑	29	7.9	62	31	
Shimizu et al[85]	1957–1990	LG > HG	S	8	3.4	25	—	.019
		O + OA	S + RT	23	7.0	74	—	
Wallner et al[86]	1940–1983	LG + HG	S	11	5.6	57	18	.09
		O	S + RT	14	11.2	80	56	

LG = low grade; HG = high grade; O = oligodendroglioma; OA = oligoastrocytoma; S = surgery; RT↓ = low-dose radiation therapy (RT) (< 50 Gy); RT↑ = high-dose RT (≥ 50 Gy); — = data not reported; NR = not reached.
*Mainly low grade.

up to several centimeters beyond tumor margin by the T2-weighted MRI scan,[52] the appropriate radiation volume should include the MRI extent of tumor with a 2- to 3-cm margin.

Regarding the potential benefit of higher doses of radiation therapy compared with lower ones, the retrospective data are mixed. Medbery and colleagues found tumor progression in 89 percent of patients receiving less than 50 Gy compared with 53 percent for those who received 50 Gy or more.[40] North and colleagues had no survivors for patients who received less than 40 Gy compared with a 5-year survival rate of 66 percent for those receiving 45 to 59 Gy and 22 percent for those who had 60 to 66 Gy.[33] The analysis of Shaw and colleagues also suggested an improvement in survival with doses of 53 Gy or more versus lower doses.[77] At least one series observed poorer survival of patients receiving greater than 50 Gy compared to less than 50 Gy.[89]

Recently, two prospective randomized clinical trials have been completed that address the issue of dose-response in adult patients with WHO grade II nonpilocytic supratentorial low-grade gliomas (diffuse astrocytomas, oligoastrocytomas, and oligodendrogliomas), one from the EORTC and the other from the North Central Cancer Treatment Group (NCCTG). The EORTC randomized 379 patients to receive low-dose radiation therapy (45 Gy) or high-dose radiation (59.4 Gy) using localized treatment fields. Initial analysis has failed to demonstrate a difference in survival between the two doses. The 5-year survival rate was 58 percent with 45 Gy and 59 percent with 59.4 Gy.[90] The NCCTG trial compared 50.4 Gy with 64.8 Gy, also using multiple localized treatment fields. Initial analysis also failed to demonstrate a difference in survival between the two doses. The 5-year survival rate was 73 percent with 50.4 Gy and 68 percent with 64.8 Gy.[91] Based on both the retrospective and prospective dose-response data, the Radiation Therapy Oncology Group (RTOG) chose a total radiation dose of 54 Gy to localized treatment fields (tumor defined by the T2-weighted MRI scan plus a 2-cm margin) for its current Intergroup study in adults with supratentorial low-grade glioma (Figure 15–5).

Other Radiation Modalities

Several other radiation modalities have been used selectively in patients with low-grade gliomas. These include stereotactic radiosurgery and brachytherapy, both interstitial and intracystic. In two series, radiosurgery for low-grade diffuse astrocytomas employing doses of 16 to 50 Gy in one or two fractions for tumors with maximum diameters of 30 to 40 mm resulted in radiographic responses in the majority of patients treated, without overt damage to normal tissue, although follow-up is short.[92,93] In another series of children with deep-seated pilocytic astrocytomas,

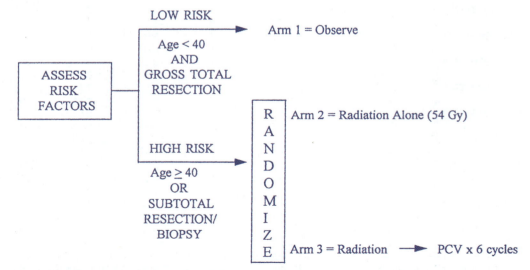

Figure 15–5. Schema of the recently activated RTOG-Intergroup low-grade glioma trial. PCV = procarbazine, CCNU (lomustine), and vincristine.

single-dose radiosurgery (15 Gy) resulted in tumor shrinkage (5 patients) or no further growth (4 patients) without early or delayed morbidity.[94] Intraoperative radiation (25 to 35 Gy, electrons) has been used in the setting of recurrent supratentorial low- to intermediate-grade gliomas with a reported 84 percent 2-year survival rate.[95] Interstitial implants, primarily with iodine-125, have been used for the treatment of some small, circumscribed, low-grade hemispheric astrocytomas. Five-year survival rates have ranged from 44 to 78 percent, which is similar to results achieved with external beam radiation therapy[96,97] (see Tables 15–6 and 15–7). Chromic phosphate (P-32) also has been used for low-grade gliomas but primarily for cystic tumors, usually of the pilocytic type, as well as for recurrent diffuse astrocytomas with cyst formation.[98]

Toxicity

There is a spectrum of radiation-induced toxicities that can occur in patients receiving brain radiation, ranging from neurocognitive sequelae, the pathogenesis of which is likely a white matter injury, to overt radiation necrosis, which is probably a consequence of vascular injury.[99,100]

Several recent studies have focused on the neurocognitive effects of radiation therapy in patients who are longer-term recurrence-free survivors, most of whom were irradiated for supratentorial low-grade gliomas. To assess the toxicity of radiation therapy, it is important to understand the neurologic and cognitive dysfunction that results from having a cerebral low-grade glioma.

In the series from Taphoorn and colleagues,[101] a subset of patients treated on the EORTC low-grade glioma trials[54,90] were assessed prospectively using serial neurologic examinations, assessment of Karnofsky Performance Status (KPS), and a battery of neuropsychological tests. Three groups of patients (about 20 patients per group) were studied. One group had histologically verified low-grade astrocytoma but did not receive postoperative radiation therapy. A second group received postoperative radiation therapy with 45 to 63 Gy, using localized treatment fields. A third control group consisted of patients with hematologic malignancies in the absence of brain involvement. With an average follow-up of 3.5 years, 93 percent of patients with low-grade astrocytoma, whether they received radiation therapy or not, had normal neurologic examinations and a KPS of 85 to 90, compared with 100 percent normal neurologic examinations and a KPS of 95 for the control group. Neuropsychological test scores were similar for the low-grade astrocytoma patients, whether they received radiation therapy or not, and were significantly worse than those of the control group, implying that the disease and not the radiation therapy was the most significant underlying cause of cognitive dysfunction. In addition, patients with left hemispheric tumors who received postoperative radiation therapy scored significantly better on several neuropsychologic tests than did patients with similarly located low-grade gliomas who did not receive radiation therapy. Other observations made in the low-grade glioma patients, independent of whether postoperative radiation therapy was given, included a higher frequency of fatigue; memory, concentration, and speech difficulties; depression; tension; and impediment of the activities of daily living as compared with the control group. The authors concluded that ". . . radiotherapy had no negative impact on neurological, functional, cognitive, and affective status."[101]

A recent report from the EORTC compared the quality of life in low-grade glioma patients who received either 45 Gy or 59.4 Gy on the dose-response trial.[90] Patients who received the higher dose reported a significantly lower level of functioning and more symptom burden, especially fatigue, malaise, and insomnia.[102]

Kleinberg and colleagues measured quality of life in 30 adult patients with hemispheric gliomas, 23 of whom had low- to intermediate-grade tumors. All patients were alive without evidence of recurrence 1 year or more after surgery and postoperative radiation therapy. Quality of life was measured by KPS, employment history, and memory function as a function of the radiation treatment field for localized brain irradiation versus whole brain treatment. None of the 14 patients treated with localized fields had a decline in KPS compared to a decline in 3 of 16 patients (19%) who received whole brain radiation. Whereas two-thirds of patients were employed prior to their diagnosis, at 1 year or more following radiation therapy, 80 percent of those who received localized treatment fields were employed compared with 38 to 46 percent who underwent whole brain irradiation. Moderate to severe memory deficits occurred in 43 percent of patients receiving whole brain irradiation as opposed to 6 percent with localized radiation therapy.[103]

In the NCCTG dose-response trial,[91] a subset of 19 of the 200 adult study patients who received either 50.4 or 64.8 Gy underwent psychometric testing prior to and up to 3 years following localized radiation therapy. No significant losses in general intellectual function, new learning function, or memory function were seen. The authors "could not document significant detrimental neurocognitive effects from brain RT [radiation therapy] in the patients with low-grade glioma evaluated prospectively over time."[104]

The incidence of overt radiation necrosis following radiation therapy for a cerebral low-grade glioma is approximately 3 percent based on data from surgical series in which reoperation data were reported.[14,33,38,42,44,47,55,56] This is consistent with findings from the NCCTG dose-response trial (50.4 Gy versus 64.8 Gy) in which the 2-year actuarial incidence of severe, life-threatening, or fatal radionecrosis was 1 percent at the 50.4 Gy dose level and 4.5 percent with 64.8 Gy.[91] Several examples of the clinical presentation, imaging changes, time course, management, and outcome of reversible and irreversible radiation toxicities seen in patients with cerebral low-grade gliomas are shown in Figures 15–6, 15–7, and 15–8.

Chemotherapy

At the present time, there is no proven role for chemotherapy in the management of newly diagnosed low-grade gliomas in adults. Eyre and colleagues reported a randomized trial performed by the Southwest Oncology Group in which patients with subtotally resected supratentorial low-grade astrocytomas were randomized to 55 Gy with localized treatment fields, either alone or with oral CCNU (lomustine) chemotherapy (100 mg/m^2). Only 54 patients were entered in the study, which failed to identify any significant differences in survival between the two treatment arms. The most significant predictor of survival was age. Median survival time was not reached for patients less than 30 years old, was 5.5 years for those 30 to 49 years old, and was 1.6 years for those 50 years of age and older.[105] Shibamoto and colleagues presented data from their retrospective series in which 19 percent of patients received chemotherapy, primarily with CCNU. Survival was not significantly affected.[57]

There are ongoing prospective studies assessing the role of the chemotherapeutic regimen PCV (procarbazine, CCNU, vincristine) in patients with cerebral low-grade glioma. The NCCTG has an ongoing phase II study for adults with low-grade astrocytoma, oligoastrocytoma, or oligodendroglioma in which six cycles of PCV are given every 8 weeks followed by localized external beam radiation therapy (54 to 59.4 Gy). Responses have been noted thus far in 8 of 29 patients (28%), and 3 patients (10%) progressed prior to their planned radiation.[106] Mason and colleagues reported a 100 percent response rate in 9 adult patients with cerebral low-grade oligodendrogliomas treated with initial PCV. Of the 8 patients who were previously untreated, radiation therapy only had to be given to 1 patient who had stable disease after receiving six cycles of chemotherapy.[107]

Figure 15–5 shows the schema of the recently activated RTOG-Intergroup low-grade glioma trial, designed for adults with supratentorial low-grade diffuse astrocytoma, oligoastrocytoma, and oligodendroglioma. Patients who are at low risk for recurrence (age < 40 years and gross-total resection) are observed. Those at high risk for recurrence (age ≥ 40 or subtotal resection/biopsy) are randomized between radiation therapy alone (54 Gy, localized treatment fields) or radiation followed by six cycles of "standard" PCV. Figures 15–9A and 15–9B show the pre- and post-chemotherapy MRI scans of a patient with a newly diagnosed low-grade oligodendroglioma who received four cycles of "intensive" PCV.

The response of recurrent, previously irradiated low-grade gliomas to chemotherapy has been variable. Response rates range from 20 percent with MOP (nitrogen mustard, vincristine, and procarbazine)[108] to 33 to 40 percent with the combination of BCNU (carmustine) and interferon-α for recur-

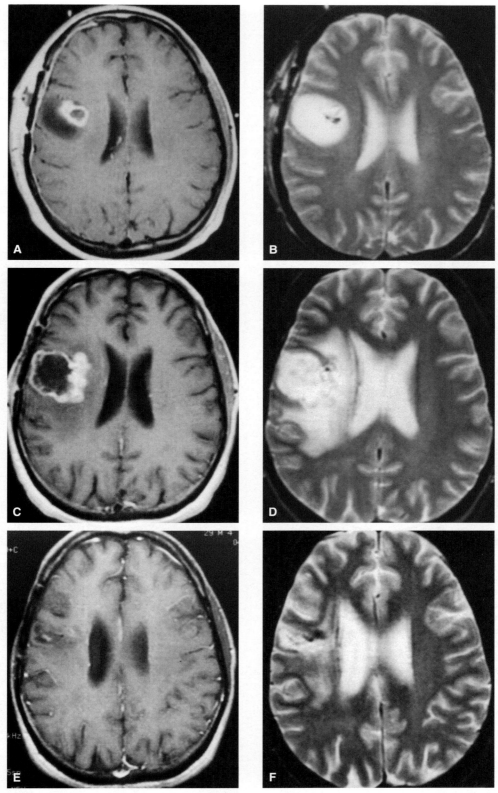

Figure 15–6. *A,* Preradiation postgadolinium T1-weighted and, *B,* T2-weighted MR images of an adult with a WHO II oligodendroglioma of the right frontotemporal lobes. Seven months following 64.8 Gy external beam radiation therapy, the patient developed headaches. *C,* Postgadolinium T1-weighted and *D,* T2-weighted MR images are shown. The differential diagnosis was recurrent tumor versus radiation necrosis. After a brief course of oral corticosteroid medications, the imaging abnormalities resolved, supporting the diagnosis of transient radiation necrosis (postgadolinium T1-weighted [*E*] and T2-weighted [*F*] MR images are shown).

rent low-grade astrocytomas or oligoastrocytomas,[109] to 90 percent with PCV for recurrent low-grade oligodendrogliomas.[110]

FAVORABLE VARIANTS

There are a group of primary CNS tumors that have a distinctly more favorable prognosis than the WHO grade II gliomas (ie, the low-grade diffuse astrocytomas, oligoastrocytomas, and oligodendrogliomas). These include the pilocytic astrocytomas (WHO grade I) and the other low-grade glioma variants including the pleomorphic xanthoastrocytomas (PXAs), subependymal giant cell astrocytomas, and subependymomas. There also are three other primary CNS tumors of neuronal or mixed neuronal-glial origin that can be grouped with the low-grade glioma variants because of their similar presentation and favorable prognosis, including the gangliogliomas, central neurocytomas, and dysembryoplastic neuroepithelial tumors. Other than the pilocytic astrocytomas, which make up approximately 20 percent of supratentorial low-grade gliomas and 80 percent of cerebellar gliomas,[13,16] the other six variants are quite uncommon, accounting for

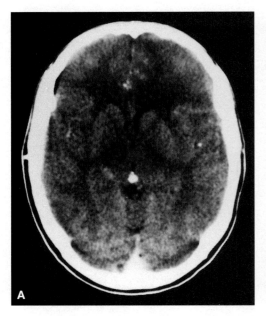
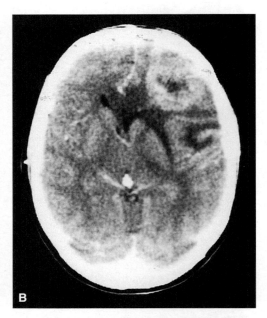
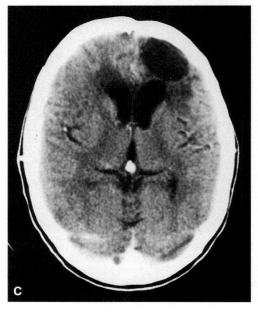

Figure 15–7. Series of contrast enhanced CT scan showing a left frontal WHO grade II astrocytoma in an adult patient, prior to 64.8 Gy external beam radiation therapy (*A*). *B*, Following radiation, the patient was symptomatic with headaches. *C*, Eighteen months following gross-total resection of what proved to be a combination of radiation necrosis and persistent low-grade astrocytoma, the patient had no evidence of further radiation necrosis or tumor.

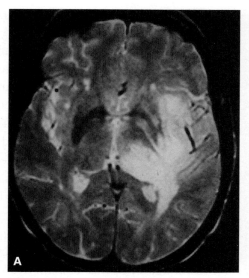
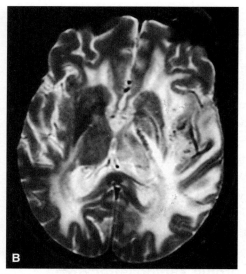

Figure 15–8. T2-weighted MRI scan of an older adult with an infiltrative, poorly defined WHO grade II astrocytoma epicentered in the left temporal lobe (*A*). Six months after completing 64.8 Gy external beam radiation therapy, the patient developed a significant decline in cognitive function and overall performance status. *B*, A repeat MRI study showed dramatic white-matter changes. The patient subsequently died. An autopsy showed diffuse demyelination, foci of radiation necrosis, and persistent low-grade astrocytoma.

approximately 1 percent or less of primary CNS tumors. From an imaging standpoint, they are typically well circumscribed, enhancing, and sometimes cystic, calcified, or both.[111,112]

Pilocytic Astrocytoma

Pilocytic astrocytoma typically occurs in children and young adults, with common locations being the cerebellum, optic pathways, hypothalamic/third ventricular region, and cerebral hemispheres. It is the most common primary brain tumor occurring in patients with type 1 neurofibromatosis.[7] The overall 10-year survival rate is 80 percent or greater, independent of location in the brain,[13,16–18,113] although, rarely, they may behave more aggressively.[15] In patients undergoing gross-total resection, the 10-year disease-free and overall survival rates approach

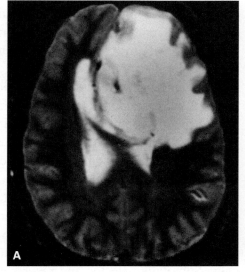
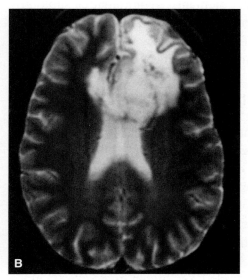

Figure 15–9. *A*, Prechemotherapy and, *B*, postchemotherapy T2-weighted MR images in a young adult with a WHO grade II oligodendroglioma of the left frontal lobe.

100 percent.[16–18,77,113] For those who have subtotal resection, particularly children, a reasonable strategy is observation with close follow-up[114] since there is no apparent survival benefit to routine postoperative radiation therapy,[76,77] and a second surgical procedure accomplishing gross-total resection appears curative.[113] Radiation therapy usually is reserved for symptomatic subtotally resected or unresectable tumors, usually in the setting of tumor recurrence. When pilocytic astrocytomas require radiation, very localized treatment fields (enhancing tumor with a 1-cm margin) and moderate doses (45 Gy to 54 Gy) are recommended.[77]

Pleomorphic Xanthoastrocytoma

Pleomorphic xanthoastrocytomas also occur in children and young adults, usually in the cerebral cortex (temporal lobes), sometimes with adjacent meningeal and, rarely, craniospinal leptomeningeal involvement. Despite their pleomorphism, they usually behave in an indolent manner.[111,112] Treatment recommendations depend on the grade of the astrocytic component. When gross-total resection has been achieved of a PXA that contains a low-grade diffuse astrocytoma (WHO grade II), observation is appropriate. Indications for radiation therapy (with doses and treatment fields similar to the more common forms of WHO grade II low-grade gliomas) include PXAs that contain an anaplastic astrocytoma or glioblastoma (WHO grade III–IV) element, symptomatic subtotally resected or unresectable tumors, or recurrent PXAs, particularly if their astrocytic component becomes more malignant in appearance.[112,115,116]

Other Favorable Variants

Gangliogliomas consist of neoplastic ganglion (neuronal) cells as well as neoplastic glial (astrocytic) cells. They can occur in children and adults, although most present in the first two to three decades of life. Whereas gangliogliomas can develop anywhere in the CNS, they tend to occur supratentorially, most often in a temporal location. Like the PXAs, the glial component can be low grade (WHO grade II) or higher grade (WHO grade III–IV).[111,112] Treatment principles are similar to those for PXAs from both a surgical and radiotherapeutic standpoint.[117]

Dysembryoplastic neuroepithelial tumors (DNTs), like gangliogliomas, contain a mixture of neuronal and glial elements, although the neuronal component is mature, and the glial component is well differentiated and astrocytic or oligodendroglial in nature. As such, they are classified as WHO I tumors. Typically, DNTs occur in a temporal location, are characteristically multinodular, and arise during the first two decades of life. Treatment principles are similar to those for pilocytic astrocytomas from both a surgical and radiotherapeutic standpoint, although radiation rarely is necessary.[111,112]

Central neurocytomas contain neuronal elements that usually are mature. They are classified as WHO grade II tumors. By definition, they arise in the ventricular system, usually as large tumors in the lateral ventricular system, and rarely have been reported to disseminate craniospinally. The typical age at presentation is in the late 20s, although they can occur in children or adults.[111,112] Treatment principles are similar to those for pilocytic astrocytomas from both a surgical and radiotherapeutic standpoint. Subtotally resected tumors have been reported to respond to radiation therapy.[118]

Subependymal giant cell astrocytomas occur in patients with tuberous sclerosis, often during their first two decades of life but sometimes later. Characterized by large astrocyte-like cells, they are classified as WHO grade I tumors, similar to pilocytic astrocytomas. Typically, they arise in an intraventricular or periventricular location (lateral ventricles, foramen of Monro).[3,113,114,119] Treatment recommendations parallel those for pilocytic astrocytomas from a surgical and radiotherapeutic standpoint. Gross-total resection is considered curative.[4,120]

Subependymomas also are classified as WHO grade I–II tumors. They contain both low-grade astrocytic and ependymal-like cells and usually arise in an intraventricular location (lateral or fourth ventricles, particularly in and around the foramen of Monro) in adults near the age of 50 years.[113,114] Treatment recommendations parallel those for pilocytic astrocytomas, both surgically and radiotherapeutically. Subtotally resected and recurrent tumors have been reported to respond to radiation therapy.[121]

RECURRENT LOW-GRADE GLIOMAS

At some point in their illness, the majority of patients with a low-grade glioma (astrocytoma, oligodendroglioma, or mixed oligoastrocytoma) likely will have the combination of progressive neurologic symptoms (and perhaps signs) and neuroimaging evidence of tumor recurrence, which usually includes the development of new contrast enhancement,[122] often with increasing edema. The clinical and radiographic features of tumor recurrence are indistinguishable from radiation necrosis, even by PET (positron emission tomography)[123] or SPECT (single-photon emission computed tomography)[124] imaging. Magnetic resonance imaging spectroscopy may prove to be more useful in this regard[125] (Figures 15–10A, 15–10B, and 15–10C). To differentiate between these diagnostic possibilities, tissue must be obtained. Data were from pooled surgical series in which 100 patients with suspected

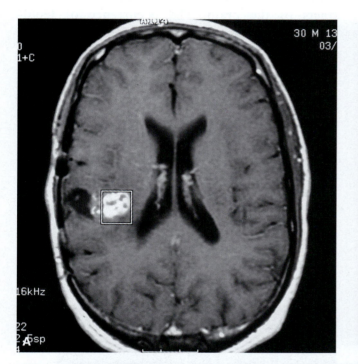

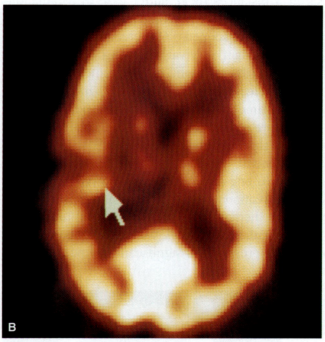

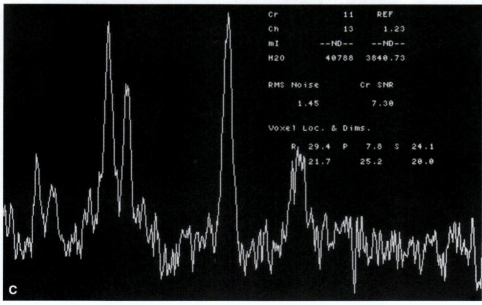

Figure 15–10. Postgadolinium T1-weighted MRI scan of a young adult with WHO grade II oligoastrocytoma status post-subtotal resection, 50.4 Gy external beam radiation therapy, and 18 Gy in 1 fraction stereotactic radiosurgery for recurrent disease at the medial edge of the resection cavity. *A*, An area of increased contrast enhancement at the site of the stereotactic radiosurgery. *B*, A PET scan using fluorodeoxyglucose showing increased uptake at the site of the contrast enhancement (*arrow*). *C*, MR spectroscopy, which is more suggestive of radiation necrosis since the choline to creatine ratio was < 2 and the NAA and lactate peaks are elevated. A subsequent biopsy demonstrated radiation necrosis.

recurrence of a cerebral low-grade astrocytoma underwent reoperation; pathology revealed low-grade tumor in 33 percent, high-grade tumor in 64 percent, and radionecrosis in 3 percent.[13,33,39,44,55,75]

In the series of Forsyth and colleagues, 51 previously irradiated patients (40 of whom had Kernohan grade I or II astrocytoma, oligoastrocytoma, or oligodendroglioma) underwent stereotactic biopsy for suspected tumor recurrence. Pathology revealed the presence of tumor only in 30 biopsies (59%), tumor plus necrosis in 17 biopsies (33%), pure radionecrosis in 3 instances (6%), and 1 case of a radiation-induced sarcoma (2%). Of the patients with tumor in their biopsy specimens, 63 percent had high-grade tumors. Median survival following biopsy was 10 months in patients found to have tumor only, which was significantly worse than the 22-month median survival time in those with tumor plus necrosis. There were no deaths among the three patients whose biopsies showed only radionecrosis.[126]

In general, survival following tumor recurrence is poor. In one series, patients who progressed following treatment with surgery and postoperative radiation therapy had a median survival time of 9.7 months with a 2-year survival rate of 29 percent.[56,77] However, prognosis is significantly impacted by the specific histologic findings at the time of biopsy or reoperation. For instance, in the recent series of Leighton and colleagues, the median survival time following recurrence was 39 months for all patients, 16 months for those with recurrent low-grade diffuse astrocytomas, and 60 months in patients with recurrent low-grade oligodendrogliomas.[43]

Several uncommon patterns of failure can occur in patients with recurrent low-grade gliomas. Figure 15–11 demonstrates the MRI appearance of tumor infiltration across the deep, dense white-matter tracts of the brain. The occurrence of leptomeningeal failure also has been reported. In one pediatric series of intracranial low-grade gliomas, its incidence was 4 percent.[127]

Treatment options for tumor recurrence include surgery, external beam radiation, brachytherapy, radiosurgery, intraoperative electron radiation, and chemotherapy. Each of these modalities has been discussed previously in this chapter.

CONCLUSION

Low-grade gliomas are a diverse group of CNS neoplasms, whose natural history depends primarily on pathologic type and patient age. Despite their having

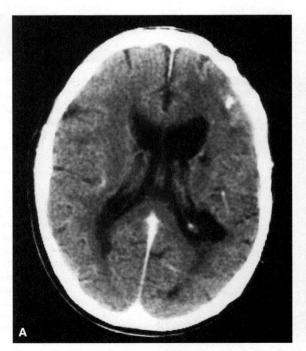 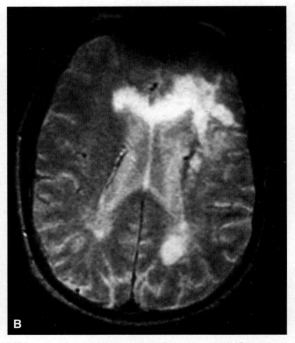

Figure 15–11. *A,* Postcontrast CT scan and, *B,* T2-weighted MRI scan of an adult patient with recurrent WHO grade II astrocytoma. The MRI shows significant ipsilateral and contralateral white-matter spread not seen on the CT scan.

been considered "benign" historically, many of these tumors behave in an aggressive manner, even following surgery and radiation therapy. The role of chemotherapy remains to be determined. Translational research, particularly studies of proliferation and molecular genetics, hopefully will provide much needed insight for the next generation of biologically based therapies.

REFERENCES

1. Greenlee RT, Hill-Harmon MB, Murray T, Thun M. Cancer statistics, 2001. CA Cancer J Clin 2001;51:15–36.
2. Okazaki H. Neoplastic and related lesions. In: Okazaki H, editor. Fundamentals of neuropathology. New York: Igaku-Shoin; 1983.
3. Kleihues P, Ohgaki H. Genetics of glioma progression and the definition of primary and secondary glioblastoma. Brain Pathol 1997;7:1131.
4. Shepherd CW, Scheithauer BW, Gomez MR, et al. Subependymal giant-cell astrocytomas—a clinical pathologic and flow cytometric study. Neurosurgery 1991;28:864–8.
5. Bailey P, Cushing H. A classification of the tumors of the glioma group on a histogenetic basis with a correlated study of prognosis. Philadelphia: JB Lippincott; 1926.
6. Cushing H. Intracranial tumors: notes upon a series of 2000 verified cases with surgical mortality percentages pertaining thereto. Springfield (IL): Charles C. Thomas; 1932.
7. Kleihues P, Burger PC, Scheithauer BW. Histologic typing of tumors of the central nervous system. 2nd ed. Berlin: Springer-Verlag; 1993.
8. Kernohan JW, Mabon RF, Svien HJ, et al. Symposium on new and simplified concept of gliomas: a classification of the gliomas. Proc Staff Meet Mayo Clin 1949;24:71–5.
9. Burger PC, Scheithauer BW, Vogel FS. Brain tumors. In: Burger PC, Scheithauer BW, Vogel FS, editors. Surgical pathology of the nervous system and its coverings. New York: Churchill-Livingstone; 1991. p. 193–437.
10. Daumas-Duport C, Scheithauer B, O'Fallon J, Kelly P. Grading of astrocytomas: a simple and reproducible method. Cancer 1988;62:2152–65.
11. Ringertz N. Grading of gliomas. Acta Pathol Microbiol Scand 1950;27:51–64.
12. Zulch KL. Histologic typing of tumors of the central nervous system. International Histologic Classification of Tumors, No. 21. Geneva: World Health Organization; 1979.
13. Shaw EG, Scheithauer BW, O'Fallon JR. Supratentorial gliomas: a comparative study by grade and histologic type. J Neurooncol 1997;31:273–8.
14. Sofietti R, Chio A, Giordana MT, et al. Prognostic factors in well-differentiated cerebral astrocytomas in the adult. Neurosurgery 1989;24:686–92.
15. Tomlinson FH, Scheithauer BW, Hayostek CJ, et al. The significance of atypia and histologic malignancy in pilocytic astrocytoma of the cerebellum. J Child Neurol 1993;9:301–10.
16. Hayostek CJ, Shaw EG, Scheithauer B, et al. Astrocytomas of the cerebellum: a comparative clinicopathologic study of pilocytic and diffuse astrocytomas. Cancer 1993;73:856–9.
17. Forsyth PA, Shaw EG, Scheithauer BW, et al. Supratentorial pilocytic astrocytomas: a clinicopathologic, prognostic, flow cytometric study of 51 patients. Cancer 1993;72:1335–42.
18. Garcia DM, Fulling DH. Juvenile pilocytic astrocytoma of the cerebrum in adults: a distinctive neoplasm with favorable prognosis. J Neurosurg 1985;63:382–6.
19. Zaprianov Z, Christov K. Histologic grading, DNA content, cell survival. Cytometry 1988;9:380–6.
20. Danova M, Giaretti W, Merlo F, et al. Prognostic significance of nuclear DNA content in human neuroepithelial tumors. Int J Cancer 1991;48:663–7.
21. Coons SW, Johnson PC, Pearl DK. Prognostic significance of flow cytometry deoxyribonucleic acid analysis of human astrocytomas. Neurosurgery 1994;35:119–26.
22. Struikmans H, Rutgers DH, Jansen GH, et al. S-phase fraction, 5-bromo-2'-deoxy-uridine labeling index, duration of s-phase, potential doubling time, and DNA index in benign and malignant brain tumors. Radiat Oncol Investig 1997;5:170–9.
23. Hoshino T, Rodriguez LA, Cho KG, et al. Prognostic implications of the proliferative potential of low-grade astrocytomas. J Neurosurg 1988;69:839–42.
24. Franzini A, Leocata F, Cajola L, et al. Low-grade glial tumors in basal ganglia and thalamus: natural history and biological reappraisal. Neurosurgery 1994;35:817–21.
25. Dudas SP, Rempel SA. Development, molecular genetics, and gene therapy of glial tumors. In: Rock J, Cairncross G, Shaw E, Rosenblum M, editors Practical management of low-grade primary brain tumors. 1st ed. Philadelphia: Lippincott-Raven; 1999. p. 193–230.
26. Lang FF, Miller DC, Pisharody S. High frequency of p53 protein accumulation without p53 gene mutation in human juvenile pilocytic, low-grade and anaplastic astrocytomas. Oncogene 1994;9:949–54.
27. Chozick BS, Pezzulo JC, Epstein MH, Finch PW. Prognostic implications of p53 overexpression in supratentorial astrocytic tumors. Neurosurgery 1994;35:831–8.
28. Ritland SR, Ganju V, Jenkins RB. Region specific loss of heterozygosity on chromosome 19 is related to the morphologic type of human glioma. Genes Chromosomes Cancer 1995;12:277–82.
29. Abdulrauf SI, Edvardsen K, Ho KL. Vascular endothelial growth factor expression and vascular density as prognostic markers of survival in patients with low-grade astrocytoma. J Neurosurg 1998;88:513–20.
30. Piepmeier JM, Fried L, Makuch R. Low-grade astrocytomas may arise from different astrocyte lineages. Neurosurgery 1993;33:627–32.
31. Piepmeier JM. Research strategies for evaluating the biological diversity of low-grade astrocytomas. Perspect Neurol Surg 1993;4:1–20.
32. Shaw EG, Scheithauer BW, Dinapoli RP. Low-grade hemispheric astrocytomas. In: Black PM, Loeffler JS, editors. Cancer of the nervous system. 1st ed. Cambridge: Blackwell Science; 1997. p. 441.

33. North CA, North RB, Epstein JA, et al. Low-grade cerebral astrocytomas: survival and quality of life after radiation therapy. Cancer 1990;66:6–14.
34. Dewit L, Van Der Schueren E, Ang KK, et al. Low-grade astrocytoma in children treated by surgery and radiation therapy. Acta Radiol 1984;23(1):1–8.
35. Bloom HJG, Glees J, Bell J. The treatment and long-term prognosis of children with intracranial tumors: a study of 610 cases, 1950–1981. Int J Radiat Oncol Biol Phys 1990;18:723–45.
36. Hoffman HJ, Soloniuk DS, Humphreys RP, et al. Management and outcome of low-grade astrocytomas of the midline in children: a retrospective review. Neurosurgery 1993;33:964–71.
37. Pollack IF, Claassen D, Al-Shboul Q, et al. Low-grade gliomas of the cerebral hemispheres in children: an analysis of 71 cases. J Neurosurg 1995;82:536–47.
38. Gajjar A, Sanford RA, Heideman R, et al. Low-grade astrocytoma: a decade of experience at St. Jude Children's Research Hospital. J Clin Oncol 1997;15:2792–9.
39. McCormack BM, Miller DC, Budzilovich GN, et al. Treatment and survival of low-grade astrocytoma in adults—1977–1988. Neurosurgery 1992;31:636–42.
40. Medbery CA III, Straus KL, Steinberg SM, et al. Low grade astrocytomas: treatment results and prognostic variables. Int J Radiat Oncol Biol Phys 1988;15:837–41.
41. Philippon JH, Clemenceau SH, Fauchon FH, Foncin JF. Supratentorial low-grade astrocytomas in adults. Neurosurgery 1993;32:554–9.
42. Piepmeier JM. Observations on the current treatment of low-grade astrocytic tumors of the cerebral hemispheres. J Neurosurg 1987;67:177–81.
43. Leighton C, Fisher B, Bauman G, et al. Supratentorial low-grade glioma in adults: an analysis of prognostic factors and timing of radiation. J Clin Oncol 1997;15:1294–301.
44. Miralbell R, Balart J, Matias-Guiu X, et al. Radiotherapy for supratentorial low-grade gliomas: results and prognostic factors with special focus on tumor volume parameters. Radiother Oncol 1993;27:112–6.
45. Lote K, Egeland T, Hager B, et al. Survival, prognostic factors, and therapeutic efficacy in low-grade glioma: a retrospective study in 379 patients. J Clin Oncol 1997;15:3129–40.
46. Laws ER Jr, Taylor WF, Clifton MB, Okazaki H. Neurosurgical management of low-grade astrocytoma of the cerebral hemispheres. J Neurosurg 1984;61:665–73.
47. Reichenthal E, Feldman Z, Cohen ML, et al. Hemispheric supratentorial low-grade astrocytomas. Neurochirurgie 1992;35:18–22.
48. Rudoler S, Corn BW, Werner-Wasik M, et al. Patterns of tumor progression after radiotherapy for low-grade gliomas. Am J Clin Oncol 1998;21(1):23–27.
49. Berger MS, Ghatan S, Haglund MM, et al. Low-grade gliomas associated with intractable epilepsy: seizure outcome utilizing electrocorticography during tumor resection. J Neurosurg 1993;79:62–9.
50. Kirkpatrick PJ, Honavar M, Janota I, Polkey CE. Control of temporal lobe epilepsy following en bloc resection of low-grade tumors. J Neurosurg 1993;78:19–25.
51. Daumas-Duport C, Scheithauer BW, Kelly PJ. A histologic and cytologic method for spatial definition of gliomas. Mayo Clin Proc 1987;62:435–49.
52. Kelly PJ, Daumas-Duport C, Scheithauer BW, et al. Stereotactic histologic correlations of computed tomography and magnetic resonance imaging–defined abnormalities in patients with glial neoplasms. Mayo Clin Proc 1987;62:450–9.
53. McGirr SJ, Kelly PJ, Scheithauer BW. Stereotactic resection of juvenile pilocytic astrocytomas of the thalamus and basal ganglia. Neurosurgery 1987;20:447–52.
54. Schuurman PR, Troost D, Verbeeten B, Bosch DA. 5-year survival and clinical prognostic factors in progressive supratentorial diffuse "low-grade" astrocytoma: a retrospective analysis of 46 cases. Acta Neurochir (Wien) 1997;139:2–7.
55. Janny P, Cure H, Mohr M, et al. Low-grade supratentorial astrocytomas: management and prognostic factors. Cancer 1994;73:1937–45.
56. Shaw EG, Scheithauer BW, Gilbertson MS, et al. Postoperative radiotherapy of supratentorial low-grade gliomas. Int J Radiat Oncol Biol Phys 1989;16:663–8.
57. Shibamoto Y, Kitakabu Y, Takahashi M, et al. Supratentorial low-grade astrocytoma: correlation of computed tomography findings with effect of radiation therapy and prognostic variables. Cancer 1992;72:190–5.
58. Silverman C, Marks J. Prognostic significance of contrast enhancement in low-grade astrocytomas of the adult cerebrum. Radiology 1981;139:211–3.
59. Recht LD, Lew R, Smith TW. Suspected low-grade glioma: is deferring treatment safe? Ann Neurol 1992;31:431–6.
60. Cairncross JG, Laperriere NJ. Low-grade glioma—to treat or not to treat? Arch Neurol 1990;46:1238.
61. Morantz RA. Radiation therapy in the treatment of cerebral astrocytoma. Neurosurgery 1987;20:975–82.
62. Recht LD, Lew R, Smith TW. Suspected low-grade glioma: is deferring treatment safe? Ann Neurol 1992;31:431–6.
63. Shaw E. The low-grade glioma debate: evidence defending the position of early radiation therapy. Clin Neurosurg 1995;42:488–94.
64. Shaw EG. Low-grade gliomas: to treat or not to treat? A radiation oncologist's viewpoint [editorial]. Arch Neurol 1990;47:1138–9.
65. Karim ABMF, Cornu P, Bleehen N, et al. Immediate postoperative radiotherapy in low-grade glioma improves progression-free survival but not overall survival: preliminary results of an EORTC/MRC randomized trial [abstract]. Proc ASCO 1998;17:400a.
66. Wilden JN, Kelly PJ. CT computerized stereotactic biopsy for low-density CT lesions presenting with epilepsy. J Neurol Neurosurg Psychiatry 1987;50:1302–5.
67. Kondziolka D, Lunsford LID, Martinez AJ. Unreliability of contemporary neurodiagnostic imaging in evaluating suspected adult supratentorial (low-grade) astrocytoma. J Neurosurg 1993;79:533–6.
68. Nicolato A, Gerosa MA, Fina P, et al. Prognostic factors in low-grade supratentorial astrocytomas: a uni- and multivariate statistical analysis in 76 surgically treated adult patients. Surg Neurol 1995;44:208–23.
69. Piepmeier J, Christopher S, Spencer D, et al. Variations in the natural history and survival of patients with supratentorial low-grade astrocytomas. Neurosurgery 1996;38:872–9.
70. Bahary JP, Villemure JG, Choi S, et al. Low-grade pure and

mixed cerebral astrocytomas treated in the CT scan era. J Neurooncol 1996;27:173–7.
71. Scerrati M, Roselli R, Iacoangeli M, et al. Prognostic factors in low-grade (WHO grade II) gliomas of the cerebral hemispheres: the role of surgery. J Neurol Neurosurg Psychiatry 1996;61:291–6.
72. Celli P, Nofrone I, Palma L, et al. Cerebral oligodendroglioma: prognostic factors and life history. Neurosurgery 1994;6:1018–35.
73. Mork SJ, Lindegaard K-F, Halvorsen TB, et al. Oligodendroglioma: incidence and biologic behavior in a defined population. J Neurosurg 1985;3:881–9.
74. Shaw EG, Scheithauer BW, O'Fallow JR. Oligodendrogliomas: the Mayo Clinic experience. J Neurosurg 1992;76:428–34.
75. Berger MS, Deliganis AV, Dobbins J, Keles GE. The effect of extent of resection on recurrent patients with low-grade cerebral hemisphere gliomas. Cancer 1994;74:1784–91.
76. Lunsford LD, Somaza S, Kondziolka D, Flickinger JC. Survival after stereotactic biopsy and irradiation of cerebral non-anaplastic, non-pilocytic astrocytoma. J Neurosurg 1995;82:523–9.
77. Shaw EG, Daumas-Duport C, Scheithauer BW, et al. Radiation therapy in the management of low-grade supratentorial astrocytomas. J Neurosurg 1989;70:853–61.
78. Westergaard L, Gjerris F, Klinken L. Prognostic parameters in benign astrocytomas. Acta Neurochir (Wien) 1993;123:1–7.
79. Bullard DE, Rawlings CE III, Phillips B, et al. Oligodendroglioma: an analysis of the value of radiation therapy. Cancer 1987;60:2179–88.
80. Chin HW, Hazel JJ, Kim TH, Webster JH. Oligodendrogliomas: 1. A clinical study of cerebral oligodendrogliomas. Cancer 1980;45:1458–66.
81. Gannett DE, Wisbeck WM, Silbergeld DL, Berger MS. The role of postoperative irradiation in the treatment of oligodendroglioma. Int J Radiat Oncol Biol Phys 1994;30:567–73.
82. Kros J, Pieterman H, van Eden CG, Avezaat CJJ. Oligodendroglioma: the Rotterdam-Dijkzigt experience. Neurosurgery 1994;34:959–66.
83. Lindegaard KF, Mørk SJ, Eide GE, et al. Statistical analysis of clinicopathological features, radiotherapy, and survival in 170 cases of oligodendroglioma. J Neurosurg 1987;67:224–30.
84. Reedy DP, Bay JW, Hahn JF. Role of radiation therapy in the treatment of cerebral oligodendroglioma: an analysis of 57 cases and a literature review. Neurosurgery 1983;13:499–503.
85. Shimizu KT, Tran LM, Mark RJ, Selch MT. Management of oligodendrogliomas. Radiology 1993;186:569–72.
86. Wallner KE, Gonzales M, Sheline GE. Treatment of oligodendrogliomas with or without postoperative irradiation. J Neurosurg 1988;68:684–8.
87. Rogers LR, Morris HH, Lupica K. Effect of cranial irradiation on seizure frequency in adults with low grade astrocytoma and medically intractable epilepsy. Neurology 1993;43:1599–601.
88. Vertosick FT, Selker RG, Arena VC. Survival of patients with well-differentiated astrocytomas diagnosed in the era of computed tomography. Neurosurgery 1991;28:496–501.
89. Rutten EH, Kazam I, Sloof JL, Walder AH. Post-operative radiation therapy in the management of brain astrocytomas—retrospective study of 142 patients. Int J Radiat Oncol Biol Phys 1981;7:191–5.
90. Karim AB, Maat B, Hatlevoll R, et al. A randomized trial on dose-response in radiation therapy of low-grade cerebral glioma: EORTC Study 22844. Int J Radiat Oncol Biol Phys 1996;36:549–56.
91. Shaw EG, Arusell R, Scheithauer B, et al. A prospective randomized trial of low- versus high-dose radiation therapy in adults with supratentorial low-grade glioma: initial report of a NCCTG-RTOG-ECOG Study [abstract]. Proc ASCO 1998;17:401a.
92. Pozza F, Colombo F, Chierego G, et al. Low-grade astrocytomas: treatment with unconventionally fractionated external beam stereotactic radiation therapy. Radiology 1989;171:565–9.
93. Souhami L, Olivier A, Podgorsak EB, et al. Fractionated stereotactic radiation therapy for intracranial tumors. Cancer 1991;68:2101–8.
94. Somoza SC, Kondziolka D, Lunsford LD, et al. Early outcomes after stereotactic radiosurgery for growing pilocytic astrocytomas in children. Pediatr Neurosurg 1996;25:109–15.
95. Hara A, Nishimura Y, Sakai N, et al. Effectiveness of intraoperative radiation therapy for recurrent supratentorial low grade glioma. J Neurooncol 1995;25:239–43.
96. Mundinger F, Ostertag CB, Birg W, Weigel K. Stereotactic treatments of brain lesions. Appl Neurophysiol 1980;43:198–204.
97. Szikla G, Schhenger M, Blond S. Interstitial and combined interstitial and external irradiation of supratentorial gliomas—results of 61 cases treated 1973–1981. Acta Neurochir (Wien) 1984;33:355–62.
98. Schomberg PJ, Kelly PJ, Earle JD, Anderson JA. Phosphorus-32 therapy of cystic brain tumors [abstract]. Int J Radiat Oncol Biol Phys 1988;15(Suppl 1):157.
99. Sheline G, Wara WM, Smith V. Therapeutic irradiation in brain injury. Int J Radiat Oncol Biol Phys 1980;6:1215–28.
100. Crossen JR, Garwood D, Glatstein E, Neuwelt EA. Neurobehavioral sequelae of cranial irradiation in adults: a review of radiation-induced encephalopathy. J Clin Oncol 1994;12:627–42.
101. Taphoorn MJB, Schiphorst AK, Snoek FJ, et al. Cognitive functions and quality of life in patients with low-grade gliomas: the impact of radiotherapy. Ann Neurol 1994;36:48–54.
102. Curran D, Kiebert GM, Aaronson NK, et al. Quality of life after radiation therapy of cerebral low-grade gliomas of the adult: results of a phase III randomized trial on dose response (EORTC Trial 22844) [abstract]. Proc ASCO 1998;17:379a.
103. Kleinberg L, Wallner K, Malkin MG. Good performance status of long-term disease-free survivors of intracranial gliomas. Int J Radiat Oncol Biol Phys 1993;26:129–33.
104. Hammack J, Shaw E, Ivnik R, et al. Neurocognitive function in patients receiving radiation therapy for supratentorial low-grade glioma: a North Central Cancer Treatment Group prospective study [abstract]. Proc ASCO 1995;14:151a.
105. Eyre HJ, Crowley JJ, Townsend JJ, et al. A randomized trial of radiotherapy versus radiotherapy plus CCNU for

105. incompletely resected low-grade gliomas: a Southwest Oncology Group study. J Neurosurg 1993;78:909–14
106. Buckner JC, Smith JS, Nelson DF, et al. Phase II trial of procarbazine, CCNU, and vincristine (PCV) as initial therapy in patients with low-grade oligodendroglioma or oligoastrocytoma: efficacy results and associations with chromosome 1p and 19q loss [abstract]. Proc ASCO 1999;18:140a.
107. Mason WP, Krol GS, DeAngelis LM. Low-grade oligodendroglioma responds to chemotherapy. Neurology 1996; 46:203–7.
108. Buckner JC, Burch PA, Schaefer PL. Phase II trial of nitrogen mustard, vincristine, and procarbazine (MOP) in patients with recurrent glioma: NCCTG Results [abstract]. Proc ASCO 1996;15:155a.
109. Buckner JC, Brown LD, Kugler JW, et al. Phase II evaluation of recombinant inteferon alpha and BCNU in recurrent glioma. J Neurosurg 1995;82:430–5.
110. Cairncross G, Macdonald D, Ludwin S, et al. Chemotherapy for anaplastic oligodendroglioma. NCIC Clinical Trials Group. J Clin Oncol 1994;12:2013–21.
111. Kleihues P, Cavanee WK. Pathology and genetics of tumours of the nervous system. Lyon (France): International Agency for Research on Cancer; 1998. p. 34–6, 53, 182–4.
112. Burger PC, Scheithauer BW, editors. Atlas of tumor pathology: tumors of the central nervous system. 3rd Series, Fascicle 10. Washington (DC): Armed Forces Institute of Pathology; 1994. p. 96–105, 133–6, 163–72, 178–87.
113. Morreale VM, Ebersold MJ, Quast LM, Parisi JE. Cerebellar astrocytoma: experience with 54 cases surgically treated at the Mayo Clinic, Rochester, Minnesota, from 1978 to 1990. J Neurosurg 1997;87:257–61.
114. Sutton LN, Cnaan A, Klatt L, et al. Postoperative surveillance imaging in children with cerebellar astrocytomas. J Neurosurg 1996;84:721–5.
115. Strom EH, Skullerud K. Pleomorphic xanthoastrocytoma—report of 5 cases. Clin Neuropathol 1982;2:188–91.
116. Whittle IR, Gordon A, Misra BK, et al. Pleomorphic xanthoastrocytoma—report of four cases. J Neurosurg 1989;70:463–8.
117. Krouwer HG, Davis RL, McDermott MW, et al. Gangliogliomas: a clinicopathological study of 25 cases and review of the literature. J Neurooncol 1993;17:139–54.
118. Kim DG, Paek SH, Kim IH, et al. Central neurocytoma: the role of radiation therapy and long term outcome. Cancer 1997;79:1995–2002.
119. Kapp JR, Paulson GW, Odom GL. Brain tumors with tuberous sclerosis. J Neurosurg 1967;26:191–202.
120. Chow CW, Klug GL, Lewis EA. Subependymal giant-cell astrocytoma in children. J Neurosurg 1988;68:880–3.
121. Lombardi D, Scheithauer BW, Meyer FB, et al. Symptomatic subependymoma: a clinicopathologic and flow cytometric study. J Neurosurg 1991;75:583–8.
122. Afra D, Müller W. Recurrent low-grade gliomas: dedifferentiation and prospects of reoperation. In: Karim ABMF, Laws ER, editors. Glioma. Berlin Heidelberg: Springer-Verlag; 1991. p. 189.
123. Francavilla TL, Miletich RS, Di Chiro G, et al. Positron emission tomography in the detection of malignant degeneration of low-grade gliomas. Neurosurgery 1989;24:1–5.
124. Kline JL, Noto RB, Glantz M. Single-photon emission CT in the evaluation of recurrent brain tumors in patients treated with gamma knife radiosurgery or conventional radiation therapy. AJNR Am J Neuroradiol 1996;17:1681–6.
125. Dillon WP, Nelson S. What is the role of MR spectroscopy in the evaluation and treatment of brain neoplasms? AJNR Am J Neuroradiol 1999;20:2–3.
126. Forsyth PA, Kelly PJ, Cascino TI, et al. Radiation necrosis or glioma recurrence: is computer assisted stereotactic biopsy useful? J Neurosurg 1995;82:436–44.
127. Civitello LA, Packer RJ, Rorke LB, et al. Leptomeningeal dissemination of low-grade gliomas in childhood. Neurology 1988;38:562–6.

Surgical Considerations in Childhood Brain Tumors

G. EVREN KELES, MD
MITCHEL S. BERGER, MD

This chapter will focus on the surgical management of the most common pediatric brain tumors: cerebellar astrocytomas, medulloblastoma, ependymoma, hemispheric low-grade gliomas, brainstem tumors, optic and diencephalic tumors, and tumors of the pineal region. Histopathologic and neuroimaging characteristics of pediatric brain tumors, as well as their clinical characteristics and oncologic management, are discussed in detail in Chapters 3, 6, and 19.

Surgical resection or biopsy is the initial therapeutic modality in the management of children with brain tumors. This applies to all pediatric brain tumors, with the following exceptions: (a) optic nerve glioma in children with excellent vision or neurofibromatosis, (b) diffuse pontine or hypothalamic glioma without exophytic components, and (c) subependymal giant cell astrocytoma without symptomatic ventriculomegaly in a child with tuberous sclerosis.

In addition to potentially removing the tumor and providing a tissue diagnosis to guide further therapy, resection permits management of increased intracranial pressure (ICP) and decompression of adjacent brain structures.

Warming pads, heated fluid bags, and an elevated room temperature are used to maintain the child's normal physiologic temperature in the operating room. As children have a larger surface-to-volume ratio than adults, their core temperature has a tendency to decrease in a cold operating room, and, subsequently, hypothermia can lead to complications, including cardiac arrhythmias and hypotension. In addition, cortical-stimulation mapping will be difficult if the patient's temperature drifts too low, especially under general anesthesia. Patients are positioned appropriately for the operation, limbs partially flexed and all pressure points padded. In children younger than 2 years of age, the head is placed on a foam headrest or padded doughnut because the skull may become deformed or fractured if pin fixation is used. The endotracheal tube is fastened into place because even the slightest pressure may dislodge it during operation, and special care should be taken to cover the endotracheal tubing with towels to prevent the skin drapes from adhering to the tubing and inadvertently dislodging the endotracheal tube when the drapes are removed.

Following skin incision, scalp bleeding is prevented by direct pressure, and the incision is continued by using electrocautery or a contact laser. Moistened sponges are placed along the edges of the scalp incision to protect the tissue and are secured in place with Michele clips. Rainey clips are usually too large for younger children, and even when they do fit, they apply excessive force and may cause local scalp necrosis.

Contemporary neurosurgical methods, including ultrasonography, functional mapping, frameless navigational resection devices, and intraoperative imaging techniques enable the neurosurgeon to achieve more extensive resections with less morbidity. Intraoperative ultrasonography provides real-time intraoperative data and is helpful in detecting the tumor, delineating its margins, and differentiating tumor from peritumoral edema, cyst, necrosis, and adjacent normal brain. Although its use is limited by artifact from blood and surgical trauma at the margin of resection, it has been shown that postresection tumor volumes based on intraoperative ultrasonography are significantly correlated with those determined by postoperative magnetic resonance imaging (MRI).[1]

Stimulation mapping techniques are essential to minimize morbidity and to achieve radical resections of tumors located in or around cortical and subcortical functionally eloquent sites.[2] The use of these techniques will be discussed later with the resection of hemispheric tumors.

Frameless navigation systems are very helpful in preoperatively planning incisions and bone flaps as well as in guiding the initial phases of the resection. Shifting of the brain contents will necessarily limit the utility of these methods when resecting gliomas because localization is based on the preoperative scan findings.[3] However, stealth images correlated with real-time sononavigation data will allow the surgeon to account for the shift.

In addition, brain shifting will not be a factor when intraoperative imaging techniques are used. Unlike frameless and frame-based systems that are limited by their reliance on preoperative imaging, both intraoperative computed tomography (CT) and magnetic resonance (MR) scanning provide intraoperative updates of data sets for navigational systems.[3] Intraoperative re-registration of target anatomy eliminates the problem of brain shift that may be caused by resection or brain retractors and allows the surgeon to achieve resection control more precisely and to modify the pre-planned surgical approach if necessary. Intraoperative MRI requires MR-compatible instruments (ie, titanium or ceramic) to minimize artifact. Surgical instruments can be tracked with the use of light-emitting diode sensors to provide image guidance during movements and interactive feedback on corresponding images.[4–6]

CEREBELLAR ASTROCYTOMAS

Astrocytomas are the most common histologic type of brain tumor seen in the pediatric patient population. They represent approximately 22 percent of all central nervous system tumors seen in this age group, and cerebellar astrocytomas account for 5 to 8 percent of all gliomas and 35 to 40 percent of all posterior fossa tumors.[7–9]

Cerebellar astrocytomas are surgically curable in the vast majority of patients. Because of their location (which is often midline or paravermian) and their indolent growth characteristics, cerebellar astrocytomas are usually associated with a certain degree of well-compensated hydrocephalus that may necessitate treatment preoperatively, intraoperatively, or postoperatively. Cystic cerebellar astrocytomas tend to be located within the hemispheres whereas midline location with possible extension into one or both cerebellar hemispheres is more common in solid cerebellar astrocytomas, when compared with the cystic varieties (Figure 16–1A). Hemispheric location, however, is more common in older patients.[10]

For most patients, dexamethasone will alleviate symptoms related to increased ICP at admission and will allow time for rehydration and nourishment of the patient who is usually dehydrated due to vomiting. Severe lethargy or stupor, however, may necessitate external ventricular drainage (EVD) to gradually drain cerebrospinal fluid (CSF). This will not be needed pre- or intraoperatively if the ventricles are not demonstrated as dilated on the preoperative neuroimaging studies. As only 30 to 40 percent of children will need a permanent shunt following complete tumor removal and unblockage of the CSF pathways (ie, fourth ventricle and aqueduct), EVD has the advantage of avoiding unnecessary shunt insertion and the risks associated with this procedure.[11] In this clinical setting, the most significant risk following shunt placement is overdrainage, which may, due to the presence of a large mass in the posterior fossa, result in upward herniation of the superior cerebellum through the incisura, causing serious upper brainstem compression.

In patients with EVD in place, the drainage system is closed preoperatively and is used during surgery if the dura appears to be tight prior to its opening. The classic prone position or the Concorde position, where the head is slightly turned to the patient's right side and flexed, allows access to lesions extending into the aqueduct or into the superior midline cerebellum and to the tectal plate. The sitting position is used less frequently and is mostly

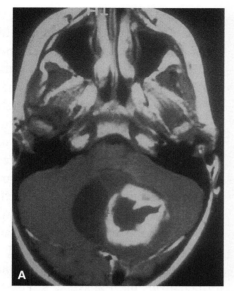 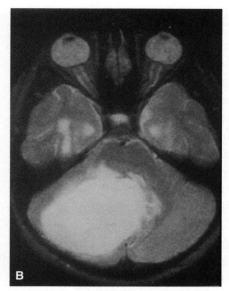

Figure 16–1. A, Contrast-enhanced T1-weighted axial magnetic resonance imaging (MRI) scan showing a large cystic cerebellar mass. It should be noted that the cyst wall does not enhance and does not contain tumor cells. B, T2-weighted axial MRI scan of a solid cerebellar astrocytoma.

limited to rostral tumors in older children or adults. A midline skin incision is used for midline or paravermian lesions, and a paramedian incision may be used for tumors confined to one cerebellar hemisphere without an extension to the midline. Following a large posterior fossa craniotomy or craniectomy extending from the inferior torcula to the foramen magnum (but not including removal of the C1 posterior arch), the dura is opened in the regular fashion, and CSF is drained from the cisterna magna if necessary due to increased pressure. For lesions that reach the cerebellar surface, an incision is made through the thinnest part of the cortex overlying the largest midportion of the tumor. For tumors located subcortically, a limited resection of the overlying cerebellar cortex may enable a better exposure and prevent possible traction injury to the vermis or cerebellar hemisphere. This approach, however, should be avoided around the inferior vermis, where surgical trauma may result in swallowing dysfunction and postoperative mutism due to damage to pathways involving oropharyngeal muscle coordination.[12]

The tumor is reddish brown and usually well demarcated from the surrounding normal tissue by compressed gliotic white matter. This is usually the case for cystic tumors with a mural nodule, lesions with a thick enhancing wall and a falsely cystic center, or those that are solid.[13,14] However, some solid tumors with midline involvement infiltrate the brain stem; in this case, a total resection becomes virtually impossible and would be associated with significant morbidity.[15] A gross total resection is usually feasible for tumors involving the cerebellar peduncles because the postoperative morbidity from operating in this area is generally mild and transient.[16] The goal of surgery is to achieve a total resection of the contrast-enhancing tumor tissue seen on preoperative imaging studies. Resection of a non-enhancing cyst wall is unnecessary as it does not contain tumor infiltration.[17] Following resection, the dura is closed in a watertight fashion with the use of autologous periosteum.

Postoperative neuroimaging studies are essential to assess the extent of resection and to detect any residual disease, in which case management options would include immediate reoperation or follow-up with reoperation at the time of documented progression. Persistent ventricular dilation following tumor removal, together with increased ICP symptoms, will often require placement of a shunt.[18] Another indication for CSF diversion is persistent pseudo-meningocele underlying the incision, which may also be treated with a lumboperitoneal or cystoperitoneal shunt.[19]

MEDULLOBLASTOMA

Medulloblastoma accounts for approximately 20 percent of all intracranial tumors in pediatric patients[20,21] (Figure 16–2). The surgical management of medulloblastoma attempts to fulfill two goals, namely, to ameliorate the symptoms of obstructive hydrocephalus and mass effect and to achieve a radical tumor resection.

Patients who present with symptoms of intracranial hypertension are often effectively managed with steroids preoperatively. If the clinical condition necessitates EVD prior to surgical decompression, drainage should not exceed 3 to 5 mL/h to avoid the risk of upward cerebellar herniation[22,23] or hemorrhage due to rapid supratentorial decompression.[24–26] Disadvantages of EVD management include traditional shunt-related complications.[22,27] Reports indicate that permanent CSF shunting should be performed if necessary in the postoperative period only. Of children with medulloblastoma, 40 to 60 percent will require permanent CSF shunting.[28,29] Concerns regarding an increased risk of systemic metastases facilitated by ventriculoperitoneal or ventriculoatrial shunting[30] have not been validated.[31] Filters have been used to minimize dissemination, but the association of these filters with shunt failure has precluded their routine use.[32]

The prone position or some variation thereof is generally preferred. This avoids the risk of serious complications such as air embolism, hypotension, and pneumocephalus and enhances visualization of the posterior fossa while reducing the surgeon's fatigue. In young children, a padded headrest shaped like a horseshoe supports the head. In older patients and in adults, the head is flexed and fixed in three points with a Mayfield clamp. In patients who have not had EVD placed preoperatively, a catheter may be inserted in the ventricle to drain CSF intraoperatively. Following a midline incision, a craniectomy is performed from the transverse sinuses to the foramen magnum. Laminectomy of CI is unnecessary for the complete resection of average-sized tumors but is often performed when the tumor is large. Laminectomies of C2 and below are typically avoided as they may cause instability and swan-neck deformity in young patients.[33] After opening, the dura is secured to the occipital periosteum to prevent torcular bleeding. Weck clips compatible with MRI are often used to occlude large dural sinuses and venous lakes at the foramen magnum. The cisterna magna is then opened, and the cerebellar surface is inspected for signs of tumor dissemination along the subarachnoid plane. The cerebellar tonsils are retracted laterally, and the inferior vermis is exposed. If the vermis is not infiltrated with tumor, it is opened in the midline until the surface of the tumor is exposed. Care is taken not to violate the inferior vermis to avoid mutism and pharyngeal dysfunction postoperatively. In the resection of tumors involving the fourth ventricle, a cerebellomedullary approach that avoids splitting the vermis and that avoids retraction on the dentate nuclei and outflow tracts may be used to decrease the frequency of postoperative cerebellar mutism syndrome.[34,35] Often, a plane can be easily developed between the medulloblastoma and surrounding parenchyma. The tumor is typically vascular and may be aspirated either with suction or with an ultrasonic aspirator. Following tumor removal (which should always include unblocking the aqueduct within the fourth ventricle, to re-establish CSF flow), the dura is re-approximated and closed in an attempted watertight

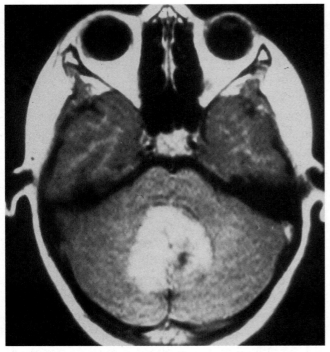

Figure 16–2. Medulloblastoma of the fourth ventricle, T1-weighted axial MRI scan.

fashion, using periosteum from the occipital region. If EVD is in place at the end of surgery, it should be elevated each day and subsequently removed at some time during the first 2 to 4 postoperative days when CSF is < 50 cc. If the patient develops headaches and lethargy, with evidence of enlarged ventricles on a CT scan during this process, a permanent shunt will almost always be necessary. Likewise, a large pseudomeningocele is cosmetically unacceptable and should be treated with a CSF diversion procedure. A postoperative scan, with and without intravenous contrast administration, should be performed within 2 to 3 days of surgery to minimize enhancement at the resection margins secondary to surgical trauma.

Postoperative mutism may be seen in 5 to 30 percent of patients who undergo surgery of the posterior fossa involving manipulation of the vermis.[36–38] The mutism and pharyngeal dysfunction are usually transient but may last up to 20 weeks. Other complications include tension pneumocephalus, Cushing's ulcers, and early postoperative seizures secondary to electrolyte abnormalities.[39]

Metastases outside of the posterior fossa are not uncommon, occurring in 5 to 15 percent of patients and involving (in decreasing order) the bone marrow, lymph nodes, and liver.[40] However, recurrence at the primary tumor site in the posterior fossa constitutes the most common pattern of failure.[41] In addition to infratentorial extension, supratentorial relapse may occur in almost half of all medulloblastoma recurrences.[41,42] Sites of intracranial dissemination include the infundibular stalk, the ventricular system, and the subfrontal subarachnoid space (although this is less common with modern radiation oncology techniques). A consensus exists that recurrences should be treated aggressively, with re-resection and adjuvant chemotherapy and radiation if the patient is eligible. Patients who relapse with leptomeningeal disease usually have a quickly progressive clinical decline despite therapy.

HEMISPHERIC TUMORS

In most pediatric series, cerebral hemisphere tumors account for 15 to 25 percent of all pediatric brain tumors and are almost twice as common in infants as in older children.[43] The most common histology among pediatric hemisphere tumors is low-grade astrocytomas, which constitute approximately half of all pediatric hemispheric tumors.[44] In addition to pilocytic and fibrillary astrocytomas, which are the most frequently encountered tumors, other histologies may be seen, such as pleomorphic xanthoastrocytoma, subependymal giant cell astrocytoma, high-grade gliomas, ganglioglioma and desmoplastic infantile ganglioglioma, primitive neuroectodermal tumors, astroblastoma, ependymoma, oligodendroglioma, choroid plexus tumors, and dysembryoplastic neuroepithelial tumors. The surgical goals are complete tumor removal, which is possible in most circumstances, and the alleviation of any associated intractable seizure disorder.

Epilepsy is a major presenting feature of pediatric patients with brain tumors.[45] The majority of patients with tumor-associated epilepsy harbor slow-growing, indolent neoplasms such as low-grade gliomas. In the majority of patients, including those patients with malignant gliomas, the seizures are infrequent and easily controlled with one antiepileptic drug. In this setting, removal of the tumor alone usually controls the epilepsy, with or without the need for additional anticonvulsants; however, children with indolent tumors may have seizure activity that is refractory to medical therapy. Optimal control of the epilepsy without postoperative anticonvulsants in this situation is provided when perioperative (ie, extraoperative or intraoperative) electrocorticographic mapping of separate seizure foci accompanies the tumor resection. When mapping is not used and a radical tumor resection is carried out with adjacent brain, the occurrence of seizures will be lessened, but most patients will have to remain on antiepileptic drugs.[46]

The operative position is dependent on the necessary exposure. In general, tumors involving the cerebral hemispheres may readily be approached in either the supine or the lateral decubitus position. The incision and underlying bone flap should be generous to allow for radical tumor resection, swelling during the procedure, and functional mapping if necessary. When a previous incision is present, care must be taken to extend the scalp opening by making perpendicular incisions from the scar lines, resulting in a wide base for each new portion of the scalp flap. The tumor is localized with intraoperative ultrasonography or surgical navigation systems. Because the dura is sensitive to pain, the area around the middle meningeal artery should be infiltrated with a lidocaine/bupivacaine mixture to alleviate discomfort while the patient is awake. As the motor cortex in children younger than 5 years of age is often resistant to electrical stimulation, the central sulcus in these children can be identified by eliciting motor or somatosensory evoked potentials although it may not be possible to map subcortical pathways.[2,47] Speech mapping is not necessary in children up to 2.5 years of age because speech function can redistribute to the contralateral hemisphere.[48]

For children with an intractable seizure disorder, preresection electrocorticography is performed. Strip electrodes are used for recordings from mesiobasal structures. In addition, recording along the hippocampus is obtained in appropriate patients following the removal of lateral temporal cortex and entry into the temporal horn of the lateral ventricle. Strip electrodes may also be used for the orbitofrontal cortex or under the bone flap if the cortical exposure is not adequate. The contact points of the electrodes are labeled with numbered tickets and photographed for permanent record. The preresection recording is carried out for 5 to 15 minutes. Intravenous infusion of methohexital (Brevital, 0.5 to 1 mg/kg) may be used to chemically induce ictal discharges if epileptiform activity is sparse.

Stimulation mapping should begin by first identifying the motor cortex (Figure 16–3). Using mul-

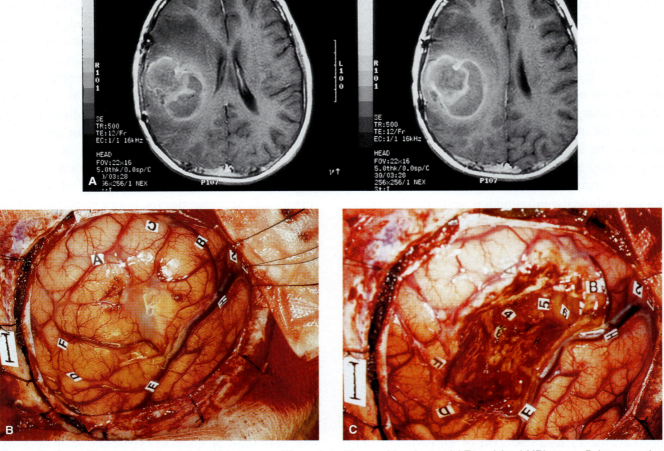

Figure 16–3. *A*, Recurrent right parietal glioblastoma multiforme in a 12-year-old patient, axial T1-weighted MRI scans. *B*, Intraoperative image, with letters demarcating the lesion. *C*, Stimulation of *1* and *2* revealed left hand movement. Numbers *4*, *5*, and *6*, are upper-extremity descending motor pathways.

tichannel electromyographic recordings in addition to visual observation of motor movements results in greater sensitivity, allowing the use of lower stimulation levels to evoke motor activity. First, the inferior aspect of the rolandic cortex is identified by eliciting responses in the face and hand. As the leg motor cortex is out of view against the falx, a strip electrode may be inserted along the falx, and stimulation using the same current applied to the lateral cortical surface may be delivered through it to evoke leg motor movements. Similarly, a subdural strip electrode may be inserted and stimulated to evoke the desired response if the craniotomy is near but not overlying the rolandic cortex. Following the identification of the motor cortex, the descending tracts may be found by using similar stimulation parameters. Descending motor and sensory pathways may be followed into the internal capsule and inferiorly to the brain stem and spinal cord. This is especially important during resection of infiltrative glial tumors because functioning motor, sensory, or language tissue can be located within macroscopically obvious tumor or surrounding infiltrated brain. A final postresection stimulation of cortical sites should be performed to confirm that the pathways are intact. This will also ensure that the underlying functional tracts have been preserved if subcortical responses have not been obtained. Even if the child's neurologic status is worse postoperatively, the presence of intact cortical and subcortical motor pathways will imply that the deficit will be transient and will resolve in days to weeks. Although somatosensory evoked potenhals (SSEPs) may be helpful in identifying the central sulcus, they do not help to localize descending subcortical motor and sensory white-matter tracts. Determination of the subcortical pathways is important while removing a deeply located tumor within or adjacent to the corona radiata, the internal capsule, the insula, the supplementary motor area, and the thalamus. As the current that is spread from the electrode contacts is minimal during bipolar stimulation, resection is stopped when movement or paresthesia is evoked.

If the tumor involves the dominant temporal, mid to posterior frontal, and mid to anterior inferior parietal lobes, identification of language sites prior to tumor removal is essential to minimize morbidity (Figure 16–4). After bone removal under propofol anesthesia, the patient is kept awake during language mapping. The electrocorticography equipment is placed on the field and attached to the skull after the motor pathways have been identified. The recording electrode–cortex contact point is stimulated using the bipolar electrode with the electrocorticography in progress. This stimulation may result in afterdischarge potentials, seen on the monitor. The presence of such afterdischarge potentials indicates that the stimulation current is too high and must be decreased by 1 to 2 mA until no afterdischarge potential is present following stimulation. At this point, the patient is asked to count from 1 to 50 while the bipolar stimulation probe is placed near the inferior aspect of the motor strip to identify Broca's area. Interruption of the counting (ie, complete speech arrest without oropharyngeal movement) localizes Broca's area. Speech arrest (eg, the complete interruption of counting) is usually localized to the area directly anterior to the face motor cortex. Using this ideal stimulation current, object-naming slides are presented and changed every 4 seconds, and the patient is expected to correctly name the object during stimulation mapping. The answers are carefully recorded. To ensure that there is no stimulation-induced error in the form of anomia and dysnomia, each cortical site is checked three times. All cortical sites essential for naming are marked on the surface of the brain with sterile numbered tickets.

A negative stimulation mapping may not provide the necessary security to proceed confidently with the resection. Therefore, it is essential to document where language is located, as well as where it is not located (if feasible). This is also the reason for having a generous exposure, not only to maximize the extent of resection but also to minimize the possibility of obtaining negative data. It has been shown that the distance of the resection margin from the nearest language site is the most important factor in determining the improvement in preoperative language deficits, the duration of postoperative language deficits, and whether the postoperative language deficits are permanent. Significantly fewer permanent language deficits occur if the distance of the resection margin from the nearest language site is > 1 cm.

A gross-total tumor resection based on ultrasonography and navigation findings, gross inspection, and frozen-section analysis of resection margins is usually attempted. Following tumor removal, postresection electrocorticography is always performed in patients with identifiable preresection seizure foci. Although obvious epileptiform foci persistent on postresection electrocorticograms are

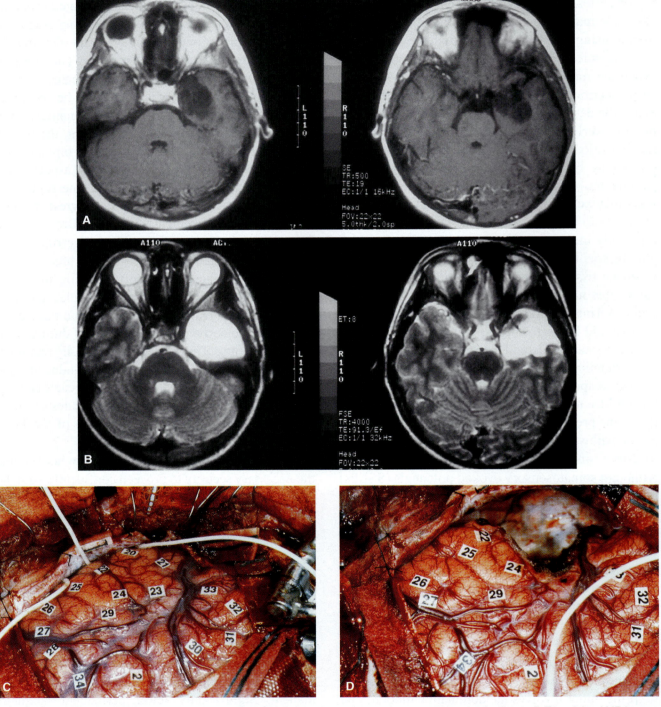

Figure 16–4. *A*, T1-weighted axial magnetic resonance (MR) images of a left mesial temporal low-grade glioma. *B*, T2-weighted MR images of same. *C*, Number *2* is the motor cortex; other numbers were tested for naming and reading functions. A strip electrode is placed under the temporal lobe to test mesial seizure activity seen on the cortex adjacent to the lesion. D, Postresection intraoperative view.

resected, occasional spike activity is not pursued, especially when it involves functional cortex. New discharging areas in postresection recordings are regarded as postresection activation phenomena unless they were independent or clearly epileptiform. Resected seizure foci are documented in regard to their relationship with the tumor nidus and are routinely submitted for histopathologic analysis. Preoperative insertion of a subdural grid electrode array that will provide ictal and interictal information may be necessary in children younger than 11 or 12 years of age.

For juvenile pilocytic astrocytomas, which are often cystic with an accompanying solid portion, it is important (in addition to removing the solid component) to resect the contrast-enhancing cyst wall, which is an extension of the tumor, to prevent recurrence.[49] Non-enhancing cyst wall is not infiltrated by the tumor, and resection is not necessary.[17]

High-grade astrocytomas and primitive neuroectodermal tumors are more vascular and more infiltrative and are approached with the intention of a gross-total resection. Subependymal giant cell astrocytomas associated with tuberous sclerosis are always located within the lateral ventricular system, usually at the level of the foramen of Monro, and are often accompanied by ventriculomegaly. If the lesion is not causing hydrocephalus, it should not be removed until symptoms develop. It can be approached through the cortex and lateral ventricle or transcallosally. Pleomorphic xanthoastrocytoma, desmoplastic infantile ganglioglioma, and astroblastoma almost always present as circumscribed masses with a pseudocapsule. The surgical goal is to achieve a complete resection. Gangliogliomas and desmoplastic infantile ganglioglioma should be approached with the same intention, which results in the greatest likelihood of long-term control.[50–52]

BRAINSTEM TUMORS

Brainstem tumors include tumors that originate from the mesencephalon, pons, and medulla and comprise approximately 10 percent of all pediatric brain tumors.[53] The tumor's location and histology direct treatment plans and prognosis. Patients with diffuse gliomas that involve the pons and other portions of the brain stem are not surgical candidates. Magnetic resonance imaging, together with clinical characteristics, is usually diagnostic.[40] Patients with focal cystic, exophytic, and cervicomedullary tumors frequently benefit from surgery. The goals of surgery are to obtain a histologic diagnosis, to reduce tumor bulk, and to re-establish CSF flow. Low-grade tumors usually displace surrounding neural structures and are therefore amenable to resection. Higher-grade tumors diffusely infiltrate functional anatomic structures, and resection will cause significant neurologic morbidity. As there is no safe surgical plane between the tumor and the brain stem, the general surgical approach is to resect from the inside of the tumor outward until the normal white matter appears.

The most common brainstem glioma is the diffuse intrinsic tumor (Figure 16–5). Surgical excision has no role in the management of these tumors. Stereotactic biopsy is usually nonpredictive, does not alter therapy, and may increase morbidity.[54,55] A stereotactic biopsy is rarely indicated only if the

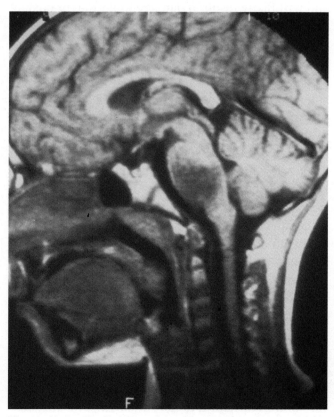

Figure 16–5. Sagittal T1-weighted magnetic resonance image depicting a diffuse infiltrative brainstem glioma.

diagnosis is questionable. This is more often the case in adults, who have a broader spectrum of pontine pathologies than children. Associated hydrocephalus is severe enough in 20 to 30 percent of cases to necessitate the placement of a shunt at the time of diagnosis.[56] These patients are candidates for conformal radiotherapy and chemotherapy.

Dorsally exophytic brainstem tumors protrude posteriorly from the floor of the fourth ventricle into the fourth ventricle. These tumors are typically low-grade astrocytomas. Surgically, they can be approached similarly to midline cerebellar neoplasms. There is a distinct boundary between the tumor and the adjacent cerebellum, but the mass arises diffusely from the floor of the fourth ventricle. The bulk of the tumor, which is the exophytic portion, can be removed, and its origins become apparent as the resection progresses. The floor of the fourth ventricle must be identified prior to resecting the ventral portions of the tumor. The exophytic portion is aspirated until a thin layer of tumor tissue remains on the ventricular floor. Resection of the part located within the brain stem is not indicated and will likely result in damage to normal brainstem structures. Progression can be treated with reoperation, chemotherapy, or radiotherapy.

Focal tumors are usually indolent and may be solid or cystic or have an exophytic component. For solid tumors, in addition to classic anatomic landmarks, mapping techniques to identify motor nuclei of the cranial nerves in the floor of the fourth ventricle are helpful in determining the point of entry.[57,58] Tissue for histologic examination is obtained initially, and the resection begins from the central portion of the tumor using the ultrasonic aspirator. The resection continues until the consistency of the tissue begins to change to normal. Focal cystic tumors are typically pilocytic astrocytomas and are treated accordingly by aspiration of the cyst material and excision of the solid component. Aspiration of the cyst alone is not sufficient as the cyst fluid will recollect and symptoms will reappear.[59] For focal brainstem tumors with an exophytic component, the excision starts from the exophytic portion and continues into the central part, with the same principles used for solid brainstem tumors. A subtemporal transtentorial route may be used for tumors of the cerebellar peduncle or for tumors located laterally. For all focal brainstem tumors, postresection bleeding control is achieved by using hemostatic agents and not by coagulating bleeding vessels located in the normal parenchyma. Although tectal tumors are rare, the majority of children with them present with hydrocephalus secondary to aqueductal stenosis and require shunting or endoscopic third ventriculostomy. The histology is typically that of pilocytic astrocytoma. These patients have a non-enhancing lesion confined to the tectal plate and are followed up with serial MR scans. No further intervention is indicated unless there is evidence of disease progression.

Cervicomedullary tumors are usually low-grade gliomas. Their growth pattern from the upper cervical cord into the medulla typically does not invade the decussating pyramidal tracts. An exophytic growth into the cisterna magna and caudal fourth ventricle may be observed. This growth pattern does not apply to higher-grade gliomas, which tend to infiltrate decussating fibers. A suboccipital craniectomy with cervical laminotomies is performed as necessary to expose the lower pole of the lesion. Intraoperative ultrasonography may be used to confirm proper exposure. The surgical approach to the intraspinal portion is through a posterior midline myelotomy. The resection proceeds caudally and rostrally, followed by excision of the intracranial portion with special attention to the posterior inferior cerebellar artery, which is usually located between the tumor, the medulla, and the inferior cerebellar hemisphere. It is also important to identify the floor of the fourth ventricle rostral to the tumor and not to extend the myelotomy beyond the obex rostrally. Spinal neurophysiologic monitoring of sensory and motor pathways may be helpful during excision of the spinal portion.

EPENDYMOMAS

Ependymomas make up between 6 and 15 percent of childhood primary brain tumors.[60–62] Approximately two-thirds of ependymomas occur in the posterior fossa, and the remaining third occur in the supratentorial compartment. Posterior fossa tumors are more common in younger children whereas supratentorial lesions tend to be more common in children over the age of 3 years. Infratentorial ependymomas frequently arise from the ependyma of the fourth ventricle but also may originate in the foramina of Luschka, the posterior cerebral aqueduct, or the lateral medullary velum. Supratentorial ependymomas are typically located adjacent to the lateral ventricles. The goals of surgery are to make a definitive tissue diagnosis, achieve a gross-total resection of the tumor, and re-establish CSF flow. Preoperative MR images are obtained for surgical planning and intraoperative frameless stereotactic-image guidance (Figure 16–6). We prefer to obtain MR images for staging spinal disease preoperatively as well to avoid the complicating factor of blood products in the subarachnoidal space, which can obscure a postoperative staging spinal MRI scan.

For infratentorial ependymomas, preoperative intravenous dexamethasone may reduce the incidence of postoperative oropharyngeal apraxia and aseptic meningitis.[12] If the patient's clinical condition warrants it, EVD may be placed to drain CSF at a controlled slow rate of 3 to 5 cc/h. The inferior extent of the tumor should be identified on the preoperative MRI scans to avoid unnecessary cervical laminectomy. Osmotic diuretics are rarely necessary when a ventriculostomy is used. Under general anesthesia and standard neuroanesthetic monitoring conditions, the child is placed in the Concorde position. In the case of lateral ependymomas arising from the lateral medullary velum or the foramen of Luschka, a lateral decubitus position, with the nose parallel to the floor, is preferred. For these lesions, adequate exposure may also be achieved in the supine position, with the head turned to the opposite side and tilted downward to minimize the amount of cerebellar tissue obscuring the lesion. For fourth ventricle ependymomas, a midline incision is made from above the inion to the midcervical region, depending on the caudal extent of the tumor. The suboccipital craniectomy should include the foramen magnum and one cervical lamina above the most caudal extent of the tumor. Removal of the inferior end of the tumor is usually possible beneath an intact lamina, and this helps to prevent postoperative swan-neck deformities, particularly in younger patients. The dura is opened in a stellate fashion based superiorly at the torcular herophili. Stay sutures are

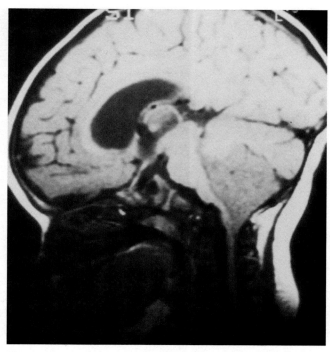

Figure 16–6. Sagittal T1-weighted magnetic resonance image of an ependymoma extending caudally through the foramen magnum.

placed superiorly to tack the dura to periosteum and are left in place at closure to prevent the formation of hematoma from sinus bleeding. For more lateral tumors, a straight retromastoid scalp incision is made with the patient in the lateral decubitus position. The dural flap is based on the transverse and sigmoid sinuses. Drainage of CSF from the cisterna magna facilitates the resection. Midline ependymomas are often initially visible in the cisterna magna as distinct gray, soft tumors with flecks of mineralization (Figure 16–7). After the portion extending into the superior cervical canal is resected, the resection continues along the floor of the fourth ventricle with gentle aspiration or with the ultrasonic aspirator on a low setting. The white floor of the fourth ventricle is identified before an attempt is made to remove the tumor from its point of attachment. It is important to avoid splitting the inferior vermis by more than 1 cm. The tumor can usually be aspirated off the cranial nerves and vascular structures without causing injury. When approaching the cerebellopontine angle, the surgeon may use a partial resection of the lateral 1 or 2 cm of the cerebellar hemisphere to facilitate exposure. Once the resection is completed, the resection cavity is inspected

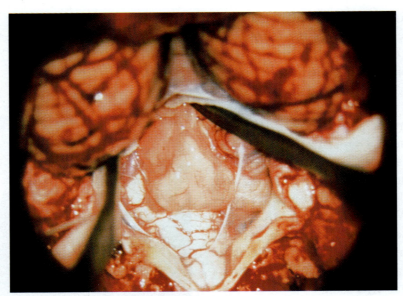

Figure 16–7. Intraoperative microscope view of an ependymoma protruding caudally and compressing the cervical spinal cord.

with small angled mirrors to identify any remaining fragments. After gentle irrigation, squares of Surgicel are used to line any exposed white matter. The inferior dura is closed primarily whereas the superior dural stay sutures are left in place to tamponade any sinus bleeding. An autogenous periosteal patch is removed and used to complete the dural closure.

For supratentorial ependymomas, the patient's position and the skin incision are dependent on the tumor location. More than half of supratentorial ependymomas are located in the periventricular areas of the cerebral hemispheres, and the location of the remainder is mostly or totally intraventricular.[63,64] Use of an image-guided frameless stereotactic system will significantly facilitate incision and bone flap planning, tumor localization, determination of the relationship of the tumor to surrounding anatomic structures, and intraoperative assessment of the extent of resection. Depending on the location of the tumor and its relationship with functionally eloquent areas, cortical and subcortical mapping techniques may be useful for minimizing morbidity.[2] Intraventricular lesions usually are more clearly encapsulated than periventricular lesions. It is important to minimize the collection of blood in the ventricular system during surgery so that postoperative chemical meningitis or hydrocephalus may be avoided. Similarly, postresection hemostasis and control of blood pressure are essential. A ventriculostomy may be placed if the resection cavity is contiguous with the ventricular system.

If a ventriculostomy was placed preoperatively or at the time of the resection, EVD is continued, with the drip chamber initially 5 cm above the eyebrow. It is then elevated by 3 to 5 cm per day until less than 50 cc of CSF is collected in a 24-hour period. If an EVD device does not provide sufficient drainage, or if a persistent pseudomeningocele develops, a ventriculoperitoneal shunt is indicated.

In patients with ependymomas, the extent of tumor resection is the single most significant prognostic factor, with gross total resections being associated with a better overall outcome.[63] An early postoperative MRI scan is obtained (within 2 to 3 days) to assess the extent of resection and to aid in postoperative therapy. Ependymoma recurrences are usually at the primary site. Disseminated disease, although seen 2 to 3 times more frequently at autopsy, is only present in 12 percent of patients at the time of initial diagnosis.[65]

OPTIC AND DIENCEPHALIC GLIOMAS

As optic and diencephalic gliomas often are not confined to a single anatomic site, naming these lesions according to their exact anatomic location may be misleading, especially for tumors with radiologically ill-defined borders. As only 10 percent of optic nerve gliomas are confined to one optic nerve and as approximately 30 percent are bilateral, the majority of optic nerve gliomas involve the chiasm or the hypothalamus[66] (Figure 16–8). Optic chiasmatic and hypothalamic gliomas are often referred to as a single entity because of their potential to infiltrate both anatomic sites regardless of the original location of the tumor (Figure 16–9).

Optic pathway gliomas account for 4 to 6 percent of all central nervous system tumors in the pediatric age group. Overall, neurofibromatosis is present in approximately one-third of patients with optic pathway tumors. Approximately 15 to 20 percent of patients with type 1 neurofibromatosis will have an optic glioma on MRI scan, but only 1 to 5 percent become symptomatic.[67] There is a higher likelihood of neurofibromatosis in patients who have multicentric optic gliomas, and there is a relatively lower incidence of neurofibromatosis in patients with chiasmatic tumors.[68]

Locally, hypothalamic and optic gliomas may extend laterally, invading the perivascular space along the arteries of the circle of Willis, and may expand posteriorly toward the brain stem as well, with rostral invagination into the third ventricle. Patients with chiasmatic and hypothalamic gliomas have an increased risk for disease dissemination along the neuraxis.[69] It has been reported that the risk of multicentric dissemination is increased approximately 20-fold in this group of patients when compared to those with low-grade gliomas located elsewhere.[70]

The only indication for resection of a unilateral optic nerve tumor is when vision is absent or nonfunctional. In addition, it is generally agreed that the exophytic portion of the lesion should be removed if vision is reasonable and that nonresectable unilateral optic nerve lesions should be decompressed at the optic canal. Regardless of the patient's neurofibromatosis status, a biopsy is not needed for chiasmatic hypothalamic mass lesions if the MRI scan is typical, that is, the chiasm or optic nerve(s) or both are affected with an expanded sella and involvement of optic tracts. For patients without neurofibromatosis who have a chiasmatic hypothalamic mass lesion and an atypical MRI scan, surgical intervention to define histopathologic type and to achieve debulking of a symptomatic large tumor is the initial approach. Some neurosurgeons limit their surgical indications to a subset of exophytic or cystic tumors with significant mass effect and hydrocephalus. However, a progressive visual deficit or progression depicted on follow-up MRI scans will necessitate surgical intervention, regardless of the presence or absence of neurofibromatosis, if there is an exophytic or cystic component. As 10 to 20 percent of children younger than 10 years of age with neurofi-

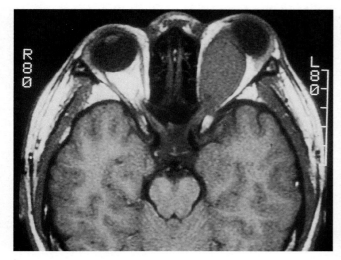

Figure 16–8. Axial T1-weighted magnetic resonance imaging scan showing a left intraorbital optic nerve glioma without extension to the chiasm.

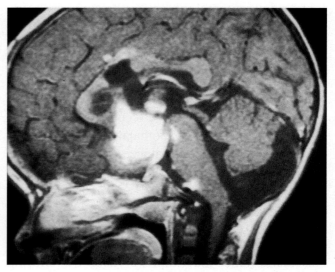

Figure 16–9. Sagittal T1-weighted contrast-enhanced MRI scan showing a diencephalic pilocytic astrocytoma with metastases.

bromatosis may have an asymptomatic low-grade glioma of the optic pathways, biopsy is not considered mandatory for asymptomatic neurofibromatosis patients with a chiasmatic or diencephalic tumor.[66,71] This subgroup of patients (ie, those with no deficit) may be followed with hormone medications and CSF shunting if necessary. In addition to general anesthesia contraindications that consider the patient's medical condition regarding a major operation, any surgery that may result in permanent neurologic morbidity should be compared with alternative treatment modalities in terms of potential benefits and risks.

The goal of surgical resection is to achieve a transient control of the disease and to alleviate symptoms caused by the tumor mass. For tumors involving one optic nerve, a frontal or frontotemporal approach may be used. With either technique, intraorbital and intracranial portions of the affected nerve as well as the chiasm should be exposed. Following craniotomy, the orbital rim may be removed. Some surgeons prefer a lumbar drain whereas others prefer to drain CSF from suprasellar cisterns. Optic chiasm and the intracranial portion of the affected optic nerve are inspected to determine a site for division, which should be more than 6 mm from the chiasm to avoid causing a contralateral superior temporal field defect. The orbital canal is drilled open, and the periorbita is divided along the optic nerve. Following division of the annulus of Zinn, the optic sheath is opened. Decompression of the tumor may first be done internally with an ultrasonic aspirator, followed by dissection of the tumor's capsule from surrounding structures and then by division and removal of the nerve. After closure of the annulus and periorbita, the orbital roof may be reconstructed if needed. Following dural closure, any open sinuses and the orbital rim should be reconstructed.

For chiasmatic and hypothalamic tumors, surgical goals should be well balanced with the risks of increased visual loss and increased hypothalamic dysfunction. Improved visual and neurologic outcomes after surgery have been reported for chiasmatic and hypothalamic gliomas.[72–74] Meticulous tumor debulking from the exophytic portion of a chiasmatic tumor may improve vision by relieving external pressure on the adjacent optic nerve. There are several surgical approaches to the chiasmatic hypothalamic region, each with certain advantages. Regardless of the approach, the aim is tumor debulking without causing additional deficit. Most surgeons prefer a frontal or pterional approach. A subtemporal approach may provide good visualization of parasellar and posterior sellar areas. The bifrontal interhemispheric approach may be preferred for adequate exposure of the pituitary stalk, both optic nerves, and the anterior half of the circle of Willis.[65] A transcallosal approach may be useful when the tumor has rostral expansion into the third ventricle. The third ventricle may also be entered by a subchoroideal trans–velum interpositum approach to minimize injury to the neural tissue. Another method of approaching intraventricular tumors is the interforniceal technique.[75]

Following an intraorbital approach, CSF leak may occur if the frontal sinus or any opened etmoid sinuses were not adequately reconstructed. Inadequate reconstruction of the orbital roof may result in pulsating proptosis. These complications are avoidable with the appropriate surgical technique. In a large series of intraorbital approaches, there were no CSF leaks, proptoses, infections, or extraocular problems.[76] Failure to repair a sectioned levator origin will result in ptosis. Surgical injury to the superior ophthalmic vein and to the nerves supplying the extraocular muscles will result in functional deficits.[77] The operative procedures for chiasmatic hypothalamic gliomas may result in significant morbidity in the form of immediate endocrinologic or neurologic deficits. Resulting sequelae may include hypothalamic or hypophyseal dysfunction, increased visual impairment, memory loss, altered consciousness, and coma.[74]

PINEAL-REGION TUMORS

Pineal tumors include a wide spectrum of histologies including germ cell tumors and pinealomas as well as gliomas, epidermoids, dermoids, meningiomas, lipomas, and craniopharyngiomas. The most frequently occurring are germ cell tumors, which include germinomas, embryonal carcinoma, yolk sac tumor, choriocarcinoma, and teratomas. Pineal parenchymal tumors include pineocytomas and pinealoblastomas.

In addition, MRI has revealed the frequent occurrence of asymptomatic cysts, which may occasionally become large enough to cause symptoms.[78,79]

Resection has the advantage of providing adequate tissue for the histologic assessment of frequently mixed tumors seen at this location and theoretically improves responses to radiation and chemotherapy. Surgical goals also include reducing the mass effect on the quadrigeminal plate and brain stem and re-establishing CSF circulation. Hydrocephalus is present in up to 90 percent of patients, and placement of EVD, if indicated, may provide adequate CSF drainage until surgery.[80] There are currently three main surgical approaches to the pineal region. The particular operative route is determined by the location of the lesion relative to surrounding critical neurovascular structures and by the size, extension, and invasiveness of the tumor.

The infratentorial supracerebellar approach allows the surgeon to work in the space created between the tentorium and the cerebellum.[81] It can be performed with the patient in the sitting or Concorde position. Following a suboccipital craniotomy exposing the entire torcula region and opening the dura, the bridging veins between the caudal surface of the tentorium and dorsal aspect of the cerebellum are divided. With the patient in the sitting position, gravity causes the cerebellum to descend, and draining CSF from the cistern helps relaxation. It is an efficient approach for midline tumors that extend into the third ventricle or posterior fossa. By approaching the tumor ventral to the deep venous system, this route minimizes the risk of venous injury. Its limitations include tumors that originate from the corpus callosum, those extending into the trigone, those that are dorsal to Galen's vein, and those with significant supratentorial extension.[82]

The occipital transtentorial approach can be performed with the patient in the sitting or "park bench" position through a nondominant hemisphere occipital craniotomy. The medial and inferior margins of the craniotomy are based on the superior sagittal and transverse sinuses, respectively. The dura is opened in an L-shaped fashion, and the occipital lobe is displaced superiorly and laterally, exposing the falx-tentorium junction. In the park bench position, gravity helps retraction of the occipital lobe. The tentorium is incised parallel to the straight sinus, and the arachnoid sheath surrounding the deep venous structures is removed. The occipital transtentorial route exposes a large area, including the pineal gland as well as the splenium, the posterior third ventricle, the quadrigeminal plate, and the vermis. The main advantage of this route over the infratentorial approach is a greater ability to mobilize and resect tumors with lateral extension. This approach, however, is not suitable for pineal tumors with significant posterior fossa extension.[82,83]

The posterior interhemispheric approach can be performed with the patient in a right lateral decubitus position, with the superior sagittal sinus parallel to the floor and then elevating the vertex 30° from the horizontal. A right paramedian occipitoparietal craniotomy with the medial side on the midline is performed, with the anterior border of the exposure depending on the extent of the tumor. The right lobe is moved away from the midline by gravity, and after dissection of the cingulum and the pericallosal arteries, the corpus callosum is incised in the midline if necessary, 1.5 cm anterior to the splenium. If a transcallosal approach is not needed, as it is in the case of lesions with caudal extension into the quadrigeminal cistern or posterior fossa rather than involvement of the posterior third ventricle, the posterior interhemispheric approach may be continued retrocallosally. The tumor is located at the falx–tentorial incisura junction and, depending on its extension, division of the falx or tentorium provides adequate exposure. This interhemispheric approach has the advantage of providing good visualization of the posterior third ventricle, quadrigeminal cistern, and pineal-region structures and allows the surgeon to revise the trajectory intraoperatively to maximize visualization and to achieve maximal tumor resection.

For pineal tumors, the retrocallosal approach is generally preferred over a transcallosal approach as it avoids damaging the corpus callosum and causing any disconnection deficit. For the minority of tumors located in the posterior segment of the third ventricle or for tumors anterior to the splenium, the transcallosal approach may be preferred. A combined retrocallosal and transcallosal approach, leaving the splenium intact, has also been described for the removal of large pineal tumors.[84]

REFERENCES

1. Hammond MA, Ligon BL, Souki R, et al. Use of intraoperative ultrasound for localizing tumors and determining the extent of resection: a comparative study with magnetic resonance imaging. J Neurosurg 1996;84:737–41.
2. Keles GE, Berger MS. Functional mapping. In: Bernstein M, Berger MS, editors. Neuro-oncology essentials. New York: Thieme Medical Publishers; 2000. p. 130–4.
3. Zakhary R, Keles GE, Berger MS. Intraoperative imaging techniques in the treatment of brain tumors. Curr Opin Oncol 1999;11:152–6.
4. Black PM, Moriarty T, Alexander E 3rd, et al. Development and implementation of intraoperative magnetic resonance imaging and its neurosurgical applications. Neurosurgery 1997; 41:831–45.
5. Steinmaier R, Fahlbusch O, Ganslandt O, et al. Intraoperative magnetic resonance imaging with the Magnetom open scanner: concepts, neurosurgical indications, and procedures: a preliminary report. Neurosurgery 1998;43:739–48.
6. Tronnier VM, Wirtz CR, Knauth M, et al. Intraoperative diagnostic and interventional magnetic resonance imaging in neurosurgery. Neurosurgery 1997;40:891–902.
7. Dohrmann GJ, Farwell JR, Flannery JT. Astrocytomas in childhood: a population based study. Surg Neurol 1985;23:64–8.
8. Hayostek CJ, Shaw EG, Scheithauer B, et al. Astrocytomas of the cerebellum: a comparative clinicopathologic study of pilocytic and diffuse astrocytomas. Cancer 1993;72:856–69.
9. Stewart AM, Lennox EL, Sanders BM. Group characteristics of children with cerebral and spinal cord tumours. Br J Cancer 1973;28:568–74.
10. Ilgren EB, Stiller CA. Cerebellar astrocytomas: clinical characteristics and prognostic indices. J Neurooncol 1987;4:293–308.
11. Culley, DJ, Berger MS, Shaw D, Geyer R. An analysis of factors determining the need for ventriculoperitoneal shunts after posterior fossa tumor surgery in children. Neurosurgery 1994;34:402–7.
12. Dailey AT, McKhann GM 2nd, Berger MS. The pathophysiology of oral pharyngeal apraxia and mutism following posterior fossa tumor resection in children. J Neurosurg 1995;83:467–75.
13. Akyol FH, Atahan L, Zorlu F, et al. Results of post-operative or exclusive radiotherapy in grade 1 and grade 2 cerebellar astrocytoma patients. Radiother Oncol 1992;23:245–8.
14. Klein DM, McCullough DC. Surgical staging of cerebellar astrocytomas in childhood. Cancer 1985;56:1810–1.
15. Undjian S, Marinov M, Georgiev K. Long-term follow-up after surgical treatment of cerebellar astrocytomas in 100 children. Childs Nerv Syst 1989;5:99–101.
16. Tomita T. Surgical management of cerebellar peduncle lesions in children. Neurosurgery 1986;18:568–75.
17. Laws ER, Bergstralh EJ, Taylor WF. Cerebellar astrocytoma in children. Prog Exp Tumor Res 1987;30:122–7.
18. Stein BM, Tenner MS, Fraser RA. Hydrocephalus following removal of cerebellar astrocytomas in children. J Neurosurg 1972;36:763–8.
19. Abdollahzadeh M, Hoffman HJ, Blazer SI, et al. Benign cerebellar astrocytoma in childhood: experience at the Hospital for Sick Children, 1980–1992. Childs Nerv Syst 1994;10:380–3.
20. Gjerris F, Agerlin N, Borgesen SE, et al. Epidemiology and prognosis in children treated for intracranial tumours in Denmark, 1960–1984. Childs Nerv Syst 1998;14:302–11.
21. Lannering B, Marky I, Nordborg C. Brain tumors in childhood and adolescence in west Sweden 1970–1984. Epidemiology and survival. Cancer 1990;66:604–9.
22. Hoffman HJ, Hendrick EB, Humphreys RP. Metastasis via ventriculoperitoneal shunt in patients with medulloblastoma. J Neurosurg 1976;44:562–6.
23. McLaurin RL. Disadvantages of the preoperative shunt in posterior fossa tumors. Clin Neurosurg 1983;30:286–92.
24. Imielinski BL, Kloc W, Wasilewski W, et al. Posterior fossa tumors in children—indications for ventricular drainage and for V-P shunting. Childs Nerv Syst 1998;14:227–9.
25. Vaquero J, Cabezudo JM, de Sola RG, Nombela L. Intratumoral hemorrhage in posterior fossa tumors after ventricular drainage. Report of two cases. J Neurosurg 1981;54:406–8.
26. Waga S, Shimizu T, Shimosaka S, Tochio H. Intratumoral hemorrhage after a ventriculoperitoneal shunting procedure. Neurosurgery 1981;9:249–52.
27. Kessler LA, Dugan P, Concannon JP. Systemic metastases of medulloblastoma promoted by shunting. Surg Neurol 1975;3:147–52.
28. Albright AL, Wisoff JH, Zeltzer PM, et al. Current neurosurgical treatment of medulloblastomas in children. A report from the Children's Cancer Study Group. Pediatr Neurosci 1989;15:276–82.
29. Berger MS, Baumeister B, Geyer JR, et al. The risks of metastases from shunting in children with primary central nervous system tumors. J Neurosurg 1991;74:872–7.
30. Tarbell NJ, Loeffler JS, Silver B, et al. The change in patterns of relapse in medulloblastoma. Cancer 1991;68:1600–4.
31. Lefkowitz IB, Packer RJ, Ryan SG, et al. Late recurrence of primitive neuroectodermal tumor/medulloblastoma. Cancer 1988;62:826–30.
32. Park TS, Hoffman HJ, Hendrick EB, et al. Medulloblastoma: clinical presentation and management. Experience at the Hospital for Sick Children, Toronto, 1950–1980. J Neurosurg 1983;58:543–52.
33. Steinbok P, Boyd M, Cochrane D. Cervical spinal deformity following craniotomy and upper cervical laminectomy for posterior fossa tumors in children. Childs Nerv Syst 1989;5:25–8.
34. Aguiar PH, Plese JP, Ciquini O, Marino R. Transient mutism following a posterior fossa approach to cerebellar tumors in children: a critical review of the literature. Childs Nerv Syst 1995;11:306–10.
35. Kellogg JX, Piatt JH Jr. Resection of fourth ventricle tumors without splitting the vermis: the cerebellomedullary fissure approach. Pediatr Neurosurg 1997;27:28–33.
36. Crutchfield JS, Sawaya R, Meyers CA, Moore BD 3rd. Postoperative mutism in neurosurgery. Report of two cases. J Neurosurg 1994;81:115–21.

37. Ferrante L, Mastronardi L, Acqui M, Fortuna A. Mutism after posterior fossa surgery in children. Report of three cases. J Neurosurg 1990;72:959–63.
38. Humphreys R. Mutism after posterior fossa surgery. Concepts Pediatr Neurosurg 1988;9:57–64.
39. Sutton LN, Phillips PC, Molloy PT. Surgical management of medulloblastoma. J Neurooncol 1996;29:9–21.
40. Anzil AP. Glioblastoma multiforme with extracranial metastases in the absence of previous craniotomy. J Neurosurg 1970;33:88–94.
41. Brust JC, Moiel RH, Rosenberg RN. Glial tumor metastases through a ventriculo-pleural shunt. Resultant massive pleural effusion. Arch Neurol 1968;18:649–53.
42. Brutschin P, Culver GJ. Extracranial metastases from medulloblastomas. Radiology 1973;107:359–62.
43. Farwell JR, Dohrmann GJ, Flannery JT. Central nervous system tumors in children. Cancer 1977;40:3123–32.
44. Berger MS. The impact of technical adjuncts in the surgical management of cerebral hemispheric low-grade gliomas of childhood. J Neurooncol 1996;28:129–55.
45. Keles GE, Berger MS. Seizures associated with brain tumors. In: Bernstein M, Berger MS, editors. Neuro-oncology essentials. New York: Thieme Medical Publishers; 2000. p. 473–7.
46. Berger MS, Ghatan S, Geyer JR, et al. Seizure outcome in children with hemispheric tumors and associated intractable epilepsy: the role of tumor removal combined with seizure foci resection. Pediatr Neurosurg 1991–92;17:185–91.
47. Berger MS, Rostomily RC. Low grade gliomas: functional mapping, resection strategies, extent of resection, and outcome. J Neurooncol 1997;34:85–101.
48. Wang EC, Geyer JR, Berger MS. Incidence of postoperative epilepsy in children following subfrontal craniotomy for tumor. Pediatr Neurosurg 1994;21:165–73.
49. Morota N, Sakamoto K, Kobayashi N, Hashimoto K. Recurrent low-grade glioma in children with special reference to computed tomography findings and pathological changes. Childs Nerv Syst 1990;6:155–60.
50. Otsubo H, Hoffman HJ, Humphries RP, et al. Detection and management of gangliogliomas in children. Surg Neurol 1992;38:371–8.
51. Silver JM, Rawlings CE III, Rossitch E, et al. Ganglioglioma: a clinical study with long-term follow-up. Surg Neurol 1991;35:261–6.
52. Vandenberg SR. Desmoplastic infantile ganglioglioma and desmoplastic cerebral astrocytoma of infancy. Brain Pathol 1993;3:275–81.
53. Albright AL. Brain stem gliomas. In: Youmans JR, editor. Youmans neurological surgery. Vol. 4. 4th ed. Philadelphia: WB Saunders; 1996. p. 2603–11.
54. Albright A, Guthkelch A, Packer R, et al. Prognostic factors in pediatric brain stem gliomas. J Neurosurg 1986;65:751–5.
55. Albright AL, Packer RJ, Zimmerman R, et al. Magnetic resonance scans should replace biopsies for the diagnosis of diffuse brain stem gliomas: a report from the Children's Cancer Group. Neurosurgery 1993;33:1026–30.
56. Sanford RA, Freeman CR, Burger P, et al. Prognostic criteria for experimental protocols in pediatric brainstem gliomas. Surg Neurol 1988;30:276–80.
57. Eisner W, Urs SD, Reulen HJ, et al. The mapping and continuous monitoring of the intrinsic motor nuclei during brainstem surgery. Neurosurgery 1995;37:255–65.
58. Straoss C, Romstock J, Nimsky C, Fahlbush R. Intraoperative identification of motor areas of the rhomboid fossa using direct stimulation. J Neurosurg 1993;79:393–9.
59. Hood TW, Gebarski SS, McKeever PE, et al. Stereotactic biopsy of intrinsic lesions of the brainstem. J Neurosurg 1986;65:172–6.
60. Duffner P, Cohen M, Myers M, Heise H. Survival of children with brain tumors: SEER program, 1973–1980. Neurology 1986;36:597–601.
61. Nazar G, Hoffman H, Becker L, et al. Infratentorial ependymomas in childhood: prognostic factors and treatment. J Neurosurg 1990;72:408–17.
62. Pollack I. Current concepts: brain tumors in children. N Engl J Med 1994;331:1500–7.
63. Berger MS, Geyer JR. Ependymomas of the fourth ventricle. In: Cohen AR, editor. Surgical disorders of the fourth ventricle. Cambridge: Blackwell Science; 1996.
64. Palma L, Celli P, Cantore C. Supratentorial ependymomas of the first two decades of life: long-term follow-up of 20 cases (including two subependymomas). Neurosurgery 1993;32:169–75.
65. Pollack IF, Gerszten PC, Martinez AJ, et al. Intracranial ependymomas of childhood: long-term outcome and prognostic factors. Neurosurgery 1995;37:655–67.
66. Hoffman HJ, Rutka JT. Optic pathway gliomas in children. In: Albright L, Pollack I, Adelson D, editors. Principles and practice of pediatric neurosurgery. New York: Thieme Medical Publishers; 1999. p. 535–43.
67. Ruggieri M. The different forms of neurofibromatosis. Childs Nerv Syst 1999;15:295–308.
68. Housepian EM. Management and results in 114 cases of optic glioma. Neurosurgery 1977;1:67–8.
69. Gajjar A, Bhargava R, Jenkins JJ, et al. Low grade astrocytoma with neuraxis dissemination at diagnosis. J Neurosurg 1995;83:67–71.
70. Mamelak AN, Prados MD, Obana WG, et al. Treatment options and prognosis for multicentric juvenile pilocytic astrocytoma. J Neurosurg 1994;81:24–30.
71. Lewis RA, Riccardi VM, Gerson LP, et al. Von Recklinghausen neurofibromatosis: II. Incidence of optic nerve gliomata. Ophthalmology 1984;91:929–35.
72. Appleton RE, Jan SE. Delayed diagnosis of optic nerve glioma: a preventable cause of visual loss. Pediatr Neurol 1989;5:226–8.
73. Bynke H, Kagstrom E, Tjernstrom K. Aspects on the treatment of gliomas of the anterior visual pathways. Acta Ophthalmol 1977;55:269–80.
74. Wisoff JH, Abbott R, Epstein F. Surgical management of exophytic chiasmatic-hypothalamic tumors of childhood. J Neurosurg 1990;73:661–7.

75. Apuzzo MLJ, Litofsky NS. Surgery in and around the anterior third ventricle. In: Apuzzo MLJ, editor. Brain surgery: complication avoidance and management. Vol 1. New York: Churchill Livingstone; 1993. p. 541.
76. Maroon JC, Kennerdell JS. Lateral microsurgical approach to intraorbital tumors. J Neurosurg 1976;44:556–61.
77. Housepian EM. Complications of transcranial orbital surgery. In: Post KD, Friedman ED, McCormick P, editors. Postoperative complications in intracranial neurosurgery. New York: Thieme; 1993. p. 87–90.
78. Lum GB, William JP, Machen BC, et al. Benign cystic pineal lesions by magnetic resonance imaging. J Comput Assist Tomogr 1987;11:228–35.
79. Mamourian AC, Towfighi J. Pineal cysts: MR imaging. AJNR Am J Neuroradiol 1986;7:1081–6.
80. Albuquerque FC, Apuzzo MLJ, Mendel E. Pineal-region masses: a unified approach. In: Apuzzo MLJ, editor. Surgery of the third ventricle. 2nd ed. Baltimore: Williams & Wilkins; 1998. p. 821–44.
81. Stein B. The infratentorial supracerebellar approach to pineal lesions. J Neurosurg 1971;35:197–202.
82. Rhoton AL, Yamamoto I, Peace DA, et al. Microsurgery of the third ventricle: part 2. Neurosurgery 1981;8:357–72.
83. Reid WS, Clark K. Comparison of the infratentorial and transtentorial approaches to the pineal region. Neurosurgery 1978;3:1–8.
84. McComb, Apuzzo MLJ. The lateral decubitus position for the surgical approach to pineal location tumors. Concepts Pediatr Neurosurg 1988;8:186–99.

17

Evaluation and Management of Pediatric Brain Tumors

CAROLYN RUSSO, MD
PHILIP V. THEODOSOPOULOS, MD
MICHAEL PRADOS, MD

Brain tumors are the most common solid tumors encountered in children (age < 20 years) and are second to leukemia in overall cancer frequency. Chapter 1 describes the incidence and epidemiology of brain tumors in detail, and the reader is encouraged to review that data concerning childhood tumors. Of the childhood brain tumors, the most common lesions encountered include low-grade tumors such as juvenile pilocytic astrocytoma, benign and malignant ependymoma, medulloblastoma and other primitive neuroectodermal tumors (PNETs), and the malignant glial neoplasms glioblastoma multiforme and anaplastic astrocytoma.[1]

EVALUATION

The evaluation of a child with a brain tumor often starts with the pediatrician or primary care doctor. The clinical presentation varies depending on the age of the child. Headache is a common presenting complaint in children with brain tumors; in a nonverbal child, the complaint of headache is unlikely to happen, and the clinical presentation may be an enlarging head size. The sutures are not fully closed, and hydrocephalus increases the skull size. Loss of developmental milestones is another presentation of a brain tumor, such as a child who was walking or cruising who is now only crawling. Another sign is motor weakness, which is often difficult to appreciate until a child is more mobile. Irritability and lethargy are signs of hydrocephalus seen in young infants. Unexplained vomiting, in particular, early morning vomiting, is a sign of hydrocephalus. One typical clinical presentation in young infants is the diencephalic syndrome.[2] These children have hypothalamic low-grade astrocytomas and often present in the first year of life with severe failure to thrive. Unlike other causes of failure to thrive, the children are often developmentally appropriate and happy. It is hypothalamic dysfunction that leads to their profound weight loss and abnormal growth.

In the older child, persistent headache is a common sign of a brain tumor, although, by far, most children with headache do not have a brain tumor. The current incidence of childhood brain tumor according to US registry data is approximately 2,200 new cases per year. Nonetheless, persistence of severe headache or headache associated with an abnormal neurologic finding should warrant a brain scan. The presence of early morning vomiting may occur with or without headache. Since many brain tumors in children occur in the infratentorial region, signs of cerebellar dysfunction are a frequent presentation. Ataxia or simply gait abnormalities also can develop insidiously, but in conjunction with headache and emesis, they lead one to suspect an intracranial tumor. New-onset seizures can be an initial presenting sign in a child with a hemispheric tumor. Low-grade tumors are frequently associated with seizures, and thus seizure presentation may be a favorable prognostic sign.

In the evaluation of a child with a brain tumor, imaging is key. At the present time, magnetic resonance imaging (MRI) with intravenous contrast is the standard of care. Myelography of the spine has been replaced by MRI in the sagittal and axial planes. In some situations, functional imaging with spectroscopy or positron emission tomography (PET) may be useful. High-quality scanning and interpretations are critical in the initial evaluation and follow-up management.

A team of health care providers is the best way to provide ideal care for a child diagnosed with a brain tumor. Treatment options should be comprehensive and derived from the input of all team members, including the pediatric neuro-oncologist, pediatric neurosurgeon, radiation oncologist, neuropathologist, neuroradiologist, pediatric neurologist, neuropsychologist, and other specialists as needed. In most centers of excellence, this process of management is accomplished in a tumor board. When feasible, consideration of appropriate clinical trials must be entertained.

MANAGEMENT

Surgical Management

In most cancer cases, a histologic diagnosis is critical to the appropriate management of the patient. Most childhood brain tumors follow this rule, but there are a few exceptions. There are specific childhood brain tumors for which an attempt at biopsy is potentially harmful. Three examples are intrinsic pontine gliomas, hypothalamic-chiasmatic tumors in infants, and neurofibromatosis type 1 (NF1) with optic tract tumors in children.

Diffusely infiltrating lesions in the pons and medulla generally do not require a pathologic diagnosis if the typical clinical and radiographic criteria are present. The typical clinical features are a short history of symptoms (usually less than 3 months) that include cranial nerve palsies, ataxia, and long tract signs. The MRI scans show an intrinsic tumor that is diffuse and may be contrast enhancing. Hydrocephalus generally is not present at diagnosis. These tumors are high-grade astrocytomas with a dismal prognosis. The median survival is 1 year with few long survivors. Since the tumor is located within the pons, surgical resection is not feasible. The tumor grade is not prognostic and thus surgery generally is not indicated. Certain situations exist when surgery and/or biopsy *should* be considered for brainstem tumors. These include (1) any atypical radiographic appearance that may indicate a degenerative process or a different tumor type such as lymphoma or primitive neuroectodermal tumor; (2) a long history of symptoms that may indicate a low-grade tumor such as juvenile pilocytic astrocytoma; (3) lesions that are exophytic or very focal; and (4) a patient with a history suspicious for infection.

Young children with hypothalamic-chiasmatic tumors may not warrant surgical management. These tumors often arise in the first several years of life and may be accompanied by the associated diencephalic syndrome with extreme failure to thrive. Unlike typical cases of failure to thrive, these children are socially and developmentally on track. Presumably these children have hypothalamic dysfunction that leads to their diminished growth. Histologically, these tumors are juvenile pilocytic astrocytomas. Given the location, attempt at complete surgical resection is not feasible. Surgical intervention is required for hydrocephalus, but the degree of surgical resection is not prognostic, and, therefore, surgical debulking generally is not indicated. Chemotherapy is the standard of care given the young age of these children at presentation. Radiation therapy is effective but is generally reserved for progressive disease or disease in older children.

Another situation that does not warrant immediate surgical management occurs in children with NF1 who present with optic tract tumors (Figure 17–1). The tumors are histologically juvenile pilocytic astrocytoma with a relatively indolent course and do not require treatment intervention if the child is asymptomatic. When clinical or radiographic progression occurs, treatment is indicated. However, since complete surgical removal is not feasible with optic tract tumors, and the response to chemotherapy is well documented, chemotherapy is the treatment of choice for this group of children. Many children with NF1 and optic tract tumors will not need treatment as the tumors do not grow or cause symptoms.

Nonsurgical Management in Infants

Chemotherapy and radiation therapy are the mainstays of nonsurgical management of pediatric brain

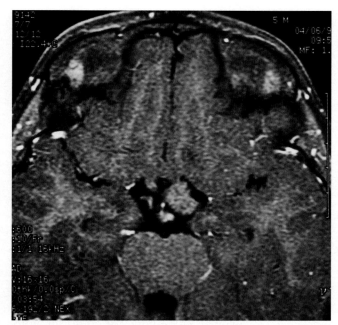

Figure 17–1. Axial T1-weighted contrast-enhanced MR image of a child with NF1 and a lesion in the optic chiasm, presumed to be a juvenile pilocytic astrocytoma.

tumors; however, novel treatments using biologic agents or gene therapy are becoming a part of the increasing armamentarium, particularly for the difficult-to-treat high-grade gliomas.

Chemotherapy has assumed a primary role in the treatment of young children (< 3 years) with malignant brain tumors since the long-term effects of radiation therapy can significantly impair normal growth and development, particularly cognition, memory and learning, and endocrine development.[3] In the 1980s, several groups used chemotherapy after surgery and before radiation therapy in infants with medulloblastoma and other PNETs. The goal was to avoid the long-term effects of radiation therapy and to attempt to prolong survival using combination chemotherapy instead of immediate irradiation. Investigators at the M.D. Anderson Cancer Center treated 9 infants of less than 36 months of age with a combination of mechlorethamine, Oncovin (vincristine), procarbazine, and prednisone (MOPP chemotherapy) following surgical resection of medulloblastoma.[4] One patient had residual tumor and 2 patients had positive cerebrospinal fluid (CSF) cytology at diagnosis. Disease recurred in 4 patients following chemotherapy, 1 in the spinal canal and 3 at the primary site. Five patients remained alive without disease recurrence with a median follow-up of 2 years. Four of 6 children were within the normal range of neuropsychological and somatic development.

This study led to several more pilot studies with the direct intent of delaying radiation therapy in children who were less than 3 years of age with malignant brain tumors. One such study used a combination of cyclophosphamide, cisplatin, vincristine, and etoposide given after surgery in children less than 2 years of age. Radiation was initiated after the last cycle of chemotherapy. In this study, tumor growth was controlled in 8 of 12 children and irradiation was delayed in 67 percent of cases.[5]

A landmark study from the Pediatric Oncology Group (POG) showed that in the cooperative group setting, the approach of postoperative chemotherapy (cyclophosphamide, cisplatin, vincristine, and etoposide) and delayed irradiation was feasible and comparable or superior to historic controls.[5] Moreover, this large study of nearly 200 children provided further understanding of the impact of treatment and demonstrated the chemosensitivity of malignant brain tumors. Neurodevelopmental function was evaluated according to the Mental Developmental Index and General Cognitive Index. Growth parameters and audiograms also were used to evaluate development. In 34 children tested at 1 year postdiagnosis, there was no significant change in the neurodevelopmental function compared to pretreatment levels, and growth was maintained. Twenty percent of children did have high-frequency hearing loss. This study was the first large group study to show encouraging results for this historically unfavorable group of children.

The Children's Cancer Group explored a similar study design with the 8-in-1 drug regimen (cisplatin, cyclophosphamide, vincristine, hydroxyurea, procarbazine, methylprednisone, cytosine arabinoside, and lomustine, all given in 1 day). The response rate and overall survival rates were inferior to the POG study.[6] Although the general treatment philosophy was similar, the dose intensity of the chemotherapy was markedly less in the Children's Cancer Group study. In addition, drugs such as cytosine arabinoside and methylprednisone have minimal efficacy against malignant brain tumors, and this likely contributed to the inferior results.

The current approach for infants with malignant brain tumors is to use chemotherapy prior to radiation therapy. The ideal time to use radiation therapy, if at all, is not clear. Active areas of investigation include dose intensification, exploration of novel agents, focal irradiation to limit the radiation field, and high-dose chemotherapy with stem cell rescue.

Primitive Neuroectodermal Tumor

Intracranial PNET accounts for 25 percent of brain tumors diagnosed in children, making it the most common malignant brain tumor in children.[7] This tumor arises from primitive neuroectoderm, although the actual cell of origin and the epidemiology are unclear.[8] It can occur anywhere within the nervous system, although the most common site is in the cerebellum, where it is commonly referred to as medulloblastoma (Figures 17–2 and 17–3). Supratentorial PNETs may occur either as pineal region tumors (pinealoblastoma) or large hemispheric tumors (cerebral PNET). Histologically, these are highly cellular malignancies, frequently composed of small, round, undifferentiated cells with hyperchromatic nuclei. Unlike glial neoplasms, all PNETs have a high propensity for leptomeningeal spread, and staging of the neuroaxis is necessary to evaluate fully the extent of disease.

Although limited cytogenetic data exist, they have not been statistically powerful enough to guide prognostication. The most frequent chromosomal abnormality detected by karyotypic analysis in PNET is a 17p deletion, which often is associated with duplication of 17q ("iso17q"), occurring in 30 to 50 percent of cases.[8,9] The prognostic value of 17p deletion is controversial. One study of 20 PNETs found that iso17q occurred more often in cerebellar PNET than in supratentorial PNET, suggesting that cerebellar and supratentorial PNETs are biologically distinct and that the presence of iso17q or 17p deletion was a survival advantage.[10] A second study of 28 PNETs showed that 29 percent had loss of heterozygosity at 17p13.1 to 13.3 and suggested that there was a survival advantage for children with deletion at 17p.[11] More research is needed to clarify and add to these data.

The major advances in the treatment of PNET have been achieved through combining surgery, radiation therapy, and chemotherapy. This approach has gradually improved disease-free survival rates for children with PNET. The goals of surgical resection are threefold. First, surgical resection establishes the

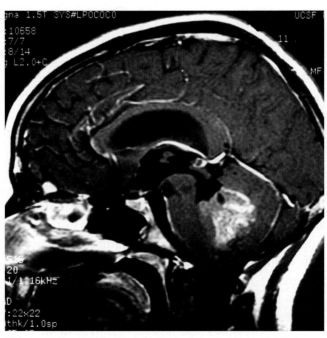

Figure 17–2. Sagittal T1-weighted contrast-enhanced MR image of a cerebellar medulloblastoma.

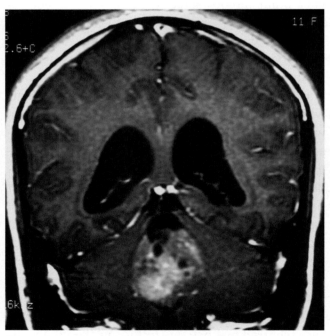

Figure 17–3. Coronal T1-weighted contrast-enhanced MR image of the same lesion, showing associated hydrocephalus.

histologic diagnosis. Second, surgical resection often will relieve obstruction of normal cerebrospinal fluid, particularly in the posterior fossa lesions, and thus usually obviates the need for a ventriculoperitoneal shunt. Last, as with most brain tumors, complete surgical resection is associated with improved response to therapy. Radiation therapy to the entire neuroaxis (brain and spine) is given following surgical resection and is responsible for the initial reports of treatment cures in children with PNET. These tumors respond to radiation as a function of dose and are very radiosensitive. Local control is not achieved with doses less than 5,000 cGy to the primary tumor, and the typical dose prescribed is at least 5,400 cGy. The remainder of the neuroaxis is treated with either 3,600 cGy if there is no obvious evidence of distant disease, or with slightly higher doses to bulky areas of tumor in other areas of the brain or spine. New studies are investigating the use of lower-dose (eg, 2,400 cGy) neuroaxis irradiation in children with standard-risk features. These studies are inconclusive, and further clinical research testing should be done before lower radiation doses are used as a standard approach. Finally, chemotherapy is effective when used in the adjuvant setting (following surgery and irradiation) in older children and neoadjuvantly (following surgery and prior to irradiation) in younger infants. Active drugs that have been reported to produce responses in vitro, in vivo, and in clinical studies include the nitrosoureas, cisplatin and carboplatin, cyclophosphamide and ifosfamide, methotrexate, and vincristine.

Patient outcome is dependent on stage. The most favorable stage is now called standard-risk disease. These children are aged 3 years and older, have had near-total or gross-total removal of all tumor in the primary site, and have no evidence of disease anywhere else within the brain, spine, or CSF. Poor-risk disease includes all other situations (eg, incomplete resection with or without dissemination elsewhere in the central nervous system [CNS], or infants with PNET). In some cases, disease is present outside the CNS, particularly in areas of bone or bone marrow. Patients with poor-risk disease are usually staged with bone scans and bone marrow examinations. The 5-year disease-free survival rate is at least 60 percent for children in the standard-risk group, with some recent studies reporting disease-free survival as high as 80 percent at 5 years.[12,13] Children in the poor-risk group have a 5-year disease-free survival rate of only 30 percent.[14] If tumor recurs, treatment generally is palliative, with few patients achieving long-term disease control. Treatment at relapse may include further surgery and re-irradiation to bulky disease and/or chemotherapy. A number of phase II studies evaluating chemotherapy for children with recurrent disease have been completed, and although high responses are noted, these typically are not durable.[15] Much more clinical research clearly is needed in this area.

Ependymoma

Ependymomas are the third most common type of childhood brain tumors. They arise from ependymal cells that line the ventricular system and spinal canal. Although these tumors can arise in many parts of the CNS, in children, they typically occur in the cerebrum or posterior fossa (Figure 17–4). Ependymomas histologically may show benign or malignant features, but the role that histology plays in prognosis is uncertain.[16,17] Treatment is based upon the extent of disease. The most important variable pre-

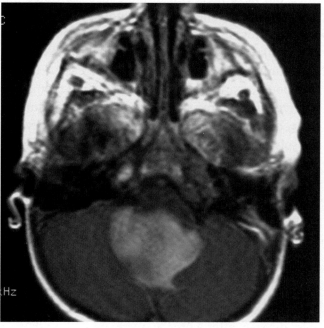

Figure 17–4. Axial T1-weighted contrast-enhanced MR image of an ependymoma in the posterior fossa of an infant.

dicting outcome is the amount of tumor remaining following surgery and, probably, the presence of an anaplastic phenotype.[18] Children with benign tumors that are completely resected without evidence of disease beyond the primary site will have the best prognosis. Incomplete resection or dissemination carries a poor prognosis. Radiation therapy usually is used to treat local disease following surgery, particularly if any residual disease is left. Most oncologists now agree that local radiation is all that is needed, rather than neuroaxis irradiation, assuming there is no evidence of dissemination.[18] There is at least one report of children treated with surgery only, without the use of radiation therapy. These children all had what appeared to be a gross-total resection of tumor, were otherwise staged negatively, and were followed up carefully.[19] These results are intriguing but need further study and longer patient follow-up.

Thus, treatment should consist of a maximum debulking surgical procedure and neuroaxis staging. Focal irradiation should be considered for all patients with incomplete resections without evidence of dissemination and probably for all patients with anaplastic features. Adjuvant chemotherapy has not been shown to increase overall survival. A variety of chemotherapeutic regimens have been advocated but have met with limited success. Since the majority of childhood ependymoma occur in the posterior fossa, the initial hope was that ependymoma, like medulloblastoma, would be a chemosensitive tumor. However, this is not the case. Like its glial counterpart, the astrocytoma, ependymoma is a relatively chemoresistant tumor. Phase II studies showed response rates using cisplatin and cyclophosphamide in ependymoma at less than 50 percent, whereas medulloblastoma response rates were consistently 70 to 100 percent. Nonetheless, chemotherapy has been investigated for children with ependymoma, particularly in the situation of the young infant in whom the use of radiotherapy is problematic. The best response data were noted in the first POG study of pre-irradiation chemotherapy for children less than 3 years of age with malignant brain tumors.[5] In this study, children with measurable disease after surgery were treated with two courses of cyclophosphamide and vincristine. In the 25 children with ependymoma, the complete and partial response rate was 48 percent, which, in this study, was the same as the response rate in children with medulloblastoma. Follow-up studies from the POG have not demonstrated a survival advantage with dose intensity of chemotherapy, which might be expected if ependymoma were, indeed, a chemoresponsive tumor. Unfortunately, other large studies of childhood ependymoma have been unable to document an advantage for adjuvant chemotherapy. In the Children's Cancer Group study of adjuvant lomustine, vincristine, and prednisone in which children were randomized to receive or not receive chemotherapy, there was no difference in outcome. A similar result was noted in a study that substituted procarbazine for prednisone, with chemotherapy not impacting survival in any way. One argument for these results could be that the most active agents were not evaluated in these studies. Platinum agents (cisplatin and carboplatin) seem to be the most active. Additional studies are ongoing with these more effective agents to evaluate response in an upfront window design.

A number of retrospective studies of intracranial ependymoma have evaluated outcome data to identify prognostic factors for progression and survival, but they have been limited by relatively low numbers of enrolled patients and conflicting results. However, several risk factors have been correlated with adverse outcomes across multiple studies. The most frequently documented statistically significant risk factor is extent of surgical resection, with patients with gross-total resections faring the best. Other factors such as lower tumor grade, adjuvant radiation therapy, and older patient age have been shown in several studies to correlate with improved outcomes.

Low-Grade Glioma

The majority of childhood gliomas tend to be of low histologic grade. A number of pathologically diverse lesions may occur within unique areas of brain, and thus the term low-grade glioma may represent many kinds of tumors. Included in this group are surgically curable lesions in the cerebellum called juvenile pilocytic astrocytoma (JPA), pure or mixed astrocytoma, oligodendroglioma, and oligoastrocytoma, as well as tumors that have a significant neuronal element such as ganglioglioma and gangliocytoma. Other less common tumors include pleomorphic xanthoastrocytoma (PXA), dysembryoplastic neuroepithelial tumors (DNET), and desmoplastic infantile glioma. Historically, patients with brain tumors have been treated with a combination of surgery and radiation therapy. However, we now know that this approach, although efficacious, may not always be the best when caring for a young child. The long-term effects of radiation therapy are age dependent. The younger the child is at the time of radiation therapy, the greater are the risks of radiation damage. For this reason, chemotherapy is playing a larger role in the treatment of certain groups of children with low-grade tumors. In some cases, surgery alone is the appropriate management. In other cases, when surgery is not possible or cannot significantly remove the tumor, chemotherapy may be needed. In some cases, such as PXA or DNET, partial resection alone may be all that is needed, with clinical and neuroimaging follow-up over time. The acute toxicity of chemotherapy has been much less severe than in the past because of advances in supportive care. Thus, chemotherapy is a reasonable option and may be associated with long-term tumor control. Clearly, long-term toxicity is a concern and an area of ongoing investigation.

The temporal lobe is a frequent site for low-grade lesions. The majority of temporal lobe tumors in children are low-grade neuronal and astrocytic tumors. Ganglioglioma and DNET are two common variants of temporal lobe tumors in children, who often will present with a chronic seizure history. The recommended treatment for these tumors is surgical resection without adjuvant therapy. Chemotherapy or radiation therapy generally is reserved for recurrent or progressive disease, which is rare in these two tumor types. The low-grade (WHO grade I and II) astrocytoma and oligodendroglioma are approached similarly, with surgery as the primary treatment modality. If a tumor is completely resected, then the child will be observed without adjuvant therapy. It is only recurrent disease or an unresectable tumor that would lead to the initiation of radiation therapy or chemotherapy.

Tumors in the hypothalamic-optic region also are frequently low-grade astrocytomas (Figures 17–5

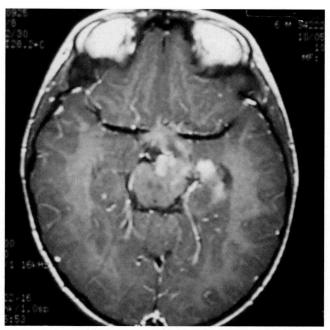

Figure 17–5. Axial T1-weighted contrast-enhanced MR image of a lesion in the hypothalamus and optic tract. This lesion was biopsied and shown to be a juvenile pilocytic astrocytoma.

and 17–6). The most common tumor type is JPA, and these lesions may be associated with NF1. Unfortunately, because of their midline location, it is much less likely that a complete surgical resection

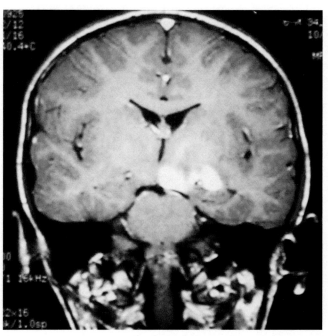

Figure 17–6. Coronal T1-weighted contrast-enhanced MR image of the lesion in Figure 17–5.

will be possible, and children are therefore more likely to be treated with other modalities. In some settings, particularly in children with NF1, treatment will be initiated without a histologic diagnosis because of the typical clinical setting and radiographic appearance of the lesion (Figure 17–7). Tumors that present anterior to the optic chiasm, within the optic nerve, often are indolent tumors that may not change in size for many years. Surgery usually is reserved in these lesions for cosmetic reasons such as proptosis.

Finally, lesions in the cerebellum typically are cystic, contrast-enhancing JPAs, and although they appear aggressive on MRI, they are slow-growing gliomas that can be cured with surgical resection. Exophytic lesions in the cervical and medullary area are also more likely to be a JPA and should be considered for resection (Figures 17–8 and 17–9). In cases where a complete resection is not possible, watchful waiting is appropriate. When tumor growth occurs clinically or radiographically, either an attempt at a repeat resection or treatment with chemotherapy or radiation therapy should be considered.

Thus, low-grade tumors are approached with surgery as the primary, and often only, treatment modality. However, in the case of a very young child with a symptomatic low-grade tumor that is incompletely resected or a child with a recurrent tumor, chemotherapy may be considered. There are several combination chemotherapy regimens available, but

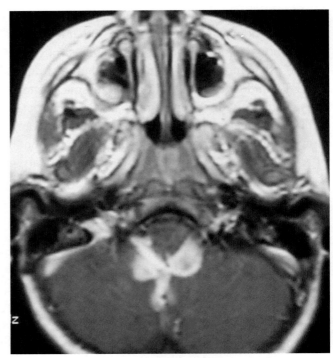

Figure 17–8. Axial T1-weighted contrast-enhanced MR image of a juvenile pilocytic astrocytoma in the cervical and medullary junction in the brain stem. A partial resection had been done earlier; here, the tumor is recurring.

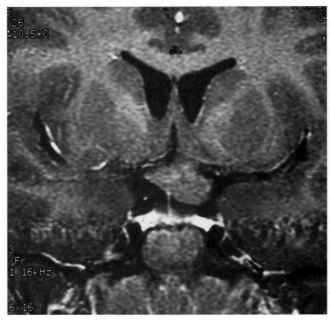

Figure 17–7. Coronal T1-weighted contrast-enhanced MR image of a lesion in the optic nerve in a child with NF1.

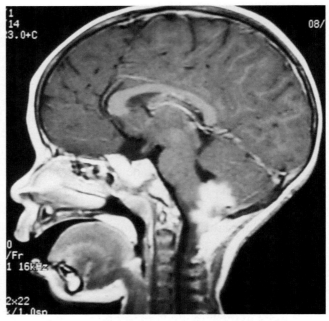

Figure 17–9. Sagittal T1-weighted contrast-enhanced MR image of the lesion in Figure 17–8.

two of the more frequently used regimens are carboplatin plus vincristine or the combination of lomustine, procarbazine, 6-thioguanine, and vincristine. The use of carboplatin and vincristine has shown promising results in children with low-grade gliomas in a report by Packer and colleagues.[20] This report examined the use of carboplatin and vincristine in 23 children with recurrent low-grade gliomas and 37 children with newly diagnosed low-grade gliomas. Response rates were determined by size of disease on MR scan after chemotherapy. In the children with recurrent disease, 12 of 23 had a complete, partial, or minor response and another 5 had stable disease. It is difficult to know what stable disease means in a tumor of indolent growth. However, the vast majority of these children had lack of disease progression for a median of approximately 2 years. The results were slightly better in the children with newly diagnosed tumors, implying that chemotherapy might hold these low-grade tumors in check for approximately 2 to 3 years. Combination chemotherapy based on the use of nitrosoureas was the focus of a similar study done at the University of California San Francisco. In this trial, children received lomustine, procarbazine, 6-thioguanine, dibromodulcitol, and vincristine. All therapy was given in the outpatient setting for a total of six treatment cycles (one cycle every 6 weeks). As with carboplatin and vincristine, objective regressions and stable disease occurred, and tumor progression was halted at a median of 2.5 years.[21] A randomized phase III study is currently under way comparing these two chemotherapy regimens in children with symptomatic low-grade gliomas.

Tumors that recur or do not respond to chemotherapy should be evaluated for radiation therapy, which should be given in a focal manner. Minimizing radiation dose to noninvolved normal brain is important to allow normal growth and development in these children.

High-Grade Astrocytoma

High-grade astrocytomas, particularly glioblastoma multiforme, generally are not curable tumors, and many novel therapies are being investigated because of the dismal prognosis (Figures 17–10, 17–11, and 17–12). The first goal of therapy is a safe complete resection since this is a critical prognostic feature of a more favorable outcome. Depending on the age of the child, radiation therapy is used following surgery. These tumors may initially respond to radiation therapy, but unfortunately the response is not durable. The data regarding adjuvant chemotherapy are mixed. Initial studies indicated a survival advantage with nitrosourea-based chemotherapy, but more recent studies, in which patient characteristics such as age, performance status, and histologic grade are stratified, have not demonstrated an advantage with adjuvant chemotherapy.[22,23] One argument is that the perfect chemotherapy has not been used or that optimal dose and schedules have not been adequately defined. The use of high-dose chemotherapy either as an adjuvant to surgery and radiation or at the time of tumor relapse has been explored in several trials in children.[24] Use of high-dose chemotherapy prior to radiation therapy in newly diagnosed children with high-grade gliomas also is being tested. Whether intensification of chemotherapy will achieve significant prolongation of survival compared to more standard therapy remains unproved at this time and will require a carefully conducted phase III study. The cur-

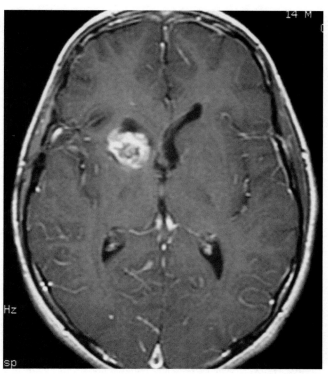

Figure 17–10. Axial T1-weighted contrast-enhanced MR image of an anaplastic astrocytoma in the inferior frontal lobe and basal ganglia.

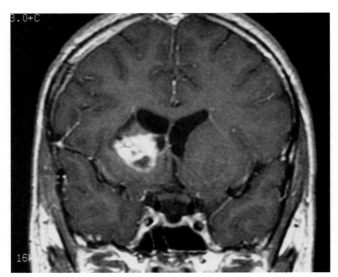

Figure 17–11. Coronal T1-weighted contrast-enhanced MR image of the lesion in Figure 17–10.

rent experimental strategies under investigation in childhood malignant glioma endeavor to find better drugs targeted to specific molecular pathways that influence growth of these tumors and to improve methods of delivery. These approaches include agents that inhibit angiogenesis, invasion, and cellular pathways that control cell-cycle regulation and growth.

Brainstem Gliomas

Magnetic resonance imaging has improved significantly our ability to diagnose and manage lesions in the brain stem and to stratify those tumors that will behave either in an indolent or slow-growing fashion or those that will grow despite aggressive therapy and cause death within 8 to 12 months. In general, focal lesions that present as an exophytic tumor lower in the medulla or focal intrinsic tumors high in the upper brain stem generally are low-grade gliomas and will respond well to chemotherapy or radiation therapy.[25–27] Lesions in the tectum, for instance, generally are not treated unless they cause obstructive hydrocephalus (Figures 17–13 and 17–14). In this situation, the hydrocephalus is treated with a shunting procedure, and the tumor is usually left alone. Exophytic lesions lower in the medulla may be partially resected and treated, if symptomatic, with either chemotherapy or radiation therapy, depending on the age of the child. Biologically, these tumors are similar to the supratentorial tumors described in the discussion of low-grade gliomas and can be referred to as good-risk brainstem gliomas.

Diffuse intrinsic lesions that arise from the pons generally are highly malignant tumors and behave in

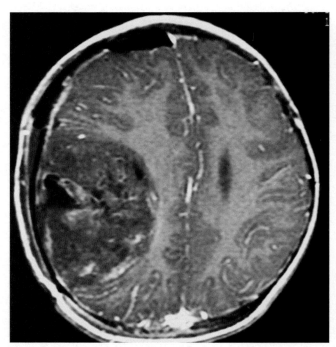

Figure 17–12. Axial T1-weighted contrast-enhanced image of a lesion in the right parietal lobe. Only a partial resection of a glioblastoma multiforme was accomplished.

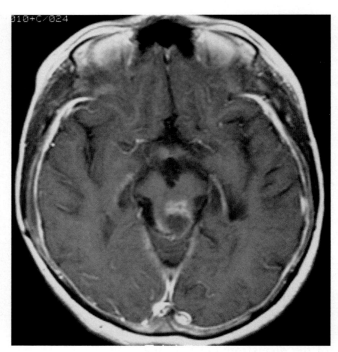

Figure 17–13. Axial T1-weighted contrast-enhanced MR image of a cystic lesion in the upper brain stem.

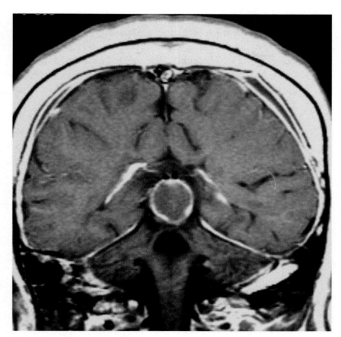

Figure 17–14. Coronal T1-weighted contrast-enhanced MR image of the lesion in Figure 17–13.

an aggressive and lethal manner. Biopsies of these tumors usually have revealed them to be astrocytic tumors, often anaplastic astrocytoma or glioblastoma multiforme. However, even those biopsied tumors called low-grade astrocytoma or grade II tumors behave in the same fashion as the higher-grade tumors. It is probable that some of these tumors were incorrectly diagnosed based on the small biopsy samples that are possible in this location. Whatever the reason, there does not appear to be a correlation with histology and outcome in characteristic lesions of the pons (as defined radiographically), and most pediatric neurosurgeons will not attempt a biopsy in this situation. This is one of the only areas of neuro-oncology in which neuroimaging is considered to be sufficiently sensitive and specific to the biology of the tumor that biopsy is no longer recommended. Unfortunately, treatment of these tumors usually will only control tumor growth for months, and most children will die of tumor progression within 8 to 12 months. Treatment includes radiation therapy, in single or multiple fractions, and, in some cases, chemotherapy.[28–33] Adjuvant chemotherapy has not been proved to alter prognosis, and most children currently treated with chemotherapy are treated according to investigational studies.

FUTURE DIRECTIONS

Physicians who treat children with brain cancer have unique challenges. One is the diversity of tumors that arise in this patient population. Unlike adults, children tend to have lower-grade astrocytic tumors, PNETs, and ependymomas. Diffuse brainstem gliomas also are seen more commonly in children than in adults. In addition, particularly in younger infants, radiation therapy is not a primary option for treatment because of the risk of radiation-associated injury and subsequent neurocognitive and neurodevelopmental delay. Newer treatment strategies include the targeting of molecular pathways that influence growth and progression of the malignant phenotype, similar to the strategies used in adult tumors. In some respects, there is no difference in this approach in children or adults. New therapies ultimately will come from laboratory efforts to understand the biology of these tumors and the translational efforts of clinical scientists to safely treat these children with specific therapies that will slow or halt tumor progression. In some tumors, such as cerebellar JPA, a cure is possible with surgical resection. In other tumors, such as PNET or disseminated ependymoma, much more work is needed to improve progression-free and overall survival. Significant improvement in therapy has occurred in recent years, particularly in the use of chemotherapy for lower-grade astrocytoma. As new strategies become available for testing in the clinic, it is important to have a team of physicians in place to ensure safety and appropriate assessment of response, and, thus, referral to specialized centers is encouraged.

REFERENCES

1. Preston-Martin S. Epidemiology of primary CNS neoplasms. Neurol Clin 1996;14:273–90.
2. Gropman AL, Packer RJ, Nicholson HS, et al. Treatment of diencephalic syndrome with chemotherapy: growth, tumor response, and long term control. Cancer 1998;83:166–72.
3. Packer RJ, Sutton LN, Atkins TE, et al. A prospective study of cognitive function in children receiving whole-brain radiotherapy and chemotherapy: 2-year results. J Neurosurg 1989;70:707–13.
4. van Eys J, Cangir A, Coody D, et al. MOPP regimen as primary chemotherapy for brain tumors in infants. J Neurooncol 1985;3:237–43.
5. Duffner PK, Horowitz ME, Krischer JP, et al. Postoperative chemotherapy and delayed radiation in children less than

three years of age with malignant brain tumors [comments]. N Engl J Med 1993;328:1725–31.
6. Geyer JR, Zeltzer PM, Boyett JM, et al. Survival of infants with primitive neuroectodermal tumors or malignant ependymomas of the CNS treated with eight drugs in 1 day: a report from the Children's Cancer Group. J Clin Oncol 1994;12:1607–15.
7. Packer RJ. Chemotherapy for medulloblastoma/primitive neuroectodermal tumors of the posterior fossa. Ann Neurol 1990;28:823–8.
8. Rorke LB, Trojanowski JQ, Lee VM, et al. Primitive neuroectodermal tumors of the central nervous system. Brain Pathol 1997;7:765–84.
9. Biegel JA, Rorke LB, Packer RJ, et al. Isochromosome 17q in primitive neuroectodermal tumors of the central nervous system. Genes Chromosomes Cancer 1989;1:139–47.
10. Cogen PH, McDonald JD. Tumor suppressor genes and medulloblastoma. J Neurooncol 1996;29:103–12.
11. McDonald JD, Daneshvar L, Willert JR, et al. Physical mapping of chromosome 17p13.3 in the region of a putative tumor suppressor gene important in medulloblastoma. Genomics 1994;23:229–32.
12. Tait DM, Thornton-Jones H, Bloom HJ, et al. Adjuvant chemotherapy for medulloblastoma: the first multi-centre control trial of the International Society of Paediatric Oncology (SIOP I). Eur J Cancer 1990;26:464–9.
13. Packer RJ. Childhood medulloblastoma: progress and future challenges. Brain Dev 1999;21:75–81.
14. Packer RJ, Sutton LN, Elterman R, et al. Outcome for children with medulloblastoma treated with radiation and cisplatin, CCNU, and vincristine chemotherapy. J Neurosurg 1994;81:690–8.
15. Packer RJ, Finlay JL. Chemotherapy for childhood medulloblastoma and primitive neuroectodermal tumors. Oncologist 1996;1:381–93.
16. Pollack IF, Gerszten PC, Martinez AJ, et al. Intracranial ependymomas of childhood: long-term outcome and prognostic factors. Neurosurgery 1995;37:655–67.
17. Hamilton RL, Pollack IF. The molecular biology of ependymomas. Brain Pathol 1997;7:807–22.
18. Horn B, Heideman R, Geyer R, et al. A multi-institutional retrospective study of intracranial ependymoma in children: identification of risk factors. J Pediatr Hematol Oncol 1999;21:203–11.
19. Awaad YM, Allen JC, Miller DC, et al. Deferring adjuvant therapy for totally resected intracranial ependymoma. Pediatr Neurol 1996;14:216–19.
20. Packer RJ, Ater J, Allen J, et al. Carboplatin and vincristine chemotherapy for children with newly diagnosed progressive low-grade gliomas. J Neurosurg 1997;86:747–54.
21. Petronio J, Edwards MS, Prados M, et al. Management of chiasmal and hypothalamic gliomas of infancy and childhood with chemotherapy. J Neurosurg 1991;74:701–8.
22. Sposto R, Ertel IJ, Jenkin RD, et al. The effectiveness of chemotherapy for treatment of high grade astrocytoma in children: results of a randomized trial. A report from the Children's Cancer Group. J Neurooncol 1989;7:165–77.
23. Finlay JL, Boyett JM, Yates AJ, et al. Randomized phase III trial in childhood high-grade astrocytoma comparing vincristine, lomustine, and prednisone with the eight-drugs-in-1-day regimen. Children's Cancer Group. J Clin Oncol 1995;13:112–23.
24. Finlay JL, Goldman S, Wong MC, et al. Pilot study of high-dose thiotepa and etoposide with autologous bone marrow rescue in children and young adults with recurrent CNS tumors. The Children's Cancer Group. J Clin Oncol 1996;14:2495–503.
25. Barkovich AJ, Krischer J, Kun LE, et al. Brain stem gliomas: a classification system based on magnetic resonance imaging. Pediatr Neurosurg 1990;16:73–83.
26. Edwards MS, Prados M. Current management of brain stem gliomas. Pediatr Neurosci 1987;13:309–15.
27. Fischbein NJ, Prados MD, Wara W, et al. Radiologic classification of brain stem tumors: correlation of magnetic resonance imaging appearance with clinical outcome. Pediatr Neurosurg 1996;24:9–23.
28. Edwards MS, Wara WM, Urtasun RC, et al. Hyperfractionated radiation therapy for brain-stem glioma: a phase I–II trial. J Neurosurg 1989;70:691–700.
29. Packer RJ, Littman PA, Sposto RM, et al. Results of a pilot study of hyperfractionated radiation therapy for children with brain stem gliomas. Int J Radiat Oncol Biol Phys 1987;13:1647–51.
30. Packer RJ, Allen JC, Goldwein JL, et al. Hyperfractionated radiotherapy for children with brainstem gliomas: a pilot study using 7,200 cGy. Ann Neurol 1990;27:167–73.
31. Packer RJ, Prados M, Phillips P, et al. Treatment of children with newly diagnosed brain stem gliomas with intravenous recombinant beta-interferon and hyperfractionated radiation therapy: a Children's Cancer Group phase I/II study. Cancer 1996;77:2150–6.
32. Packer RJ, Boyett JM, Zimmerman RA, et al. Outcome of children with brain stem gliomas after treatment with 7800 cGy of hyperfractionated radiotherapy. A Children's Cancer Group phase I/II trial. Cancer 1994;74:1827–34.
33. Prados MD, Wara WM, Edwards MS, et al. The treatment of brain stem and thalamic gliomas with 78 Gy of hyperfractionated radiation therapy [comments]. Int J Radiat Oncol Biol Phys 1995;32:85–91.

18

Meningiomas

MICHAEL W. McDERMOTT, MD, FRCSC
ALFREDO QUINONES-HINOJOSA, MD
ANDREW W. BOLLEN, DVM, MD
DAVID A. LARSON, PHD, MD
MICHAEL PRADOS, MD

An intracranial meningioma is one of the three most common primary brain tumors to be treated surgically, and great progress has been made in this area in the last 15 years. Much of the surgical treatment of intracranial meningiomas in the first 70 years of the twentieth century was based on the 1938 publication on the subject by Cushing and Eisenhardt.[1] Since that time, there have been many advances in the microsurgical and anesthetic techniques used for the excision of these benign tumors. Major advances have been made in understanding the molecular biology of meningiomas and the biology of signal transduction from the cell surface to the nucleus.[2-8] As these cellular mechanisms are further worked out, new targets for therapy will be developed, improving the treatment of recurrent tumors after standard surgical and radiation therapy.

Some issues from the clinic have not been completely resolved by these scientific advances. Examples are the associations between the female sex and the increased incidence of meningiomas, the rare case of worsening of clinical symptoms in a pregnant patient who harbors a meningioma, and the association (if any) between breast cancer and meningiomas.[9-12] This chapter will briefly review some of the more recent information on the epidemiologic, pathologic, biologic, clinical, and surgical information about meningiomas. After this brief review, the reader will realize that there is still much that needs to be done to improve outcomes for patients harboring these seemingly simple tumors.

INCIDENCE

Meningiomas account for between 15 and 25 percent of all primary intracranial tumors; incidences range from 0.08 to 13.72 per 100,000 population.[13-16] In the 1997 report from the Central Brain Tumor Registry of the United States, meningiomas accounted for 24 percent of primary brain tumors, second only to astrocytomas and other gliomas combined, and well ahead of pituitary tumors.[13] Two recent studies from the Kumamoto Prefecture in Japan (population, 1.85 million) provided longitudinal follow-ups of from 5 to 7 years on meningiomas.[17,18] One report found that overall, meningiomas were the most common primary brain tumor in this population group: the age-adjusted incidence was 2.76 per 100,000, with the highest incidence being 13.02 per 100,000 among women aged 70 to 79 years. With 2 more years of data, a second report from the same group showed that meningiomas accounted for 32.2 percent of all primary tumors and that 38.9 percent of these tumors were asymptomatic. In other studies, approximately one-third of incidental intracranial tumors found at autopsy are meningiomas. Asymptomatic meningiomas occur most often in women, particularly women in the seventh or eighth decade. Intracranial meningiomas are almost twice as common in women as in men; in the spine, this ratio rises to 20:1. This preponderance in women suggests a role for sex hormones in the predisposition or development of these tumors. Meningiomas are a rare form of primary brain tumor in children, and there does not appear to be any sex predilection for females (in fact, these ratios can be reversed).[19] Multiple meningiomas appear in about 10 percent of patients with sporadic meningiomas, and multiple meningiomas are commonly seen in the setting of neurofibromatosis type 2 (NF2). Atypical meningiomas account for 5 to 7 percent of all meningiomas. Anaplastic or malignant meningiomas account for between 1 and 3 percent.[20]

LOCATION

Meningiomas are thought to arise from arachnoid cap cells. Cushing and Eisenhardt pointed out that they "adhere to and involve the dura even though they do not actually arise from it."[1] Therefore, one would expect tumors to be most common at sites where these cap cells are involved with the formation of arachnoid granulations, the sites where cerebrospinal fluid is returned to the venous system. These granulations are concentrated along the basal and convex venous sinuses. As a result, two of the more common locations are in a parasagittal (superior sagittal sinus) or sphenoid wing (sphenoparietal and cavernous sinus) location. In the largest clinical series, the most common locations were parasagittal, falx, convexity, and sphenoid wing (Table 18–1).[1,21–23] The posterior fossa is the location of 3 to 16 percent of tumors. Intraventricular meningiomas are uncommon and account for less than 10 percent of all tumors. When a meningioma does occur within the lateral ventricle, it is more often on the left than on the right, and it usually occurs in the atrium. Tumors within the third and fourth ventricles are rare. Atypical and anaplastic meningiomas are more common on the falx and lateral convexity. When metastases disseminate from a malignant meningioma they most commonly spread to lung, liver, and bone.[24]

ETIOLOGY

Radiation

In spite of the fact that radiation therapy is recommended for recurrent benign meningiomas and for all malignant meningiomas, meningiomas are known to be induced by both low- and high-dose irradiation. For a tumor to be considered radiation induced, it must meet the following criteria: (1) the tumor must occur within the irradiated field, (2) it must not be present prior to radiation treatment, (3) there must be a reasonable latent interval between irradiation and development of the new tumor, (4) the new tumor should be verified histologically, and (5) the new tumor should differ from the original tumor.[25] The experience with low-energy, low-dose irradiation of tinea capitus in the 1940s did much to confirm this relationship. In a group of Israeli children treated with 250 cGy of low-energy cobalt-60 irradiation, meningiomas were the most common brain tumor seen, and the risk of these children developing the tumor was increased by a factor of 9.5.[26,27] It has also been shown that the higher the radiation dose, the shorter the latent interval to the development of the tumor in the range of 10 to 40 years. Hug and colleagues reported that for low (< 1,000 cGy), moderate (1,000 to 2,000 cGy), and high (> 2,000 cGy) doses, the mean intervals for a diagnosis of radiation-induced meningioma were 35.2 years, 26.1 years, and 19.5 years, respectively.[28] Reviewing the experience in Slovenia over a 31-year period, Strojan and colleagues found that in 445 children younger than 16 years of age, the cumulative actuarial risk of a secondary meningioma at 10, 20, and 25 years was 0.53

Table 18–1. COMMON LOCATIONS FOR MENINGIOMAS					
		Location (% of Meningiomas Occurring)			
Clinical Series	No. of Patients	Convexity	Parasagittal	Sphenoid Wing	Posterior Fossa
Cushing and Eisenhardt[1]	295	18	22	18	8
Jaaskelainen[21]	657	25	21	12	3
Kallio et al[22]	935	22	27	23	10
Stafford et al[23]	581	16.8	18.6	15.3	13.6

percent, 1.2 percent, and 8.18 percent, respectively.[29] Radiation-induced meningiomas are more likely to behave aggressively or to be pathologically atypical or malignant. They tend to occur in a younger age group, compared to sporadic benign meningiomas, and they are frequently multiple.

Trauma

Trauma has long been implicated as a factor in the development of meningiomas. Cushing and Eisenhardt found that in 24 percent of their cases of meningioma with a history of trauma, the injured area corresponded to the site of the development of tumor.[1] Subsequent studies were not as compelling. In a study of 2,953 head injuries, Annegers and colleagues found that meningiomas did not occur more frequently in this group than in the general population. In addition, the location of the injury had no influence on the site of tumor development.[30] A more recent international review of 1,178 glioma patients and 330 meningioma patients, matched with 2,236 controls, found that the risk for ever having had a head injury was highest for males with meningioma, but the risk for having had serious head injuries was lower compared to controls.[31] Among males, a latency of 15 to 24 years increased the risk of developing a meningioma, and the risk was highest in those involved in sports most often associated with head injury. Unlike blunt trauma, penetrating trauma that injures the dura and arachnoid might be expected to be associated with a small increased risk. In the spectrum of all craniotomies done for a variety of pathologies where the dura and arachnoid are surgically incised, this increased risk related to penetrating trauma is exceedingly small.

Viruses

A large number of deoxyribonucleic acid (DNA) and ribonucleic acid (RNA) viruses are known to cause oncogenic transformation in laboratory settings with the creation of primary brain tumors in rodents. As yet, there is no virus that can cause the de novo formation of a typical dural-based meningioma in rodents. Previous work with human tumor samples has focused on looking for homology in the tumor DNA of meningiomas with known oncogenic DNA viruses. Candidates have included simian virus 40 (SV40) and the human papovavirus. In a recent study by Weggen and colleagues, a polymerase chain reaction assay with fluorescent labeled primers found SV40 sequences in only 1 of 131 meningiomas, a result that argues against a significant role for DNA viruses in the development of meningiomas.[32]

Hormones and Peptides

Conflicting clinical studies either support or refute a role for sex steroid hormones in the development of meningiomas. The majority of benign sporadic meningiomas are estrogen receptor negative and progesterone receptor positive.[33] In one study (by Schlehofer and colleagues), menopausal women had a greatly reduced risk of meningiomas; this reduced risk was most pronounced when menopause had been produced surgically at a younger age.[34] Oophorectomy beyond menopause did not appear to influence the risk of the development of meningioma, and there was no association found between parity and the development of a meningioma.[34] Since menopause was associated with the cessation of estrogen production, the authors felt that these findings support the role of this hormone in the development of the tumor.[34] Lambe and colleagues concluded the opposite: from 1,088 patients with meningiomas, they selected 5 age-matched controls from a fertility registry in Sweden and found that parity and the age of the women when they first gave birth were unrelated to the risk of meningioma development.[35] There was no evidence that unopposed estrogen activity was associated with an increased risk of developing meningiomas.[35]

The growth of meningiomas during pregnancy is taken as evidence of hormonal stimulation of meningioma growth, yet there are other physiologic changes that may also affect the presentation of these patients. In a recent literature review of 62 cases of pregnancy-related symptomatic meningiomas, Roelvink and colleagues felt that if a causal relationship between pregnancy and meningiomas existed, the number of cases reported should be higher and their incidence should be higher in the reproductive years.[36,37] The incidence of meningiomas is, however, higher during the fifth, sixth, and seventh decades of a woman's life. During these times, progestins and estradiol levels are low if not absent, but peripheral tissues such as adipose cells are still producing esterone. As well, if progestins and estrogens are important in stimulating the growth of meningiomas, antagonists for these receptors might be expected to have an equally marked inhibitory effect on growth, but (as is noted later) this is not the case.

A possible link supporting a role for hormones in the development of meningiomas is the reported clinical association between meningiomas and breast cancer. Does this suggest a causal link between an uncommon tumor (meningioma) and a very common one (breast cancer), or is this related to chance? In a study of 283 patients with meningiomas, Jacobs and colleagues indentified all other tumors in the same patients and then compared these rates to the expected numbers by using age- and sex-matched cancer incidence data. They found that the number of breast cancers in the meningioma group was not significantly higher than that predicted for age and sex.[9] Beyond the role for sex hormones, cytogenetic studies have shown that both meningiomas and breast cancers show a loss of the long arm or all of chromosome 22. Sulman and colleagues found that 34 percent also had a loss of heterozygosity in the short arm of the chromosome 1p32 region in meningiomas, the same region that has been reported for breast carcinoma, melanoma, and other cancers.[12] Other studies, however, have failed to find a genetic link between meningiomas and breast cancer. Kirsch and colleagues examined sporadic meningiomas for the putative tumor-suppressor genes *BRCA1* and *BRCA2*, which are associated with familial and sporadic forms of breast and ovarian cancer. The study found no alterations of these genes in the meningiomas to suggest a common pathogenesis for these tumors.[10]

An ever-increasing number of receptors have been indentified on the surface of meningioma cells. A number of peptides have been shown to have stimulatory effects on meningioma cells in culture through their interactions with such receptors. Targeting these same receptors with antagonists may have the corresponding inhibitory effect on tumor cell growth. Epidermal growth factor (EGF) is one cytokine that has been shown by (Weisman and colleagues) to increase DNA synthesis and cell growth in primary cultures of meningioma cells. The EGF receptor (EGFR) in meningiomas was characterized by the same workers, and they suggested the involvement of this growth factor in the proliferation and/or differentiation of meningioma cells.[38] Several studies have also suggested that the growth of meningiomas may be mediated by platelet-derived growth factor (PDGF). The PDGF ligand is found in two subunits (A and B), and there are two isoforms of the receptors (α and β). The β-receptor is functionally involved in meningioma growth, and when it is activated, c-fos oncogene levels and meningioma cell division are increased. These findings support the hypothesis that PDGF-BB acts as a growth factor in meningiomas.[39–41]

There are several studies that evaluate the cause of peritumoral vasogenic edema in meningiomas. The exact cause of the edema is not known, but the edema is thought to result from increased microvascular permeability of brain adjacent to tumor and from the extravasation of proteinaceous and plasma fluid into the adjacent peritumoral space. Several studies have confirmed the importance of the production (by meningiomas) of vascular endothelial growth factor (VEGF), a 40- to 46-kDa protein that is 10,000 to 50,000 times more potent than histamine in increasing vascular permeability, in stimulating tumorigenesis, and in neovascularization. To confirm the link between VEGF messenger ribonucleic acid (mRNA) expression and peritumoral edema in meningiomas, 31 meningioma specimens were subjected to Northern blot analysis, hybridization with a complementary DNA VEGF probe, and laser densitometry to determine the relative levels of VEGF mRNA expression. Magnetic resonance imaging features were assessed in a double-blind fashion to grade the extent of preoperative peritumoral edema and to correlate these with the VEGF expression by meningiomas. The investigators found that meningiomas with peritumoral edema exhibited 3.4 times the level of VEGF mRNA as compared to those without edema.[42] These data suggest that VEGF expression may be an important factor in the development of edema around meningiomas. The regulation of VEGF expression by meningiomas has also been studied in vitro. Tsai and colleagues demonstrated that epidermal and basic fibroblast growth factors induce VEGF secretion by meningioma cells to 160 percent above baseline. The sex hormones estradiol, progesterone, and testosterone did not stimulate or inhibit VEGF secretion, whereas dexamethasone decreased VEGF secretion to 32 percent of baseline.[43] This study suggests that growth factors and corticosteroids (but not sex hormones) may regulate VEGF secretion and provides another explanation for the beneficial effect of corticosteroids in alleviating peritumoral brain edema in meningiomas.

Whereas VEGF stimulates angiogenesis, both VEGF and other mitogens cause the activation of the *ras* signaling pathway. Inhibition of *ras* activity may therefore control both tumor mitotic and angiogenic growth. Shu and colleagues studied the *ras* pathway by using nine primary meningioma cell cultures infected with the recombinant adenovirus Ad-rasN17 (encoding the dominant-negative ras protein that inhibits the function of all endogenous cellular ras proteins) or with control adenovirus Ad-pAC.[44] The results demonstrated that transfection of meningioma cells with Ad-rasN17 increased the expression levels of the rasN17 mutant protein and inhibited phosphorylation of the mitogen-activated protein kinases.[44] Suppression of ras proteins inhibited the proliferation of all exponentially growing and growth-arrested meningioma cells stimulated with serum, suggesting that proliferation of primary meningioma cells is dependent on the presence of functional ras proteins. Inhibiting the *ras* pathway may be of great value in preventing growth factor–stimulated proliferation of meningioma cells.

PATHOLOGY

Grading and Macro- and Microscopic Features

In 1922, Cushing coined the term "meningioma" to describe a frequently benign and globular tumor arising from the meninges.[45] Subsequently, a variety of histopathologic schemes were used; most recently, the World Health Organization (WHO) published its classification scheme (Table 18–2).[46] Hemangiopericytoma is now recognized as a separate entity, and melanocytic tumors (diffuse melanocytosis, melanocytoma, and primary meningeal malignant melanoma) are those with different biologic behaviors and are also classified separately. Previously, we have used the grading system developed at the University of Helsinki (Table 18–3).[14,20,21] Points from 0 to 3 are assigned for each of five cellular features: 0 for the feature being absent and 1, 2, and 3 for increasing degrees associated with a more malignant phenotype. The fifth feature, brain invasion, is either absent (0) or present (3). It should be noted that in the new WHO grading, brain invasion alone is not sufficient for the histopathologic diagnosis of malig-

Table 18–2. GROUPING OF MENINGIOMAS BY PROBABLE RECURRENCE AND GRADE*

Histopathologic Subtype	Risk of Recurrence / Aggressive Growth[†]	WHO Grade
Meningothelial	Low	I
Fibrous	Low	I
Transitional	Low	I
Psammomatous	Low	I
Angiomatous	Low	I
Microcystic	Low	I
Secretory	Low	I
Lymphoplasmacyte-rich	Low	I
Metaplastic	Low	I
Atypical	Moderate	II
Clear cell	Moderate	II
Chordoid	Moderate	II
Rhabdoid	High	III
Papillary	High	III
Anaplastic	High	III

*World Health Organization grading system, 2000.
[†]Higher for any subtype with high proliferation index and/or brain invasion.
Adapted from Kleihues P, Cavenee WK, International Agency for Research on Cancer, editors. Pathology and genetics of tumours of the nervous system. Lyon: IARC Press; 2000.

Table 18–3. HELSINKI GRADING SYSTEM

Histologic Feature	Points
Increased cellularity	0–3
Nuclear pleomorphism	0–3
Loss of architecture	0–3
Mitotic figures	0–3
Necrosis	0–3
Brain infiltration	0 = Absent
	3 = Present
Total Points	**Grade/Description**
0–3	I/Benign
4–6	II/Atypical
7–11	III/Anaplastic
12–18	IV/Sarcomatous

nancy. One advantage of the Helsinki system is that it provides documentation of the grading of histologic features used to assess anaplasia. In a report of 935 meningiomas graded by using the Helsinki system, 94.3 percent were grade I, 4.7 percent were grade II, and 1 percent were grade III.[20]

An assessment of the proliferation index of meningiomas can now be readily determined, as with other tumors. Hoshino had done much of the pioneering work in this area and had relied on the preoperative administration of bromodeoxyuridine.[47,48] A MIB-1 labeling index is now used, derived by the immunostaining of paraffin-embedded material and a manual count of stained cells in a high-power field.

The three classic histopathologic types of meningioma are meningothelial, transitional, and fibroblastic. Certain histologic subtypes are associated with less favorable clinical behavior. The recent WHO grading system reclassifies meningiomas on the basis of their likelihood of recurrence and also applies a grade based on the subtype.[46]

Meningiomas of the convexity dura are globular masses with discrete edges (Figure 18–1). Hypervascular tissue is seen in the dura at the edge of larger tumors and likely accounts for the so-called dural tail sign on magnetic resonance imaging studies. Tumors of the falx, tentorium, and basal dura tend to have a wider dural attachment; the "en plaque" variant is the extreme example. As meningiomas arise from arachnoid cap cells, they tend to push the surrounding normal arachnoid and brain away, excavating a cavity similar to their shape. The softer tumors are generally beefy red, and the fibrous tumors are whitish-tan. Hyperostotoic bone of the convexity tends to be softer and less dense than the same type of bone in the skull base (Figure 18–2). Cysts that are within or at the edge of the tumor are rare.

The microscopic features of meningiomas are best reviewed under their WHO grades and their descriptive subtypes, listed below.[46] On immunohistochemical staining, most meningiomas are vimentin positive and most benign tumors are positive for epithelial membrane antigen (EMA). Other stains with variable degrees of positivity are laminin, fibronectin, cytokeratin, S-100, and carcinogenic embryonic antigen (CEA).

Specific Subtypes of Meningioma

Meningiomas with Low Risks of Recurrence and Aggressive Growth (Grade I)

Meningothelial Meningioma. In this subtype, cells are uniform in nature and are arranged in sheets. The nuclei are large and centrally located. Cellular whorls are frequent. The tumor cells form lobules that are surrounded by collagenous septa.[46]

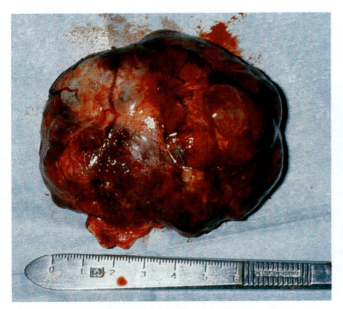

Figure 18–1. Lobular convexity meningioma, removed in total due to preserved arachnoid planes. Tumor "fell out" with circumferential dural incision. Note the beefy red color in this non-embolized meningioma.

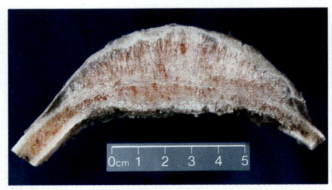

Figure 18–2. Cross-section of hyperostotic bone removed before excision of underlying falx and parasagittal meningioma. Decalcification and sectioning confirms tumor within diploic space and cortical bone. Note the loss of a distinct line of inner and outer table of skull. The defect was repaired with a combination of titanium mesh and methylmethacrylate.

Fibrous Meningioma. Tumors of this type contain bundles of spindle-shaped shells with long and narrow nuclei. Whirl formation and psammoma bodies are infrequent. There is an abundant interlacing matrix of collagen and reticulan.[46] Intraventricular meningiomas are commonly of this subtype.

Transitional (Mixed) Meningioma. This tumor has features of both meningothelial and fibrous meningiomas—hence their name. Meningothelial cells forming cellular whirls are separated by spindle-shaped cells. Psammoma bodies are frequent and are typically found in the center of cellular whirls (Figure 18–3).[46]

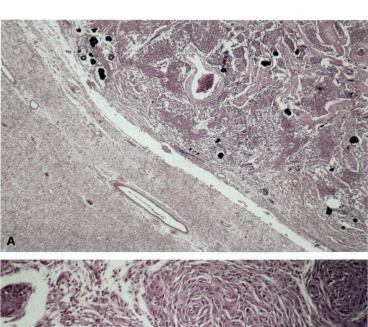
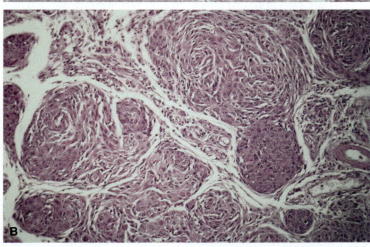
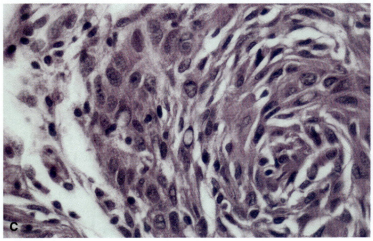

Figure 18–3. *A*, Low-power view of a transitional meningioma at the interface with the brain (×25 original magnification). *B*, Lobular and fascicular arrangement of tumor with whorls (×100 magnification). *C*, High-power view of the same tumor, with whorl formation evident and with cytoplasmic nuclear inclusions (×250 magnification) (H & E stain).

Psammomatous Meningioma. A psammamatous meningioma resembles a transitional tumor, in which numerous psammoma bodies are found in the center of cellular whorls. The psammoma bodies may become confluent, forming irregular or confluent calcified masses. Although most commonly found in the thoracic spinal region as intradural and extramedullary tumors, they are also seen in the olfactory groove intracranially (Figure 18–4).[46]

Angiomatous Meningioma. This tumor should not be confused with "angioblastic meningioma" (a previous designation) or hemangiopericytoma, which has a much different clinical behavior and appearance. Angiomatous meningiomas contain numerous blood vessels on a background of a benign meningioma. Although the vessels can vary in size, most are small, with hyalinized walls.[46]

Microcystic Meningioma. This tumor contains cells with loose cytoplasm and elongated processes. This type of tumor occurs intracranially and within the spinal canal. Previously, it was referred to as "humid" because of the apparent cystic change seen microscopically.[46]

Secretory Meningioma. Secretory meningioma cells show focal epithelial differentiation with an accumulation of eosinophilic material (so-called pseudopsammoma bodies). These bodies stain for CEA and may be associated with elevated serum levels of the same marker. Peritumoral edema may be prominent.[46]

Lymphoplasmacyte-Rich Meningioma. Lymphoplasmacyte-rich meningiomas are meningiomas with an extensive plasma cell infiltrate and lymphoid follicles. They tend to occur in the posterior fossa and may be associated with hematologic abnormalities.[46]

Metaplastic Meningioma. Focal osseous, lipomatous, or myxoid changes may be seen within meningiothelial, fibrous, and transitional meningiomas. The clinical significance is unclear, but these tumors follow a benign course.[46]

Menigiomas with Aggressive Behavior (Grades II and III)

Chordoid Meningioma. This tumor has areas that resemble chordoma, interspersed with typical areas of meningioma. These regions may contain chronic inflammatory cells and areas with trabeculae of eosinophilic vacuolated cells in a myxoid background. They are classified as WHO grade II.[46]

Clear Cell Meningioma. Clear cell menigiomas contain periodic acid–Schiff (PAS)–positive cells with cytoplasmic clearing secondary to glycogen. The cells are polygonal in shape and do not assume any particular pattern or structure. More common in the cerebellopontine angle and cauda equina, they are classified as WHO grade II when they occur intracranially.[46]

Atypical Meningioma. This tumor has four or more mitoses per 10 high-power fields and three or more of the following features: areas of necrosis, increased cellularity, high nuclear/cytoplasmic ratio, prominent nucleoli, and sheetlike growth. Atypical meningiomas have a high labeling index and are classified as WHO grade II (Figure 18–5).[46]

Papillary Meningioma. This meningioma shows a perivascular pseudopapillary pattern and has a high rate of recurrence. It is more common in children and is classified as WHO grade III.[46]

Rhabdoid Meningioma. Rhabdoid meningiomas contain areas or sheets of rhabdoid tumor cells with eccentric nuclei and eosinophilic cytoplasm composed of whorled intermediate filaments. These rhabdoid cells resemble those described in other areas of the body. Rhabdoid meningiomas are classsifed as WHO grade III.[46]

Anaplastic Meningioma. Also called malignant meningiomas, anaplastic meningiomas have malignant features to a much greater degree than atypical meningiomas. Invasion of the brain alone is not sufficient for the diagnosis. There are usually 20 or

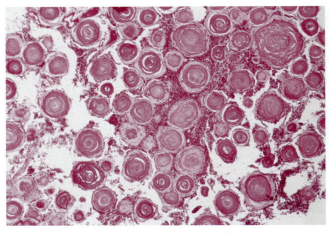

Figure 18–4. Psammomatous meningioma (H & E stain; ×40 magnification) with an area of confluent bodies and a small amount of intervening meningiothelial cells.

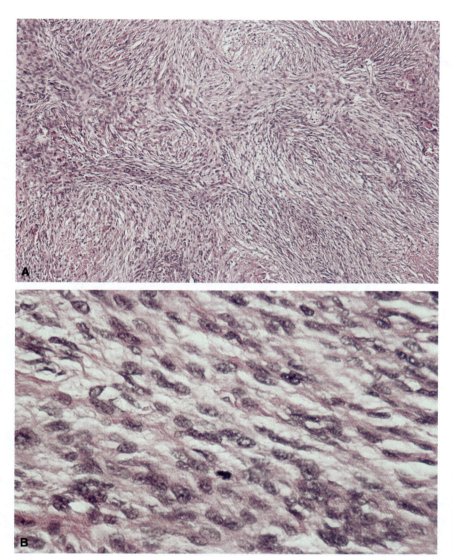

Figure 18–5. *A,* An atypical fibroblastic meningioma seen at low power, revealing a loss of architecture and more sheetlike growth (×100 magnification). *B,* Same tumor, showing mitosis, small cells, nuclear and cytoplasmic atypia, and prominent nucleoli (×250 magnification) (H & E stain).

more mitoses per 10 high-power fields, and they may resemble sarcomas. They are classified as WHO grade III (Figure 18–6).[46]

MOLECULAR BIOLOGY

The most consistent and characteristic karyotypic change in meningiomas is deletion of the long arm or all of chromosome 22.[49,50] The tumor-suppressor gene NF2 resides in this region. With the use of restriction fragment length polymorphisms (RFLPs), the locus for the gene has been localized on the long arm of chromosome 22, between the myoglobin locus and the 22q12.3-qter.[51] Mutations of the NF2 gene are seen in up to 60 percent of sporadic meningiomas, and the common effect is a truncated and presumably nonfunctional merlin protein. Merlin, or schwannomin, is a member of the band 4.1 superfamily of proteins that have been shown to play important roles in linking the cell membrane proteins with the cytoskeleton, a site of activation of tumor-suppressor genes in humans. Lee and colleagues showed that schwannomin is expressed as a protein of approximately 66 kDa and that its expression was severely reduced in almost 60 percent of primary sporadic meningiomas.[52] All six meningotheliomatous meningiomas in their analysis had normal schwannomin expression, suggesting the involvement of other oncogenes or tumor-suppressor genes

The next most frequent karyotypic changes are in the short arm of chromosome 1. In one study by Sulman and colleagues, loss of heterozygosity (LOH)

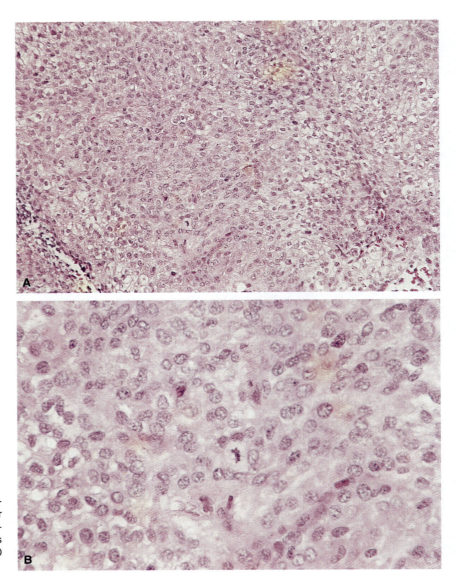

Figure 18–6. *A*, Low-power view of a malignant meningioma with increased cellularity over atypical tumor (×100 magnification). *B*, High-power view of the same tumor, showing mitoses and a high nuclear-cytoplasmic ratio (×250 magnification) (H & E stain).

appeared on the short arm of chromosome 1 (more specifically, in the 1P32 region) in 34 percent of cases.[12] In addition, the 1P32 LOH was associated with chromosome 22 deletions.[12] These and other karyotypic abnormalities tend to be more extensive in atypical and anaplastic meningiomas. Losses of 6Q, 10Q, 14Q, 17P, and 18Q have also been identified and associated with a more aggressive type of meningioma.[53,54]

CLINICAL SYMPTOMATOLOGY

Meningiomas generally present with headache, seizures, progressive focal neurologic deficit, and/or change in personality. As many of these tumors grow slowly, the onset of symptoms is rarely abrupt, except for the largest tumors, in which the ability to accommodate the increasing tumor mass has been exceeded. Symptoms referable to the delayed effects of chronic increased intracranial pressure, such as deteriorating vision from papilledema or double vision from sixth cranial nerve palsies, occur only with the largest tumors.[55]

Olfactory groove meningiomas arise in the midline adjacent to the crista galli in front of the planum sphenoidale. These tumors usually present when they are moderately large, compressing the inferior frontal lobe, and patients usually have a slow onset of change in mental status, depressed mood and impaired insight, judgment, and motivation. It is rare for patients to complain of these changes; family members usually notice a change in personality first. Patients may complain of headaches and reduced vision but rarely complain of a loss of sense of smell.[55] The Foster Kennedy syndrome includes the triad of anosmia, unilateral optic atrophy, and contralateral papilledema.

Posterior to the the olfactory groove are two other locations for meningiomas to develop: regions of the planum sphenoidale (Figure 18–7) and the tuberculum sellae (Figure 18–8). Tumors of the planum usually present with headache, seizures, change of mental status, or visual impairment related to compression of the optic chiasm. Tumors of the tuberculum sellae (the bone on the anterior aspect of the sella turcica) present with a progressive visual loss that is usually asymmetric. Visual field findings may resemble those of pituitary adenoma with a bitemporal field defect. Changes in personality are uncommon. Tumors at this site are more common in women than in men and typically present in the fifth or sixth decades of life.[55]

Meningiomas of the sphenoid wing are some of the most common intracranial, supratentorial meningiomas. Typically, they arise along the course of the sphenoid wing, from medial to the lateral. They are thus referred to by location as clinoid, middle, and lateral sphenoid wing meningiomas. Patients with medial clinoid meningiomas usually have slow progressive unilateral visual loss, headaches, and seizures. Patients with tumors of the middle third sphenoid wing present with headaches, seizures, and mild proptosis. Lateral sphenoid wing meningiomas present with headaches, seizures, and fullness in the region of the temporal fossa. Hyperostotic en plaque meningiomas of the sphenoid wing are characteristically found in middle-aged women with a history of slowly increasing unilateral exophthalmos and fullness in the temporal region. Involvement of the posterolateral orbit and lateral rectus muscle can produce diplopia, and medial extension into the optic canal can reduce visual acuity.[55]

Patients with meningiomas of the cavernous sinus present with double vision, facial numbness, and headache. The fact that the third, fourth, and fifth cranial nerves lie within the lateral wall of the cavernous sinus explains the double vision and facial numbness that these patients can develop late in their course. Seizures are uncommon unless there is a large exophytic middle fossa component to the tumor.[55]

Parasagittal meningiomas (Figure 18–9) are those meningiomas that fill the space between the convexity dura and the midline falx. Patients with these tumors present with headache and focal motor (or sensory) seizures. When the tumors are in the middle third of the distance between the glabella and inion, the seizures begin in the lower extremity and progress up into the body, arm, and face. Frequently, these patients will have interictal unilateral upper-motoneuron signs or cortical sensory disturbance.[55]

Meningiomas can be described as *falcine* when they are covered on their superior aspects by cortical tissue of the frontal, parietal, or occipital lobes. Clinical symptoms are related to tumor position along this interhemispheric dural fold. Patients with anterior-third falx meningiomas may present with headache, seizure, and change of mental status; those with middle-third falx meningiomas may present with headache, seizures, and focal motor sensory deficit. Patients with posterior-third falx meningiomas present with headache and visual loss or irritative visual phenomena with visual hallucinations.[55]

Convexity meningiomas (Figures 18–10 and 18–11) are the most straightforward meningiomas to deal with surgically. They can arise in the dura over the frontal, temporal, parietal, or occipital lobes and are frequently asymptomatic. However, patients with large tumors present with headache, seizures, and focal neurologic deficit, depending on whether

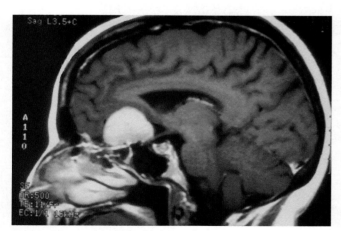

Figure 18–7. Sagittal T1-weighted magnetic resonance imaging (with contrast) of a planum sphenoidale meningioma.

the tumor is on the right or left and whether it is over the speech, motor, sensory, or occipital cortex. Tumors over the nondominant frontal or parietal lobe can reach large sizes, and these patients present only with symptoms and signs of increased intracranial pressure.[55]

Intraventricular (Figure 18–12) meningiomas are uncommon and can reach large sizes before diagnosis. In the series of Cushing and Eisenhardt, patients with tumors within the atrium of the lateral ventricle typically presented with headache, nausea, vomiting, seizures, and speech disturbance.[1] Those with third and fourth ventricular meningiomas present with symptoms of increased intracranial pressure.[55]

Patients with tentorial meningiomas present most often with headache, extremity or gait ataxia, nausea, and vomiting. Seizures are uncommon because most of these tumors project inferiorly from their origin, but upward tumor growth can indent the undersurface of the temporal lobe. Clinical findings include evidence of papilledema; deficits of cranial nerves four, five, and six; and extremity ataxia. The more medial and anterior the tentorial meningioma, the more likely the patients are to have extraocular muscle disturbance. A meningioma involving the junction of the falx cerebri and tentorium is referred to as a falcotentorial meningioma (Figure 18–13). The straight sinus is often occluded, and patients typically present with symptoms of increased intracranial pressure but without focal neurologic deficit.[55]

Meningiomas that occur along the petrous face with extension medially in front of the pons are referred to as petroclival meningiomas (Figure 18–14). Patients with these tumors usually have an

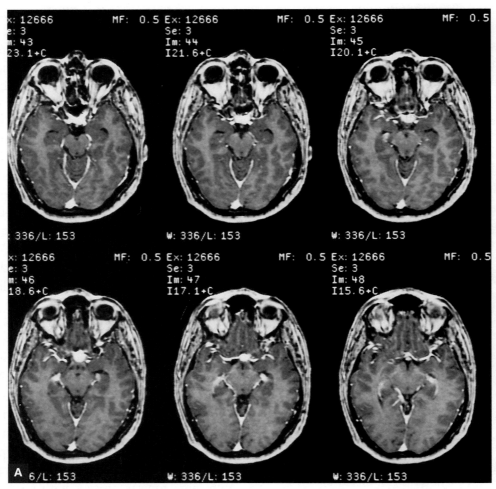

Figure 18–8. *A,* Axial and, *B,* coronal preoperative T1-weighted MRI scans of a small tuberculum meningioma that presented with bitemporal hemianopsia.

insidious onset of headache, gait disturbance, double vision, reduced hearing, and vertigo. Clinical signs include cranial neuropathy of nerves four, five, six, and eight. Papilledema, ataxia, and cerebellar dysmetria can also occur with larger tumors. Sami and Ammirati distinguished between the symptoms of tumors arising along the petrous face anterior to the internal auditory canal (IAC) and the symptoms of tumors arising posterior to the canal.[56] Patients with anterior tumors present with reduced hearing and facial pain or numbness.[56] Those with posterior tumors present with cerebellar signs and gait disturbance (Figure 18–15). A tumor in this location can be confused with a vestibular schwannoma except that (1) there is usually no enlargement of the IAC and (2) meningiomas show the "dural tail" along the petrous face.

Meningiomas at other sites within the posterior fossa are less common, but many patients with these have similar symptoms and signs. Patients with meningiomas of the cerebellar convexity usually present with symptoms and signs of increased

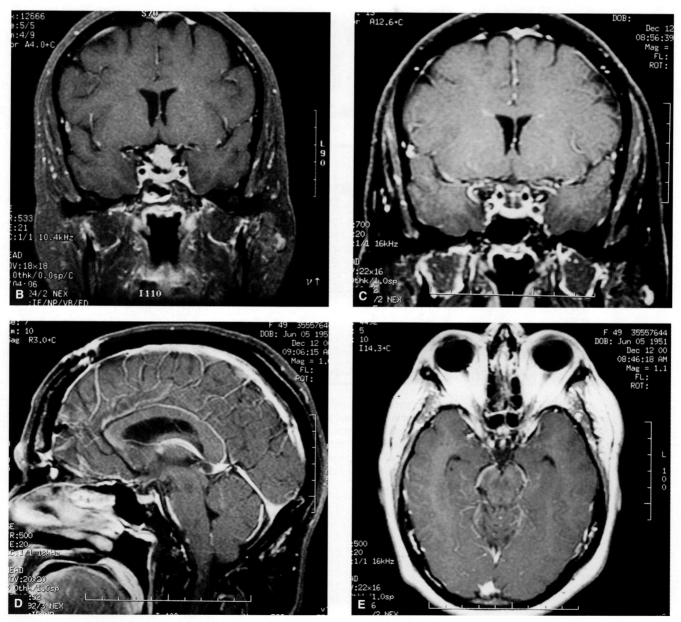

Figure 18–8. *C,* Postoperative coronal, *D,* sagittal, and, *E,* axial images after a bifrontal extended frontal craniotomy.

intracranial pressure, hydrocephalus, or cerebellar dysfunction ipsilateral to the tumor. Patients with meningiomas of the foramen magnum have a history of neck and suboccipital pain that is worse with flexion and Valsalva's maneuver. Motor and sensory deficits usually develop first in the arm and then in the legs; eventually, all extremities may be involved, to the point of spastic quadraparesis. In a clinical

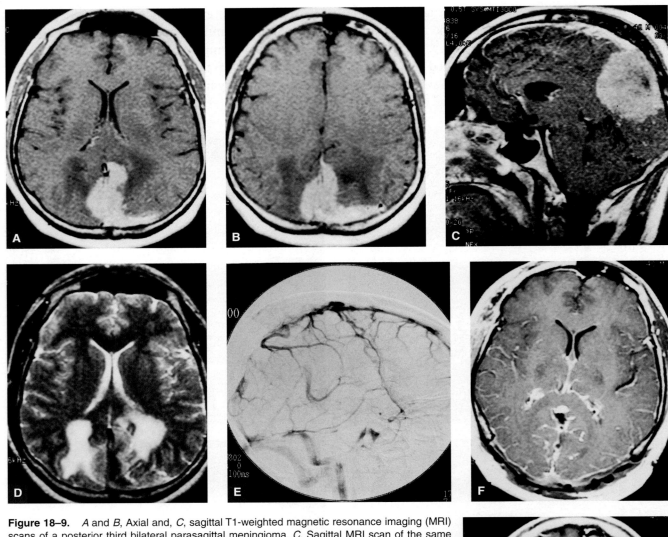

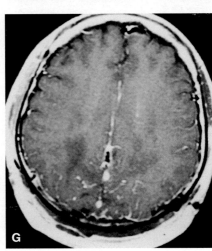

Figure 18–9. *A* and *B*, Axial and, *C*, sagittal T1-weighted magnetic resonance imaging (MRI) scans of a posterior third bilateral parasagittal meningioma. *C*, Sagittal MRI scan of the same meningioma. *D*, T2-weighted axial image showing associated vasogenic edema and low signal intensity of a posterior left-sided tumor that proved to be a malignant meningioma. *E*, Late venous-phase sagittal angiography confirms the occlusion of the superior sagittal sinus, which was excised with the tumor. *F, G*, Postoperative axial postcontrast MRI confirms total removal.

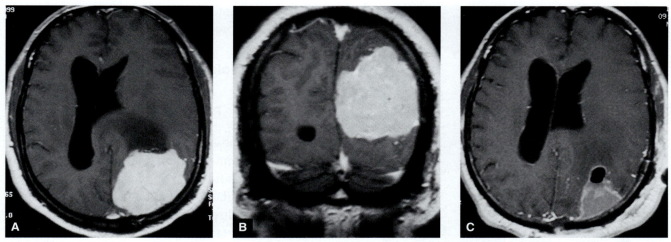

Figure 18–10. *A,* Axial magnetic resonance imaging (MRI) scan of a large left-sided convexity meningioma. *B,* Coronal scan of same tumor. The patient presented with complex language disturbance and with blurred vision from hemorrhagic papilledema. On the axial scan, note the edema at the deepest tumor-brain interface, where at surgery, the arachnoid plane was absent. *C,* Postoperative axial MRI with contrast. The patient was discharged on the third postoperative day.

series of foramen magnum meningioma patients from the Mayo Clinic, 94 percent of patients complained of upper-extremity dysesthesia, 75 percent of suboccipital or neck pain, 49 percent of upper-extremity weakness, 47 percent of gait disturbance, and 42 percent of clumsiness of the hands.[57] The differential diagnosis in these patients included demyelinating disease, syringomyelia, and intramedullary cervical spinal cord tumors. Patients with meningiomas occurring near the confluence of the superior sagittal, straight, transverse, and occipital sinuses (the torcular Herophili) present with symptoms of increased intracranial pressure. In the series of Cushing and Eisenhardt, patients complained of visual impairment, headache, and neck pain. The authors noted that the visual field defects tended to involve the lower quadrants of the visual field before they involved the upper quadrants and that the recovery of deficits proceeded in the reverse direction.[1] The last location for meningiomas of the posterior fossa is the fourth ventricle. The radiographic differential for tumors in this location includes choroid plexus papillomas and ependymomas in adults. Patients with these tumors usually present

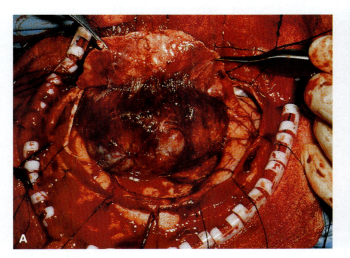
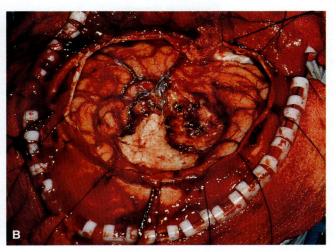

Figure 18–11. *A,* Right frontal temporal, parietal convexity meningioma being removed with a cuff of hypervascular dura that was consistent on MRI, with a "dural tail." *B,* Tumor has been removed (gross specimen is seen in Figure 18–1), with preservation of all but the most medial arachnoid plane. The white tissue in the depths of the cavity is subcortical white matter.

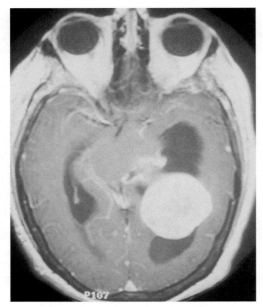

Figure 18–12. A large left atrial intraventricular meningioma, seen by T1-weighted magnetic resonance imaging with contrast. The left temporal and occipital horns are trapped by an atrial tumor, producing obstructive hydrocephalus.

only with symptoms of obstructive hydrocephalus and increased pressure.

Radiologic Imaging Studies

Plain Radiography

In the past, radiographic evidence of punctate or homogeneous intracranial calcification, hyperostosis of the sphenoid wing or calvarium, displacement of the pineal gland, or enlarged vascular channels was used as indirect supportive evidence of the presence of a long-standing vascular tumor attached to the dura or invading the bone. This modality is now rarely used, having been superceded by computed tomography (CT) and magnetic resonance imaging (MRI). Preoperatively, plain radiography may be helpful in delineating the extent of prior craniotomy or craniectomy, which may assist with operative planning and cranial-pin fixation. We rely on CT for

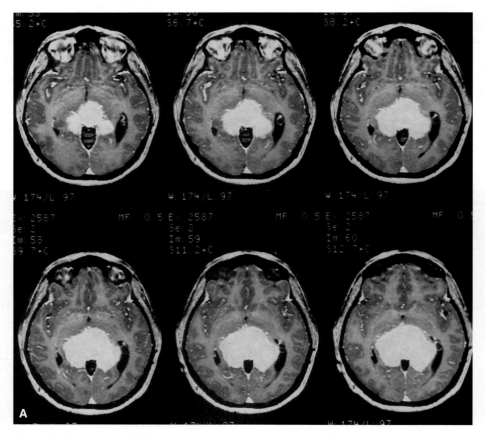

Figure 18–13. *A* and *B*, Falcotentorial meningioma removed via a bilateral occipital craniotomy for interhemispheric approach. The images show the tumor over an extended vertical dimension imaged in the axial plain by T1-weighted magnetic resonance imaging (MRI) with contrast.

bony detail and three-dimensional reconstructions to determine the extent of bone removal around the skull base.

Computed Axial Tomography

On noncontrast CT scans, meningiomas appear isodense to slightly hyperdense. Intratumoral calcification can be punctate or confluent. Kuratsu and colleagues, in evaluating the clinical features of asymptomatic meningiomas, found that those patients with evidence of tumoral calcification on CT scans had a significantly lower likelihood of tumor growth in more than 1 year of follow-up ($p = .008$).[17] Optic-nerve-sheath meningiomas, which have an indolent course clinically, may show a "tram track" linear calcification outlining the orbital course of the optic nerve.[58] When hyperostosis of surrounding bone related to direct tumor invasion is extensive, the bone can be hyperdense and white on images or it

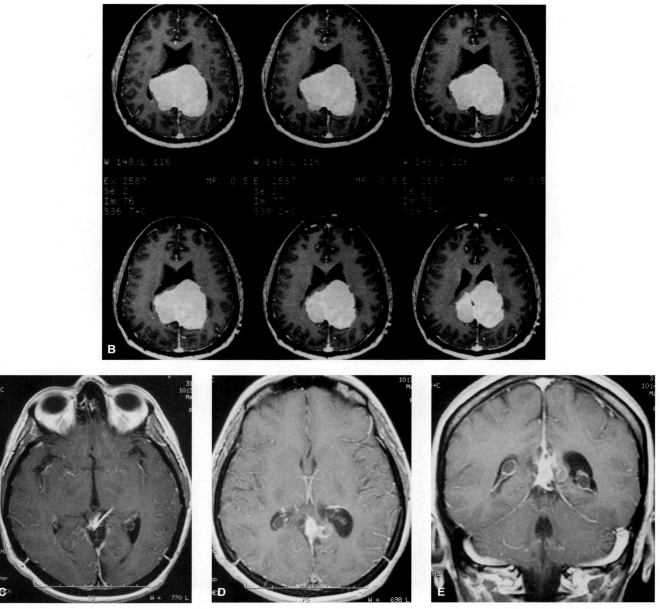

Figure 18–13. *C*, Surgical removal in a single session lasting for over 20 hours produced near-total removal, with normal visual fields 6 weeks postoperatively. Residual tumor above Galen's vein was treated with radiosurgery. The image shows the patient imaged lower down in the axial plain by T1-weighted MRI with contrast. *D*, Image of same but higher up in the axial plain, *E*, Coronal image of same.

can have a mottled, mixed-density appearance. Hyperostosing sphenoid wings produce dense hyperostosis of the greater wing, producing exophthalmos. Computed tomography is superior to MRI for defining the extent of bony hyperostosis but is inferior to MRI for delineating soft-tissue details of both the meningioma and the surrounding brain. Pathologic studies have demonstrated that hyperostotic bone contains meningiothelial cells, and failure to remove this involved bone may lead to later recurrence of a soft-tissue tumor or progression primarily within bone. In the series from the Mayo Clinic, 6 percent (35 of 581 patients) had bone involvement, and this was of borderline significance ($p = .054$) in predicting decreased progression-free survival.[23] Computed tomography may be used now with image-guided surgical systems to help define the margins of bony hyperostosis intraoperatively.

With the intravenous administration of iodinated contrast, meningiomas usually enhance homogeneously. The dural tail reported with MRI is not seen well on CT because of proximity to the underlying bone. Peritumoral edema is hypodense and is thought to be related in some ways to pial blood supply to the tumor. In one series (135 patients), peritumoral brain edema found by CT was used for predicting the probability for recurrence of meningiomas.[59] Edema grade was linearly related to edema volume by digi-

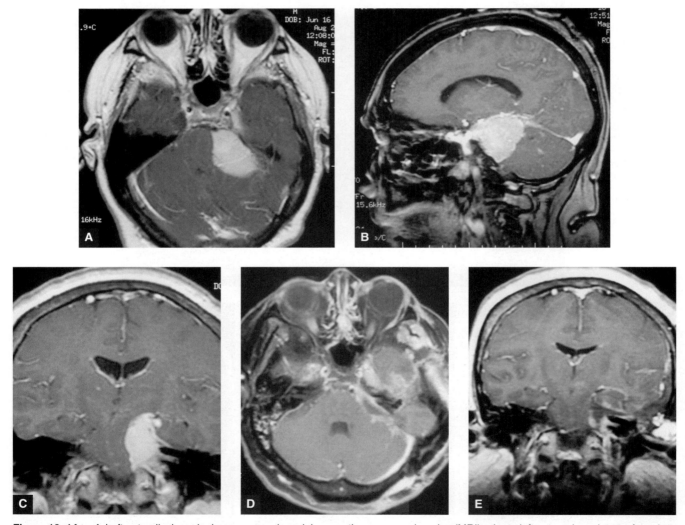

Figure 18–14. *A,* Left petroclival meningioma as seen by axial magnetic resonance imaging (MRI) prior to left petrosal craniotomy for subtotal removal. *B,* Sagittal image of same. *C,* Coronal image of same. *D,* Postoperative axial fat-suppressed MRI shows residual tumor in cavernous sinus. *E,* Coronal image suggests persistent enhancement of the dura of the internal auditory canal. The patient was treated postoperatively with external irradiation.

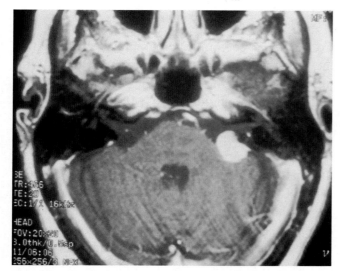

Figure 18–15. Posterior petrous-face meningioma in a patient who presented with tinnitus and dizziness.

tizing the CT scans. The authors found that the three predictors of recurrence were resection completeness, edema grade, and brain invasion.[59] The chance of recurrence within 10 years after complete resection was exponentially related to the maximum linear dimension of surrounding peritumoral edema. The chance of recurrence also increased by approximately 10 percent for each centimeter grade increase in the amount of edema. The likelihood of histopathologic documentation of brain invasion increased by 20 percent per centimeter of edema on the CT scan.[59] Even the simplest imaging study can obtain valuable information that may influence treatment and outcome.

Multiplanar imaging with CT is limited. Direct coronal imaging without much artifact is limited to the anterior and middle cranial fossa, and direct sagittal imaging cannot be achieved. Three-dimensional reconstructions available from image-guided system workstations give bony spatial resolution and detail superior to that of MRI. Current image fusion technologies available with image-guided systems allow the surgeon to use MRI data for delineating soft-tissue margins and to then switch to CT-based images for the resection of tumor-involved bone.

Magnetic Resonance Imaging

Meningiomas are typically dural-based lesions. On T1-weighted MRI scans, approximately 60 percent of these tumors are isointense and 30 percent are hypointense. When the tumor extends into normal marrow, there is a loss of marrow signal hyperintensity, and both the tumor and diploic space are isointense with brain (Figure 18–16). On T2-weighted studies, intensities may vary from hypo- to hyperin-

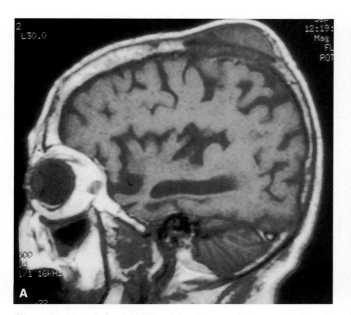
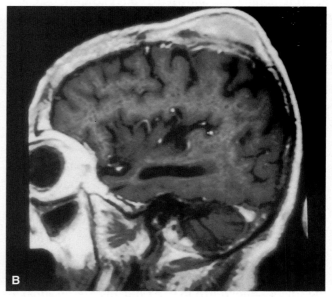

Figure 18–16. *A*, Sagittal T1-weighted magnetic resonance imaging without contrast shows a loss of diploic-space signal hyperintensity due to invasion by meningioma. *B*, Postcontrast image confirms the enhancement of tumor in bone producing a "tower skull." Surgical excision specimen is the same as that seen in Figure 18–2.

tense, and a hypointense signal that surrounds the edge of a meningioma may represent the compressed but preserved arachnoid plane between brain and tumor. Hypointensity within the tumor on T1-weighted imaging may relate to cystic change or to intratumoral calcification. Zee and colleagues evaluated the MRI features of 15 cystic meningiomas, classifying them into three different types. Type I cystic meningiomas were those with cysts wholly within the tumor, type II were those with cysts at the periphery but still within the margins of the tumor, and type III were cysts peripheral to the tumor in adjacent brain.[60] Enhancement of cyst walls was seen in type II cystic meningiomas, and the authors recommended surgical excision of the enhancing wall. They also found that the pathology in these cystic meningiomas tended to be of a more aggressive nature.[60] The dural tail is an imaging feature that is thought to represent hypervascularity of the dura and not infiltration by tumor. The relationship between peritumoral edema (as evidenced by hyperintensity on T2-weighted images) and the cleavage plane between tumor and surrounding brain has been evaluated by Ildan and colleagues. They found that increasing degrees of peritumoral edema on T2-weighted images correlated significantly with a more difficult surgical cleavage plane between tumor and surrounding brain and with increased pial arterial supply as shown by angiography.[61] Thus, MRI findings may preoperatively predict the difficulty of microsurgical dissection.

Magnetic resonance imaging is used most often for image-guided surgical systems that can help with planning skin flaps, bony openings, and the extent of removal as surgery proceeds. The use of image-guided surgical systems in 100 patients with meningiomas was evaluated by Paleologos and colleagues. These patients were compared with 170 patients who were operated on without the use of intraoperative navigational systems. Surgical times were shorter, blood loss was less, mean hospital days were less, and surgical complications (either permanent neurologic deficits or those complications requiring an additional surgical procedure) were significantly less for the image-guided group.[62] At our institution, image-guided surgical systems are the standard for operations on large convexity or skull-based meningiomas.

Cerebral Angiography

Conventional cerebral angiography is still used in the preoperative evaluation of some patients with meningiomas, even with the development of magnetic resonance angiography (MRA) and magnetic resonance venography (MRV). Angiographic information about tumor blood supply and the displacement of major arteries and their relative position to the margins of the tumor assists the surgeon with surgical planning. The venous phase of angiography is still the "gold standard" for determining whether or not a major venous sinus is patent. The position of major cortical veins relative to the tumor is important as well because these veins must be preserved. Embolization of very hypervascular tumors may assist with surgical removal and reduce intraoperative blood loss. Bendszus and colleagues tried to evaluate the benefit of preoperative embolization of meningiomas in a nonrandomized noncontrolled study. Sixty consecutive patients in two different neurosurgical centers were operated on and observed.[63] In one facility, no embolization was performed; in the other center, all patients underwent embolization. There was one new permanent neurologic deficit related to embolization (3%). Mean tumor sizes and mean blood losses from surgery did not differ between centers, but in the subgroup of patients who had devascularization of more than 90 percent of the tumor with embolization, blood loss was significantly less when compared to the subgroup of patients who were not embolized ($p < .05$).[63] There were no differences between the two groups with respect to tumor consistency or intratumoral necrosis.[63] At our institution, preoperative embolization is preserved for the largest meningiomas even if the external carotid supply can be accessed easily during exposure of the tumor. A variety of embolic agents have been used, including Gelfoam powder, polyvinyl alcohol foam, and platinum coils. It has been our practice to embolize these large meningiomas on the day before operation, without waiting for further thrombosis to occur. In the principal author's experience, there has been only one complication related to peritumoral hemorrhage in over 100 surgical cases. In this case, the hematoma encircled the tumor dissecting the arachnoid plane, and this facilitated tumor removal. Embolization may also compromise the blood supply to the scalp, and this should be considered when planning skin incisions.

TREATMENT OPTIONS

Observation

Not every patient with an intracranial meningioma requires surgical intervention. One of the first questions to ask when a tumor is found on imaging studies is whether the imaged tumor is responsible for the patient's symptoms and signs. If not, and if the imaging features are consistent with a benign tumor (homogeneous enhancement, smooth rounded margins, no associated brain edema, and no satellite lesions), then a period of observation is recommended. Typically the first follow-up image is done at 4 months and then (if stable) again at 6 months. Another year of follow-up at 6-month intervals is reasonable until moving to annual examinations. In this way, an interval of nearly 2 years is available for comparison of the first and last imaging study. Asymptomatic meningiomas come to neurosurgical attention more often through imaging studies done for some other reason. In one study by Olivero and colleagues, 57 patients with meningiomas were observed over an average of 32 months (range, 6 months to 15 years), and none of the patients became symptomatic from their enlarging tumor during this follow-up period.[64] In only 10 (22%) of 45 patients who had imaging was tumor growth noted, and the average growth in these patients was a 0.24-cm increase in maximum diameter per year.[64] In another study, Kuratsu and colleagues observed 109 patients; of these, 63 (57.7%) had imaging follow-ups of over 1 year. Thirty-one percent of this subgroup showed tumor growth over an average follow-up period of 27.8 months (range, 12 to 87 months). Tumors that did not grow were more likely to be shown as calcified on CT or as hypointense on T2-weighted MRI, consistent with intratumoral calcification.[17] Clearly, then, not all tumors grow under observation, and intervention can be deferred until there is documented growth or until the patient becomes symptomatic.

Surgery

For symptomatic meningiomas, surgery is the mainstay of diagnosis and the first step in treatment. The surgeon must consider indications for surgery, risks associated with surgery, reasonable goals of surgery, and projected outcomes for expected or unexpected pathologies. Patient factors such as age, life expectancy, neurologic condition, and associated medical conditions are considered. With surgical removal, there is no delay in "tumor response," as with other forms of therapy. Symptoms related to increased intracranial pressure or to local compression of brain can be improved quickly. As an example, Chozick and colleagues found that 39.9 percent of 158 patients with meningiomas had preoperative seizures and that 88.9 percent of these patients had complete control of seizures after tumor removal.[65]

In some locations, such as the cavernous sinus, complete removal of all microscopic tumor tissue is very difficult if not impossible. Larson and colleagues documented microscopic invasion by tumor into cranial nerves in surgical specimens from patients with cavernous sinus meningiomas.[66] In six patients with benign meningiomas of the cavernous sinus who were examined at autopsy, Sen and Hague found a tendency for infiltration of the carotid artery, the pituitary gland, the trigeminal nerve and ganglion, and the connective tissue between fascicles of nerves.[67] Clinical experience with neurologic morbidity and recurrence of these tumors after surgery, along with pathologic studies such as these, has prompted a more conservative surgical approach regarding tumor locations, treating residual or recurrent disease with radiotherapy.

The degree of surgical removal is also related to the risk of recurrence, and this was outlined in the seminal paper by Donald Simpson (Table 18–4).[68] Failure to remove both tumor-infiltrated bone and simple coagulation of the tumor's dural attachment (rather than excision) increase the risk of recurrence. A number of large modern-day series have confirmed Simpson's earlier findings. Condra and colleagues classified "total excision" (gross-total resection [GTR]) as a Simpson grade I, II, or III excision and found that in 174 (76%) of 229 patients with this degree of excision, the local control rates were 93 per-

Grade	Tumor Removal			Dural Attachment			Bone / Sinus Excised	
	Complete	Partial	Biopsy	Excised	Coagulated	Neither	Yes	No
I	X	—	—	X	—	—	X	—
II	X	—	—	—	X	—	X	—
III	X	—	—	—	—	X	—	X
IV	—	X	—	—	—	X	—	X
V	—	—	X	—	—	X	—	X

Table 18–4. SIMPSON CLASSIFICATION OF TUMOR GRADE BY EXTENT OF EXCISION OF TUMOR, DURA, AND BONE OR VENOUS SINUS

cent, 80 percent, and 76 percent at 5, 10, and 15 years, respectively.[69] In contrast, the "subtotal excision" (subtotal resection [STR], Simpson grade IV) results for equivalent time periods were 53 percent, 40 percent, and 30 percent.[69] These authors felt that STR alone was inadequate therapy. In the Mayo Clinic series of 581 patients operated on for intracranial meningioma, the 5- and 10-year progression-free survival rates were 88 percent and 75 percent, respectively, for those who had GTR, compared to 61 percent and 39 percent for those who had STR.[23] Multivariate modeling of factors important for decreased progression-free survival revealed the following factors as significant: age < 40 years, male sex, tumor removal less than GTR, and intracranial optic-nerve or orbital involvement.[23] In contrast, in reporting their results for the removal of 38 petroclival meningiomas, Jung and colleagues felt that STR (with or without radiation) was an option for patients with petroclival meningiomas.[70] They found that the median progression-free survival was 66 months after subtotal excision and that the growth rate was slow: 0.37 cm per year, with a mean tumor-doubling time of 8 years.[70] Couldwell and colleagues reported an experience with 109 petroclival meningioma patients, many of whom had STR of the posterior cavernous sinus component.[71] In 69 percent, GTR was achieved, with a recurrence rate of only 13 percent over a 6.1-year mean follow-up. Of the 20 patients with known STR of the cavernous sinus component, however, 12 (60%) demonstrated progression on radiography and went on to further treatment.[71]

Complications of surgery for meningiomas depend on a number of factors, such as the surgeon's experience, the patient's age, and the tumor's location. For patients operated on at the Mayo Clinic between 1978 and 1988, the mortality rates at 10, 30, and 90 days were 1.6 percent, 2.4 percent, and 3.7 percent, respectively.[23] In the series of patients with asymptomatic meningiomas that were surgically removed (reported by Kuratsu and colleagues), perioperative morbidity for those over the age of 70 years was 23.3 percent versus 3.5 percent for those less than 70 years of age. The neurologic, medical, and surgical morbidity rates in the entire group were 6.9 percent, 3.4 percent, and 2.3 percent, respectively.[17] In a series of 109 patients with petroclival meningiomas (reported by Couldwell and colleagues), permanent new cranial nerve deficits developed in 33 percent.[71]

During surgery, meningiomas are seen as attached to the dura, displacing the adjacent arachnoid and brain. In small- and moderate-sized tumors showing no abundant edema on preoperative MRI, the "arachnoid plane" is preserved, and it assists the surgeon with the separation of tumor from brain. There are two common practices employed during meningioma surgery: (1) debulking the tumor centrally first and then dissecting the tumor-brain interface (rather than retracting the brain to define the tumor margin) and (2) resecting the arachnoid membranes that help separate tumor from the adjacent brain, blood vessels, and cranial nerves. In the last 10 to 15 years, a variety of devices have been developed that have facilitated better surgical and patient outcomes, including the operating microscope, neurophysiologic monitoring, image-guided surgical navigation systems, and ultrasonic aspirators. Lasers are used for only the deepest tumors and are inefficient for tissue removal. Intraoperative MRI is being developed for many academic centers and may assist with the removal of the most difficult tumors. For many of the complex skull base tumors, a team approach is taken, combining the skills of neurosurgeons and neuro-otologists. For very long operations, this allows the surgeons to rest between operative sessions of 2 to 4 hours, thus maintaining concentration and stamina.

Several general comments can be made about the surgical removal of meningiomas. For meningiomas in the supratentorial compartment, common locations include convexity, falx/parasagittal, sphenoid wing, and parasellar locations. Convexity meningiomas are straightforward when small, but when they are very large, the most medial surface may have a poor brain-tumor interface, even with benign pathology. For tumors in these locations, Kinjo and colleagues have coined the term "grade zero excision" for when a 2-cm cuff of normal dura is included in the excision of dura around the tumor base (see Figure 18–11).[72] We use image-guided surgical systems to mark out the location of the tumor on the scalp for the skin incision and reconfirm this on the skull and then dura to plan for a margin of normal dural excision. Surgical planning for falx/parasagittal meningiomas may require the preoperative assessment of the venous sinuses and parasagittal draining veins with MRV or MRA. In the middle third of the falx, care must be taken to preserve parasagittal draining veins to avoid risk of venous infarction in the postoperative period. For elderly patients, it is often best to leave a small residual of benign tumor on these veins or on the lateral wall of the sinus to avoid a significant hemiparesis or hemiplegia. Sufficient data exist to support radiotherapy for small residual or recurrent benign tumors with prolonged tumor control, as will be presented next. Image-guided surgical navigation systems have become almost routine for the surgery of these tumors. For meningiomas of the sphenoid wing and parasellar region, the routine use of skull base approaches with orbitozygomatic osteotomies, combined with removal of the roof and the lateral walls of the orbit, limits the amount of brain retraction, reducing brain retraction injury. In a similar manner, a bifrontal and extended frontal (bilateral supraorbital osteotomy) craniotomy provides excellent exposure with the least brain retraction for large olfactory-groove, planum sphenoidale, and tuberculum meningiomas. Microdissection of the olfactory nerves for tumors of the planum and tuberculum can be done to preserve the patient's sense of smell.

In the posterior fossa tentorial, petroclival and petrous meningiomas of the cerebellopontine angle are the most common tumors. Petroclival tumors and medial anterior tentorial tumors with extension into Meckel's cave or into the posterior cavernous sinus are best approached with a petrosal craniotomy. In this approach, a low temporal craniotomy is combined with a presigmoid retrolabyrinthine craniectomy to avoid cerebellar retraction and to preserve hearing. Physiologic monitoring of the fifth, sixth, and seventh to eleventh cranial nerves is routine. For several months after operation, all patients will have some degree of conductive hearing loss related to fluid accumulation within the mastoid air cells and the middle ear. For foramen magnum meningiomas, a far lateral transcondylar approach is used to remove bone and avoid spinal cord or brain retraction. In this approach, after the suboccipital craniotomy and C-1 hemilaminectomy, the posterior third of the occipital condyle is drilled off; the dura is then opened in a curvilinear fashion, just medial to the entry of the vertebral artery into the posterior fossa dura. With intraoperative monitoring of cranial nerves IX to XII, internal debulking of the tumor allows (1) displacement of the capsule away from the nerves, brain stem, and upper spinal cord and (2) coagulation of the dural attachments anteriorly. Using this approach, Arnautovic and colleagues reported GTRs in 12 of 18 patients.[73]

Radiotherapy

External Beam Irradiation

Radiation therapy for residual benign meningiomas is still somewhat controversial although there is good evidence that subtotal excision plus radiotherapy gives superior local control and overall survival than subtotal removal alone. In an evaluation of factors associated with meningioma patient survival (data from the National Cancer Data Base) McCarthy and colleagues found that the administration of radiation was a significant factor associated with improved survival for patients with benign meningiomas (N = 8,891; $p < .0001$) as well as for those with malignant meningiomas (N = 771; $p < .001$).[16] The problems of arachnoid scarring (created by radiotherapy) that make reoperation for recurrence more difficult, as well as the very low chance of malignant degeneration or secondary tumors, need to be balanced against the risk of earlier recurrence. Current techniques of delivering external irradiation (external radiation therapy [XRT]) using three-dimensional treatment planning limit the amount of dose to surrounding normal brain. Intensity-modulated radiation therapy (IMRT), using multileaf collimators to shape beams and to vary the intensity of dose over space and time, provides for even greater dose conformity. Combined with inverse treatment planning to minimize the volume of normal tissue included in the high-dose field, the toxicity and side effects of XRT should be lower than in the past.

The effects of radiation on tumor cells (reproductive and apoptotic cell death) and tumor vasculature produce the excellent clinical control observed for meningiomas. Incident photons produce an indirect form of DNA damage that results from the ionization of water and the production of free-radical species, and this mechanism accounts for about 80 percent of the observed clinical effect. Since any DNA damage produced will be manifest when cells attempt to divide, there is a latent interval following treatment, before the slowly proliferating tumors start to shrink. Several studies that document the effectiveness of this treatment have been published, and some of the largest series are included in Table 18–5.[69,74–78] Goldsmith and colleagues (from the University of California San Francisco [UCSF]) reported 5- and 10-year progression-free survival (PFS) rates of 89 percent and 77 percent, respectively, for patients with residual benign meningiomas treated with XRT.[74] Frontal and olfactory locations resulted in slightly higher recurrence rates, and the risk of recurrence increased 2.2-fold for every 100-cm^2 increase in tumor size. A dose-response effect on tumor control was observed for benign and malignant tumors: doses > 5,200 cGy for benign tumors and > 5,300 cGy for malignant tumors were associated with significantly improved local control.[74] In the Mayo Clinic series reported by Stafford and colleagues, when 43 patients treated for recurrence were considered, the 2-year PFS rate was 76 percent for patients who had XRT with or without surgical treatment and 54 percent for those treated with surgery alone (p = .0582).[23] Of the 41 patients who received XRT sometime during their course, 2 had complications. One patient developed a dry-eye syndrome; another developed bilateral radiation retinopathy where the dose to the frontal fossa had been 5,760 cGy.[23] Condra and colleagues reported the experience with 262 patients at the University of Florida.[69] They divided the patients into treatment groups of total excision (TE), subtotal excision (SE), and subtotal excision plus radiotherapy (SE + RT). The median follow-up for the entire group was 8.2 years. Of the 25 patients with SE alone who recurred, salvage therapy of any type was less successful in regaining long-term tumor control. Local control (LC) and cause-specific survival (CSS) at 15 years were significantly reduced after SE alone (30% LC;

Table 18–5. EXTERNAL IRRADIATION FOR MENINGIOMAS: RESULTS OF STUDIES SINCE 1994

Author	Pathology	No. of Patients	Dose (Gy)	Control Rate (%)/(yr)
Goldsmith et al[74]	Benign	117	54*	89/5 77/10
	Malignant	23	54*	48/5
Maire et al[76]	Mixed†	91	50.9‡	91/5§ 72/10§
Milosevic et al[77]	Atypical	17	50‖	51§
	Malignant	42		27§
Condra et al[69]	Benign	21	53.3*	87/15 86/15§
Maguire et al[75]	Mixed †	28	53.1*	81/8
Nutting et al[78]	Benign	82	55–60	92/5 83/10

*Median dose.
†The majority of tumors are benign.
‡Mean dose.
§Cause-specific survival.
‖Range of 40 to 60 Gy.

51% CSS) compared with SE + RT (87% LC; 86% CSS) ($p = .0001$ for LC; $p = .0003$ for CSS).[69] In the period of follow-up, no radiation-induced malignancy was reported as a complication of treatment. Nutting and colleagues published their results with fractionated external irradiation for skull base meningiomas, proposing these as a baseline for the evaluation of new treatment strategies.[78] There were 82 patients with histologically confirmed benign meningiomas; the median follow-up period was 9 years. The 5- and 10-year PFS rates were 92 percent and 83 percent, respectively. Tumor location at the sphenoid ridge resulted in a higher recurrence rate than parasellar locations (31% vs 10%).[78] Complication of treatment occurred in only one patient with radiation retinopathy, and (similarly to other series) there were no cases of secondary tumor development.

With respect to the time interval from treatment, toxicity of external irradiation is usually described as acute (hours to days), early-delayed (weeks to months), and late-delayed (months to years). In the series of 140 patients reported by Goldsmith and colleagues, only 5 (3.6%) had permanent (late-delayed) complications of treatment. Three patients had sudden blindness 20 to 22 months after the completion of radiation therapy; as a result, the authors made separate recommendations for the treatment of meningiomas around the optic apparatus. Two patients developed cerebral necrosis 13 and 30 months after treatment.[74] In the series (reported by Nutting and colleagues) of 82 patients with cavernous sinus meningiomas, 6 patients (9.8%) had visual impairment, 5 from cataracts and 1 from retinopathy. Three patients (4.9%) developed hypopituitarism, and 4 (6.5%) had impairment of short-term memory.[78] It is possible that radiosurgery for small localized meningiomas farther than 4 mm from the optic apparatus may further reduce the incidence of pituitary and hypothalamic failure.

Radiosurgery

Radiosurgery delivers a high dose of radiation to a defined intracranial target by using stereotactic methods in a single treatment session and by using a stereotactic frame applied to the patient's skull. Radiosurgery can be carried out with a specially adapted linear accelerator or gamma-knife unit. The ability to deliver a high dose of radiation in a single session relies on a steep dose gradient outside the edge of the target, presumably limiting effects on normal tissue. Radiosurgery for small meningiomas is an accepted form of treatment now, and published results confirm stabilization or shrinkage of tumors after treatment (Table 18–6).[79–86] The major limitations to treatment are (1) proximity to the optic pathways and/or to the brain stem and (2) tumor size > 3 cm in diameter.

For meningiomas located outside the cranial base, complete excision of the tumor and dural attachments is the goal. For some tumor locations (parasagittal, cavernous sinus, parasellar, and petroclival), achieving this goal is not possible without an increased risk of neurologic morbidity. Kondziolka and colleagues reported the results of a multicenter study of radiosurgery for benign parasagittal meningiomas in 203 patients, with a median follow-up of 3.5 years.[81] The mean tumor volume was 10 cc, and the 5-year overall tumor control rate was 67 percent ± 8.77 percent. The in-field control rate for the targeted lesion was 85 ± 6.2 percent at 5 years. Some patients had radiosurgery as the primary mode of

Table 18–6. RADIOSURGERY FOR MENINGIOMAS: RESULTS OF SELECTED SERIES, 1998				
Author	Pathology	No. of Patients	Dose (Gy)	Control Rate (%)/(yr)
Kondziolka et al[81]	Benign	185	15*	85/5
Hakim et al[79]	Benign	106	15*	89/5
Subach et al[86]	Benign	62	15†	87/8
Shafron et al[85]	Benign	38	12.7†	100/2
Iwai et al[80]	Benign	24	10.6*	100/1.5
Morita et al[82]	Benign	88	16*	95/5
Roche et al[84]	Benign	92	15*	93/5
Ojemann et al[83]	Malignant	22	15.5*	48/2

*Median marginal dose.
†Mean marginal dose.

therapy, without biopsy, and had a better control rate than those who had undergone prior resection (93% vs 60%; p = .08).[81] This may be explained by a change in the biology of the recurrent tumors. In multivariate analyses, predictors of tumor progression were the preexisting neurologic deficit and a tumor volume > 7.5 cc. Of those with deficit prior to radiosurgery, 65 percent were improved or stable, compared with a rate of 83 percent for those without deficit prior to treatment. There was no dose-response relationship above a marginal dose of 15 Gy, so higher doses were not associated with improved tumor control. The delayed complication rate was low, with both 3- and 5-year actuarial rates of symptomatic edema of 16 ± 3.8 percent. Patients felt their treatment was effective, and in 99 patients who underwent radiosurgery for meningiomas, 96 percent of those surveyed believed that radiosurgery provided a satisfactory outcome and 93 percent required no further treatment.[81]

Hakim and colleagues reported similar results in 127 patients with 155 meningiomas treated by using a linear accelerator, with a median follow-up of 31 months.[79] One hundred six tumors were benign, 26 were atypical, and 18 were malignant. The tumor control rates for benign meningiomas at 1, 2, 3, 4, and 5 years were 100 percent, 92 percent, 92 percent, 92 percent, and 92 percent, respectively. Very similar results were achieved for benign meningiomas located at the skull base. The median time to progression was 24.4 months for atypical meningiomas and 13.9 months for malignant meningiomas. The 2- and 4-year survival rates following radiosurgery were 94.8 percent and 91 percent for benign meningiomas, 83.3 percent and 83.3 percent for atypical meningiomas, and 64.6 percent and 21.5 percent for malignant meningiomas. Complications occurred in 6 patients (4.7%); of these, 2 patients died, 1 from cerebral infarction and 1 from hypothalamic dysfunction.[79]

Skull base meningiomas that extend into the cavernous sinus are rarely ever completely removed. Radiosurgery is an ideal form of adjuvant treatment for these tumors, but conformal treatment plans are a must to keep complications at acceptable levels. Chang and Adler reported their preliminary results with linear accelerator (LINAC) radiosurgery for 55 patients with skull base meningiomas.[87] The 2-year actuarial control rate was 98 percent. Of these controlled tumors, 29 percent decreased in size and 69 percent remained stable. Twelve patients (22%) developed new cranial nerve deficits 6 to 12 months after treatment; these deficits were transient in 10 patients and permanent in 2.[87] In two of the largest series of cavernous sinus meningiomas treated with radiosurgery, results appear to be equal to those of XRT, with acceptable side effects. In the series reported by Roche and colleagues (N = 80), with a median follow-up of 30.5 months, the actuarial 5-year PFS rate was 92.8 percent.[84] No new oculomotor deficit was observed.[84] Morita and colleagues reported a series of 88 skull base meningiomas treated with radiosurgery; in this study, the risk of trigeminal neuropathy was associated with doses ≥ 19 Gy, and the optic apparatus appeared to tolerate doses > 10 Gy.[82] Iwai and colleagues achieved similar control rates in other series over a shorter term of follow-up (median, 17.1 months), with a much lower marginal median prescription dose of 10.6 Gy.[80] Only 1 of the 24 patients in their series developed a worsening of a preexisting cranial nerve deficit, and no patient had a new deficit.[80] Clearly, a low dose of radiation will control some benign meningiomas, but a follow-up of 5 to 10 years will be required to truly assess the results.

Interstitial Brachytherapy

Interstitial brachytherapy is an irradiation technique reserved most often for the salvage of patients with aggressive recurrent benign or malignant meningiomas. The most common technique employed is the implantation of permanent iodine-125 (I-125) sources at open craniotomy. These low-activity implants have a half-life of 60 days and produce low-energy photons (27 to 35 keV) with a half-value thickness of 20 mm in tissue. The continuous irradiation produced by permanent sources has many theoretic biologic advantages for tumor control. The low dose rate allows for the repair of sublethal damage by normal tissue. In addition, the brain stem or spinal cord can be protected from irradiation at open operation by placing a small amount of sterile gold foil between the implant site and the surrounding neural tissue.

One of the first series of interstitial brachytherapy for recurrent skull base tumors was reported by Gutin and colleagues.[88] In this series (which included other pathologies), there were 6 meningiomas, 3 benign and 3 malignant. From 5 to 36 sources were implanted at open operations, delivering 80 to 150 Gy to the periphery of the tumors over the lifetime of the sources. Two patients had recurrences outside the implanted volume, 1 surviving only 8 months and the other surviving only 9 months. The remaining 4 patients were stable in follow-up of from 2+ to 54+ months.[88] In contrast to the open implant technique, Kumar and colleagues treated 15 patients who had primary and recurrent skull base meningiomas, using stereotactic implantation of I-125 sources. The median follow-up was 29 months. The authors reported an impressive 73 percent complete radiographic response rate, and no patients developed early- or late-delayed radiation toxicity.[89] The largest experience with interstitial brachytherapy is by Vuorinen and colleagues. In their series, 25 parasellar-clival meningiomas and 19 globoid meningiomas were implanted stereotactically in elderly patients.[90] Doses to the margins of the tumors ranged from 100 to 150 Gy. In the parasellar-clival group, followed for a median of 19 months, 16 percent were moderately smaller, 52 percent were slightly smaller, and 20 percent were stable in size. Of the 17 patients with third, fifth, and sixth cranial nerve neuropathy prior to treatment, 36 percent had improvement, and only 1 patient suffered a new nerve deficit (cranial nerve III). Facial numbness developed or increased in 47 percent of patients.[90] For recurrent benign or malignant meningiomas undergoing reoperation, the advantage of brachytherapy is that the adjuvant treatment can be administered at the same time, without a need for immediate follow-up procedure. Results with this technique will need further evaluation.

Chemotherapy

Hormone Receptor Antagonists

A number of cell surface and nuclear receptors have been identified in meningiomas, but only a few of these have been targeted clinically. Hormone receptor antagonists have received the most attention as laboratory work has shown that estrogen receptors are present at reduced levels, compared to progesterone. Unfortunately, clinical trials of the antiestrogen agent tamoxifen have not been encouraging. Six patients with recurrent inoperable meningiomas were treated with tamoxifen over a 6- to 12-month period by Markwalder and colleagues. Over a short period of follow-up, 1 patient appeared to show an initial tumor response, 2 patients had stabilization of tumor, and 3 had disease progression.[91] Similarly, the Southwest Oncology Group found that after a median follow-up of 15.1 months in 21 patients treated with tamoxifen, 32 percent had no tumor growth and 53 percent had disease progression.[92] Given that progesterone receptors are more abundant in meningiomas, other investigators targeted these receptors. The antiprogestational agent medroxyprogesterone acetate (MPA), given preoperatively to patients with recurrent meningiomas, could reduce the level of tumor progesterone receptor (PR) as compared with historical controls. In 4 of 5 women who took the drug once a week for 17 to 29 weeks, it did not produce a radiographic response.[93] There is one recent case report by Oura and colleagues that shows a 73 percent volume reduction in a presumed meningioma after 2 years of treatment with MPA. Another trial, in which the antiprogestational drug RU-486 (mifepristone) was given to 14 patients with recurrent and unresectable meningiomas, produced some response in 4 patients who showed a minor decrease in tumor size on imaging studies and in 1 other patient who had an improved visual-field examination.[94] Lamberts and colleagues, using the same dosage of 200 mg per day, noted that of 12 patients, 3 (25%) had transient tumor regression, but only 1 patient had a response.[95] As more specific and potent antagonists for PRs become available, there seems to be some laboratory evidence that future trials should be pursued.

Cytotoxic Chemotherapy

The treatment of recurrent benign or malignant meningiomas with standard alkylating agents has been largely unsuccessful. From our institution, Wilson reported the experience of using cyclophosphamide, doxorubicin (Adriamycin), and vincristine in 11 patients for malignant meningiomas recurrent after surgery and radiation therapy; 73 percent of patients showed progression at 1 year, and 100 percent showed progression at 2 years.[8] Chamberlain reported the results of using the same agents after radiotherapy in 14 patients.[96] Those who had GTR received three cycles of chemotherapy, and those with subtotal removal received six cycles of treatment. There were 3 partial responses, and 11 patients had stable disease. The median time to tumor progression was 4.6 years, and the median survival was 5.3 years.[96] Schrell and colleagues reported on 4 patients with reductions in tumor volumes of 15 to 74 percent after treatment with 1,000 to 1,500 mg/day of hydroxyurea over a period of 5 to 24 months.[97] We have not observed any objective tumor volume reductions with this agent. The use of intra-arterial or intravenous infusions of drugs such as cisplatin, doxorubicin, and dacarbazine have not produced dramatic results. Kaba and colleagues reported on the use of interferon-α-2b in 6 patients at a dosage of 4 mU/m^2/day, 5 days per week for 4 to 14+ months.[98] Five patients showed radiographic responses, 4 with stabilization of disease and 1 with a slight tumor reduction. One of the responding patients had progression of tumor on two occasions after stopping treatment.[98] Further investigations with this agent and other biologic response modifiers seem indicated.

MALIGNANT MENINGIOMA

Malignant meningiomas (MMs) generally account for fewer than 10 percent of all meningiomas and are some of the most difficult primary brain tumors to control. Palma and colleagues found that 8.6 percent of intracranial meningiomas were atypical or malignant,[99] and in the personal series of Wilson from UCSF, the incidence was 12 percent.[8] There does not appear to be the same predominance of female sex, and this is supported by Younis and colleagues, who found that 67 percent of MMs occurred in males.[100] Survivals from a number of clinical series that all include surgery and irradiation range from 2 to 9 years (Table 18–7).[28,77,79,83,99,100]

The clincial presentation of MM is no different than that of benign meningioma, except that the duration of symptoms is shorter. Systemic metastases have been documented in up to 24 percent of patients prior to death, and common sites for metastases are the lungs, the liver, and bone. On imaging studies, these tumors reflect their aggressive nature with irregular borders, "mushrooming" of tumor nodules directed away from the main tumor mass, surrounding edema, and nonhomogeneous contrast enhancement. Radiology reviews report that 50 percent of these tumors show indistinct margins, 41 percent show mushrooming, and 33 percent have soft-tissue involvement. As expected, they almost never show any intratumoral calcification, a feature of slow-growing psammomatous meningiomas.

As with benign meningiomas, the mainstay of therapy for these tumors is surgical removal, and there is a relationship between the extent of removal and the time to progression and survival. In their series, Palma and colleagues found that of patients with atypical meningiomas, those with a Simpson grade I excision did significantly better than those with Simpson grade II or III excisions ($p < .0071$).[99] For MM, patients with tumors of the convexity did significantly better than those with basal and parasagittal malignant tumors. In multivariate analysis, convexity location proved to be a positive factor for survival.[67]

Following surgical excision, external irradiation is the standard therapy. Goldsmith and colleagues found a dose-response relationship for external irradiation, with a 5-year PFS rate of 63 percent for those receiving a dose of ≥ 53 Gy versus 17 percent for those receiving < 53 Gy.[74] Milosevic and colleagues also found a significant relationship between CSS and dose above or below 50 Gy ($p = .0005$), suggesting that with fractionated therapy, doses used for malignant gliomas seem appropriate.[77] One recent report from the Harvard proton therapy unit suggests that boosting the radiation dose of the primary tumor site for MMs may significantly improve local control.[28] Actuarial 5- and 8-year survival rates for patients with MM were significantly improved with proton over photon therapy and with doses > 60 Gy.

Radiosurgery has been used in a number of centers to treat MM, most often for recurrent disease. Hakim and colleagues treated 26 atypical meningiomas and 18 MMs with radiosurgery, from an overall series of 127 patients in which 51 percent

Table 18-7. RECURRENCE RATES AND SURVIVAL FOR MALIGNANT AND ANAPLASTIC MENINGIOMA*

Author	No. of Patients	Pathology	Recurrence Rate	Survival
Younis et al[100]	6	Atypical	67% at 2 yr	50% at 5 yr
	12	Malignant	44% at 2 yr	62% at 5 yr
Milosevic et al[77]	17	Atypical	66%	28% at 5 yr
	42	Malignant	All patients	All patients
Palma et al[99]	42	Atypical	52% at 5 yr	95% at 5 yr
	29	Malignant	84% at 5 yr	64.3% at 5 yr
Hakim et al[79]	26	Atypical	24.4 mo†	83.3% at 4 yr
	18	Malignant	13.9 mo†	21.5% at 4 yr
Hug et al[28]	15	Atypical	62% at 5 yr	93%
	16	Malignant	48% at 5 yr	38% (mean: 59 mo)
Ojemann et al[83]	22	Malignant	68% at 2 yr; 74% at 5 yr	75% at 2 yr; 40% at 5 yr

*Selected series since 1995.
†Median freedom from progression.

were being treated for recurrence.[79] The median time to tumor progression was 24.4 months for atypical meningiomas and 13.9 months for MMs. Five-year disease-specific survival rates were 83.3 percent for atypical meningiomas and 21.5 percent for MMs.[79] From our institution, Ojemann and colleagues reported the results of radiosurgery for malignant meningioma in 22 patients, 3 of whom were treated in a boost setting.[83] Nineteen patients were treated for recurrence and had 37 lesions treated in 30 sessions. For the 31 MMs treated, the 2- and 5-year PFS rates were 48 percent and 34 percent, respectively. On multivariate analysis, factors affecting time to tumor progression were age < 50 years ($p = .003$) and tumor volume < 8 cc ($p < .05$). Twenty-three percent of patients developed radiation necrosis as a complication of treatment, with a median time to onset of 77 weeks after treatment (range, 15 to 120 weeks).[83] As with malignant gliomas (for which the external irradiation dose is at the tolerance level, using standard fractionation), radiosurgery for recurrence of MMs has some toxicity, and boosting the radiation dose of the primary tumor site immediately after XRT should be done with caution.

CONCLUSION

Meningiomas are one of the three most common primary brain tumors in adults, and in spite of recent advances in surgery and radiotherapy, they have a not insignificant recurrence rate. Developments in molecular biology may provide information about the mechanisms of oncogenesis in these tumors and about possible future targets for therapy. The hormone receptor antagonists for future trials will target not only the sex steroid hormone nuclear receptors but also other cell surface receptors for small peptides shown in the laboratory to have an influence on tumor cell growth. For the time being, surgery will remain the standard first step in treatment. Already, results for radiosurgery used as the primary modality are impressive. Patients with recurrent and malignant meningiomas need therapies that are more effective and have acceptable side effects soon, and it is hoped that well-coordinated trials of novel agents will provide improved outcomes, if not a cure.

REFERENCES

1. Cushing H, Eisenhardt L. Meningiomas: their classification, regional behavior, life history and surgical end-results. Springfield (IL): Charles C. Thomas; 1938.
2. Carroll RS, Black PM, Zhang J, et al. Expression and activation of epidermal growth factor receptors in meningiomas. J Neurosurg 1997;87:315–23.
3. Carroll RS, Schrell UM, Zhang J, et al. Dopamine D1, dopamine D2, and prolactin receptor messenger ribonucleic acid expression by the polymerase chain reaction in human meningiomas. Neurosurgery 1996;38:367–75.
4. Carroll RS, Zhang J, Black PM. Expression of estrogen receptors alpha and beta in human meningiomas. J Neurooncol 1999;42:109–16.
5. Carroll RS, Zhang J, Dashner K, et al. Progesterone and glucocorticoid receptor activation in meningiomas. Neurosurgery 1995;37:92–7.
6. Carroll RS, Zhang J, Dashner K, et al. Androgen receptor expression in meningiomas. J Neurosurg 1995;82:453–60.

7. Katsuyama J, Papenhausen PR, Herz F, et al. Chromosome abnormalities in meningiomas. Cancer Genet Cytogenet 1986;22:63–8.
8. Wilson CB. Meningiomas: genetics, malignancy, and the role of radiation in induction and treatment. The Richard C. Schneider Lecture. J Neurosurg 1994;81:666–75.
9. Jacobs DH, Holmes FF, McFarlane MJ. Meningiomas are not significantly associated with breast cancer. Arch Neurol 1992;49:753–6.
10. Kirsch M, Zhu JJ, Black PM. Analysis of the BRCA1 and BRCA2 genes in sporadic meningiomas. Genes Chromosomes Cancer 1997;20:53–9.
11. Rubinstein AB, Schein M, Reichenthal E. The association of carcinoma of the breast with meningioma. Surg Gynecol Obstet 1989;169:334–6.
12. Sulman EP, Dumanski JP, White PS, et al. Identification of a consistent region of allelic loss on 1p32 in meningiomas: correlation with increased morbidity. Cancer Res 1998;58:3226–30.
13. Central Brain Tumor Registry in the United States (CBTRUS). Statistical report: primary brain tumors in the United States, 1992–1997. In: Central Brain Tumor Registry of the United States. Chicago: CBTRUS; 2000. p. 11–26.
14. Jaaskelainen J, Haltia M, Laasonen E, et al. The growth rate of intracranial meningiomas and its relation to histology. An analysis of 43 patients. Surg Neurol 1985;24:165–72.
15. Longstreth WT Jr, Dennis LK, McGuire VM, et al. Epidemiology of intracranial meningioma. Cancer 1993;72:639–48.
16. McCarthy BJ, Davis FG, Freels S, et al. Factors associated with survival in patients with meningioma. J Neurosurg 1998;88:831–9.
17. Kuratsu J, Kochi M, Ushio Y. Incidence and clinical features of asymptomatic meningiomas. J Neurosurg 2000;92:766–70.
18. Kuratsu J, Ushio Y. Epidemiological study of primary intracranial tumors: a regional survey in Kumamoto prefecture in the southern part of Japan. J Neurosurg 1996;84:946–50.
19. Germano IM, Edwards MS, Davis RL, et al. Intracranial meningiomas of the first two decades of life. J Neurosurg 1994;80:447–53.
20. Jaaskelainen J, Haltia M, Servo A. Atypical and anaplastic meningiomas: radiology, surgery, radiotherapy, and outcome. Surg Neurol 1986;25:233–42.
21. Jaaskelainen J. Seemingly complete removal of histologically benign intracranial meningioma: late recurrence rate and factors predicting recurrence in 657 patients. A multivariate analysis. Surg Neurol 1986;26:461–9.
22. Kallio M, Sankila R, Hakulinen T, et al. Factors affecting operative and excess long-term mortality in 935 patients with intracranial meningioma. Neurosurgery 1992;31:2–12.
23. Stafford SL, Perry A, Suman VJ, et al. Primarily resected meningiomas: outcome and prognostic factors in 581 Mayo Clinic patients, 1978 through 1988. Mayo Clin Proc 1998;73:936–42.
24. Kepes JJ, MacGee EE, Vergara G, et al. A case report. Malignant meningioma with extensive pulmonary metastases. J Kans Med Soc 1971;72:312–6.
25. Harrison MJ, Wolfe DE, Lau TS, et al. Radiation-induced meningiomas: experience at the Mount Sinai Hospital and review of the literature. J Neurosurg 1991;75:564–74.
26. Ron E, Modan B, Boice JD Jr. Mortality after radiotherapy for ringworm of the scalp. Am J Epidemiol 1988;127:713–25.
27. Ron E, Modan B, Boice JD Jr, et al. Tumors of the brain and nervous system after radiotherapy in childhood. N Engl J Med 1988;319:1033–9.
28. Hug EB, Devries A, Thornton AF, et al. Management of atypical and malignant meningiomas: role of high-dose, 3D-conformal radiation therapy. J Neurooncol 2000;48:151–60.
29. Strojan P, Popovic M, Jereb B. Secondary intracranial meningiomas after high-dose cranial irradiation: report of five cases and review of the literature. Int J Radiat Oncol Biol Phys 2000;48:65–73.
30. Annegers JF, Laws ER Jr, Kurland LT, et al. Head trauma and subsequent brain tumors. Neurosurgery 1979;4:203–6.
31. Preston-Martin S, Pogoda JM, Schlehofer B, et al. An international case-control study of adult glioma and meningioma: the role of head trauma. Int J Epidemiol 1998;27:579–86.
32. Weggen S, Bayer TA, von Deimling A, et al. Low frequency of SV40, JC and BK polyomavirus sequences in human medulloblastomas, meningiomas and ependymomas. Brain Pathol 2000;10:85–92.
33. Black PM. Hormones, radiosurgery and virtual reality: new aspects of meningioma management. Can J Neurol Sci 1997;24:302–6.
34. Schlehofer B, Blettner M, Wahrendorf J. Association between brain tumors and menopausal status. J Natl Cancer Inst 1992;84:1346–9.
35. Lambe M, Coogan P, Baron J. Reproductive factors and the risk of brain tumors: a population-based study in Sweden. Int J Cancer 1997;72:389–93.
36. Roelvink NC, Kamphorst W, August H, et al. Literature statistics do not support a growth stimulating role for female sex steroid hormones in haemangiomas and meningiomas. J Neurooncol 1991;11:243–53.
37. Roelvink NC, Kamphorst W, van Alphen HA, et al. Pregnancy-related primary brain and spinal tumors. Arch Neurol 1987;44:209–15.
38. Weisman AS, Raguet SS, Kelly PA. Characterization of the epidermal growth factor receptor in human meningioma. Cancer Res 1987;47:2172–6.
39. Black PM, Carroll R, Glowacka D, et al. Platelet-derived growth factor expression and stimulation in human meningiomas. J Neurosurg 1994;81:388–93.
40. Shamah SM, Alberta JA, Giannobile WV, et al. Detection of activated platelet-derived growth factor receptors in human meningioma. Cancer Res 1997;57:4141–7.
41. Todo T, Adams EF, Fahlbusch R, et al. Autocrine growth stimulation of human meningioma cells by platelet-derived growth factor. J Neurosurg 1996;84:852–9.
42. Kalkanis SN, Carroll RS, Zhang J, et al. Correlation of vascular endothelial growth factor messenger RNA expression with peritumoral vasogenic cerebral edema in meningiomas. J Neurosurg 1996;85:1095–101.
43. Tsai JC, Hsiao YY, Teng LJ, et al. Regulation of vascular endothelial growth factor secretion in human meningioma cells. J Formos Med Assoc 1999;98:111–7.
44. Shu J, Lee JH, Harwalkar JA, et al. Adenovirus-mediated gene transfer of dominant negative Ha-Ras inhibits proliferation of primary meningioma cells. Neurosurgery 1999;44:579–87.
45. Cushing H. The meningiomas (dural endotheliomas): their

source, and favoured seats of origin. Brain 1922;45: 282–316.
46. Kleihues P, Cavenee WK, International Agency for Research on Cancer, editors. Pathology and genetics of tumours of the nervous system. Lyon: IARC Press; 2000.
47. Lee KS, Hoshino T, Rodriguez LA, et al. Bromodeoxyuridine labeling study of intracranial meningiomas: proliferative potential and recurrence. Acta Neuropathol 1990;80:311–7.
48. Shibuya M, Hoshino T, Ito S, et al. Meningiomas: clinical implications of a high proliferative potential determined by bromodeoxyuridine labeling. Neurosurgery 1992;30:494–8.
49. Dumanski JP, Carlbom E, Collins VP, et al. Deletion mapping of a locus on human chromosome 22 involved in the oncogenesis of meningioma. Proc Natl Acad Sci U S A 1987;84:9275–9.
50. Seizinger BR, de la Monte S, Atkins L, et al. Molecular genetic approach to human meningioma: loss of genes on chromosome 22. Proc Natl Acad Sci U S A 1987;84:5419–23.
51. Peyrard M, Seroussi E, Sandberg-Nordqvist AC, et al. The human LARGE gene from 22q12.3-q13.1 is a new, distinct member of the glycosyltransferase gene family. Proc Natl Acad Sci U S A 1999;96:598–603.
52. Lee JH, Sundaram V, Stein DJ, et al. Reduced expression of schwannomin/merlin in human sporadic meningiomas. Neurosurgery 1997;40:578–87.
53. Smith DA, Cahill DW. The biology of meningiomas. Neurosurg Clin N Am 1994;5:201–15.
54. Vagner-Capodano AM, Grisoli F, Gambarelli D, et al. Correlation between cytogenetic and histopathological findings in 75 human meningiomas. Neurosurgery 1993;32:892–900.
55. McDermott M, Wilson C. Meningiomas. In: Youmans J, editor. Neurological surgery. Vol 4. 4th ed. Philadelphia: WB Saunders; 1996. p. 2782–825.
56. Samii M, Ammirati M. Cerebellopontine angle meningiomas (posterior pyramid meningiomas). In: Al-Mefty O, editor. Meningiomas. New York: Raven Press; 1991. p. 503–15.
57. Yasuoka S, Okazaki H, Daube JR, et al. Foramen magnum tumors. Analysis of 57 cases of benign extramedullary tumors. J Neurosurg 1978;49:828–38.
58. Johns TT, Citrin CM, Black J, et al. CT evaluation of perineural orbital lesions: evaluation of the "tram-track" sign. AJNR Am J Neuroradiol 1984;5:587–90.
59. Mantle RE, Lach B, Delgado MR, et al. Predicting the probability of meningioma recurrence based on the quantity of peritumoral brain edema on computerized tomography scanning. J Neurosurg 1999;91:375–83.
60. Zee CS, Chen T, Hinton DR, et al. Magnetic resonance imaging of cystic meningiomas and its surgical implications. Neurosurgery 1995;36:482–8.
61. Ildan F, Tuna M, Gocer AP, et al. Correlation of the relationships of brain-tumor interfaces, magnetic resonance imaging, and angiographic findings to predict cleavage of meningiomas. J Neurosurg 1999;91:384–90.
62. Paleologos TS, Wadley JP, Kitchen ND, et al. Clinical utility and cost-effectiveness of interactive image-guided craniotomy: clinical comparison between conventional and image-guided meningioma surgery. Neurosurgery 2000;47:40–8.
63. Bendszus M, Rao G, Burger R, et al. Is there a benefit of preoperative meningioma embolization? Neurosurgery 2000;47:1306–12.
64. Olivero WC, Lister JR, Elwood PW. The natural history and growth rate of asymptomatic meningiomas: a review of 60 patients. J Neurosurg 1995;83:222–4.
65. Chozick BS, Reinert SE, Greenblatt SH. Incidence of seizures after surgery for supratentorial meningiomas: a modern analysis. J Neurosurg 1996;84:382–6.
66. Larson JJ, van Loveren HR, Balko MG, et al. Evidence of meningioma infiltration into cranial nerves: clinical implications for cavernous sinus meningiomas. J Neurosurg 1995;83:596–9.
67. Sen C, Hague K. Meningiomas involving the cavernous sinus: histological factors affecting the degree of resection. J Neurosurg 1997;87:535–43.
68. Simpson D. The recurrence of intracranial meningiomas after surgical treatment. J Neurol Neurosurg Psychiatry 1957; 20:22–39.
69. Condra KS, Buatti JM, Mendenhall WM, et al. Benign meningiomas: primary treatment selection affects survival. Int J Radiat Oncol Biol Phys 1997;39:427–36.
70. Jung HW, Yoo H, Paek SH, et al. Long-term outcome and growth rate of subtotally resected petroclival meningiomas: experience with 38 cases. Neurosurgery 2000;46:567–75.
71. Couldwell WT, Fukushima T, Giannotta SL, et al. Petroclival meningiomas: surgical experience in 109 cases. J Neurosurg 1996;84:20–8.
72. Kinjo T, Al-Mefty O, Kanaan I. Grade zero removal of supratentorial convexity meningiomas. Neurosurgery 1993; 33:394–9.
73. Arnautovic KI, Al-Mefty O, Husain M. Ventral foramen magnum meninigiomas. J Neurosurg 2000;92:71–80.
74. Goldsmith BJ, Wara WM, Wilson CB, et al. Postoperative irradiation for subtotally resected meningiomas. A retrospective analysis of 140 patients treated from 1967 to 1990 [published erratum appears in J Neurosurg 1994; 80:777]. J Neurosurg 1994;80:195–201.
75. Maguire PD, Clough R, Friedman AH, et al. Fractionated external-beam radiation therapy for meningiomas of the cavernous sinus. Int J Radiat Oncol Biol Phys 1999;44:75–9.
76. Maire JP, Caudry M, Guerin J, et al. Fractionated radiation therapy in the treatment of intracranial meningiomas: local control, functional efficacy, and tolerance in 91 patients. Int J Radiat Oncol Biol Phys 1995;33:315–21.
77. Milosevic MF, Frost PJ, Laperriere NJ, et al. Radiotherapy for atypical or malignant intracranial meningioma. Int J Radiat Oncol Biol Phys 1996;34:817–22.
78. Nutting C, Brada M, Brazil L, et al. Radiotherapy in the treatment of benign meningioma of the skull base. J Neurosurg 1999;90:823–7.
79. Hakim R, Alexander E 3rd, Loeffler JS, et al. Results of linear accelerator-based radiosurgery for intracranial meningiomas. Neurosurgery 1998;42:446–54.
80. Iwai Y, Yamanaka K, Yasui T, et al. Gamma knife surgery for skull base meningiomas. The effectiveness of low-dose treatment. Surg Neurol 1999;52:40–5.
81. Kondziolka D, Flickinger JC, Perez B. Judicious resection and/or radiosurgery for parasagittal meningiomas: outcomes from a multicenter review. Gamma Knife Meningioma Study Group. Neurosurgery 1998;43:405–14.
82. Morita A, Coffey RJ, Foote RL, et al. Risk of injury to cranial nerves after gamma knife radiosurgery for skull base

82. ...meningiomas: experience in 88 patients. J Neurosurg 1999;90:42–9.
83. Ojemann SG, Sneed PK, Larson DA, et al. Radiosurgery for malignant meningioma: results in 22 patients. J Neurosurg 2000;93(Suppl 3):62–7.
84. Roche PH, Regis J, Dufour H, et al. Gamma knife radiosurgery in the management of cavernous sinus meningiomas. J Neurosurg 2000;93(Suppl 3):68–73.
85. Shafron DH, Friedman WA, Buatti JM, et al. LINAC radiosurgery for benign meningiomas. Int J Radiat Oncol Biol Phys 1999;43:321–7.
86. Subach BR, Lunsford LD, Kondziolka D, et al. Management of petroclival meningiomas by stereotactic radiosurgery. Neurosurgery 1998;42:437–45.
87. Chang SD, Adler JR Jr. Treatment of cranial base meningiomas with linear accelerator radiosurgery. Neurosurgery 1997;41:1019–27.
88. Gutin PH, Leibel SA, Hosobuchi Y, et al. Brachytherapy of recurrent tumors of the skull base and spine with iodine-125 sources. Neurosurgery 1987;20:938–45.
89. Kumar PP, Patil AA, Syh HW, et al. Role of brachytherapy in the management of the skull base meningioma. Treatment of skull base meningiomas. Cancer 1993;71:3726–31.
90. Vuorinen V, Heikkonen J, Brander A, et al. Interstitial radiotherapy of 25 parasellar/clival meningiomas and 19 meningiomas in the elderly. Analysis of short-term tolerance and responses. Acta Neurochir (Wien) 1996;138:495–508.
91. Markwalder TM, Waelti E, Konig MP. Endocrine manipulation of meningiomas with medroxyprogesterone acetate. Effect of MPA on receptor status of meningioma cytosols. Surg Neurol 1987;28:3–9.
92. Goodwin JW, Crowley J, Eyre HJ, et al. A phase II evaluation of tamoxifen in unresectable or refractory meningiomas: a Southwest Oncology Group study. J Neurooncol 1993;15:75–7.
93. Jaaskelainen J, Laasonen E, Karkkainen J, et al. Hormone treatment of meningiomas: lack of response to medroxyprogesterone acetate (MPA). A pilot study of five cases. Acta Neurochir (Wien) 1986;80:35–41.
94. Grunberg SM, Weiss MH, Spitz IM, et al. Treatment of unresectable meningiomas with the antiprogesterone agent mifepristone. J Neurosurg 1991;74:861–6.
95. Lamberts SW, Tanghe HL, Avezaat CJ, et al. Mifepristone (RU 486) treatment of meningiomas. J Neurol Neurosurg Psychiatry 1992;55:486–90.
96. Chamberlain MC. Adjuvant combined modality therapy for malignant meningiomas. J Neurosurg 1996;84:733–6.
97. Schrell UM, Rittig MG, Anders M, et al. Hydroxyurea for treatment of unresectable and recurrent meningiomas. II. Decrease in the size of meningiomas in patients treated with hydroxyurea. J Neurosurg 1997;86:840–4.
98. Kaba SE, DeMonte F, Bruner JM, et al. The treatment of recurrent unresectable and malignant meningiomas with interferon alpha-2B. Neurosurgery 1997;40:271–5.
99. Palma L, Celli P, Franco C, et al. Long-term prognosis for atypical and malignant meningiomas: a study of 71 surgical cases. J Neurosurg 1997;86:793–800.
100. Younis GA, Sawaya R, DeMonte F, et al. Aggressive meningeal tumors: review of a series. J Neurosurg 1995;82:17–27.

19

Spinal Tumors

WILLIAM S. ROSENBERG, MD
PHILIP V. THEODOSOPOULOS, MD

Tumors involving the spinal cord and its coverings are uncommon. They represent approximately 10 percent of all central nervous system neoplasms. Nevertheless, knowledge of their presentation, pathophysiology, and treatment is important to the clinician since many tumors are curable and their consideration is important in the differential diagnosis of a new neurologic deficit referable to the spinal cord.

A variety of neoplastic processes may involve the spine. Primary intraspinal tumors may arise from astrocytes, ependymal and Schwann cells, neurons, meningeal cells, and displaced mesenchymal and melanoma cells. The presentation and clinical outcomes of this diverse group of tumors vary significantly according to histology and location. Tumors can present either in the epidural space or in the subdural space. In the latter case, they can then be described as being intramedullary (involving the spinal cord parenchyma) or extramedullary (outside of the spinal cord but still within the dura). The cell of origin often determines the location. Astrocytomas and ependymomas usually are intramedullary, whereas nerve sheath tumors such as neurofibromas and schwannomas are intradural and extramedullary. Meningiomas may be epidural or intradural extramedullary, depending on their relationship to the dura. Technical advances have allowed for a more aggressive surgical approach to these tumors with better functional results and outcomes. Adjuvant therapies play a role in attempting to control the growth of more malignant neoplasms.

CLINICAL PRESENTATION

Most spinal tumors present with the onset of new neurologic deficits, which can range from isolated sensory changes to weakness, including complete paralysis. Symptoms often correlate more with the growth rate than the size of the tumor; slower-growing tumors allow the spinal cord to adapt to compression and often have minimal or no neurologic consequences. Rapidly growing tumors such as high-grade gliomas often have significant neurologic deficits on presentation.

The somatotopic organization of the spinal cord is important in understanding the neurologic manifestations of tumor growth. As sensory tracts ascend, new fibers entering the spinal cord are added to the medial aspect of the long tracts. This results in a displacement of the sacral sensory fibers toward the periphery of the cord. Intramedullary tumors arising within the central portion of the spinal cord therefore often spare sacral sensation. In the case of nerve sheath tumors, an asymmetric location results in differential lateral impingement on the neural elements. This asymmetry can result in a form of Brown-Séquard's syndrome, with a contralateral pain/temperature sensory loss and ipsilateral motor deficit.

Back or radicular pain is not uncommon with spinal tumors. Direct nerve root compression, particularly in the case of extramedullary intradural tumors, results in radiculopathy. Axial back pain, which can be hard to differentiate from that caused by musculoskeletal etiologies, often is more difficult to diagnose and can result in a long interval between presentation and treatment.

IMAGING

Magnetic resonance imaging (MRI) currently is the mainstay for the evaluation of any spinal mass. The use of gadolinium intravenous contrast allows for clear visualization of the extent of enhancing tumors and evaluation of scar formation in cases of reoperation. Sagittal and axial planes of imaging give a clear and accurate anatomic delineation of the neoplasm and the involvement of bone, neural foramina, and the extraspinal space (Figures 19–1 and 19–2). In addition, MRI evaluation provides information necessary to exclude other disease processes involving the spine that may mimic tumors in their clinical presentation.

One of the most useful features allowing differentiation of intramedullary tumors from other diagnoses is spinal cord expansion. It has been noted that these tumors almost always increase the axial dimension of the spinal cord. In contrast, nontumoral etiologies (eg, inflammations, infections) tend to produce lesions within the cord parenchyma without such an expansion. However, in the presence of concomitant spinal stenosis, a common disease process, laminectomy and intraoperative ultrasonic examination may be required.

Other modalities of imaging include computed tomography (CT) and plain radiography of the spine. Computed tomography is used less frequently than MRI, but it can prove helpful for the assessment of bony infiltration or erosion. Spinal instability and the need for intraoperative fixation often are evaluated with plain radiography and CT scanning. Flexion/extension views often can diagnose any gross preoperative instability. Indications of the presence of a spinal tumor such as widening of a neural foramen are sometimes seen on radiographs obtained for other reasons.

DIFFERENTIAL DIAGNOSIS

The clinician caring for a patient with new neurologic deficits attributable to the spinal cord needs to be familiar with the gamut of spinal pathologies that can account for such symptoms. Although most spinal cord tumors cause a neurologic deficit, the list of possible etiologies causing such a deficit is extensive and often imaging provides incomplete information. Conditions that mimic the clinical presentation of a spinal cord tumor include infectious, inflammatory, degenerative, traumatic, and vascular pathologies.

Conditions That Can Mimic Spinal Cord Tumor

Transverse Myelitis

Transverse myelitis is defined as an acutely evolving inflammatory or demyelinating lesion that involves all of the elements of the spinal cord in a transverse plane. Frequently, the severity of disease is unevenly distributed, resulting in incomplete and asymmetric lesions. Transverse myelitis commonly presents shortly after a viral infection or antiviral vaccination, and it is thought to be caused by an autoimmune mechanism. A number of viral infections have been associated with this disease, including Epstein-Barr virus (EBV), cytomegalovirus (CMV), and hepatitis B, as well as mycoplasma bacterial infection. Other etiologies of transverse myelitis include demyelinating disease, lupus vasculitis, and paraneoplastic syndrome. Transvese myelitis can be differentiated from a spinal cord neoplasm by its rapid onset (often within hours) of progressive painful paraparesis and its temporal association with a viral syndrome, vaccination, or inflammatory disorder exacerbation.

Infection

Epidural abscess, the most common spinal infection causing a neurologic deficit, may present with paraparesis, sensory loss, and back pain. Signs of meningeal irritation, fever, malaise, laboratory values consistent with significant infection, and abnormal cerebrospinal fluid (CSF) studies (elevated cell counts and elevated protein) can be helpful in making the appropriate diagnosis. Hypoglycorrhachia indicates probable meningitis, as does the parameningeal focus of infection (epidural abscess). Conversely, an epidural abscess that does not communicate with the CSF may not produce the usual findings of meningitis. Epidural abscess can develop within hours and can be fatal if not treated in a timely fashion.

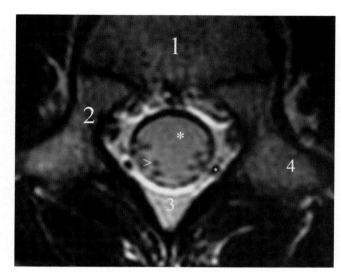

Figure 19–1. Axial MRI cross-sectional scan at the level of a lumbar pedicle (2). The vertebral body (1), transverse process (4), epidural fat (3), exiting nerve root (*small star*), CSF (*large star*), and a nerve root of the cauda equina (*arrowhead*) are shown.

True focal, intradural infection such as intramedullary abscess is quite rare and is suggested by a ring-enhancing lesion within the spinal cord on MRI, a dense neurologic deficit, and clinical signs of infection.

Syringomyelia

Post-traumatic syringomyelia is a well-described phenomenon of dilation of the central canal (or a closely related structure) following significant injury to the spinal cord, sometimes occurring months to years later. It is chronic and progressive over many months and results in areas of myelomalacia and cavitation. Neurologic deficits are caused by a combination of neuronal loss and enlargement of the syrinx. Abnormal CSF dynamics, presumably associated with the formation of scar and arachnoidal adhesions, cause the rostrocaudal extension of the syrinx that is often seen. Intraparenchymal spinal tumors also may be associated with cysts; an appropriate history of trauma and a long progression of symptoms may help in the diagnosis of syringomyelia. Interruption of crossing sensory fibers near the central canal results in loss of pain and temperature sensation at the level of the syrinx with preservation of those sensations below the syrinx. In addition, a true post-traumatic syrinx should not enhance after administration of gadolinium on MRI scan.

Vascular Malformations

Vascular malformations of the spine consist of abnormal, direct connections between the arterial and venous systems without an intervening capillary bed. There are four types of spinal vascular malformation, depending on the location and size of the fistulous connection: (1) a simple fistula, within the dura, causes symptoms due to venous hypertension and intramedullary edema or ischemia; (2) intramedullary malformations (arteriovenous or cavernous) may cause symptoms due to the shunting of blood away from normal spinal cord parenchyma or direct hemorrhagic injury; (3) large, complex, arteriovenous malformations, with multiple feeding vessels, can involve musculoskeletal structures in addition to the spinal cord and may resemble tumors on imaging studies; (4) intradural extramedullary malformations, also called perimedullary fistulae that may exhibit high or low blood flow. Presentation depends on the mechanism by which the vascular malformation becomes clinically apparent. Hemorrhage is often catastrophic, presenting with a rapidly precipitous course of severe neurologic deficits that may improve over several weeks. Venous hypertension can account for a long, subtle, and extended course of slowly progressive neurologic deficit and is often

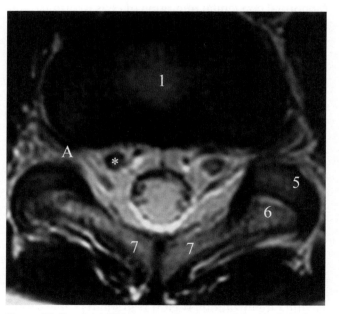

Figure 19–2. Axial MRI cross-sectional scan at the level of a lumbar foramen (*A*). The disc (1), superior (6) and inferior (5) facets, laminae (7), and nerve root (*star*) are illustrated.

difficult to diagnose unless vascular etiology is entertained. Although tumors may be associated with a hemorrhage, the absence of intramedullary expansion and the presence of abnormal vessels differentiate these two entities. Spinal angiography often is necessary for definitive determination.

Others

Other conditions such as metastasis, lymphoma, sarcoidosis, amyloid angiopathy, tuberculosis, histiocytosis, and histoplasmosis also may mimic a primary spinal tumor (Figure 19–3).[1–3] Given the high incidence of metastatic lesions to the spine, a systemic work-up may be instrumental in their diagnosis (Figure 19–4). In a large series of 212 intramedullary spinal cord lesions, Lee and colleagues found non-neoplastic conditions to represent 4 percent of diagnoses.[4] In this retrospective analysis, such conditions were found to expand the spinal cord less frequently on preoperative MRI studies.

Intradural Extramedullary Tumors

Tumors arising from cells within the dura, but outside of the spinal cord parenchyma are classified as intradural extramedullary. These can be divided into meningioma (meningeal cell), nerve sheath tumor (Schwann cell), epidermoid/dermoid/teratoma/lipoma (abnormal congenital migration of cells of origin), and primary spinal melanoma.

Meningiomas

Meningiomas occur most commonly in women and represent approximately 25 to 47 percent of primary intraspinal tumors and 40 percent of tumors in an intradural extramedullary location. These tumors arise from arachnoidal cells, usually in the region of the nerve sheath, displacing the spinal cord. They occur at any level, most commonly presenting in the thoracic spine. Meningiomas may appear as multiple lesions in the setting of neurofibromatosis. En plaque spinal meningioma, a rare form, is a diffuse, collar-like mass that surrounds the cord. Atypical meningiomas are rare, aggressive tumors (World Health Organization [WHO] II grade II; Table 19–1) that exhibit frequent mitoses, increased cellularity, necrosis, and high nucleus-to-cytoplasm ratio.

Meningiomas often can be completely resected, usually with preservation of the pial plane between the tumor and the spiral cord. A safe dissection plane often can be found at surgery, allowing complete extirpation of the tumor without involving the spinal cord. Removal of the dural attachment from which the meningioma arises is necessary for gross-total resection, which is curative. Approximately 8 percent of spinal meningiomas are extradural, necessitating a combination of intradural and extradural approaches for a gross-total resection. In a large series of patients with spinal meningiomas, Levy and colleagues found an 83 percent rate of gross-total resection. Neurologic improvement was observed in 85 percent of the patients.[5] Three patients had recurrences at 8, 13, and 16 years postoperatively. No clear outcome studies or guidelines for the routine use of adjuvant irradiation in the treatment of meningiomas exist. However, adjuvant irradiation has been advocated in the treatment of incompletely resected malignant meningiomas.

Nerve Sheath Tumors

Nerve sheath tumors are tumors of a common Schwann cell origin and are divided into two distinct entities: schwannoma and neurofibroma. Schwannoma (neurinoma, neurilemoma) contains a preponderance of Schwann cells. Histologically, they consist of elongated bipolar cells that are arranged in compact palisading formations (Antoni A pattern) alternating with looser areas (Antoni B pattern). Macroscopically, schwannomas present as an eccentric enlargement of the nerve root.

Neurofibromas consist of Schwann cells admixed with perineural cells and fibroblasts. These ovoid curved cells surrounded by collagen matrix tend to cause fusiform nerve enlargement. Neurofibromas have a high incidence in neurofibromatosis type 1, and they often diffusely involve multiple nerve roots and nerves ("plexiform tumors").

Nerve sheath tumors predominantly arise from the sensory rootlets. They are evenly distributed throughout the spine. In approximately 10 to 15 percent of cases, these tumors extend through the spinal foramen into the extraspinal space ("dumbbell tumors") (Figures 19–5 and 19–6). Only 2.5 percent of these tumors are malignant, and about half of these present in patients with neurofibromatosis.

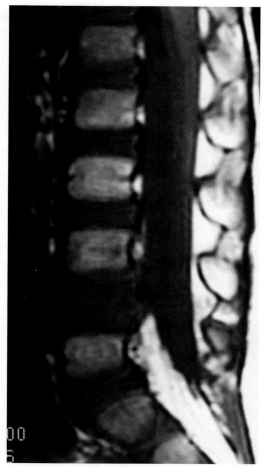

Figure 19–3. Sagittal T1-weighted MR image of the lumbar spine with an enhancing intradural mass at the sacrococcygeal region consistent with histiocytosis.

Seppälä and colleagues have reported a series of 187 gross-total resections of schwannomas and showed a life expectancy similar to that of the general population.[6] Combined late postoperative complications of cystic myelopathy, arachnoiditis, and pain were present in 15 percent of the patients. In a study of 86 patients with spinal schwannomas who underwent gross-total resection, Kim and colleagues found that the involved root was sacrificed in 31 patients; however, related neurologic symptoms developed only in 23 percent of them.[7]

Neurofibromas usually are associated with worse outcome than schwannomas. In their series of patients with spinal neurofibromas, Seppälä and colleagues reported a 75 percent root sacrifice rate and a worse overall survival rate than the general population, presumably secondary to comorbidities of neurofibromatosis type 1.[8] Levy and colleagues showed a 60 percent complete functional recovery after resection of spinal neurofibromas.[9] Similar results also have been reported for surgical resection of plexiform dumbbell nerve sheath tumors. Several studies have reported 90 percent rates of gross-total resection, both in the cervical and thoracic spine, with good functional results and minimal recurrence.[10,11]

Tumors of Disordered Congenital Cell Migration

Epidermoid and dermoid cysts are rare tumors, comprising 1 percent of primary spinal tumors. They arise from ectodermal elements trapped at the time of closure of the neural groove. They usually are associated with congenital bony defects of the spine and also

Nerve sheath tumors often are amenable to surgical resection. For schwannomas, it is well accepted that gross-total resection is the goal of treatment.

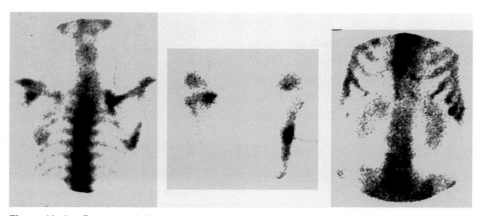

Figure 19–4. Bone scan indicating multiple bone lesions throughout the skeleton in a patient with lymphoma and an epidural mass.

Table 19–1. TUMOR GRADING SYSTEMS

WHO		St. Anne/Mayo	
Grade	Designation	Designation	Criteria
I	Pilocytic astrocytoma	—	—
II	Astrocytoma (low grade, diffuse)	Astrocytoma grade 1	Zero criteria
		Astrocytoma grade 2	One criterion, usually nuclear atypia
III	Anaplastic astrocytoma	Astrocytoma grade 3	Two criteria, usually nuclear atypia and mitotic activity
IV	Glioblastoma multiforme	Astrocytoma grade 4	Three criteria, usually nuclear atypia, mitoses, endothelial proliferation, and/or necrosis

WHO = World Health Organization.
Adapted from Kleihues P, Cavenee KW, editors. Pathology and genetics: tumours of the nervous system. Lyon: International Agency for Research on Cancer; 1997. p. 2.

occasionally with lumbar punctures. Dermoids are more frequent than epidermoids in the spine. Dermoids usually present within the first two decades of life, whereas epidermoids come to clinical attention in patients in the third and fourth decades of life.

Lipomas represent 1 percent of all intraspinal tumors. They frequently are subpial but occasionally may be intramedullary. Histologically, these tumors consist of adipose tissue interdigitated with normal neural elements. These tumors often present with symptoms of tethered cord syndrome, including back pain, lower extremity weakness, and urinary incontinence. The adipocytes are metabolically normal, resulting in the potential for symptomatic changes with weight gain or loss.

Epidermoid and dermoid cysts are adherent to the spinal cord and nerve roots. The intimate involvement of lipomas with normal neural tissue makes their total removal impossible and undesirable; debulking and spinal cord untethering are the usual surgical goals. Fortunately, these lesions are not true tumors, and their potential for continued growth is small.

Teratomas are rare lesions that contain ectodermal, mesodermal, and endodermal elements. They most often present in the sacrococcygeal region and infrequently are intramedullary. Unlike the other lesions of disordered cell migration, these tumors have the potential for malignancy. They can be difficult to remove surgically.

Primary Spinal Melanoma

Primary spinal melanoma is a rare tumor that may arise from melanoblasts within the arachnoid, from pial sheaths of vascular bundles, or from neuroectodermal congenital rests. They most often involve the meninges but may present as intramedullary lesions.

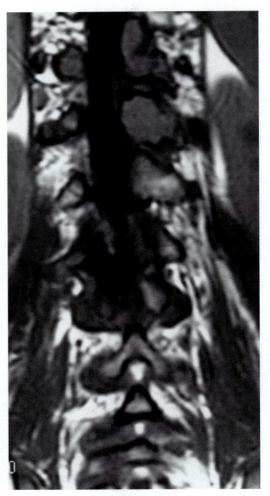

Figure 19–5. Coronal T1-weighted MR image of the lumbar spine demonstrating multiple variable-size intraforaminal enhancing masses in a patient with neurofibromatosis.

Immunohistochemical staining with S-100 and HMR-45 facilitates their diagnosis.

Primary melanoma of the spine may be treated with resection followed by radiation therapy.[12–14] Dacarbazine has been used with successful reduction in CSF melanoma cell counts with no recurrence or metastases for 1 year.[12]

Intramedullary Tumors

The common tumors within the parenchyma of the spinal cord arise from glial cells (astrocytoma, ependymoma) or vascular components (hemangioblastoma).

Glial Tumors

Astrocytomas and ependymomas are the most common intramedullary tumors, comprising approximately 20 percent of all intraspinal tumors. Astrocytomas present more frequently in children than adults, in whom they account for 90 percent of all intramedullary neoplasms. According to the WHO II classification, they are divided into four grades (I to IV), with higher grades characterizing tumors of increased malignant potential as defined histologically by the presence of nuclear atypia, frequent mitoses, necrosis, and endothelial proliferation.

Most spinal astrocytomas are low grade (grades I and II), with only 10 to 15 percent being high grade (grades III and IV).

Ependymomas are tumors arising from the ependymal lining of the cerebral ventricles and the central canal remnants of the spinal cord (Figure 19–7). They usually are intramedullary or in the region of the filum terminale. These tumors usually arise in children and young adults, and the incidence is equal in males and females. According to the WHO II classification, ependymomas present in three histologic subtypes: ependymoma, anaplastic ependymoma, and sacral myxopapillary ependymoma. The most common ependymal neoplasm of the spine, ependymoma, is a grade II tumor. They usually demonstrate moderate cellularity with monotonous nuclei. Characteristically, they have areas of perivascular rosettes and ependymal rosettes. They also may contain areas of necrosis, myxoid degeneration, and calcification as well as areas of cartilage and bone formation. The presence of nuclear polymorphism, giant cells, mitoses, and endothelial proliferation are key characteristics of anaplastic ependymoma. As a process restricted to cauda equina ependymomas, myxomatous degeneration is thought to be caused by pressure atrophy.

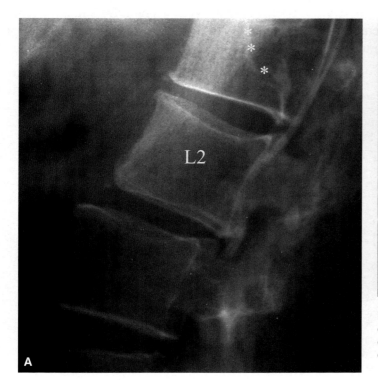
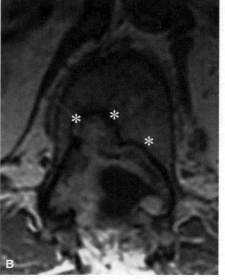

Figure 19–6. *A*, A plain lateral lumbar radiograph and, *B*, a T1-weighted axial MR image of the same level showing a schwannoma (*) eroding the body of L1.

Surgical resection is the primary mode of treatment for intramedullary tumors. The potential for gross-total resection is dependent on the presence of a dissection plane between the mass and the functional neural tissue. Tumors that are infiltrating in character, such as astrocytomas, usually have no useful plane around them and blend into the normal neural tissue. Well-delineated circumscribed lesions, such as ependymomas, usually allow for complete resection. Several studies have shown a lack of recurrence after gross-total resection of ependymomas without any adjuvant therapy, with follow-up ranging from 24 to 62 months. In cases of subtotal resection (STR) or anaplastic histology, radiation therapy can provide effective disease control with an overall survival of 69 percent at 5 years and 62 percent at 10 years.[15] A survival improvement has been shown repeatedly with gross-total resection over STR for spinal ependymomas.[15–17]

Astrocytomas tend to be more infiltrating than ependymomas and, as such, are more difficult to completely resect. There appears to be no added survival benefit for gross-total resection over STR.[16–18] Astrocytomas have a worse prognosis than ependymomas, with a 5-year overall survival after resection and radiation therapy of 58 to 91 percent in patients with low-grade tumors and 0 to 14 percent in patients with high-grade lesions.[19] The main predictive factor for survival in spinal astrocytomas is histology.[21] In general, low-grade tumors tend to have low recurrence rates and survival periods of several years,[16,20,21] whereas high-grade tumors have poor prognosis with mean survival after resection ranging between 5 and 16 months, regardless of the use of adjuvant therapy.[16,20,22–24] Incomplete resection and higher tumor grade have been factors associated with the decision for radiation therapy, the main goal of which is local control; the radiation field usually includes the tumor area with a 1- to 2-cm margin.

Chemotherapy has not been widely used for spinal cord tumors, and little is known regarding its efficacy. Allen and colleagues used the "8-in-1" combination regimen in children with high-grade spinal astrocytomas. Chemotherapy was started immediately following resection and was supplemented by radiation therapy. They showed 5-year progression-free survival of 46 percent and an overall survival of 54 percent, with 5 responses, 4 stabilizations, and 1 failure.[25] In a study of adult high-grade spinal astrocytomas, Cohen and colleagues used carmustine (BCNU), procarbazine, lomustine, vincristine (PCV), or "8-in-1" chemotherapy as adjuvant treatment after resection and radiation therapy. Despite this aggressive regimen, mean survival was 6 months.[24]

Vascular Tumors

Hemangioblastomas account for 3 to 8 percent of all intramedullary spinal cord tumors. The origin of these tumors remains obscure. Histologically, they

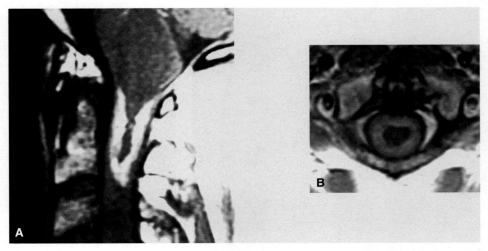

Figure 19–7. *A*, Sagittal and, *B*, axial T1-weighted MR image after the administration of gadolinium contrast demonstrating a large cystic cervicomedullary junction tumor with peripheral intense enhancement at its inferior aspect, consistent with an ependymoma.

consist of large cells filled with lipid vesicles surrounded by variable-size vascular channels. They are most commonly found in the thoracic spine but may be multiple (von Hippel-Lindau disease). They often involve the dorsal aspect of the cord and cause pain and sensory loss. These tumors usually are well-encapsulated lesions with a clear tissue plane that comes to the dorsal surface of the spinal cord. They can be completely resected for cure (Figure 19–8).

GENERAL PRINCIPLES OF TREATMENT

Surgery is the mainstay of treatment for all spinal cord tumors. Surgical outcomes have been shown to be encouraging in several studies with approximately 50 percent neurologic improvement and another 25 to 35 percent stabilization of neurologic function across the variety of primary spinal tumors.[16,22,23,26] The most common approach is a simple laminectomy. This involves the removal of the posterior part of the vertebral body arch, the lamina, thus exposing the contents of the spinal canal. The laminectomy can be extended laterally to include the removal of a facet joint or even the removal of a pedicle (transpedicular approach), allowing access to more ventrally positioned tumors without unsafe retraction of the spinal cord. For intradural tumors, intraoperative ultrasonography can be used to localize the tumor and guide the placement of the myelotomy.

Surgical technique requires the use of the operating microscope to develop a clear plane between tumor and neural tissue. Careful coagulation and hemostasis are crucial to avoid postoperative hematoma formation. Watertight dural closure and tension-free wound closure are necessary steps to avoid a postoperative CSF leak that may complicate the care of these patients by causing the development of meningitis and local wound infections.

For incompletely resected tumors, adjuvant therapy often is indicated, usually in the form of radiation therapy or, less commonly, chemotherapy. Spinal cord irradiation usually is limited to less than 50 Gy, secondary to its side effects, particularly postradiation myelitis. Injury to adjacent organs such as the lungs, kidneys, and intestines are less common toxicities.

A number of trials currently are under way that are assessing the efficacy of different chemotherapeutic agents and modalities in the treatment of spinal tumors. In a phase I/II trial, irinotecan is being used for recurrent malignant ependymomas (North American Brain Tumor Consortium [NABTC]-9801). Patients are being actively recruited for several phase

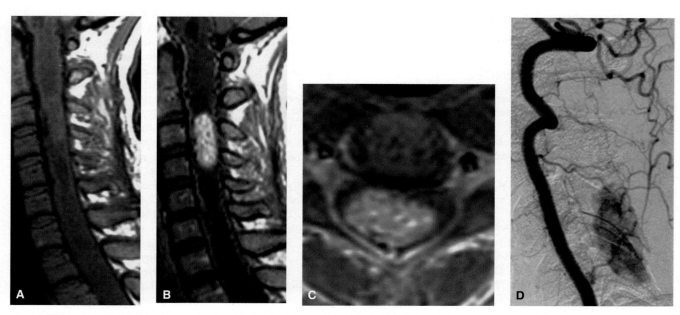

Figure 19–8. *A* and *B*, Midsagittal and, *C*, axial cervical T1-weighted MR image showing a large intramedullary brightly enhancing homogeneous mass occupying more than 90 percent of the spinal canal. *D*, Angiogram of the vertebral artery in lateral projection shows the tumor blush of this hemangioblastoma.

II studies, including temozolamide for recurrent high-grade gliomas (SPRI-C96-348), irinotecan for primary malignant gliomas (Duke University Medical Center [DUMC]-981-98-6R2), thymidine and carboplatin combination for malignant gliomas (NABTC-9705), etoposide and cisplatin in patients with recurrent ependymomas (Mayo Clinic [MAYO]-907253), pre-irradiation combination chemotherapy for disseminated ependymoma (E4397), hydroxyurea for progressive recurrent meningiomas (DUMC-1236-98-8R1), and ifosfamide for aggressive meningeal tumors (South West Oncology Group [SWOG]-9624). A phase III randomized double-blind study of mifepristone versus placebo also is under way for unresectable meningiomas (SWOG-9005).

The efficacy of chemotherapy as adjuvant treatment in spinal tumors remains unclear. The results of the ongoing studies will be necessary to establish histologic and other indications for the use of chemotherapy.

CONCLUSION

It is important to recognize the important role of spinal cord tumors in causing neurologic deficit referable to the spinal cord. This diagnosis can easily be missed, to the detriment of the patient. Once the tumor has been found, expeditious evaluation for surgery, competent postoperative management, and proper adjuvant therapy will help to minimize fixed neurologic deficit and to optimize outcome.

REFERENCES

1. Levivier M, Brotchi J, Balériaux D, et al. Sarcoidosis presenting as an isolated intramedullary tumor. Neurosurgery 1991;29:271–6.
2. Rhoton AL, Ballinger WE Jr, Quisling R, Sypert GW. Intramedullary spinal tuberculoma. Neurosurgery 1988;22:733–6.
3. Voelker JL, Muller J, Worth RM. Intramedullary spinal *Histoplasma* granuloma. Case report. J Neurosurg 1989;70:959–61.
4. Lee M, Epstein FJ, Rezai AR, Zagzag D. Nonneoplastic intramedullary spinal cord lesions mimicking tumors. Neurosurgery 1998;43:788–94.
5. Levy WJ Jr, Bay J, Dohn D. Spinal cord meningioma. J Neurosurg 1982;57:804–12.
6. Seppälä MT, Haltia MJ, Sankila RJ, et al. Long-term outcome after removal of spinal schwannoma: a clinicopathological study of 187 cases. J Neurosurg 1995;83:621–6.
7. Kim P, Ebersold MJ, Onofrio BM, Quast LM. Surgery of spinal nerve schwannoma. Risk of neurological deficit after resection of involved root. J Neurosurg 1989;71:810–4.
8. Seppälä MT, Haltia MJ, Sankila RJ, et al. Long-term outcome after removal of spinal neurofibroma [published erratum appears in J Neurosurg 1995;83:186]. J Neurosurg 1995;82:572–7.
9. Levy WJ, Latchaw J, Hahn JK, et al. Spinal neurofibromas: a report of 66 cases and a comparison with meningiomas. Neurosurgery 1986;18:331–4.
10. McCormick PC. Surgical management of dumbbell tumors of the cervical spine. Neurosurgery 1996;38:294–300.
11. McCormick PC. Surgical management of dumbbell and paraspinal tumors of the thoracic and lumbar spine. Neurosurgery 1996;38:67–75.
12. Yamasaki T, Kikuchi H, Yamashita J, et al. Primary spinal intramedullary malignant melanoma: case report. Neurosurgery 1989;25:117–21.
13. Ozden B, Barlas O, Hacihanefioglu U. Primary dural melanomas: report of two cases and review of the literature. Neurosurgery 1984;15:104–7.
14. Larson TC, Houser OW, Onofrio BM, Piepgras DG. Primary spinal melanoma. J Neurosurg 1987;66:47–9.
15. Whitaker SJ, Bessell EM, Ashley SE, et al. Postoperative radiotherapy in the management of spinal cord ependymoma. J Neurosurg 1991;74:720–8.
16. Cooper PR. Outcome after operative treatment of intramedullary spinal cord tumors in adults: intermediate and long-term results in 51 patients. Neurosurgery 1989;25:855–9.
17. Samii M, Klekamp J. Surgical results of 100 intramedullary tumors in relation to accompanying syringomyelia. Neurosurgery 1994;35:865–73.
18. Guidetti B, Mercuri S, Vagnozzi R. Long-term results of the surgical treatment of 129 intramedullary spinal gliomas. J Neurosurg 1981;54:323–30.
19. Larson D. Radiation therapy of tumors of the spine. In: Youmans J, editor. Neurological surgery. Philadelphia: WB Saunders; 1996. p. 3168–74.
20. Epstein FJ, Farmer JP, Freed D. Adult intramedullary astrocytomas of the spinal cord. J Neurosurg 1992;77:355–9.
21. Rossitch E Jr, Zeidman SM, Burger PC, et al. Clinical and pathological analysis of spinal cord astrocytomas in children. Neurosurgery 1990;27:193–6.
22. Cristante L, Herrmann HD. Surgical management of intramedullary spinal cord tumors: functional outcome and sources of morbidity. Neurosurgery 1994;35:69–76.
23. Cooper PR, Epstein F. Radical resection of intramedullary spinal cord tumors in adults. Recent experience in 29 patients. J Neurosurg 1985;63:492–9.
24. Cohen AR, Wisoff JH, Allen JC, Epstein F. Malignant astrocytomas of the spinal cord. J Neurosurg 1989;70:50–4.
25. Allen JC, Aviner S, Yates AJ, et al. Treatment of high-grade spinal cord astrocytoma of childhood with "8-in-1" chemotherapy and radiotherapy: a pilot study of CCG-945. Children's Cancer Group. J Neurosurg 1998;88:215–20.
26. Brotchi J, Dewitte O, Levivier M, et al. A survey of 65 tumors within the spinal cord: surgical results and the importance of preoperative magnetic resonance imaging. Neurosurgery 1991;29:651–7.

20

Metastatic Brain Tumors

PENNY K. SNEED, MD

Brain metastases are a common occurrence responsible for significant morbidity and mortality among cancer patients. Major advances have been made over the past several decades in the imaging and treatment of brain metastases. In addition, much attention has been focused on prognostic factors to provide the background information needed for clinicians to appropriately individualize treatment selection.

EPIDEMIOLOGY

Brain metastases tend to be grossly under-reported. In reality, they represent the most common intracranial tumor, significantly surpassing primary brain tumors in incidence. Autopsy series estimate that up to 25 percent of cancer patients develop intracranial metastases.[1,2] Males and females are affected equally and experience peak incidence in the fifth to seventh decades.[2] The most common primary sites of origin in adults include the lung, breast, skin (melanoma), colon, and kidney (renal cell carcinoma),[3,4] and the most common solid tumor primary sites in children are sarcomas and germ cell tumors.[5]

ANATOMY

Most intracranial metastases occur via arterial hematogenous spread to the brain parenchyma and, less often, to the dura or leptomeninges. There is a predilection for metastases to arise at the gray-white junction where the vasculature narrows and to terminal "watershed" areas at the borders of the territories of major cerebral vessels.[4,6] Much less commonly, the central nervous system (CNS) can become involved via direct extension of skin cancer or head and neck cancer through bone or along cranial nerves. A variety of routes have been implicated for development of leptomeningeal metastases: arterial spread, venous spread through Batson's plexus (the vertebral venous system), direction extension from an adjacent bone or parenchymal metastasis, and intraoperative spread at the time of resection of a metastasis. There is a higher risk of leptomeningeal dissemination from posterior fossa metastases than from supratentorial metastases.[7,8] Also, leukemias and lymphomas are more likely to metastasize to the leptomeninges than to the brain parenchyma, unlike solid primary malignancies.[2]

The distribution and number of brain metastases were described in a series of 288 patients imaged with computed tomography (CT).[4] Eighty percent of lesions were located in the cerebral hemispheres, 15 percent in the cerebellum, and 5 percent in the basal ganglia. Single metastases were more common from breast, pelvic, or abdominal primary sites than from melanoma or lung cancers; posterior fossa metastases occurred more frequently in association with prostate, uterine, or gastrointestinal primary tumors than other primary tumors ($p < .001$). A single metastasis was seen in 49 percent of patients, two metastases in 21 percent, three in 13 percent, four in 6 percent, and at least five in the remaining 11 percent. However, this study was based on CT scans, and it is clear that higher numbers of metastases are identified on magnetic resonance imaging (MRI) than CT imaging[9] and on triple-dose compared with single-dose gadolinium-enhanced MRI.[10,11]

PATHOLOGY

Grossly, metastases tend to be fairly spherical and well circumscribed. They may be cystic due to necrosis, deposits of degenerating keratin squamous cell carcinomas, or extensive mucin secretion in adenocarcinomas, and hemorrhage may be seen in metastases from melanoma, renal cell carcinoma, bronchogenic carcinoma, or choriocarcinoma.[2,12] On histopathologic examination, metastases tend to be well demarcated, but there may be infiltration into surrounding parenchyma, especially in the case of small cell carcinomas and malignant melanomas, or microscopic nests of cells in surrounding tissue that cannot be appreciated grossly. Although well-differentiated tumors are easily identified as metastases, immunohistochemistry and electron microscopy may be needed for poorly differentiated metastases to distinguish them from primary brain tumors and to indicate likely sites of origin. For instance, mucin or keratin stains may be positive in carcinomas, whereas the glial fibrillary acid protein (GFAP) stain should be negative in carcinomas but positive in primary gliomas. Changes in surrounding brain tissue may include extensive edema as well as reactive gliosis and vascular proliferation.

CLINICAL PRESENTATION

Brain metastases may be synchronous, found at the time of primary diagnosis, but they are more commonly metachronous, detected subsequent to the primary diagnosis and often subsequent to the development of extracranial metastases. The term "solitary metastasis" indicates one metastasis in the absence of other extracranial disease, whereas the term "single metastasis" does not imply extracranial control.

Specific symptoms and signs depend on the location of the metastases, but the most common presenting complaints include headache, focal weakness, impaired mentation, and cerebellar dysfunction. Focal or generalized seizures occur in about 15 to 20 percent of patients.[3,13] The percentage of asymptomatic patients depends on the aggressiveness of screening for brain metastases.

DIAGNOSTIC STUDIES

Diagnostic imaging of the brain has improved dramatically over the past several decades with the advent of CT and then MRI. On noncontrast CT scans, brain metastases generally appear hypodense or isodense in comparison with normal brain parenchyma, and there is surrounding low-attenuation edema. However, hemorrhagic metastases appear hyperdense, and melanomas and tumors with a high nuclear-to-cytoplasmic ratio may appear hyperdense in the absence of hemorrhage. Brain metastases generally enhance brightly after administration of iodinated contrast because of blood-brain barrier breakdown and tumor neovascularity.

Magnetic resonance imaging is the most sensitive imaging modality at present. Most metastases appear hypointense or isointense on noncontrast T1-weighted images, and there is a surrounding low signal corresponding to edema. Melanomas may appear hyperintense secondary to high-signal melanin, and adenocarcinomas may appear hyperintense for unclear reasons. Characteristics of hemorrhagic metastases evolve depending on the age of the hemorrhage. On T2-weighted images, most metastases appear hyperintense but not as bright as surrounding areas of edema, except that adenocarcinomas tend to be hypointense. Most metastases densely enhance after the administration of gadolinium contrast; the pattern of enhancement may be homogeneous, heterogeneous, or ring-like. Figure 20–1 shows the appearance of parenchymal brain metastases on a T2-weighted image and a contrast-enhanced T1-weighted image.

Brain metastases may be difficult to distinguish from other types of lesions. Ring enhancement usually is thicker and more irregular in tumors than in abscesses, demyelinating lesions, or resolving hematomas. In comparison with primary tumors,

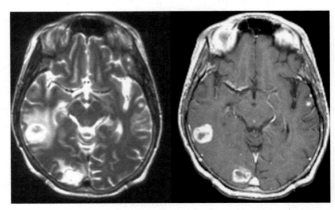

Figure 20–1. Multiple parenchymal brain metastases shown on T2-weighted (*left*) and gadolinium-enhanced T1-weighted (*right*) magnetic resonance imaging.

metastases are more likely to be multiple and less likely to have edema extending into the corpus callosum or gray matter, but it is frequently not possible to distinguish metastases from primary brain tumors based on imaging characteristics alone. Other entities that can be confused with brain metastases include granuloma, infection, cerebral infarction, and radiation necrosis; hemorrhagic metastases may be mistaken for non-neoplastic hemorrhagic lesions and vice versa. Particularly in the absence of other metastatic disease, a biopsy may be indicated to make a definitive diagnosis and to avoid inappropriate therapy. Eleven percent of patients enrolled in a randomized trial of biopsy + whole brain radiotherapy (WBRT) versus resection + WBRT for single brain metastases had to be excluded because lesions thought to be brain metastases were found to be glioma, abscess, or inflammation.[14] In a stereotactic biopsy series of 100 patients with multifocal brain lesions and no known primary malignancy or systemic disease explaining the brain lesions, only 15 percent of patients were found to have brain metastases.[15]

Triple-dose gadolinium significantly improves the sensitivity of MRI in detecting small metastases, although this may only be cost-effective in cases for which management potentially could change based on results.[10,11] Van Dijk and colleagues imaged 39 patients with brain metastases before and after 0.1-, 0.2-, and 0.3-mmol gadolinium-complex per kg body weight.[10] Compared with a dose of 0.1 mmol/kg, the number of metastases detected increased by 15 percent using 0.2 mmol/kg and by 43 percent using 0.3 mmol/kg. In a multicenter study involving 49 patients with abnormal MRI findings, the number of metastases visualized increased by 51 percent using 0.3 mmol/kg compared with 0.1 mmol/kg ($p = .0001$).[11] In addition, 8 of 49 patients thought to have a single metastasis on a single-dose gadolinium-enhanced MRI were found to have multiple metastases on triple-dose, gadolinium-enhanced MRI, and 2 patients with normal single-dose gadolinium-enhanced MRI had lesions identified on triple-dose gadolinium-enhanced MRI.

Screening for brain metastases in patients without neurologic symptoms is controversial. Older reports of CT screening found brain metastases in approximately 10 percent of asymptomatic lung cancer patients,[16] but the yield is likely to be higher with MRI. It is rational to perform screening for primary disease sites with a propensity for brain metastases in patients for whom the management would be different based on the findings.

Metabolic imaging modalities that may be useful, particularly to distinguish between active tumor and necrosis post-treatment, include positron emission tomography (PET), single-photon emission computed tomography (SPECT), and magnetic resonance spectroscopy (MRS). On PET imaging, tumors may be visualized as a region of increased ^{18}F-fluorodeoxyglucose (FDG) uptake because of their higher rate of glucose use, whereas necrosis appears as a "cold" region of decreased FDG uptake. An advantage of PET imaging is that whole body images are readily obtained, potentially providing whole body staging information. A disadvantage of PET is that the relatively high metabolic activity of normal brain cortex may make it difficult to discriminate tumor from brain tissue. Alignment of MRI and PET images can aid in the interpretation of PET images.[17] On SPECT imaging, thallium-201 or another radiotracer that localizes in tumor creates a region of increased uptake in tumor and decreased uptake in necrosis. Proton MRS is a different technique that provides spectra characterizing metabolites in one or multiple voxels in conjunction with MRI. Metastases tend to have increased choline and decreased N-acetylaspartate (NAA, a neuronal marker) compared with normal brain tissue, and larger metastases also may have lipid and/or lactate resonances that are not detectable in normal brain tissue.[18]

PROGNOSTIC FACTORS

An understanding of prognostic factors is useful for decision-making in the management of patients with brain metastases. These factors are complex, depending on primary site, patient parameters, and both intracranial and extracranial disease burden. The number of metastases is not the most important parameter, although patients with a single metastasis tend to fare better than those with multiple metastases, and those with a solitary metastasis have the best prognosis.

Gaspar and colleagues used recursive partitioning analysis (RPA) to analyze prognostic factors in

1,200 evaluable patients treated on three successive Radiation Therapy Oncology Group (RTOG) trials for brain metastases from 1979 to 1993.[19] Based on this analysis, they defined three prognostic groupings. Class 1 patients (Karnofsky Performance Scale [KPS] ≥ 70, age < 65 years, controlled primary disease, and no extracranial metastases; 20 percent of patients) had a median survival time of 7.1 months and class 3 patients (KPS < 70; 15 percent of patients) had a median survival time of 2.3 months. All other patients were grouped into class 2 and had a median survival time of 4.2 months.

Univariate and multivariate analyses of 12 factors were performed among 1,292 patients managed for brain metastases at the Daniel Den Hoed Cancer Center in Rotterdam from 1981 to 1990.[20] The median survival times were 1.3 months for patients treated with steroids only, 3.6 months for WBRT, and 8.9 months for surgery + WBRT. The most important prognostic factors included treatment approach, performance status, extent of systemic disease, response to steroids, serum lactate dehydrogenase, and age (< 70 vs ≥ 70 years). Lesser prognostic factors included primary site and number of metastases. The "good prognosis" subset (23 percent of all patients) had a median survival time of 6.3 months and included patients with a KPS ≥ 70, no or limited systemic tumor activity, and good response to steroids. The "poor prognosis" subgroup, with a median survival time of only 1.3 months, included the 9 percent of patients with a KPS < 70, limited or extensive systemic tumor activity, and little response to steroids. The remaining patients had a median survival time of 3.4 months.

Among patients treated with radiosurgery (RS), favorable prognostic factors also include absence of extracranial metastases, a higher KPS, age ≤ 60 to 70 years, and control of the primary tumor; an additional important parameter is smaller total tumor volume.[21,22]

TREATMENT

Medical Management

Brain Edema

Vasogenic brain edema secondary to disruption of the blood-brain barrier frequently accounts for or aggravates brain dysfunction associated with metastases. Although they are associated with numerous undesirable side effects, glucocorticoids have been the mainstay of treatment for vasogenic brain edema since the 1960s, resulting in symptomatic improvement in approximately 75 percent of patients,[20] beginning within hours of institution of steroid therapy and reaching full effect within 24 to 72 hours. Dexamethasone often is prescribed with a starting dose of 10 mg and then 4 mg four times daily, although lower doses may be just as effective. Steroids generally should be reduced to the lowest effective dose, maintained during treatment, and then tapered and hopefully discontinued, as symptoms permit. Because of the adverse effects of prolonged steroid therapy, other steroid formulations such as corticotropin-releasing factor (CRF) and 21-aminosteroids are under evaluation.

Severe, life-threatening increased intracranial pressure from edema may be managed with hyperventilation or osmotherapy, most commonly with mannitol. Hyperventilation decreases Pco_2, causing cerebral vasoconstriction in undamaged brain tissue, decreasing cerebral blood volume, and thus decreasing intracranial pressure. Mannitol increases the osmolality in the blood, drawing water out of the brain in areas where the blood-brain barrier is intact.

Seizure Activity

Seizures are a presenting sign in 15 to 20 percent of patients with brain metastases and occur at some point in 30 to 40 percent of patients.[3,13,23] Anticonvulsant therapy should be instituted in patients who have experienced a seizure; phenytoin is the initial drug of choice, followed by carbamazepine, phenobarbital, and valproate. The empiric use of anticonvulsants in patients who have not had a seizure is controversial and has fallen out of favor; several retrospective and randomized trials have failed to show a benefit of prophylactic anticonvulsant therapy.[24]

Whole Brain Radiotherapy

Whole brain radiotherapy is the mainstay of treatment for most patients with brain metastases. It results in good short-term palliation without the use of sophisticated equipment or techniques. However, in patients with a longer life expectancy, the usefulness of WBRT is limited by poor long-term local control and by potential radiation-induced dementia.

Technique

Lateral opposed fields are used to encompass the whole brain; care is taken to include the entire temporal lobe and to block the eyes (except when intraocular involvement is present). Some practitioners angle each field posteriorly by 5° to help avoid the contralateral retina. Port films are taken with eye markers to demonstrate adequate eye blocking and adequate coverage of intracranial contents (Figure 20–2). Extra margin may be desirable at the skull base for patients with cranial nerve involvement, and fields may be extended to include the spinal cord down to the C2 level in patients considered to be at significant risk for spinal canal dissemination. Megavoltage radiotherapy is administered using a cobalt 60 teletherapy unit or linear accelerator with photon peak energies ranging from about 4 to 10 MV. Very high energies may be undesirable because of potential underdosing of the brain surface.

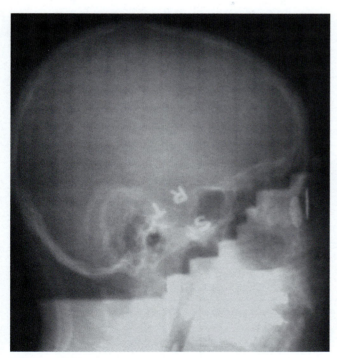

Figure 20–2. Double-exposed radiation therapy portal image of a whole brain radiotherapy field (*darker region*) and surrounding shielded tissues (*lighter region*). Markers placed on the eyelids demonstrate adequate blocking of the eyes.

Symptomatic Response

Careful analyses of symptomatic improvement from WBRT (plus steroids in 70 percent of patients) were reported by Borgelt and colleagues for 1,812 evaluable patients treated in two randomized RTOG trials conducted from 1971 to 1976.[3] The WBRT regimens used included 20 Gy in 5 fractions, 30 Gy in 10 or 15 fractions, and 40 Gy in 15 or 20 fractions. Four neurologic function classes were defined, and change to a higher functional class was scored as improvement. The overall rate of improvement was 49 percent. Relief of specific neurologic symptoms also was evaluated. Complete response and overall (complete + partial) response rates ranged from 35 to 72 percent and 64 to 85 percent, respectively, for headaches, motor weakness, impaired mentation, cerebellar dysfunction, cranial nerve deficits, and seizures (Table 20–1). Overall, 80 percent of patients' remaining survival time was spent in an improved or stable neurologic state, and 50 percent of patients had improved or stable neurologic status at the time of death. Steroids resulted in more rapid symptomatic response but did not appear to affect the duration of response. Results were similar among the five dose-fractionation schemes used.

Ultra-rapid regimens involving 10 Gy in one fraction or 12 Gy in two fractions were evaluated at a limited number of institutions participating in the first two RTOG studies of WBRT for brain metastases. Compared with the other regimens studied, the ultra-rapid regimens yielded similar rates of symptomatic response and morbidity but resulted in fewer complete responses and a shorter duration of improvement.[25]

Table 20–1. SYMPTOMATIC RESPONSE TO WBRT IN THE FIRST TWO RTOG TRIALS

Symptom	Number of Patients (%)	Complete Response (%)	Complete + Partial Response (%)
Headache	982 (54)	60	82
Motor deficit	910 (50)	35	67
Impaired mentation	780 (43)	44	70
Cerebellar dysfunction	477 (26)	45	69
Cranial nerve deficit	459 (25)	42	64
Seizures	327 (18)	72	85

WBRT = whole brain radiotherapy; RTOG = Radiation Therapy Oncology Group.
Adapted from Borgelt B, Gelber R, Kramer S, et al. The palliation of brain metastases: final results of the first two studies by the Radiation Therapy Oncology Group. Int J Radiat Oncol Biol Phys 1980;6:1–8.

Survival

Multiple successive randomized trials to evaluate various radiation dose fractionation schemes have been performed by the RTOG, beginning in 1971, the pre-CT era. These trials are summarized in Table 20–2. The first two trials compared five different WBRT regimens—20 Gy in 5 fractions, 30 Gy in 10 or 15 fractions, and 40 Gy in 15 or 20 fractions—with stratification by primary site (lung, breast, other) and by presence or absence of extracranial metastases.[3] All five regimens yielded similar results in terms of symptomatic response, duration of response, and survival, with median survival times ranging from 3.7 to 4.8 months for the first study and 3.4 to 4.1 months for the second study.[26] Given equal efficacy of all five schemes, the authors recommended the shorter, more cost-effective regimens of 20 Gy in 5 fractions over 1 week or 30 Gy in 10 fractions over 2 weeks. The most commonly accepted WBRT regimen has become 30 Gy delivered in 10 fractions over 2 weeks.

After the first two RTOG brain metastasis trials, multiple other protocols were designed to try to improve upon the results. One reason for difficulty in distinguishing efficacy of various treatment regimens is that many patients die of extracranial disease within several months after WBRT. To test whether higher doses of radiotherapy could result in better survival in "good prognosis" patients, the RTOG conducted a trial comparing 50 Gy in 20 fractions over 4 weeks with 30 Gy in 10 fractions over 2 weeks in patients with controlled primary tumor, no evidence of extracranial metastases, and a KPS $\geq$ 50.[27] Contrary to the expectation, higher radiation dose yielded no survival advantage; median survival times were 3.9 months in the 50 Gy arm and 4.1 months in the 30 Gy arm, and uncontrolled brain metastases were the cause of death in 52 percent and 54 percent of patients,

Table 20–2. PROSPECTIVE, RANDOMIZED TRIALS OF WHOLE BRAIN RADIOTHERAPY ALONE FOR BRAIN METASTASES

Protocol	Years of Study	No. of Patients	Scheme	Median Survival (mo)
RTOG 6901*	1971–1973	233	30 Gy/10 fx/2 wk	4.8
		217	30 Gy/15 fx/3 wk	4.1
		233	40 Gy/15 fx/3 wk	4.1
		227	40 Gy/20 fx/4 wk	3.7
RTOG 7361†	1973–1976	447	20 Gy/5 fx/1 wk	3.4
		228	30 Gy/10 fx/2 wk	3.4
		227	40 Gy/15 fx/3 wk	4.1
RTOG 6901‡	1971–1973	26	10 Gy/1 fx/1 day	3.4
RTOG 7361‡	1973–1976	33	12 Gy/2 fx/2 days	3.0
RTOG 7606§	1976–1979	130	30 Gy/10 fx/2 wk	4.1
		125	50 Gy/20 fx/4 wk	3.9
RTOG 8528‖	1986–1989	30	48.0 Gy at 1.6 Gy bid	4.9
		53	54.4 Gy at 1.6 Gy bid	5.4
		44	64.0 Gy at 1.6 Gy bid	7.2
		26	70.4 Gy at 1.6 Gy bid	8.2
RTOG 9104#	1991–1995	213	30 Gy/10 fx/2 wk	4.5
		216	54.4 Gy at 1.6 Gy bid	4.5
RTOG 7916**	1979–1983	193	30 Gy/10 fx/2 wk	4.5
		200	30 Gy/6 fx/3 wk	4.1
		196	30 Gy/6 fx + miso	3.1
		190	30 Gy/10 fx + miso	3.9
RTOG 8905††	1989–1993	36	37.5 Gy/15 fx/3 wk	6.1
		34	37.5 Gy/15 fx + BUDR	4.3

RTOG = Radiation Therapy Oncology Group; fx = fractions; WBRT = whole brain radiotherapy; miso = misonidazole; BUDR = 5-bromodeoxyuridine.
*"First study"; Borgelt et al[3] and Coia.[26]
†"Second study"; Borgelt et al[3] and Coia.[26]
‡"Ultra rapid"; Borgelt et al.[25]
§"Favorable patients"; Kurtz et al.[27]
‖Accelerated hyperfractionation for unresected single metastases; Epstein et al.[28]
#Accelerated hyperfractionation vs standard WBRT; Murray et al.[30]
**Misonidazole; Komarnicky et al.[31]
††BUDR; Phillips et al.[32]

respectively. It appears that the selection criteria and/or staging evaluation were inadequate to select a good prognosis population and that 50 Gy in 20 fractions was not an adequate dose to significantly improve intracranial control.

Another attempt to improve intracranial control with higher radiation dose involved accelerated hyperfractionation. An initial phase I/II dose-escalation RTOG study gave WBRT to 32 Gy at 1.6 Gy twice daily followed by a boost to 48.0, 54.4, 64.0, or 70.4 Gy at 1.6 Gy twice daily in patients with a KPS ≥ 70 and unresected single brain metastasis (153 patients) or multiple brain metastases (181 patients).[28,29] Half of the patients had extracranial metastases and/or uncontrolled primary disease. A dose escalation advantage was seen in patients with single but not multiple metastases. Among the patients with single metastasis, median survival times for the 48.0, 54.4, 64.0, or 70.4 Gy strata were 4.9, 5.4, 7.2, and 8.2 months, respectively, and survival was significantly improved comparing the 48 Gy arm to the arms receiving at least 54.4 Gy ($p = .05$).[28] Unfortunately, a subsequent randomized phase III study in patients with single or multiple brain metastases and a KPS ≥ 70 showed no advantage for accelerated hyperfractionation overall for patients with single metastases or for RPA class 1 patients; it compared WBRT with 30 Gy in 10 daily fractions to WBRT to 32 Gy at 1.6 Gy twice daily followed by a boost to a total dose of 54.4 Gy at 1.6 Gy twice daily.[30]

Other prospective, randomized trials evaluating WBRT ± radiation sensitizers have failed to demonstrate any survival advantage for misonidazole,[31] 5-bromodeoxyuridine,[32] or lonidamine.[33]

Despite improvements in brain imaging and other advances in cancer management over the past several decades, the prognosis of most patients with brain metastases has improved little. The most commonly accepted dose-fractionation scheme remains 30 Gy in 10 fractions over 2 weeks, resulting in an expected median survival time of about 3 to 4 months. Slower dose-fractionation regimens of about 40 Gy at 2 Gy per fraction tend to be given in patients with a life expectancy of at least 6 to 12 months because of concern about potential late effects of WBRT. In addition, a partial brain boost may be considered to encompass a single or dominant metastasis, although the usefulness of an external beam radiotherapy boost has not been proven.

Local Control

Because routine follow-up imaging often is not obtained and life expectancy frequently is limited, relatively few data have been available regarding response and freedom from progression of brain metastases after WBRT. Nieder and colleagues analyzed response in patients followed up with CT imaging every 3 months after WBRT, including 164 patients treated with 30 Gy in 10 fractions and 39 patients treated with total doses of 40 to 60 Gy.[34] Among the 138 of 164 patients with follow-up imaging, the best local result was complete response of all brain metastases in 12 percent of patients, partial response in 32 percent, no change in 47 percent, progression in 7 percent, and "no consistent behavior" of multiple metastases in 3 percent. For the higher-dose group, 13 percent of patients had complete response, 64 percent partial response, 18 percent no change, and 5 percent mixed response. Response rates were higher in patients with breast cancer or small cell lung cancer. The median survival time was only 3 months, and actuarial probability of freedom from progression of brain metastases was not presented.

Time to local progression or recurrence was evaluated in a randomized trial of biopsy + WBRT versus resection + WBRT for patients with a single metastasis.[14] Crude local recurrence rates were 12/23 (52%) for biopsy + WBRT versus 5/25 (20%) for resection + WBRT ($p < .02$), and actuarial freedom from local tumor recurrence was significantly shorter for biopsy + WBRT than resection + WBRT ($p < .0001$; median, 4.8 months vs > 13.6 months; relative risk = 7.1 with 95 percent confidence interval [CI] 2.4 to 21.5). At 1 year after biopsy + WBRT, the actuarial freedom from local tumor recurrence probability was very poor—approximately 15 percent. New brain metastases or leptomeningeal dissemination (with or without local recurrence) occurred in 20 percent of patients treated with resection + WBRT and 13 percent of those who underwent biopsy + WBRT.

Toxicity

Side effects and complications of WBRT may be divided into acute, early-delayed, and late. Acute sequelae of WBRT occurring in essentially all patients during the course of treatment include epilation, fatigue (ranging from mild to severe), and mild to moderate scalp erythema and/or hyperpigmentation. Less commonly, external otitis or otitis media may occur. Headache, nausea, and vomiting from increased intracranial pressure rarely occur during WBRT, perhaps because most patients with symptomatic edema are started on steroids before WBRT and are continued on steroids during WBRT.

Ultra-rapid WBRT schemes of 10 Gy in one fraction or 15 Gy in two fractions appear to be associated with more acute morbidity than standard regimens. In an early report, 3 of 54 patients (6%) died within 48 hours after receiving 10 Gy in one fraction to the whole brain, possibly due to herniation, although these 3 patients had poor performance status prior to WBRT.[35] In another trial, 83 patients were treated with 15 Gy in two fractions, resulting in a median survival time of only 1.9 months and a 49 percent incidence of complications (fever, headache, nausea, vomiting, herniation, lethargy, or agitation), including a 7 percent incidence of cerebral herniation.[36]

Early-delayed radiation reactions occurring a few weeks to 2 to 3 months after WBRT have not been described by most authors but may include transient neurologic deterioration[37] or the somnolence syndrome, especially in children, consisting of somnolence, anorexia, and irritability.[38] The mechanism of early-delayed reaction may be temporary inhibition of myelin synthesis by oligodendroglial cells.

Data regarding late toxicity of WBRT are limited because of the relatively short life expectancy of most patients. However, long-term survivors are at risk for serious late effects, particularly diffuse white matter changes associated with varying degrees of dementia (Figure 20–3). DeAngelis and colleagues described 12 patients who had long-term intracranial control but severe dementia after WBRT to total doses of 25 to 39 Gy using 3-, 5-, and/or 6-Gy fractions.[39] Late effects began 5 to 36 months after WBRT with dizziness, fatigue, mild headache, and decreased short-term memory, progressing to severe dementia and disabling ataxia. Brain atrophy, ventricular dilation, and diffuse hypodense white matter were seen on CT imaging. Contrast enhancement typical of radiation necrosis was seen in 3 cases. The authors estimated the incidence of WBRT-induced dementia to be 2 to 5 percent, but only severely affected patients were identified in this retrospective review. To determine the full range of late toxicities and the actuarial risk at various points in time, patients must be followed up and tested prospectively before and at various intervals after WBRT. Such studies are under way as part of some ongoing phase III clinical trials.

Radiation fraction size, total dose, patient age, chemotherapy agents used (if any), and sequencing and timing of chemotherapy are all determinants of late effects of WBRT.[40,41] The patients with severe dementia reported by DeAngelis and colleagues were treated with radiation fractions of at least 3 Gy,[39] and Sundaresan and colleagues reported cases of brain necrosis occurring with daily fractions > 2.5 Gy.[42] The risk of cognitive deficits is higher in young children and in older adults than in older children and young adults. The risk of damage also appears to be higher in leukemia and small cell lung cancer patients treated with chemotherapy and WBRT, particularly when chemotherapy is concurrent with WBRT.[41] Methotrexate given during or after WBRT has been implicated specifically, but other agents also may enhance CNS toxicity of WBRT.

To minimize the risk of serious late neurotoxicity of WBRT, patients with a life expectancy of at least 6 to 12 months who require WBRT should be treated with 40 Gy at 2.0 Gy per fraction or 45 Gy at 1.8 Gy per fraction. Although diffuse white-matter damage has been described after 40 Gy at 2 Gy per daily fraction,[43] the incidence and severity of damage should be less using 1.8 to 2.0 Gy per daily fraction than 3.0 Gy or more per fraction. Partial brain radiotherapy could be used in place of WBRT for a single metastasis, but it is not standard treatment. Unlike RS, partial brain radiotherapy compromises the ability to give later WBRT or to treat the remainder of the brain if multiple metastases develop at a later date.

Re-irradiation

Because of the high failure rate of brain metastases after WBRT alone, patients who live long enough

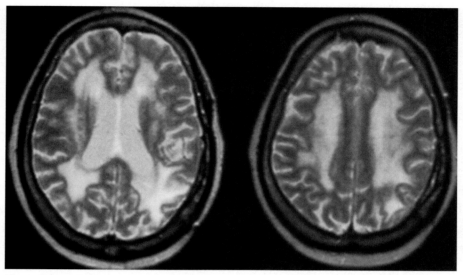

Figure 20–3. T2-weighted magnetic resonance images showing diffuse white-matter changes and ventricular dilation 1 year after whole brain radiotherapy with 30 Gy in 10 fractions over 2 weeks.

may present with recurrent brain metastases. Depending upon the number of metastases, patient performance status, and multiple other factors, treatment options may include surgery, brachytherapy,[44] focal brain re-irradiation, RS, or repeat WBRT. Patients with numerous brain metastases or a limited expected life span who require palliative treatment may benefit from repeat WBRT. As shown in Table 20–3, a variety of re-irradiation schemes have resulted in symptomatic improvement in 27 to 75 percent of patients, with a duration of response of about 2.5 months and median survival times ranging from 1.8 to 4.0 months after re-irradiation.[45–49] Typically, doses of 20 to 25 Gy were given in 10 fractions over 2 weeks. In cases in which late toxicity is of potential concern, there may an advantage to hyperfractionated WBRT of approximately 30 Gy at 1 Gy twice daily.

Surgery

Biopsy may be indicated in patients with single or multiple brain metastases to obtain a histologic diagnosis, and surgical resection may be indicated in selected patients with a single, dominant, or small number of brain metastases for a variety of reasons: to obtain a histologic diagnosis; to promptly relieve mass effect (Figure 20–4), edema, or obstructive hydrocephalus; or to improve the likelihood of long-term local control, survival, and functionally independent survival. As discussed in the section "Diagnostic Studies," lesions such as brain abscesses or primary brain tumors may be mistaken for brain metastases. In particular, single lesions in patients with a history of cancer and single or multiple lesions in patients without a known cancer diagnosis may warrant histologic proof. Of 54 patients with suspected single brain metastases entered in a randomized trial of surgical removal or biopsy followed by WBRT, 11 percent had to be excluded because their lesion proved to be a primary brain tumor or an infectious or inflammatory process.[14] It is also important to obtain histologic material in patients with multiple lesions without a known cancer. In a stereotactic biopsy series of 100 such patients, brain metastases accounted for only 15 percent of the diagnoses; the most common other diagnoses included malignant glioma (37%), CNS lymphoma (15%), low-grade glioma (12%), infectious disease (10%), and ischemic lesions (6%).[15]

Three prospective, randomized trials of WBRT ± surgery have been performed in patients with potentially resectable single brain metastases (Table 20–4). In a trial reported by Patchell and colleagues, 48 eligible patients with a KPS ≥ 70 and a single metastasis were randomized between biopsy + WBRT versus resection + WBRT (36 Gy in 12 fractions).[14] Patients who underwent resection had sig-

Table 20–3. RETROSPECTIVE REVIEWS OF REPEAT WBRT FOR RECURRENT BRAIN METASTASES

Authors	N	Treatment	% with Improved Symptoms	Duration of Response (mo)	Median Survival (mo)
Shehata et al[45]	35	NS	69	2.6	NS
Kurup et al[46]	56	20 Gy/10 fx	75	2.5	3.5
Hazuka and Kinzie[47]	44	6–36 Gy at 2–4 Gy/fx	27	NS	1.8
Cooper et al[48]	52	~25 Gy/10 fx	42	NS	3.7
Wong et al[49]	86	Median 20 Gy/10 fx	70	NS	4.0

WBRT = whole brain radiotherapy; NS = not stated; fx = fractions.

nificantly longer survival (median, 9.2 months vs 3.4 months; $p < .01$) and duration of functional independence (median, 8.7 months vs 1.8 months; $p < .005$). Noordijk and colleagues randomized 63 evaluable patients to WBRT (40 Gy at 2 Gy bid) ± surgery and found a benefit in the 43 patients with stable or absent systemic disease (median survival time, 12 months for 22 patients treated with WBRT

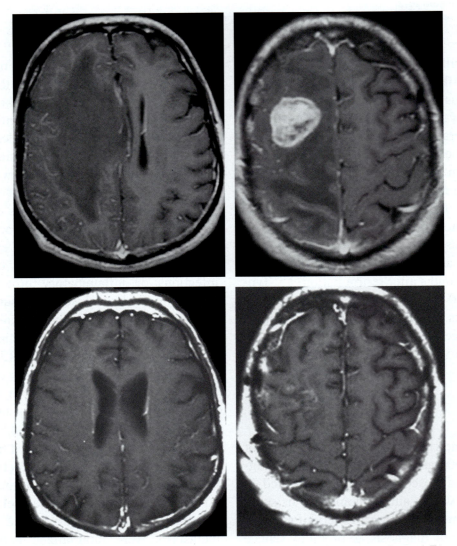

Figure 20–4. Preoperative (*above*) and postoperative (*below*) contrast-enhanced T1-weighted magnetic resonance images showing resection of a large brain metastasis resulting in relief of mass effect.

+ surgery vs 7 months for 21 patients treated with WBRT; $p = .02$) but not in the 20 patients with progressive systemic disease (median survival time, 5 months in both arms).[50] Overall, the median survival times were 10 months for WBRT + surgery versus 6 months for WBRT alone ($p = .04$). In the randomized trial reported by Mintz and colleagues, many of the 143 eligible patients declined the study; 84 patients were randomized to WBRT (30 Gy in 10 fractions) ± surgery.[51] Of these 84 patients, 45 percent of patients had extracranial metastases and 21 percent had a KPS < 70. The median survival times were unusually long for WBRT alone (6.3 months) and unusually short for surgery + WBRT (5.6 months). This may have been caused in part by an imbalance between the arms in terms of primary site, with more good-prognosis breast cancer patients in the WBRT-alone arm and more poor-prognosis colon cancer patients in the WBRT + surgery arm. Also, 23 percent of patients on the "WBRT-alone" arm underwent surgery before or after WBRT. The operative morbidity and 30-day mortality rates reported for the resection + WBRT arms in these three randomized trials ranged from 8 to 12.5 percent and 4 to 10 percent, respectively; the 30-day mortality rate in the WBRT-alone arms ranged from 0 to 7 percent.[14,50,51]

Surgical resection of multiple metastases is even more controversial than resection of a single metastasis, but Bindal and colleagues reported encouraging results of a retrospective review of patients who underwent resection for multiple brain metastases.[52] Among the 26 patients who had all lesions resected, the median survival time was 14 months; symptoms improved in 83 percent and worsened in 6 percent of patients; and the morbidity and 30-day mortality rates were 9 percent and 4 percent, respectively.

Postoperative Whole Brain Radiotherapy

Multiple investigators have addressed the question of whether adjuvant WBRT is warranted after resection of a single brain metastasis. The two largest retrospective reviews suggested a benefit for postoperative WBRT. DeAngelis and colleagues reported results in patients who had complete resection of a single brain metastasis at Memorial Sloan-Kettering Cancer Center from 1978 to 1985. The median survival time was 21 months in 79 patients who underwent WBRT versus 14 months in 19 patients who did not.[8] Smalley and colleagues retrospectively reviewed 229 patients with or without systemic disease who underwent subtotal resection (STR) or gross-total resection (GTR) of a single brain metastasis at the Mayo Clinic from 1972 to 1982, with or without adjuvant postoperative WBRT.[53] Adjuvant WBRT was associated with significantly longer median survival among patients without evidence of systemic disease: 1.3 years versus 0.7 years comparing 46 patients who had GTR + adjuvant WBRT to 73 patients who had GTR alone ($p < .001$) and 1.1 years versus 3 months comparing 20 patients who had STR + adjuvant WBRT to 8 patients who had STR alone ($p < .001$). Multivariate analysis adjusting for other prognostic parameters confirmed the association between adjuvant WBRT and improved survival ($p < .001$). Of note, there was a 21 percent 5-year survival probability among the 46 patients who had no systemic disease and GTR of a solitary brain metastasis followed by adjuvant WBRT.

It is likely that these retrospective studies were biased by selection factors. Therefore, a prospective trial was performed from 1989 to 1997, randomizing patients with complete resection of a single brain metastasis to observation versus adjuvant postoperative WBRT (50.4 Gy in 28 fractions over 5½ weeks) (see Table 20–4).[54] Of 146 eligible patients, 51 did not enter the study because of patient refusal or physician preference. Intracranial control was significantly longer for the 49 patients randomized to postoperative WBRT than for the 46 patients randomized to observation, although survival was not significantly different for the two study arms. The crude incidence of local recurrence was 46 percent in the observation arm versus 10 percent in the WBRT arm, and the median freedom from recurrence of the original brain metastasis was > 12.0 months for WBRT vs 6.2 months for observation ($p < .001$; relative risk [RR] 6.03; 95% CI 2.48 to 14.65). The median time to development of new brain metastases or leptomeningeal disease was 12.2 months in the observation arm versus 50.6 months in the WBRT arm ($p = .04$; RR = 2.77; 95% CI 1.16 to 6.59). The median survival time was 11.0 months for WBRT versus 9.9 months for obser-

Authors	Years of Study	Number of Patients	Treatment	Median Local FFP (mo)	Median FI Survival (mo)	Median Survival (mo)
Patchell et al[14]	1985–1988	23	Biopsy + WBRT	4.8	1.8	3.4
		25	Resection + WBRT (36 Gy/12 fx)	>13.6 ($p < .0001$)	8.7 ($p < .005$)	9.2 ($p < .01$)
Noordijk et al[50]	1985–1990	31	WBRT	NS	3.5	6
		32	Resection + WBRT (40 Gy at 2 Gy bid)	NS NS	7.5 ($p = .06$)	10 ($p = .04$)
Mintz et al[51]	1989–1993	43	WBRT	NS	NS	6.3
		41	Resection + WBRT (30 Gy/10 fx)	NS NS	NS NS	5.6 ($p = .24$)
Patchell et al[54]	1989–1997	46	Resection	6.2	8.0	9.9
		49	Resection + WBRT (50.4 Gy/28 fx)	>12.0 ($p < .001$)	8.5 ($p = .61$)	11.0 ($p = .39$)

FFP = freedom from progression; FI = functionally independent; WBRT = whole brain radiotherapy; fx = fractions; NS = not stated.

vation ($p = .39$), and the duration of functional independence also was similar in the two arms: 8.5 months for WBRT versus 8.0 months for observation. The percentage of deaths due to neurologic causes was 44 percent in the observation group versus 14 percent in the WBRT group ($p = .003$). The authors pointed out that a reduction in death due to neurologic causes is all that can be expected from therapies directed at the brain, and they concluded that routine postoperative WBRT is indicated after resection of a single brain metastasis to reduce the number of neurologic deaths.

Stereotactic Radiosurgery

Radiosurgery is a relatively new modality for the management of brain metastases. A single fraction of highly focused radiation is precisely targeted to deliver a dose of about 15 to 22 Gy to one or more metastases using multiple arcs in the case of a linear accelerator adapted for RS or 201 convergent cobalt 60 beams in the case of the Gamma Knife® (Figure 20–5). Tumor shrinkage occurs over weeks or months, so RS is not a good alternative to surgery if immediate relief of mass effect is necessary. In addition, RS generally is considered applicable only in metastases up to 3 cm in diameter. Advantages of RS are that it can be applied in surgically inaccessible locations and is more easily applicable to multiple lesions than surgery.

Retrospective reviews of RS ± WBRT for newly diagnosed or recurrent brain metastasis are summarized in Table 20–5. Survival times range from 11 to 12.9 months after RS for patients with newly diagnosed or recurrent single metastases[55,56] and from 7.4 to 10.5 months after RS for single or multiple newly diagnosed or recurrent brain metastases.[21,22,57–59] One-year actuarial freedom from progression of treated metastases ranged from 76 to 88 percent on lesion analysis[21,22] and 61 percent as analyzed by patients,[22] which still compares favorably to results of WBRT alone. The incidence of symptomatic radiation necrosis ranged from 0 to 6 percent in the series with mean or median prescribed RS dose ≤ 18.5 Gy and 13 to 17 percent in the two series with mean prescribed RS doses of 26.6 to 27 Gy (see Table 20–5).

A disadvantage of RS is higher cost in comparison with WBRT alone. However, given the longer survival time associated with RS, a cost-effectiveness analysis concluded that the cost per month of survival time was lower for WBRT + RS than for WBRT alone.[60] Three analyses found RS + WBRT to be more cost effective than surgery + WBRT.[60–62]

Because of concern about potential dementia from WBRT, some investigators have questioned the routine use of adjuvant WBRT in patients undergoing RS for newly diagnosed brain metastases. To date, no prospective, randomized trial addressing this issue has been reported, but a retrospective review was performed by Sneed and colleagues comparing patients with newly diagnosed brain metastases managed initially with RS alone or RS + adjuvant WBRT.[63] Survival and freedom from progression of treated brain metastases (local FFP) were similar for the two groups, with median survival times of 11.3 versus 11.1 months and 1-year local FFP probabilities of 71 percent versus 79 percent, respectively. The risk of developing new brain metastases was twofold higher after RS alone compared with RS + WBRT (hazard ratio = 2.0; median time to developing new brain metastases, 8.5 vs 16.8 months; $p = .03$). However, after allowing for successful salvage of a first failure with WBRT, RS, and/or surgery, there was no significant difference between the two groups (median brain control, 19.8 months for RS alone vs 18.1 months for RS + WBRT; $p = .31$). A prospective, randomized trial is needed to compare survival, quality of life, and cost of care in good-prognosis patients with brain metastases managed initially with RS or RS + WBRT.

Chemotherapy

Chemotherapy may be useful for the treatment of patients with brain metastases from chemosensitive tumors, especially if chemotherapy is indicated for the treatment of the primary tumor or extracranial metastases and the brain metastases are not very symptomatic. Encouraging results recently were reported for a prospective trial of up-front cisplatin and etoposide chemotherapy conducted from 1986 to 1993 in 107 evaluable patients with brain metastases who were not amenable to surgery and who were not pretreated with radiotherapy.[64] Cisplatin was given at 100 mg/m^2 on day 1, and etoposide was given at 100 mg/m^2 on days 1, 3, and 5 or days 4, 6, and 8 every 3 weeks. The protocol allowed for WBRT after six cycles of chemotherapy or for salvage at the time of progression, but data regarding WBRT were not reported. Overall response rates (complete + partial responses) and median survival times were 38 percent and 7.1 months among the 56 breast cancer patients, 30 percent and 7.4 months among the 43 non–small cell lung cancer patients, and 0 percent and 3.9 months among 8 malignant melanoma patients, respectively. The authors recommended a randomized study comparing WBRT alone to this chemotherapy regimen followed by WBRT in patients with brain metastases from breast cancer or non–small cell lung cancer not amenable to surgery or RS.

SUMMARY

Approximately one-quarter of cancer patients develop brain metastases at some point in the course of their disease. Brain metastases generally appear as

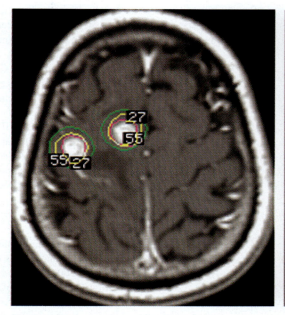 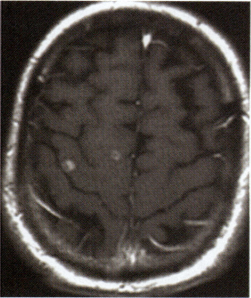

Figure 20–5. Contrast-enhanced T1-weighted magnetic resonance images on the day of radiosurgery with superimposed radiation isodose lines (*left*) and 6 months after radiosurgery (*right*), showing partial response of two metastases treated with 18.0 Gy at the 55% isodose line.

Table 20–5. RESULTS OF RADIOSURGERY ± WHOLE BRAIN RADIOTHERAPY FOR NEWLY DIAGNOSED OR RECURRENT BRAIN METASTASES

Authors	Number of Metastases/Patients	Mean or Median Dose (Gy)	% Local Control by Lesion	% Necrosis	Median Survival (mo)
Auchter et al[55§]	122/122	17.0	86*	0	12.9
Flickinger et al[56§]	116/116	17.5	85*/~75†	4‡	11.0
Flickinger et al[57‖]	229/157	16.0	89*	0	10.0
Joseph et al[58‖]	189/120	26.6	~95*	17	7.4
Kihlstrom et al[59‖]	235/160	27.0	94*	13	—
Moriarty et al[21‖]	643/353	15.0	88†	3–6	10.5
Shu et al[22‖]	248/116	18.5	76†	3	9.2

*Crude estimate.
†1-year actuarial estimate.
‡2-year actuarial estimate.
§Single metastases.
‖Single or multiple metastases.

fairly well-circumscribed, contrast-enhancing masses on CT or MRI. Most patients are managed with WBRT, often given to a total dose of 30 Gy in 10 fractions over 2 weeks. Whole brain radiotherapy significantly palliates symptoms in 50 to 80 percent of patients and extends median survival time from approximately 1 to 2 months to 3 to 4 months, with 80 percent of patients' remaining survival time spent in an improved or stable neurologic state. After WBRT, 25 to 50 percent of deaths result from uncontrolled brain metastases. When a patient's life expectancy is limited by progressive primary disease or extracranial metastases, short-term palliation is more important than long-term intracranial control. However, patients with a life expectancy of at least 6 to 12 months may benefit from more protracted WBRT regimens, such as 40 Gy in 20 fractions, to reduce the risk of radiation-induced cognitive deficits. Furthermore, good-prognosis patients with limited intracranial disease may benefit from more aggressive treatment strategies involving surgical resection or RS of single or multiple metastases, with or without adjuvant WBRT. Selected patients treated with surgery or RS have median survival times of 9 to 11 months, and, occasionally, patients are cured.

REFERENCES

1. Posner JB, Chernik NL. Intracranial metastases from systemic cancer. Adv Neurol 1978;19:579–92.
2. Hojo S, Hirano A. Pathology of metastases affecting the central nervous system. In: Takakura K, Sano K, Hojo S, et al, editors. Metastatic tumors of the central nervous system. Tokyo: Igaku-Shoin; 1982. p. 5-35.
3. Borgelt B, Gelber R, Kramer S, et al. The palliation of brain metastases: final results of the first two studies by the Radiation Therapy Oncology Group. Int J Radiat Oncol Biol Phys 1980;6:1–8.
4. Delattre JY, Krol G, Thaler HT, Posner JB. Distribution of brain metastases. Arch Neurol 1988;45:741–4.
5. Graus F, Walker RW, Allen JC. Brain metastases in children. J Pediatr 1983;103:558–61.
6. Hwang TL, Close TP, Grego JM, et al. Predilection of brain metastasis in gray and white matter junction and vascular border zones. Cancer 1996;77:1551–5.
7. Mirimanoff RO, Choi NC. Intradural spinal metastases in patients with posterior fossa brain metastases from various primary cancers. Oncology 1987;44:232–6.
8. DeAngelis LM, Mandell LR, Thaler HT, et al. The role of postoperative radiotherapy after resection of single brain metastases. Neurosurgery 1989;24:798–805.
9. Sze G, Milano E, Johnson C, Heier L. Detection of brain metastases: comparison of contrast-enhanced MR with unenhanced MR and enhanced CT. AJNR Am J Neuroradiol 1990;11:785–91.
10. Van Dijk P, Sijens PE, Schmitz PI, Oudkerk M. Gd-enhanced MR imaging of brain metastases: contrast as a function of dose and lesion size. Magn Reson Imaging 1997;15:535–41.
11. Yuh WTC, Fisher DJ, Runge VM, et al. Phase III multicenter trial of high-dose gadoteridol in MR evaluation of brain metastases. AJNR Am J Neuroradiol 1994;15:1037–51.
12. France LH. Contribution to the study of 150 cases of cerebral metastases. II. Neuropathological study. J Neurosurg Sci 1975;19:189–210.
13. Posner JB. Management of central nervous system metastases. Semin Oncol 1977;4:81–91.
14. Patchell RA, Tibbs PA, Walsh JW, et al. A randomized trial of surgery in the treatment of single metastases to the brain. N Engl J Med 1990;322:494–500.
15. Franzini A, Leocata F, Giorgi C, et al. Role of stereotactic biopsy in multifocal brain lesions: considerations on 100 consecutive cases. J Neurol Neurosurg Psychiatry 1994;57:957–60.
16. Salbeck R, Grau HC, Artmann H. Cerebral tumor staging in

patients with bronchial carcinoma by computed tomography. Cancer 1990;66:2007–11.
17. Nelson SJ, Day MR, Buffone PJ, et al. Alignment of volume MR images and high resolution [18F]fluorodeoxyglucose PET images for the evaluation of patients with brain tumors. J Comput Assist Tomogr 1997;21:183–91.
18. Sijens PE, Levendag PC, Vecht CJ, et al. 1H MR spectroscopy detection of lipids and lactate in metastatic brain tumors. NMR Biomed 1996;9:65–71.
19. Gaspar L, Scott C, Rotman M, et al. Recursive partitioning analysis (RPA) of prognostic factors in three Radiation Therapy Oncology Group (RTOG) brain metastases trials. Int J Radiat Oncol Biol Phys 1997;37:745–51.
20. Lagerwaard FJ, Levendag PC, Nowak PJCM, et al. Identification of prognostic factors in patients with brain metastases: a review of 1292 patients. Int J Radiat Oncol Biol Phys 1999;43:795–803.
21. Moriarty TM, Loeffler JS, Black PM, et al. Long-term follow-up of patients treated with stereotactic radiosurgery for single or multiple brain metastases. In: Kondziolka D, editor. Radiosurgery 1995. Vol 1. Basel: Karger; 1996. p. 83–91.
22. Shu H-KG, Sneed PK, Shiau C-Y, et al. Factors influencing survival after gamma knife radiosurgery for patients with single and multiple brain metastases. Cancer J Sci Am 1996;2:335–42.
23. Cohen N, Strauss G, Lew R, et al. Should prophylactic anticonvulsants be administered to patients with newly-diagnosed cerebral metastases? A retrospective analysis. J Clin Oncol 1988;6:1621–4.
24. Batchelor T, DeAngelis LM. Medical management of cerebral metastases. Neurosurg Clin N Am 1996;7:435–46.
25. Borgelt B, Gelber R, Larson M, et al. Ultra-rapid high dose irradiation schedules for the palliation of brain metastases: final results of the first two studies by the Radiation Therapy Oncology Group. Int J Radiat Oncol Biol Phys 1981;7:1633–8.
26. Coia LR. The role of radiation therapy in the treatment of brain metastases. Int J Radiat Oncol Biol Phys 1992;23:229–38.
27. Kurtz JM, Gelber R, Brady LW, et al. The palliation of brain metastases in a favorable patient population: a randomized clinical trial by the Radiation Therapy Oncology Group. Int J Radiat Oncol Biol Phys 1981;7:891–5.
28. Epstein BE, Scott CB, Sause WT, et al. Improved survival duration in patients with unresected solitary brain metastasis using accelerated hyperfractionated radiation therapy at total doses of 54.4 Gray and greater. Cancer 1993;71:1362–7.
29. Sause WT, Scott C, Krisch R, et al. Phase I/II trial of accelerated fractionation in brain metastases RTOG 85-28. Int J Radiat Oncol Biol Phys 1993;26:653–7.
30. Murray K, Scott C, Greenberg H, et al. A randomized phase III study of accelerated hyperfractionation versus standard fractionation in patients with unresected brain metastases: a report of Radiation Therapy Oncology Group (RTOG) 9104 [abstract]. Int J Radiat Oncol Biol Phys 1996;36(Suppl 1):193.
31. Komarnicky LT, Phillips TL, Martz K, et al. A randomized phase III protocol for the evaluation of misonidazole combined with radiation in the treatment of patients with brain metastases (RTOG-7916). Int J Radiat Oncol Biol Phys 1991;20:53–8.
32. Phillips TL, Scott CB, Leibel SA, et al. Results of a randomized comparison of radiotherapy and bromodeoxyuridine with radiotherapy alone for brain metastases: report of RTOG trial 89-05. Int J Radiat Oncol Biol Phys 1995;33:339–48.
33. DeAngelis LM, Currie VE, Kim J-H, et al. The combined use of radiation therapy and lonidamine in the treatment of brain metastases. J Neurooncol 1989;7:241–7.
34. Nieder C, Berberich W, Nestle U, et al. Relation between local result and total dose of radiotherapy for brain metastases. Int J Radiat Oncol Biol Phys 1995;33:349–55.
35. Hindo WA, DeTrana FAI, Lee M-S, Hendrickson FR. Large dose increment irradiation in treatment of cerebral metastases. Cancer 1970;26:138–41.
36. Young DF, Posner JB, Chu F, Nisce L. Rapid-course radiation therapy of cerebral metastases: results and complications. Cancer 1974;34:1069–76.
37. Boldrey E, Sheline GE. Delayed transitory clinical manifestations after radiation treatment of intracranial tumors. Acta Radiol 1966;5:5–10.
38. Littman P, Rosenstock J, Gale G, et al. The somnolence syndrome in leukemic children following reduced daily dose fractions of cranial radiation. Int J Radiat Oncol Biol Phys 1984;10:1851–3.
39. DeAngelis LM, Delattre JY, Posner JB. Radiation-induced dementia in patients cured of brain metastases. Neurology 1989;39:789–96.
40. Sheline GE, Wara WM, Smith V. Therapeutic irradiation and brain injury. Int J Radiat Oncol Biol Phys 1980;6:1215–28.
41. Crossen JR, Garwood D, Glatstein E, Neuwelt EA. Neurobehavioral sequelae of cranial irradiation in adults: a review of radiation-induced encephalopathy. J Clin Oncol 1994;12:627–42.
42. Sundaresan N, Galicich JH, Deck MDF, Tomita T. Radiation necrosis after treatment of solitary intracranial metastases. Neurosurgery 1981;8:329–33.
43. Asai A, Matsutani M, Kohno T, et al. Subacute brain atrophy after radiation therapy for malignant brain tumor. Cancer 1989;63:1962–74.
44. McDermott MW, Cosgrove GR, Larson DA, et al. Interstitial brachytherapy for intracranial metastases. Neurosurg Clin N Am 1996;7:485–95.
45. Shehata WM, Hendrickson FR, Hindo WA. Rapid fractionation technique and re-treatment of cerebral metastases by irradiation. Cancer 1974;34:257–61.
46. Kurup P, Reddy S, Hendrickson FR. Results of re-irradiation for cerebral metastases. Cancer 1980;46:2587–9.
47. Hazuka MB, Kinzie JJ. Brain metastases: results and effects of re-irradiation. Int J Radiat Oncol Biol Phys 1988;15:433–7.
48. Cooper JS, Steinfeld AD, Lerch IA. Cerebral metastases: value of reirradiation in selected patients. Radiology 1990;174:883–5.
49. Wong WW, Schild SE, Sawyer TE, Shaw EG. Analysis of outcome in patients reirradiated for brain metastases. Int J Radiat Oncol Biol Phys 1996;34:585–90.
50. Noordijk EM, Vecht CJ, Haaxma-Reiche H, et al. The choice of treatment of single brain metastasis should be based on

extracranial tumor activity and age. Int J Radiat Oncol Biol Phys 1994;29:711–7.
51. Mintz AH, Kestle J, Rathbone MP, et al. A randomized trial to assess the efficacy of surgery in addition to radiotherapy in patients with a single cerebral metastasis. Cancer 1996;78:1470–6.
52. Bindal RK, Sawaya R, Leavens ME, Lee JJ. Surgical treatment of multiple brain metastases. J Neurosurg 1993;79:210–6.
53. Smalley SR, Laws ER Jr, O'Fallon JR, et al. Resection for solitary brain metastasis: role of adjuvant radiation and prognostic variables in 229 patients. J Neurosurg 1992;77:531–40.
54. Patchell RA, Tibbs PA, Regine WF, et al. Postoperative radiotherapy in the treatment of single metastases to the brain: a randomized trial. JAMA 1998;280:1485–9.
55. Auchter RM, Lamond JP, Alexander E III, et al. A multiinstitutional outcome and prognostic factor analysis of radiosurgery for resectable single brain metastasis. Int J Radiat Oncol Biol Phys 1996;35:27–35.
56. Flickinger JC, Kondziolka D, Lunsford LD, et al. A multiinstitutional experience with stereotactic radiosurgery for solitary brain metastasis. Int J Radiat Oncol Biol Phys 1994;28:797–802.
57. Flickinger JC, Lunsford LD, Somaza S, Kondziolka D. Radiosurgery: its role in brain metastasis management. Neurosurg Clin N Am 1996;7:497–504.
58. Joseph J, Adler JR, Cox RS, Hancock SL. Linear accelerator-based stereotaxic radiosurgery for brain metastases: the influence of number of lesions on survival. J Clin Oncol 1996;14:1085–92.
59. Kihlstrom L, Karlsson B, Lindquist C. Gamma knife surgery for cerebral metastases. Implications for survival based on 16 years experience. Stereotact Funct Neurosurg 1993;61(Suppl 1):45–50.
60. Noyes WR, Auchter RM, Craig B, et al. Cost analysis of radiosurgery versus resection for single brain metastases. In: Kondziolka D, editor. Radiosurgery 1995. Vol 1. Basel: Karger; 1996. p. 172–9.
61. Sperduto PW, Hall WA. The cost-effectiveness for alternative treatments for single brain metastases. In: Kondziolka D, editor. Radiosurgery 1995. Vol 1. Basel: Karger; 1996. p. 180–7.
62. Rutigliano MJ, Lunsford LD, Kondziolka D, et al. The cost effectiveness of stereotactic radiosurgery versus surgical resection in the treatment of solitary metastatic brain tumors. Neurosurgery 1995;37:445–55.
63. Sneed PK, Lamborn KR, Forstner JM, et al. Radiosurgery for brain metastases: is whole brain radiotherapy necessary? Int J Radiat Oncol Biol Phys 1999;43:549–58.
64. Franciosi V, Cocconi G, Michiara M, et al. Front-line chemotherapy with cisplatin and etoposide for patients with brain metastases from breast carcinoma, nonsmall cell lung carcinoma, or malignant melanoma. Cancer 1999;85:1599–605.

21

Diagnosis and Treatment of Neoplastic Meningitis

MARC C. CHAMBERLAIN, MD

Neoplastic meningitis (NM) is a common problem in neuro-oncology, occurring in approximately 5 percent of all patients with cancer. Notwithstanding frequent focal signs and symptoms, NM is a disease affecting the entire neuraxis, and, therefore, staging and treatment need to encompass all cerebrospinal fluid (CSF) compartments. Central nervous system (CNS) staging of NM includes contrast-enhanced cranial computed tomography (CE-CT) or magnetic resonance imaging (MRI-Gd), contrast-enhanced spine MRI (S-MRI), or CT myelography (CT-M) and radionuclide CSF flow study (FS). Treatment of NM consists of involved-field radiotherapy of bulky or symptomatic disease sites and intra-CSF drug therapy. The inclusion of concomitant systemic therapy may benefit patients with NM and may obviate the need for intra-CSF chemotherapy. At present, intra-CSF drug therapy is confined to three chemotherapeutic agents (ie, methotrexate, cytosine arabinoside, and thiotepa) administered in a variety of schedules either by intralumbar or intraventricular drug delivery. Although treatment of NM is palliative, with an expected median patient survival of 2 to 6 months, it often affords stabilization and protection from further neurologic deterioration.

PREVALENCE

Neoplastic meningitis is a common clinical problem both for the oncologist and neurologist. Several clinical series have estimated NM to occur in 4 to 15 percent of patients with solid tumors, 7 to 15 percent of patients with lymphomas, 5 to 15 percent of patients with leukemias, and 1 to 2 percent of patients with primary brain tumors.[1–7] Solid tumors are disproportionately represented in clinical series of patients with NM due to their high frequency of occurrence wherein breast (range of occurrence [RO], 12 to 34%), lung (RO, 10 to 26%), melanoma (RO, 17 to 25%), and gastrointestinal (RO, 4 to 14%) cancers are most frequently encountered. Carcinomas of unknown primary constitute 1 to 7 percent of all cases of NM, a range similar to that found in patients with other metastatic complications of the CNS.[1–7] In more contemporary series, 10 to 32 percent of NM patients had primary brain tumors, reflecting both institutional biases and the not infrequent dissemination of primary brain tumors.[7–12] Acquired immunodeficiency syndrome [AIDS]-related lymphomatous meningitis, as a result of either systemic lymphomas that metastasize or primary CNS lymphomas with CSF dissemination, is increasingly frequent and constitutes nearly one-third of all NM seen at the University of California San Diego.[13]

Autopsy studies of patients with cancer both from the Memorial Sloan-Kettering Cancer Center and the National Cancer Institute demonstrate a high prevalence of NM exceeding that seen in clinical series. In the Memorial Sloan-Kettering Cancer Center experience of 2,375 patients with cancer and postmortem CNS analysis, an 8 percent prevalence of NM was demonstrated.[8] Similarly, in the National Cancer Institute study of small cell lung cancer, an 11 percent prevalence of NM was seen antemortem compared to a 25 percent prevalence seen postmortem.[14]

CLINICAL PRESENTATION

Neoplastic meningitis is pleomorphic in its clinical presentation as it affects all levels of the CNS.[1-7] In general, three domains of neurologic disturbance are characterized as affected by NM including (1) the cerebral hemispheres, (2) the cranial nerves, and (3) the spinal cord and roots. The common symptoms of cerebral hemispheric dysfunction are headache and mental status change, as illustrated in Table 21–1. Signs found in patients with NM and cerebral hemisphere disturbance encompass mental status changes including confusion and dementia, seizures, and hemiparesis.

Symptoms referable to disturbance of cranial nerve dysfunction include double vision, hearing loss, facial numbness, and loss of vision (Table 21–2). Signs of cranial nerve dysfunction include ophthalmoplegia, with abducens palsy seen more frequently than oculomotor dysfunction and oculomotor palsies seen more frequently than trochlear palsies, trigeminal sensory or motor loss, cochlear dysfunction, and optic neuropathy.

Spinal symptoms are referable to either the spinal cord or exiting nerve roots and the spinal meninges (Table 21–3). These symptoms include weakness (more often in the leg than arm), numbness, and pain (neck, back, or radicular patterns). Common signs of spinal cord dysfunction include weakness of extremities and dermatomal or segmental sensory loss.

With progression of NM, new signs and symptoms appear, often affecting CNS domains not previously involved; in addition, preexisting findings worsen. As in the initial examination, neurologic findings in patients with progressive disease exceed patient symptoms. The most useful instrument in diagnosing NM is recognizing the pleomorphic clinical manifestations of NM and maintaining a high clinical suspicion of NM in an appropriate clinical context.

LABORATORY FINDINGS

The most useful laboratory test in diagnosing NM is an examination of the CSF, usually obtained by lumbar puncture.[1-7,15] In nearly all patients with NM, the CSF is abnormal, regardless of the results of CSF cytology (Table 21–4). Cerebrospinal fluid cytology positive for malignant cells is the standard method by which NM is diagnosed, notwithstanding the results of postmortem analysis discussed below. The variable results of CSF analysis in patients with NM are partially explained by the results of a study by Murray and colleagues, who demonstrated variable CSF levels of protein, glucose, and malignant cells at different levels of the neuraxis in the absence of blockage to CSF flow.[16] These findings emphasize the multifocal nature of NM, wherein CSF obtained from a site distant from pathologically involved meninges may be misleading as to disease presence or response to therapy.

In a clinical series reported by Wasserstrom and colleagues, approximately 5 percent of patients demonstrated to have positive CSF cytology were positive only from CSF examined from either the ventricles or cisterna magna.[5] Two important points are derived from this series: first, there is a subgroup of patients with NM and persistently negative CSF cytology, regardless of the level from which CSF is withdrawn, and second, there is a subgroup of patients with NM who manifest positive cytology only if CSF is examined from cisternal or ventricular compartments.

Table 21–1. LEPTOMENINGEAL METASTASES FROM SOLID TUMORS IN 90 PATIENTS: CEREBRAL SYMPTOMS AND SIGNS AT PRESENTATION*			
Symptoms	No. of Patients (%)	Signs	No. of Patients (%)
Headache	30 (75)	Mental status change	28 (62)
Mental change	15 (33)	Seizures	5 (11)
Difficulty walking	12 (27)	Focal	5 (11)
Nausea/vomiting	10 (22)	Generalized	3 (6)
Unconsciousness	2 (4)	Sensory disturbance	5 (11)
Dysphagia	2 (4)	Diabetes insipidus	2 (4)
Dizziness	2 (4)	Hemiparesis	1 (2)

*Cerebral symptoms and signs were present in 45 (50%) of the 90 patients.

Table 21–2. LEPTOMENINGEAL METASTASES FROM SOLID TUMORS IN 90 PATIENTS: CRANIAL NERVE SYMPTOMS AND SIGNS AT PRESENTATION*

Symptoms	No. of Patients (%)	Signs (Nerve[s])	No. of Patients (%)
Diplopia	18 (30)	Ocular motor paresis (III, IV, VI)	18 (30)
Hearing loss	7 (12)	Facial weakness (VII)	16 (27)
Visual loss	5 (8)	Diminished hearing (VIII)	8 (13)
Facial numbness	5 (8)	Optic neuropathy (II)	5 (8)
Decreased hearing	3 (5)	Trigeminal neuropathy (V)	5 (8)
Tinnitus	2 (3)	Hypoglossal neuropathy (XII)	5 (8)
Hoarseness	2 (3)	Blindness (II)	3 (5)
Dysphagia	1 (2)	Diminished gag (IX, X)	3 (5)
Vertigo	1 (2)		

*Cranial nerve symptoms and signs were present in 60 (67%) of the 90 patients.

In the series reported by Wasserstrom and colleagues, which included only patients with carcinomatous meningitis due to metastatic spread from systemic solid tumors, lumbar CSF examination was cytologically positive in 55 percent of patients initially and increased to 80 percent following a second CSF examination.[5] Little benefit was seen in performing multiple lumbar punctures following the initial two lumbar CSF examinations. By contrast, in a series by Kaplan and colleagues that included patients with carcinomatous, leukemic, and lymphomatous meningitis, a high positive cytologic yield (> 90%) following one or two lumbar punctures was demonstrated.[6] Kaplan and colleagues also emphasized the frequent disassociation between CSF cell count and malignant cytology wherein 29 percent of cytologically positive CSF examinations had concurrent CSF leukocyte counts less than 4/mm^3.

In the largest postmortem analysis of patients with NM, Glass and colleagues demonstrated 41 percent of patients with autopsy-proven NM had negative antemortem CSF cytology.[15] Furthermore, Glass and colleagues demonstrated that in patients with pathologically focal NM, the occurrence of cytologically false-negatives was greater than 50

Table 21–3. LEPTOMENINGEAL METASTASES FROM SOLID TUMORS IN 90 PATIENTS: SPINAL SYMPTOMS AND SIGNS AT PRESENTATION*

Symptoms	No. of Patients (%)	Signs	No. of Patients (%)
Lower motor neuron weakness	34 (46)	Reflex asymmetry	64 (86)
Paresthesias	31 (42)	Weakness	54 (73)
Radicular pain	19 (26)	Sensory loss	24 (32)
Back/neck pain	23 (31)	Straight leg raising	11 (15)
Bladder/bowel dysfunction	12 (16)	Decreased rectal tone	10 (14)
Upper motor neuron weakness	11 (14)	Nuchal rigidity	7 (9)

*Spinal symptoms and signs were present in 74 (82%) of the 90 patients.

Table 21–4. LEPTOMENINGEAL METASTASES: FINDINGS ON INITIAL AND TOTAL LUMBAR CSF EXAMINATIONS

	Authors			
CSF Findings	Olson et al[1]	Theodore and Gendelman[4]	Wasserstrom et al[5]	Kaplan et al[6]
Pressure > 150 mm of H$_2$O (I/T)	57/72	30/61	50/71	—/44
WBC > 4 mm^3 (I/T)	57/77	58/79	57/72	—/64
Protein > 50 mg/dL (I/T)	74/91	73/79	81/89	—/83
Glucose 60 < mg/dL (I/T)	—/77	55/61	31/41	—/47
Positive cytology (I/T)	45/77	73/100	54/91	71/100

I/T = % positive on initial lumbar puncture/% positive on total lumbar punctures performed; WBC = white blood (cell) count.

percent, emphasizing the frequent co-occurrence of patients with NM and negative CSF cytology.

A variety of biochemical markers of NM have been studied in CSF including β-glucuronidase, carcinoembryonic antigen, β-microglobulin, phosphohexoseisomerase, cancer-specific monoclonal antibodies, lactate dehydrogenase (LDH; both isoenzymes and the LDH 5:1 ratio), oligoclonal bands, the immunoglobulin G (IgG) index, the CSF-to–serum albumin ratio, polyamines, α-fetoprotein, and β-human chorionic gonadotropin.[17–22] These biochemical markers serve as adjunctive diagnostic tests that are most useful when used serially and, in particular, when following response to treatment in patients with NM.

Another adjunct to CSF cytologic examination is the evaluation of deoxyribonucleic acid (DNA) abnormalities by flow cytometry, which permits an estimation of aneuploidy and the number of cells in S, G_2, and M phases of the cell cycle.[23] Cibas and colleagues suggested that flow cytometry is capable of detecting tumor cells not found by conventional CSF cytology.[23] This appears to be particularly true in instances of lymphomatous or leukemic meningitis, in which differentiating malignant lymphocytes from background mononuclear cells may be difficult. Several other authors have suggested the use of B cell marker monoclonal antibodies to differentiate leukemic and lymphomatous meningitis from the normal or reactive T-cell CSF lymphocyte population.[24–26]

A variety of neuroradiographic methods are available to evaluate patients with suspected NM including cranial CT, brain and S-MRI, computed tomographic myelography, and radionuclide CSF flow studies. Cranial CE-CT is abnormal in 25 to 56 percent of patients with NM.[27] Abnormalities seen on CE-CT include parenchymal volume loss (93%), sulcal-cisternal enhancement (21%), ependymal or subependymal enhancement (75%), irregular tentorial enhancement (7%), cisternal or sulcal obliteration (14%), subarachnoid-enhancing nodules (29%), intraventricular-enhancing nodules (10%), and communicating hydrocephalus (10%). In addition, 30 to 60 percent of patients with NM will have coexistent parenchymal brain metastases.[7,8,27–30]

Qualitatively similar abnormalities are detected by brain MRI-Gd; however, MRI-Gd appears to have a greater specificity and sensitivity (1.5- to 2.0-fold increase in lesion detection) when compared with CE-CT in the evaluation of patients with NM and would therefore appear to be the preferred imaging modality.[27–31] Despite the superiority of cranial MRI-Gd to CE-CT in the evaluation of NM, both studies have a high incidence of false-negatives (30% by MRI-Gd and 58% by CE-CT). Normal studies by either methodology do not exclude a diagnosis of NM in patients with negative CSF cytologies; however, positive MRI-Gd or CE-CT both may be suggestive and diagnostic of NM.[27] In the majority of patients with NM, MRI-Gd and CE-CT are most useful in demonstrating bulky disease, a pattern of disease most responsive to radiotherapy and least responsive to intra-CSF chemotherapy (see below).

A number of studies have evaluated patients with NM by spine imaging, usually employing either CT-M or S-MRI.[32–39,40] However, relatively few studies have compared both CT-M and S-MRI in patients with NM. Myelographic features characteristic of NM include parallel longitudinal striations due to thickened nerve roots in the cauda equina, nerve root filling defects, widening of the spinal cord, varying degrees of CSF flow block, subarachnoid nodules, and scalloping of the subarachnoid membranes.[32,33,37] Similar findings are seen with S-MRI in addition to pial enhancement of the spinal cord, a finding termed by Kramer and colleagues as sugar-coating.[34–36,38,39] In a recent study, 61 patients with NM were studied sequentially by both CT-M and S-MRI.[40] Thirty-three percent of patients had abnormal CT-M and 34 percent of patients demonstrated abnormalities by S-MRI. Computed tomographic myelography demonstrated nerve root thickening and cord enlargement, whereas subarachnoid nodules, intraparenchymal cord tumor, and coexistent epidural spinal cord compression were better demonstrated by S-MRI. Few discordant results were seen in comparing CT-M and S-MRI in this study (less than 10%), and, in general, CT-M and S-MRI were complementary. The differences seen usually were quantitative and not qualitative. Given the noninvasive nature of S-MRI, its greater acceptability by patients, and its low rate of morbidity, S-MRI is the preferable spine imaging modality for patients with NM.

Radionuclide CSF FSs or so-called radionuclide ventriculography provides a safe physiologic assessment of the functional anatomy of the CSF spaces.[7,24,40–45] In prior reports, FSs have demonstrated superiority in detecting interruption of CSF flow in patients with NM when compared with CT-M and S-MRI.[7,40,44,45] However, FSs are informative only with respect to compartmentalization of CSF and provide no information regarding bulky leptomeningeal disease, an aspect of NM best addressed by CT-M or S-MRI. In addition, though infrequently demonstrated, CT-M and S-MRI are clearly superior to FS in detecting epidural spinal cord compression or intraparenchymal spinal cord metastases—two CNS complications of metastatic systemic cancer requiring emergent radiotherapy. Notwithstanding these limitations, FSs provide the best radiographic assessment of CSF circulation and are abnormal in 30 to 40 percent of patients with NM. As seen in Table 21–5, normal times of radionuclide appearance in various CSF compartments following intraventricular administration of ^{111}In DTPA are indicated. Failure of radionuclide to appear in a given CSF compartment is operationally defined as CSF flow block. Similarly, normal times of radionuclide appearance in various CSF compartments following intralumbar administration of radioisotope are seen (Table 21–6). In the study discussed above, 20 of 61 (33%) patients demonstrated abnormal FS.[40] These abnormalities most commonly were seen at the base of the brain, at the spinal subarachnoid space (in particular, at the level of the conus medullaris or cauda equina), and over the cerebral convexities. Abnormalities of CSF flow as demonstrated by FS are addressed therapeutically by administering involved-field radiotherapy to the obstructed site of CSF flow. Approximately 50 percent of patients with an intracranial disturbance of CSF flow and 30 percent of patients with a disturbance of CSF flow intraspinally will have restored normal CSF flow as assessed by postradiotherapy FS.[7]

PATHOLOGY AND PATHOPHYSIOLOGY

Diffuse infiltration of the leptomeninges is the characteristic pattern of tumor growth in NM.[1,46,47] Tumor grows in a sheath-like fashion along the surface of the brain and spinal cord, at times exciting an inflammatory response. These changes are prominent along the ventricular surface, especially in the

Table 21–5. LEPTOMENINGEAL METASTASES: NORMAL COMPARTMENTAL APPEARANCE OF ^{111}INDIUM DTPA CSF FLOW STUDIES FOLLOWING INTRAVENTRICULAR ADMINISTRATION

Time to Appearance (min)	Cerebrospinal Fluid Compartment						
	Ventricular System	Cisterna Magna/Basal Cisterns	Cervical Cord*	Thoracic Cord*	Lumbar Cord*	Cistern of Fossa of Sylvius	Cerebral Convexities
Median	1	5	15	20	30	50	720–1440
Range	0–5	5–15	5–20	10–20	25–50	35–90	720–1440

DTPA = pentetic acid; CSF = cerebrospinal fluid.
*Spinal subarachnoid compartments.

Table 21–6. LEPTOMENINGEAL METASTASES: NORMAL COMPARTMENTAL APPEARANCE OF ^{111}INDIUM DTPA CSF FLOW STUDIES FOLLOWING INTRALUMBAR ADMINISTRATION

Time to Appearance (min)	Cerebrospinal Fluid Compartment						
	Lumbar Cord*	Thoracic Cord*	Cervical Cord*	Cisterna Magna/Basal Cisterns	Cistern of Fossa of Sylvius	Ventricular System	Cerebral Convexities
Median	1	22.5	32.5	37.5	65	720–1440	720–1440
Range	0–1	20–25	30–35	35–40	60–70	720–1440	720–1440

DPTA = pentetic acid; CSF = cerebrospinal fluid.
*Spinal subarachnoid compartments.

chiasmatic and infundibular cisterns, the contiguous medial sulcus of the temporal lobes, and the interpeduncular, ambient, and cerebellopontine cisterns. Hydrocephalus may be present due to either ependymal nodules or sheets of tumor cells obstructing CSF outflow channels, particularly at the level of the fourth ventricle or basal cisterns. In the spinal cord, tumor infiltration is more common over the dorsal surface of the spinal cord and cauda equina. A high incidence of coexistent CNS metastases is found in patients with NM including parenchymal brain metastases (RO, 25 to 40%), dural metastases (RO, 16 to 37%), epidural spinal cord compression (RO, 1 to 5%), and leptomeningeal nodular disease (RO, 10 to 15%).[1,5,7]

Numerous clinicians have speculated on the route by which cancer cells reach the leptomeninges.[46,47] These speculations include (1) a vascular mechanism, either by arterial (associated with parenchymal or choroid plexus metastases) or venous routes (metastases spread through the plexus of Batson); (2) spread from adjacent bone metastases either by venous anastomoses or direct extension; (3) spread by contiguity from adjacent primary or secondary foci of tumor; (4) migration along perivascular spaces; or (5) spread along perineural spaces. In an autopsy study by Kokkoris, a sequential centripetal mode of NM invasion was demonstrated to occur by either skull or vertebral body metastases moving centrally by way of perivenous spaces through dural or arachnoid nerve sleeves and subsequently infiltrating the leptomeninges.[46] When cancer cells enter the subarachnoid space, these cells appear to spread along the leptomeninges, surround or invade nerve roots, form perivascular cuffs and enter the Virchow-Robin spaces, or penetrate the pia to involve the superficial layers of the CNS parenchyma. The arterial route of NM invasion, a less common mode of CSF contamination in the study by Kokkoris, is more likely when NM is associated with CNS parenchymal metastases. Following a hematogenous metastasis to brain parenchyma, NM occurs either by rupture of the pia or ependyma or by centrifugal extension along perivascular spaces. Occasionally, especially in tumors of the head and neck, spread from a contiguous focus of tumor occurs by way of perivascular or perineural spaces.

STAGING EXTENT OF DISEASE

Patients with suspected NM should undergo a sequential method of evaluation including (1) CSF analysis for pathologic confirmation—at least two lumbar punctures followed by either a ventricular or cisternal CSF examination are sufficient to confirm the presence or absence of malignant cells in CSF; (2) CE-CT or MRI-Gd to define bulky disease including both dural-based and intraparenchymal metastatic disease and, in addition, documentation of the presence or absence of hydrocephalus; (3) CT-M or S-MRI in patients with spinal cord dysfunction to define bulky disease including intradural tumor nodules and extradural tumor that may result in epidural spinal cord compression; (4) FS performed either by intraventricular or intralumbar radionuclide injection; (5) spine imaging (either CT-M or S-MRI) in patients with spinal cord CSF flow block documented by FS (if not previously performed for symptomatic spinal cord dysfunction); (6) serial FS, which may be useful in evaluating both response to treatment and disease progression during treatment; and (7) serial CSF cytology examinations in patients with positive CSF cytology; these are useful in evaluating both response to treatment and disease progression during treatment.[7,24,27,40,44,45]

Diagnosis of NM can be made in two clinical contexts. In the first, patients are demonstrated to have tumor cells by CSF cytology; these patients have pathologically defined NM regardless of results of corroborating tests (cranial or spinal MRI, cranial CT, or CT myelography). In the second, patients are considered to have NM if they have pathologically proven cancer, negative CSF cytology, and a clinical syndrome consistent with NM with or without corroborating neuroradiographic tests. A clinical syndrome consistent with NM includes a patient with known cancer and the development of communicating hydrocephalus, cranial nerve palsy(-ies), or cauda equina syndrome. This group of cytologically negative patients constitutes 40 to 50 percent of all patients with NM. The majority of patients with cytologically negative NM will, however, have abnormalities demonstrated by CSF analysis (see Table 21–4). The rationale for diagnosing patients with NM despite negative CSF cytology is from the autopsy data of Glass and colleagues, wherein 40 percent or more of patients with autopsy-proven NM had negative antemortem CSF examinations.[15] Therefore patients suspected of having NM should undergo (1) one or two lumbar punctures for CSF cytology and, if negative, proceed to undergo either a ventricular or lateral cervical CSF analysis; (2) contrast-enhanced cranial imaging (MRI preferred over CT); (3) contrast-enhanced S-MRI (in patients with spinal symptoms); and (4) CSF FS by either lumbar or ventricular radioisotope administration.

TREATMENT

The treatment of NM varies as there are no well-accepted treatments and all established and published treatments are palliative. Because NM involves the entire neuraxis, treatment is designed to encompass the entire subarachnoid space including the ventricular system, base-of-brain cisterns, and the spinal subarachnoid space[1-7] (Tables 21–7 and 21–8 and Figure 21–1). After achieving a diagnosis of NM, deciding whom to treat and in what manner is problematic. As discussed below, the majority of patients are poor candidates for aggressive therapy and are best offered supportive care (see Figure 21–1). In patients selected for treatment, the timing of the various therapies as performed at our institution is as follows. Initially patients undergo cranial, and when indicated, S-MRI. Subsequently, an intraventricular catheter and subgaleal reservoir are placed and a radioisotope ventricular CSF FS is performed. These studies usually can be performed within 7 to 10 days of diagnosis. Next, patients are treated with radiotherapy, as discussed below, followed by administration of chemotherapy. Radiotherapy usually is completed within 10 to 15 days.

Radiotherapy

Neoplastic meningitis sometimes coexists with bulky metastatic disease, which, irrespective of location (subarachnoid nodules, dural lesions, or parenchymal metastases), is best managed by involved-field radiotherapy regardless of whether the disease is clinically symptomatic or asymptomatic.[1-7] Radiotherapy of bulky disease is indicated as intra-CSF chemotherapy has limited tumor nodule penetration diffusing only 2 to 3 mm from the brain- or tumor-CSF interface.[48] Notwithstanding the utility of craniospinal radiation for the treatment of leukemic meningitis, craniospinal irradiation is difficult technically and is associated with significant systemic toxicity, in particular, myelosuppression and radiation esophagitis or colitis. Furthermore, patients with NM frequently have received radiotherapy to various regions of the CNS, thereby further compromising applications of radiation therapy.

When NM is evaluated by FS, CSF flow abnormalities sometimes are documented that result in compartmentalization or loculation of CSF pathways.[7,24,27,40,44,45] As a consequence of CSF compartmentalization, homogeneous distribution of intra-CSF administered chemotherapy is not possible.

Table 21–7. LEPTOMENINGEAL METASTASES: TREATMENT MODALITIES

Chemotherapy
  Regional
    Antimetabolites: methotrexate, ara-C
    Alkylators: thiotepa, ACNU, mafosphamide, 4-HC, AZQ
  Systemic
    High-dose IV methotrexate, ara-C, thiotepa
Regional immunotherapy
  Interferon
  Monoclonal antibody ± radioactive ligand
  Interleukin-2
  Gene therapy
Radiotherapy
  Limited field
  Craniospinal
Surgery
  CSF diversion
  CSF reservoir and intra-CSF catheter

ara-C = cytarabine; ACNU = nimustine; 4-HC = 4-hydroperoxy-cyclophosphamide; AZQ = diaziquone; IV = intravenous, CSF = cerebrospinal fluid.

Table 21–8. STANDARD THERAPY FOR NEOPLASTIC MENINGITIS

Radiotherapy to sites of symptomatic and bulky disease and to sites of CSF flow obstruction
Intra-CSF chemotherapy (one of the following may be used sequentially in patients failing prior therapy)
  Methotrexate (10–15 mg twice weekly or 2 mg/d for 5 d every other week) given in conjunction with oral folinic acid (5–10 mg q6h × 2 or 3 following intra-CSF methotrexate)
  Cytarabine (25–100 mg two or three times weekly)
  Thiotepa (10 mg two or three times weekly)
Concurrent systemic treatment of primary tumor

CSF = cerebrospinal fluid.

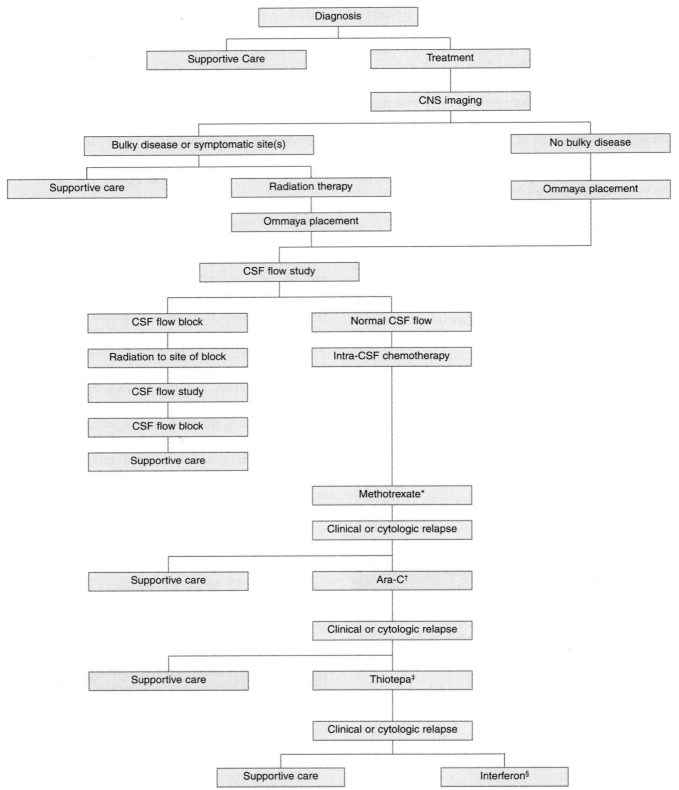

Figure 21–1. Treatment algorithm for neoplastic meningitis. CNS = central nervous system; CSF = cerebrospinal fluid; ara-C = cytarabine. *Methotrexate dosage: induction: 2 mg/d × 5 every other week × 4; consolidation: 2 mg/d × 5 every other week × 2; maintenance: 2 mg/d × 5 q month. †Ara-C dosage: induction: 30 mg/d × 3 weekly × 4; consolidation: 30 mg/d × 3 every other week × 2; maintenance: 30 mg/d × 3 q month. ‡Thiotepa dosage: induction: 10 mg/d × 3 weekly × 4; consolidation: 10 mg/d × 3 qow × 2; maintenance: 10 mg/d × 3 q month. §Interferon dosage: induction: 1×10^6 u qod tiw weekly × 4; consolidation: 1×10^6 u qod tiw every other week × 2; maintenance: 1×10^6 u qod 3 times a week q month.

These CSF flow abnormalities may be corrected by involved-field radiotherapy or may necessitate administration of intra-CSF chemotherapy from both the intraventricular and lumbar routes to ensure homogeneous distribution of intra-CSF administered drug. However, the administration of intra-CSF chemotherapy by both lumbar and ventricular routes is difficult and is not of proven value. The majority of patients with CSF flow blocks following involved-field radiotherapy are best managed with supportive care only (see Figure 21–1).

Systemic Chemotherapy

Systemic chemotherapeutic treatment of NM often fails due to poor CSF penetration of nearly all chemotherapeutic agents and the difficulty in achieving a significant intra-CSF drug exposure interval.[49–51] Exceptions are seen with systemic high-dose intravenous methotrexate, cytarabine, and thiotepa, all of which result in cytotoxic CSF levels and have been used successfully to treat NM.[49–51] By way of contrast, intra-CSF chemotherapy spares systemic dose-limiting toxicity and therefore achieves systemic rescue. Furthermore, intra-CSF drug therapy results in high intra-CSF drug levels that may be maintained by frequent intra-CSF drug administrations.[13,52,53] Notwithstanding the theoretic limitations of systemic chemotherapy in the treatment of patients with NM, several authors contend that this therapy may be sufficient to obviate the need for intra-CSF chemotherapy (discussed further in "Conclusion").

Surgery

The role of surgery is limited to performance of two procedures: (1) CSF diversion using ventriculoperitoneal shunting in patients with symptomatic hydrocephalus and (2) placement of intraventricular catheters and subgaleal reservoirs to facilitate intra-CSF chemotherapy administration. Most oncology centers are able to place an intraventricular catheter and subgaleal reservoir within a week of diagnosis of NM if the patients are considered candidates for aggressive NM-directed therapy. In patients with symptomatic hydrocephalus due to NM, initial treatment, if clinically possible, is base-of-brain or whole brain radiotherapy. Irradiation of brain to sites of CSF outflow obstruction may convert a patient with symptomatic hydrocephalus to a nonobstructed asymptomatic patient, obviating the need for CSF shunting. If shunting is necessary, however, consideration should be given to placing an in-line on/off valve and a reservoir, permitting a ventriculoperitoneal shunt to be used for administration of intra-CSF chemotherapy. When in use, the off valve is activated, thereby allowing intra-CSF-administered drug to circulate in the CSF. Most patients can tolerate the shunt being in the off position for several hours to days. In patients with persistent blockage of ventricular CSF following brain irradiation, a lumbar catheter and reservoir (or serial lumbar punctures) may be placed in addition to a ventricular catheter to permit treatment of the spine with intra-CSF drugs. Fortunately, this occurs infrequently. These patients are best managed by a team including a neurosurgeon, a neurologist, and an oncologist. As mentioned previously, patients with CSF flow blocks not restored to normal following involved-field radiotherapy are best managed with supportive care, as there are no data demonstrating that combined intraventricular and intralumbar intra-CSF drug administration is of value.

Regional Chemotherapy

Only three chemotherapeutic agents are used routinely for intra-CSF drug administration in patients with NM: methotrexate, cytosine arabinoside, (ara-C or cytarabine), and thiotepa[3,54–59] (see Table 21–8). A number of investigational agents are being explored including DepoFoam encapsulated cytarabine, mafosphamide (a derivative of cyclophosphamide), diaziquone, 4-hydroperoxy-cyclophosphamide (another derivative of cyclophosphamide), interferon, monoclonal antibodies, gene therapy, and interleukin-2[60–66] (see Table 21–7). However, these agents are available only in an experimental protocol setting and are therefore unattainable for most patients with NM. At present, there are no compelling data to suggest an improved response when using multiple-agent versus single-agent intra-CSF drug therapy or when using single-agent methotrexate versus thiotepa in the treatment of NM.[67,69] Pharmacokinetic studies of intra-CSF drug administration in NM demonstrate sustained cytotoxic lumbar and ventricular chemotherapeutic drug levels following administration by the ventricular route; similar studies of drug administration by the lumbar route are highly inconsistent with respect to cytotoxic ventricular chemotherapeutic drug levels.[54,65,66] Despite the pharmacokinetic advantages of intraventricular CSF drug administration. there are no studies that document this method of administration resulting in improved patient survival when compared to intralumbar drug administration.

Disadvantages of intralumbar intra-CSF drug administration include the pain and inconvenience associated with the multiple lumbar punctures necessary to deliver drugs frequently and to achieve cytotoxic concentrations, the inadvertant administration of drugs in either the subdural or epidural space in up to 12 percent of cases, and limited and variable distribution of drugs into the cranial CSF compartments.[3,5–7,13,52–55] As a result, the majority of North American neuro-oncologists treat patients with NM by intraventricular drug administration using an intraventricular catheter and subgaleal reservoir. A variety of drug schedules exist; most commonly, drug is administered in a bolus manner twice a week (see Table 21–8).[52–59] Folinic acid often is given orally following methotrexate administration to mitigate systemic myelosuppression (see Table 21–8). Alternatively, following the placement of an intraventricular catheter and subgaleal reservoir, treatment of NM by intraventricular drug administration permits the use of a concentration-times-time (C x T) approach based on pharmacokinetic principles.[52–55] Accordingly, methotrexate may be administered as 2 mg/d for 5 consecutive days every other week for 4 treatment weeks (total 8 weeks); ara-C may be delivered 25 mg/d for 3 consecutive days weekly for 4 weeks (total 4 weeks); and thiotepa may be administered 10 mg/d for 3 consecutive days weekly for 4 weeks (total 4 weeks) as induction therapies. However, no comparative phase III studies exist comparing differing intra-CSF drug schedules or drug doses in the treatment of NM. Our institution uses a C x T method of drug delivery by the ventricular route, which we believe results in (1) a lower frequency of neurotoxicity, (2) improved tumor cell killing based on prolonged exposure to intra-CSF chemotherapeutics, and (3) better palliation and patient survival. Whether to give intra-CSF chemotherapy concurrently is problematic. The only published prospective randomized trials of NM permitted concurrent radiotherapy and intra-CSF chemotherapy.[68,69] This approach, similar to that at our institution, may result in an increased risk of delayed neurotoxicity as discussed below.

Complications of intra-CSF drug therapy are not infrequent and may profoundly affect patients with NM (Table 21–9).[70,71] Complications of placing intraventricular catheters and subgaleal reservoirs are well known and, fortunately, are infrequent. Misplacement of the catheter tip may be circumvented by performance of postoperative plain skull films, CT or MRI, and radionuclide ventriculography. Clinically significant hemorrhage is distinctly uncommon in occurrence, primarily because of meticulous attention to preoperative coagulation parameters. Unfortunately, infection is a difficult problem seen at the time of intraventricular catheter placement or as a consequence of its use and occurs in up to 8 percent of patients. In both circumstances, skin flora and primarily *Staphylococcus epidermidis* contaminate the system and result in iatrogenic bacterial meningitis. Our institution's policy when such an infection occurs is to treat the patient with a combination of intravenous, oral, and intraventricular antibiotics, with the intraventricular catheter tube in situ. In the majority of instances we have been successful in preserving the intraventricular system and thereby avoiding Ommaya system removal and, ultimately, reoperation.

Table 21–9. COMPLICATIONS OF INTRAVENTRICULAR CHEMOTHERAPY*	
Complication	Patients (%)
Meningitis	52 (43)
Aseptic/chemical	52 (43)
Bacterial (catheter infection)	9 (8)
Myelosuppression	21 (18)
Transfusion-requiring myelosuppression	6 (5)
Unidirectional catheter obstruction	5 (4)
Catheter misplacement	2 (2)
Reservoir exposure	2 (2)
Chemotherapy-related leukoencephalopathy	2 (2)
Chemotherapy-related myelopathy	1 (1)

*As seen in 120 patients receiving a total of 1,110 cycles of intraventricular chemotherapy (median = 10) and undergoing a total of 4,400 Ommaya punctures (median = 46).

Infrequently, patients with intraventricular catheter and subgaleal reservoirs develop pressure necrosis of the skin overlying the reservoir, resulting in reservoir exposure and necessitating its removal and, if clinically appropriate, its replacement. The most common complication of intraventricular catheter use or installation of intra-CSF chemotherapy relates primarily to the toxicity of administering drugs directly into the CNS. The majority of these complications are inflammatory and transient in nature and are best characterized as aseptic chemical meningitis. The latter is manifested by fever, headache, nausea, vomiting, meningismus, photophobia, and, occasionally, dehydration. This complication may easily be managed in the outpatient setting with oral antipyretics, antiemetics, and steroids. Overall, serious complications requiring surgery are infrequent (6%) and most often secondary to catheter infections, Ommaya reservoir exposure, or initial catheter misplacement.

Rarely, direct neurotoxicity occurs as a manifestation of intra-CSF drug administration, which may result in either chemotherapy-related leukoencephalopathy or myelopathy. These complications may be idiosyncratic, or, in some instances, related to total intra-CSF drug dose and delayed drug clearance. In patients with prolonged survival, such as patients with leukemic or lymphomatous meningitis, the incidence of treatment-related delayed neurotoxicity, manifested primarily as a leukoencephalopathy, is considerably higher and may approach 30 percent. This delayed neurotoxicity, defined by either neuroradiographic or clinical criteria, reflects the combined effects of radiotherapy and intra-CSF chemotherapy and, at present, is an unavoidable consequence of treatment. The majority of patients treated with partial or whole brain radiotherapy develop neuroradiographic evidence of leukoencephalopathy, which, fortunately, is clinically apparent in only a minority. Data from the literature regarding the treatment of childhood leukemia suggest that delayed neurotoxicity may be mitigated by administering intra-CSF methotrexate prior to the application of cranial irradiation. The issue of timing of radiotherapy and methotrexate administration is more problematic in patients with NM as radiotherapy most often is used initially to treat symptomatic or bulky intracranial disease, as discussed above.

Symptomatic Therapy

A variety of medical therapies are used in the care of patients with NM irrespective of whether the patients are offered aggressive NM-directed therapy. A minority of patients will manifest seizures as a consequence of NM, and the use of nonsedating anticonvulsant drugs is appropriate for this group of patients. Patients with difficult-to-control pain may be managed with narcotics, or in the instance of neuropathic pain, either anticonvulsant drug or tricyclic antidepressant drug therapy. Antidepressants (especially tricyclic agents) also are useful for chronic insomnia and for the symptomatic treatment of depression. Steroids are most useful to control vasogenic edema secondary to parenchymal brain or epidural metastases, but they have limited use in the management of NM-related neurologic symptoms. Steroids additionally may be useful in patients with raised intracranial pressure or with chronic nausea or vomiting. Nausea or vomiting also may be managed by antiemetics. Weight loss and cancer-related anorexia may be mitigated by concurrent steroids, megestrol acetate, or cannabinols. Finally, decreased attention and somnolence, common side effects of whole brain irradiation, may be improved modestly by the use of psychostimulants such as dextroamphetamine.

CONCLUSION

Neoplastic meningitis is a complicated disease for a variety of reasons. First, most reports concerning carcinomatous meningitis treat all subtypes as being equivalent with respect to CNS staging, treatment, and outcome. However, clinical trials in oncology are based on specific tumor histologies. Comparing responses in patients with carcinomatous meningitis due to breast cancer to patients with non–small cell lung cancer outside of investigational new drug trials may be misleading. A general consensus is that breast cancer is inherently more chemosensitive than non–small cell lung cancer or melanoma, and, therefore, survival following chemotherapy is likely to be different. This observation has been substantiated in patients with systemic metastases, although comparable data regarding CNS metastases and, in particular, NM are meager.[72,73]

A second complicating feature of NM is deciding whom to treat.[74–79] Not all patients warrant aggressive CNS-directed therapy; however, few prognostic guidelines exist to help determine appropriate choice of therapy (Table 21–10). Previous studies have indicated that performance status and extent of systemic cancer influence outcome in patients with NM. An additional consideration is the extent of the disease in the CNS.[77,78] A coassociation with epidural spinal cord compression, parenchymal brain metastases, or bulky subarachnoid nodules may identify patients who are poor candidates for intraventricular chemotherapy; however, this issue has been addressed only recently. Extent of CNS disease is reflected in the performance of radionuclide ventriculography, which assesses CSF compartmentalization. Blockage of CSF flow as demonstrated by radionuclide ventriculography is a result of leptomeningeal cancerous adhesions that prevent homogeneous distribution of intraventricular- or intralumbar-administered chemotherapy. Interruption of normal CSF flow demonstrated by radioisotope ventriculography may have a neuroradiographic correlative abnormality. The supposition of cancerous adhesions causing CSF flow block as demonstrated by radioisotope ventriculography in patients with normal neuroradiography is supported by a postmortem study of two patients who were demonstrated (at our institution) to have tumor-related subarachnoid adhesions. This issue remains controversial pending further data. Additionally, it has recently been demonstrated that patients with interrupted CSF flow not responding to radiotherapy do poorly as compared to patients with normal or restored CSF flow.[74,77] Radionuclide ventriculography may therefore be useful both for prognosis and treatment of patients with NM. Based on the clinically determined prognostic variables and the extent of disease, a majority of patients are not candidates for aggressive NM-directed therapy. Supportive comfort care only (radiotherapy to symptomatic disease, antiemetics, and narcotics) is offered to patients with NM who are considered poor candidates for aggressive therapy (see Figure 21–1).

Third, optimal treatment of NM remains poorly defined. Notwithstanding aggressive treatment of NM, depending upon tumor histology, survival ranges from 2 to 6 months, and in all cases of NM, therapy is palliative[52–55,72,73,75,76] (Table 21–11). A provocative study by Siegal and colleagues suggests that a subset of patients with NM, predominantly patients with lymphoma or breast cancer, may respond to standard-dose systemic chemotherapy without the inclusion of intra-CSF therapy.[80] Similar conclusions were reached by Boogerd and colleagues and Fizazi and colleagues, suggesting the importance of systemic chemotherapy in treating patients with NM.[81,82]

Fourth, since progression of systemic cancer accounts for 50 to 60 percent of NM deaths, and treatment-related complications account for another 0.5 to 1.0 percent, it is difficult to assess response rates or duration of responses for those patients with truly progressive NM.[1–7,24,71] Treatment of NM today usually is palliative and rarely is curative with a median patient survival of 2 to 3 months, based on data of the two prospective randomized trials in this disease.[68,69] However, palliative therapy of NM often affords the patient protection from further neurologic deterioration and, consequently, an improved neurologic quality of life. No studies to date have attempted an economic assessment of the treatment of NM and, therefore, no information is available regarding a cost-benefit analysis as has been performed for other cancer-directed therapies.

Table 21–10. LEPTOMENINGEAL METASTASES: PROGNOSTIC VARIABLES

Performance status (function of neurologic disability)
Tumor histology
Status of systemic disease
CSF compartmentalization
Coexistent bulky metastatic CNS disease
Use of concurrent systemic chemotherapy

CSF = cerebrospinal fluid; CNS = central nervous system.

Table 21–11. LEPTOMENINGEAL METASTASES: SURVIVAL

Treatment and Histology	Median Survival (mo)
Untreated	1.0
Treated but not responding	2.0
Primary tumor histology*	
Melanoma	4.0
Non–small cell lung cancer	6.0
AIDS-related lymphoma	6.0
Breast cancer	7.5
Non-AIDS-related lymphoma	10.0

AIDS = acquired immunodeficiency syndrome.
*Data from our institution, based on selected patients.

Fifth, in patients with NM, the response to treatment is a function primarily of CSF cytology and secondarily of clinical improvement of neurologic signs and symptoms.[1–7,68,69,75,76] Aside from CSF cytology and perhaps biochemical markers, no other CSF parameters predict response. Furthermore, because CSF cytology may manifest a rostrocaudal disassociation, consecutive negative cytologies (defined as a complete response to treatment) require confirmation by both ventricular and lumbar CSF cytologies. In general, only pain-related neurologic symptoms improve with treatment. Neurologic signs such as confusion, cranial nerve deficit(s), ataxia, and segmental weakness minimally improve or stabilize with successful treatment.

Finally, there are a number of potential causes for the failure of regional chemotherapy to control NM including (1) de novo or acquired drug resistance; (2) incomplete distribution of drug within CSF spaces; (3) inability to achieve adequate CSF drug levels; (4) failure to control primary tumor; (5) toxicity (both neurologic and systemic toxicity of regional chemotherapy); (6) concurrent CNS metastatic disease (parenchymal brain, dural, and epidural spinal cord metastases); (7) patients' limited capacity for treatment; and (8) disseminated systemic disease.[7,24,65,69,70,74,77,83,84] In general, the majority of patients die due to progressive systemic disease occurring either in isolation or in combination with progressive neoplastic meningitis. However, a significant majority of patients die of isolated progressive neoplastic meningitis, which attests to our modest therapeutic impact on this disease.

ACKNOWLEDGMENTS

The authors acknowledge the invaluable assistance of Barbara F. Bailey and Nanette Mosley for providing secretarial assistance in the preparation of this manuscript.

REFERENCES

1. Olson M, Chernik N, Posner J. Infiltration of the leptomeninges by systemic cancer. A clinical and pathologic study. Arch Neurol 1974;30:122–37.
2. Little J, Dale A, Okazaki H. Meningeal carcinomatosis: clinical manifestations. Arch Neurol 1974;30:138–43.
3. Shapiro W, Posner J, Ushio Y, et al. Treatment of meningeal neoplasms. Cancer Treat Rep 1977;61:733–43.
4. Theodore WH, Gendelman S. Meningeal carcinomatosis. Arch Neurol 1981;38:696–9.
5. Wasserstrom W, Glass J, Posner J. Diagnosis and treatment of leptomeningeal metastases from solid tumors: experience with 90 patients. Cancer 1982;49:759–72.
6. Kaplan J, DeSouza T, Farkash A, et al. Leptomeningeal metastases: comparison of clinical features and laboratory data of solid tumors, lymphomas and leukemias. J Neurooncol 1990;92:25–9.
7. Chamberlain M, Corey-Bloom J. Leptomeningeal metastases: ^{111}indium-DTPA CSF flow studies. Neurology 1991;41:1765–9.
8. Posner J, Chernik N. Intracranial metastases from systemic cancer. Adv Neurol 1978;19:579–91.
9. Packer R, Siegel K, Sutton L, et al. Leptomeningeal dissemination of primary central nervous system tumors of childhood. Ann Neurol 1985;18:217–21.
10. Yung W, Horten B, Shapiro W. Meningeal gliomatosis: a review of 12 cases. Ann Neurol 1980;8:605–8.
11. Awad I, Bay J, Rogers L. Leptomeningeal metastasis from supratentorial malignant gliomas. Neurosurgery 1986;19:247–51.
12. Civitello L, Packer R, Rorke L, et al. Leptomeningeal dissemination of low-grade gliomas in childhood. Neurology 1988;38:562–6.
13. Chamberlain M, Dirr L. Involved field radiotherapy and intra-Ommaya methotrexate/ara-C in patients with AIDS-related lymphomatous meningitis. J Clin Oncol 1993;11:1978–84.
14. Rosen S, Aisner J, Makuch R, et al. Carcinomatous leptomeningitis in small cell lung cancer: a clinicopathologic review of the National Cancer Institute experience. Am J Med 1982;61:45–53.
15. Glass J, Melamed M, Chernik N, et al. Malignant cells in cerebrospinal fluid (CSF): the meaning of a positive CSF cytology. Neurology 1979;29:1369–75.
16. Murray J, Greco F, Wolff S, et al. Neoplastic meningitis: marked variations of cerebrospinal fluid composition in the absence of extradural block. Am J Med 1983;75:289–94.
17. Schold S, Wasserstrom W, Fleisher M, et al. Cerebrospinal fluid biochemical markers of central nervous system metastases. Ann Neurol 1980;8:597–604.
18. Ernerudh J, Olsson T, Berlin G, et al. Cerebrospinal fluid immunoglobulins and β$_2$-microglobulin in lymphoproliferative and other neoplastic diseases of the central nervous system. Arch Neurol 1987;44:915–20.
19. Klee G, Tallman R, Goellner J, et al. Elevation of carcinoembryonic antigen in cerebrospinal fluid among patients with meningeal carcinomatosis. Mayo Clin Proc 1986;6:19–23.
20. Schipper H, Bardosi A, Jacobi C, et al. Meningeal carcinomatosis: origin of local IgG production in the CSF. Neurology 1988;38:413–6.
21. Newton H, Fleisher M, Schwartz M, et al. Glucosephosphate isomerase as a CSF marker for leptomeningeal metastasis. Neurology 1991;41:395–8.
22. Malkin M, Posner J. Perspectives and commentaries: cere-

23. Cibas E, Malkin M, Posner J, et al. Detection of DNA abnormalities by flow cytometry in cells from cerebrospinal fluid tumor markers for the diagnosis and management of leptomeningeal metastases. Eur J Cancer Clin Oncol 1986;22:387–92.
23. Cibas E, Malkin M, Posner J, et al. Detection of DNA abnormalities by flow cytometry in cells from cerebrospinal fluid. Am J Clin Pathol 1987;88:570–7.
24. Grossman S, Moynihan T. Neurologic complications of systemic cancer: neoplastic meningitis. Neurol Clin 1991; 9:843–56.
25. Recht L. Neurologic complications of systemic cancer: neurologic complications of systemic lymphoma. Neurol Clin 1991;9:1001–15.
26. Walker R. Neurologic complications of systemic cancer: neurologic complications of leukemia. Neurol Clin 1991;9:989–99.
27. Chamberlain M, Sandy A, Press G. Leptomeningeal metastasis: a comparison of gadolinium-enhanced MR and contrast-enhanced CT of the brain. Neurology 1990;40:435–8.
28. Jaeckle K, Krol G, Posner J. Evolution of computed tomographic abnormalities in leptomeningeal metastases. Ann Neurol 1985;17:85–9.
29. Lee Y, Glass J, Geoffray A, et al. Cranial computed tomographic abnormalities in leptomeningeal metastasis. AJR Am J Roentgenol 1984;143:1035–9.
30. Ascherl G Jr, Hilal S, Brisman R. Computed tomography of disseminated meningeal and ependymal malignant neoplasms. Neurology 1981;31:567–74.
31. Sze G, Soletsky S, Bronen R, et al. MR imaging of the cranial meninges with emphasis on contrast enhancements and meningeal carcinomatosis. AJNR Am J Neuroradiol 1989;10:965–75.
32. Kim K, Ho S, Weinberg P, et al. Spinal leptomeningeal infiltration by systemic cancer myelographic features. AJR Am J Roentgenol 1982;139:361–5.
33. Krol G, Sze G, Malkin M, et al. MR of cranial and spinal meningeal carcinomatosis comparison with CT and myelography. AJNR Am J Neuroradiol 1988;9:709–14.
34. Kramer E, Rafto S, Packer R, et al. Comparison of myelography with CT follow-up versus gadolinium MRI for subarachnoid metastatic disease in children. Neurology 1991; 41:46–50.
35. Sze G, Abramson A, Krol G, et al. Gadolinium-DTPA in the evaluation of intradural extramedullary spinal disease. AJNR Am J Neuroradiol 1988;9:153–63.
36. Lim V, Sobel D, Zyroff J. Spinal cord pial metastases MR imaging with gadopentetate dimeglumine. AJNR Am J Neuroradiol 1990;11:975–82.
37. Pedersen A, Paulson O, Gyldensted C. Metrizamide myelography in patients with small cell carcinoma of the lung suspected of meningeal carcinomatosis. J Neurooncol 1985;3:85–9.
38. Wiener M, Boyko O, Friedman H, et al. False-positive spinal MR findings for subarachnoid spread of primary CNS tumor in postoperative pediatric patients. AJNR Am J Neuroradiol 1990;11:1100–3.
39. Rippe D, Boyko O, Friedman H, et al. Gd-DTPA-enhanced MR imaging of leptomeningeal spread of primary CNS tumor in children. AJNR Am J Neuroradiol 1990;11:329–32.
40. Chamberlain MC. Comparative spine imaging in leptomeningeal metastases. Neurooncology 1995;23:233–8.
41. Larson S, Johnston G, Ommaya A, et al. The radionuclide ventriculogram. JAMA 1973;224:853–7.
42. Di Chiro G, Hammock M, Bleyer A. Spinal descent of cerebrospinal fluid in man. Neurology 1976;26:1–8.
43. Lyons M, Meyer F. Subject review: cerebrospinal fluid physiology and the management of increased intracranial pressure. Mayo Clin Proc 1990;65:684–707.
44. Chamberlain M. Pediatric leptomeningeal metastasis [111]indium-DTPA CSF flow studies. J Child Neurol 1994;9:150–4.
45. Chamberlain M. Spinal [111]indium-DTPA CSF flow studies in leptomeningeal metastasis. J Neurooncol 1995;25:135–41.
46. Kokkoris C. Leptomeningeal carcinomatosis: how does cancer reach the pia-arachnoid? Cancer 1983;51:154-60.
47. Gonzalez-Vitale J, Garcia-Bunuel R. Meningeal carcinomatosis. Cancer 1976;37:2906–11.
48. Blasberg R, Patlak C, Fenstermacher J. Intrathecal chemotherapy brain tissue profiles after ventriculo-cisternal perfusion. Pharm Exp Ther 1975;195:73–83.
49. Slevin M, Piall E, Aherne G, et al. Effect of dose and schedule on pharmacokinetics of high-dose cytosine arabinoside in plasma and cerebrospinal fluid. J Clin Oncol 1983;1:546–51.
50. Lopez J, Nassif E, Vannicola P, et al. Central nervous system pharmacokinetics of high-dose cytosine arabinoside. J Neurooncol 1985;3:119–24.
51. Ackland S, Schilsky R. Review article; high-dose methotrexate: a critical reappraisal. J Clin Oncol 1987;5:2017–31.
52. Balis F, Poplack D. Central nervous system pharmacology of antileukemic drugs. Am J Pediatr Hematol Oncol 1989; 11:74–86.
53. Collins J. Pharmacokinetics of intraventricular administration. J Neurooncol 1983;1:283–91.
54. Shapiro W, Young D, Mehta B. Methotrexate distribution in cerebrospinal fluid after intravenous, ventricular and lumbar injections. N Engl J Med 1975;293:161–6.
55. Bleyer W. Current status of intrathecal chemotherapy for human meningeal neoplasms. NCI Monogr 1977;46:171–8.
56. Gutin P, Weiss H, Wiernik P, et al. Intrathecal N, N', N"-triethylenethiophosphoramide [thio-TEPA (NSC 6369)] in the treatment of malignant meningeal disease; phase I–II study. Cancer 1976;38:1471–5.
57. Gutin P, Levi J, Wiernik P, et al. Treatment of malignant meningeal disease with intrathecal thio-TEPA: a phase II study. Cancer Chemother Rep 1977;61:885–7.
58. Fulton D, Levin V, Gutin P, et al. Intrathecal cytosine arabinoside for the treatment of meningeal metastases from malignant brain tumors and systemic tumors. Cancer Chemother Pharmacol 1982;8:285–91.
59. Strong J, Collins J, Lester C, et al. Pharmacokinetics of intraventricular and intravenous N, N', N"-triethylenethiophosphoramide (thiotepa) in rhesus monkeys and humans. Cancer Res 1986;46:6101–4.
60. Jaeckle K, Lukes S, Krown S, et al. Phase I study of intraventricularly administered human interferon in patients with leptomeningeal tumor. Ann Neurol 1983;14:138–9.
61. Blacklock J, Grimm E, Loudon W, et al. CNS tumors: 362 intraventricular interleukin-2 in the treatment of leptomeningeal melanomatosis, phase I clinical trial and kinetic study. Proc ASCO 1989;8:93.

62. Lashford L, Davies G, Richardson R, et al. A pilot study of ^{131}I monoclonal antibodies in the therapy of leptomeningeal tumors. Cancer 1988;61:857–68.
63. Berg S, Balis F, Zimm S, et al. Phase I/II trial and pharmacokinetics of intrathecal diaziquone in refractory meningeal malignancies. J Clin Oncol 1992;10:143–8.
64. Arndt C, Colvin O, Balis F, et al. Intrathecal administration of 4-hydroperoxycyclo-phosphamide in rhesus monkeys. Cancer Res 1987;47:5932–4.
65. Chamberlain M, Khatibi S, Kim J, et al. Leptomeningeal metastasis with intraventricular depo/ara-C: a phase I study. Arch Neurol 1993;50:261–4.
66. Kim S, Chatelut E, Kim J, et al. Extended CSF cytarabine exposure following intrathecal administration of DTC 101. J Clin Oncol 1993;11:2186–93.
67. Giannone L, Greco F, Hainsworth J. Combination intraventricular chemotherapy for meningeal neoplasia. J Clin Oncol 1986;4:68–73.
68. Hitchens R, Bell D, Woods R, et al. A prospective randomized trial of single-agent versus combination chemotherapy in meningeal carcinomatosis. J Clin Oncol 1987;5:1655–62.
69. Grossman SA, Finkelstein DM, Ruckdeschel JC, et al. Randomized prospective comparison of intraventricular methotrexate and thiotepa in patients with previously untreated neoplastic meningitis. J Clin Oncol 1993;11:561–9.
70. Chamberlain MC, Kormanik PA. Complications associated with intraventricular chemotherapy in patients with leptomeningeal metastases. J Neurosurg 1997;87:694–9.
71. Lishner M, Perrin R, Feld R, et al. Complications associated with Ommaya reservoirs in patients with cancer. Arch Intern Med 1990;150:173–6.
72. Chamberlain MC, Kormanik P. Leptomeningeal metastases due to melanoma: combined modality therapy. Int J Oncol 1996;9:505–10.
73. Chamberlain MC, Kormanik PA. Carcinomatous meningitis secondary to breast cancer: combined modality therapy. J Neurooncol 1997;35:55–64.
74. Glantz M, Hall WA, Cole BF, et al. Diagnosis, management, and survival of patients with leptomeningeal cancer based on cerebrospinal fluid-flow studies. Cancer 1995;75:2919–31.
75. Grant R, Naylor B, Greenberg HS, et al. Clinical outcome in aggressively treated meningeal carcinomatosis. Arch Neurol 1994;51:457-61.
76. Balm M, Hammack J. Leptomeningeal carcinomatosis. Arch Neurol 1996;53:626–32.
77. Chamberlain MC, Kormanik P. Prognostic significance of ^{111}indium-DTPA CSF flow studies. Neurology 1996;46:1674–7.
78. Chamberlain MC, Kormanik PA. Prognostic significance of co-existent bulky metastatic CNS disease in patients with leptomeningeal metastases. Arch Neurol 1997;54:1364–8.
79. Freilich RJ, Krol G, DeAngelis LM. Neuroimaging and cerebrospinal fluid cytology in the diagnosis of leptomeningeal metastasis. Ann Neurol 1995;38:51–7.
80. Siegal T, Lassos A, Pfeffer MR. Leptomeningeal metastases: analysis of 31 patients with sustained off-therapy response following combined-modality therapy. Neurology 1994;44:1463–9.
81. Boogerd W, Hart AAM, Van der Sande JJ, et al. Meningeal carcinomatosis in breast cancer. Prognostic factors and influence of treatment. Cancer 1991;67:1685–95.
82. Fizazi K, Asselain B, Vincent-Salomon A, et al. Meningeal carcinomatosis in patients with breast carcinoma. Cancer 1996;77:1315–23.
83. Dedrick R, Zaharko D, Bender R, et al. Pharmacokinetic considerations on resistance to anticancer drugs. Cancer Chemother Rep 1975;59:795–804.
84. Grossman S, Trump D, Chen D, et al. Cerebrospinal fluid flow abnormalities in patients with neoplastic meningitis. Am J Med 1982;73:641–7.

22

Paraneoplastic Syndromes

FRANK S. LIEBERMAN, MD

Neurologic dysfunction is a major cause of morbidity and diminished quality of life for patients with systemic cancer.[1] Whereas metastatic disease and, unfortunately, the neurologic toxicities of cancer therapies cause the majority of neurologic problems in patients with systemic cancer, paraneoplastic syndromes are increasingly recognized as causes.[2] Neurologic diseases are defined as paraneoplastic when they occur in increased frequency in patients with cancer and are not related to metastatic disease, infection, metabolic abnormalities, or toxicity of therapy. Astute clinical neurologists identified paraneoplastic syndromes in the 1950s, and novel syndromes are still being described. The molecular and immunologic techniques of the past two decades have partially elucidated the mechanism of cell injury or dysfunction in most of the defined syndromes.[3] Elucidation of the mechanisms of cell injury in paraneoplastic syndromes has provided insight into nervous system function and dysfunction. The majority of paraneoplastic syndromes are associated with disordered humoral and/or cellular immunity.[4]

Although these syndromes are relatively rare, accurate and expeditious diagnosis is important for several reasons. The diagnosis of a neurologic paraneoplastic syndrome may be the first indication of an occult malignancy, and it affords an opportunity for early detection. When a paraneoplastic syndrome is misdiagnosed as a metastatic complication or as a result of radiation or chemotherapy, inappropriate treatment decisions may be made. Finally, early diagnosis may allow time for immunosuppressive treatment before irreversible neurologic injury occurs.

In current practice, paraneoplastic syndromes are diagnosed by the identification of stereotypic clinical syndromes and confirmatory laboratory studies, which demonstrate evidence of autoimmunity. Autoantibodies against specific neural antigens characterize several neurologic disorders (Figure 22–1).[3] In some disorders, for instance Lambert-Eaton syndrome (LES) associated with small cell lung cancer (SCLC)[5], or myasthenia gravis associated with thymoma,[6] the antibodies are clearly important to the pathogenesis of the disease, and immunosuppression is therapeutically effective.[7,8] For other disorders such as encephalomyeloneuritis associated with SCLC, the role of the antibody response in producing neurologic dysfunction is less clear.[8–10]

Paraneoplastic syndromes may involve any part of the central or peripheral nervous systems. For patients without a known malignancy prior to the appearance of the paraneoplastic syndrome, recognition of a clinical syndrome and the detection of the appropriate autoantibodies lead to diagnosis. Appropriate imaging or other diagnostic studies must exclude metastatic disease. Infectious and metabolic disorders are excluded by the appropriate investigations.

The classification of these syndromes is based on the clinical features and associated immunologic abnormalities. Over the past four decades, different investigators have identified and reported these disorders using a variety of names. As the immunologic abnormalities associated with several of the syndromes were defined, investigators realized the part of the nervous system most affected might vary among patients harboring antibodies against the same target antigen. In the discussion of the specific syndromes, this chapter will follow the nosology used by Posner.[2]

SUBACUTE SENSORY NEURONOPATHY-ENCEPHALOMYELONEURITIS

Most frequently associated with SCLC, subacute sensory neuronopathy-encephalomyeloneuritis (SSN-EMN) may affect multiple sites within the central and peripheral nervous systems.[11,12] When SSN-EMN occurs in patients with SCLC, an antibody called anti-Hu is usually present in the serum (see Figure 22–1). A high titer of antibodies to the Hu antigen is almost never seen in patients without SCLC.[13] Diagnosis of SSN-EMN and documentation of anti-Hu antibodies should lead to the search for an SCLC. The neurologic syndrome may antedate the appearance of the SCLC on a chest radiograph or CT scan by months to several years. The SCLC is often localized at the time of diagnosis, and the neurologic disorder, rather than metastatic complications of the SCLC, is the cause of death.

One group of patients with the anti-Hu antibody presents with a pure sensory neuropathy.[14] Subacute sensory neuronopathy usually begins with dysesthesia and sensory loss involving all sensory modalities. The sensory loss usually begins distally and is relentlessly progressive over days to weeks. The loss of position and kinesthetic sense may cause sensory ataxia. Reflexes are lost, but muscle strength is preserved. Neurophysiologic testing shows sensory nerve action potentials are diminished in amplitude or lost.[15] The cerebrospinal fluid (CSF) usually demonstrates increased protein and a lymphocytic pleocytosis.

In SSN associated with the anti-Hu antibody (Figure 22–2), the dorsal root ganglia show lymphocytic infiltration and loss of neurons. Dorsal roots, posterior columns, and peripheral nerves may be involved as the disorder worsens.[16,17] At postmortem examination, inflammatory changes in other regions of the nervous system have been seen in approximately half of SSN patients studied.

Only a minority of SSN patients have cancer. Most cases are associated with other autoimmune disorders, and anti-Hu antibodies are absent.[18] Small cell lung cancer is the cancer associated most commonly, but other malignancies also may occur.

The paraneoplastic disorder usually is relentlessly progressive and frequently disabling, most often

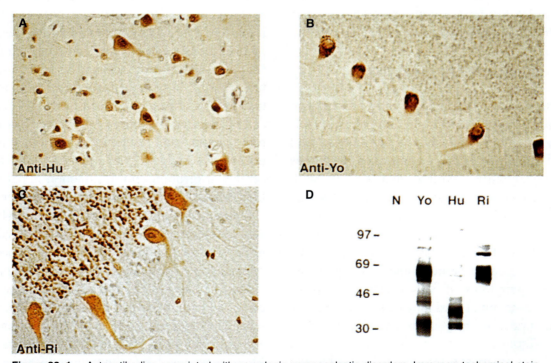

Figure 22–1. Autoantibodies associated with neurologic paraneoplastic disorders. Immunocytochemical staining of target cell populations is shown for anti-Hu (A), anti-Yo (B), and anti-Ri (C) antisera. D, Western blots using homogenates of normal human cerebellum (for anti-Yo) and normal human cortexes (for anti-Hu and anti-Ri) illustrate the apparent molecular weights of the target antigens when prepared using denaturing conditions (H & E stain; ×100 original magnification). (Photo courtesy of Dr. Jerome B. Posner.)

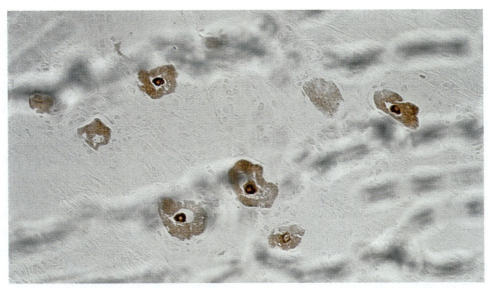

Figure 22–2. Immunocytochemical staining of human dorsal root ganglion cells by human anti-Hu immunoglobulin G (H & E stain; ×100 original magnification). (Photo courtesy of Dr. Jerome B. Posner.)

because of sensory ataxia. Immunosuppression has shown disappointing results.[8,19] Spontaneous remission may occur. When possible, the associated tumor should be eradicated; neurologic improvement may occur after successful treatment of SCLC.[3,8] Treatment of Hodgkin's disease with chemotherapy was followed by clinical improvement in one patient.[20]

LIMBIC ENCEPHALITIS

Limbic encephalitis (LE) may initially present as a progressive disturbance of mood and behavior, followed by memory disturbance, agitation, and seizures.[14] The disorder may be mistaken for herpes simplex encephalitis, which also occurs with increased frequency in patients with cancer. Usually patients are afebrile, but magnetic resonance imaging (MRI) scans may show mesial temporal contrast enhancement or T2-signal hyperintensities.[21] The CSF shows increased protein and a lymphocytic pleocytosis. Symptoms of SSN or involvement of the brain stem or spinal cord may be present. Biopsy of the temporal lobe may show perivascular lymphocytic infiltrates. In autopsy specimens, neuronal loss and gliosis are most prominent in the limbic and insular cortices.[22,23]

Limbic encephalitis is one example of a syndrome in which molecular characterization of the abnormal immune response has subdivided patients with a similar clinical picture into distinguishable diseases. Patients with testicular cancer and LE manifest a distinct antibody.[24] In a series reported from Memorial Sloan-Kettering Cancer Center, 10 of 13 patients with testicular cancer and limbic or brainstem dysfunction harbored antibodies that recognized a novel onconeural antigen, named Ma2. Ma2 is a 40-kD protein found in testis and normal brain tissue. Immunohistochemical studies suggest that Ma2 is widely expressed in the normal human central nervous system (CNS) as well as in dorsal root ganglia. Ma2 resembles a previously identified onconeural antigen, Ma1, that is associated with cerebellar or brainstem dysfunction in patients with lung, breast, parotid gland, or colon cancer.[25]

Immunosuppressive therapy of anti-Hu-associated LE is usually ineffective.[8,19] Occasional patients improve after treatment of SCLC.[26,27] Spontaneous remission also may occur. Although the number of reported cases is small, the anti-Ma2-associated disorder appears to have a better prognosis. Orchiectomy and aggressive treatment of residual disease appear to be the most effective treatments for anti-Ma2-associated LE.[24] Immunosuppressive therapy was largely ineffective, but one patient improved after treatment with corticosteroids and intravenous immunoglobulin G (ivIgG).

Patients with LE should be tested for the anti-Hu antibody; male patients should undergo examination of the testes and be tested for anti-Ma2 antibodies. Detection of anti-Hu or anti-Ma antibodies indicates the likelihood of SCLC or testicular cancer, respectively.

BRAINSTEM ENCEPHALITIS-MYELITIS

Brainstem encephalitis (BSE) usually occurs in association with LE.[13] Patients develop subacutely progressive, relentless cranial nerve and bulbar dysfunction. The lower brain stem seems to be preferentially affected, and dysphagia and aspiration are common problems in advanced disease.[28,29]

Myelitis usually occurs in conjunction with BSE. Progressive weakness with fasciculations, autonomic dysfunction, and sensory loss may occur. Examination of CSF reveals an inflammatory profile. Magnetic resonance imaging should exclude spinal cord compression from metastatic tumor. The majority of cases of paraneoplastic myelitis have been associated with the anti-Hu antibody, and inflammatory infiltrates in the anterior and posterior horns were seen.[13] Rare patients may have other autoantibodies.[30] Paraneoplastic myelitis usually is relentlessly and rapidly progressive and unresponsive to immunosuppression.

AUTONOMIC NEUROPATHY

A pure paraneoplastic autonomic neuropathy (AN) is rare, but approximately 25 percent of patients with anti-Hu syndrome and SSN-EMN have autonomic dysfunction.[13] Progressive paraneoplastic autonomic failure may rarely be the first manifestation of an occult malignancy. Bladder dysfunction, bowel immotility and obstipation, and postural hypotension may be disabling.[31] The disorder usually is associated with SCLC, and some patients have had autoantibodies that react with neurons in the myenteric plexus.[32]

SIGNIFICANCE OF ANTI-Hu ANTIBODY

The presence of anti-Hu antibody in significant titer characterizes a significant percentage of patients with SSN, EMN, progressive cerebellar degeneration (PCD), and paraneoplastic autonomic failure. Many patients present with a multisystem disorder combining features of the separate entities. Why some patients develop disease at one site in preference to others has not been explained by demonstrating molecular heterogeneity in the target antigen or in antibody specificity. The Hu antigens are a family of ribonucleic acid (RNA)-binding proteins, related to the *Drosophila* protein Elav, that may play a role in the regulation of translation.[33] (Figures 22–1 and 22–3). Whereas low-titer immunoreactivity may be seen in patients with no neurologic illness and without cancer, high-titer anti-Hu antibody in serum is almost always associated with SCLC and paraneoplastic neurologic dysfunction.[13]

In patients with paraneoplastic EMN, intrathecal synthesis of the anti-Hu antibody is demonstrable.[34] At postmortem, inflammatory infiltrates may be seen, consistent with an immune-mediated destructive process.[23] The anti-Hu-associated neurologic syndromes are an example of a large class of disorders in which an autoantibody directed against an intracellular antigen is hypothesized to cause cell injury.[9] The anti-Hu antibodies will internalize and bind to antigen in cells that express Hu, and antibody translocation to the nuclear locus of Hu can be demonstrated. However, it is unclear whether the antibodies are cytotoxic.

Attempts to produce the disorder by active immunization in mice or rats using recombinant Hu antigen have failed. Investigators have searched with limited success for cytotoxic T cell activity in patients with anti-Hu.[3] The precise pathophysiology of the anti-Hu-associated neurologic disorders remains to be identified. Pragmatically, the identification of the anti-Hu antibody in the serum of a patient with a neurologic disorder should lead to a search for an underlying malignancy—usually SCLC. Although results of treatment with immunosuppression have been disappointing, most neuro-oncologists treat patients intensively with plasmapheresis, intravenous γ-globulin, or high-dose corticosteroids if the disorder is identified early in its course.[8,19] There are reports of spontaneous remission and partial recovery after treatment of the underlying tumor.[26,27] Unfortunately, in most patients, treatment of the lung cancer does not halt

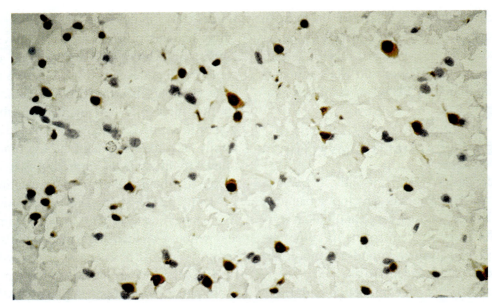

Figure 22–3. Anti-Hu antibodies react with neurons from normal human cortex (H & E stain; ×100 original magnification). (Photo courtesy of Dr. Jerome B. Posner.)

progression of the neurologic disorder, and bulbar dysfunction, respiratory failure, and autonomic failure are the causes of death.

PROGRESSIVE CEREBELLAR DEGENERATION

Subacute cerebellar degeneration in an adult without a family history of cerebellar disease should prompt an investigation to determine whether the disorder is associated with a malignancy.[2] It is important to classify PCD with respect to the underlying tumor type and the presence or absence of an associated autoantibody. Clinical and immunologic variants appear to have different prognoses.[35,36]

Patients usually complain first of difficulty with walking that progresses over weeks to months. Diplopia and vertigo may be early symptoms. Dysarthria, loss of dexterity, and oscillopsia associated with nystagmus occur. The disorder may stabilize but usually not before patients are unable to write or use a word processor, speak intelligibly, or walk without assistance.[37,38]

Neurologic findings are usually symmetric and limited to the cerebellum and related pathways, but subtle findings indicating motor system or cognitive dysfunction may be present.[35,37,39] There is controversy regarding the frequency of associated dementia; mental status testing and neuropsychological evaluation may be complicated by the profound difficulties with communication. Magnetic resonance images usually are unremarkable in the early stages of disease and later show diffuse cerebellar atrophy.[40] Contrast-enhancing lesions or lesions with mass effect are not part of PCD and suggest metastatic or infectious etiologies. Examination of the CSF usually reveals a lymphocytic pleocytosis and a mildly elevated protein content during the early phase of the disorder; oligoclonal bands in the CSF have been reported.[40] The most common pathologic finding is diffuse, extensive loss of cerebellar Purkinje cells.[39,41] Frequently, inflammatory changes are modest or absent, perhaps because the majority of patients have been studied after the inflammatory component of the disorder has exhausted itself and only neuronal loss remains. When present, inflammation usually is relatively minimal in the Purkinje cell layer and more prominent in the surrounding white matter, leptomeninges, or the region of the dentate nucleus.

Posner[2] has classified PCD into subcategories based on the underlying tumor, associated clinical features, and the presence of specific associated autoantibodies. Although the number of patients in each of the categories is small, this system may have prognostic implications and may guide treatment decisions in the future.

Anti-Yo PCD is associated most commonly with ovarian or breast carcinoma[40,42] (see Figures 22–1, 22–4, and 22–5). Patients are almost exclusively women. Frequently, the neurologic disorder antedates the discovery of the tumor. The disorder is subacute in onset and is usually progressive. Most patients develop downbeating nystagmus, oscillopsia, and diplopia. Progressive cerebellar degeneration renders patients unable to walk, and dysarthria is frequently severe. Once the disorder reaches this stage, treatment with immunosuppression or effective treatment of the underlying malignancy rarely produces significant improvement. Early recognition of the syndrome may allow more effective attempts at immunosuppressive therapy.

Progressive cerebellar degeneration associated with Hodgkin's disease (HD) differs from anti-Yo PCD in several respects. Patients are predominantly male and are younger than the females with anti-Yo PCD.[35] The disorder frequently develops in patients already treated for HD.

Antibodies against a novel onconeural antigen, Tr, have been found in patients with HD and PCD.[36,43,44] Immunohistochemical studies with anti-Tr antisera demonstrate staining of dendritic spines of rat Purkinje cells.[44] Although the number of patients reported is small, PCD associated with HD appears to have a better prognosis for recovery than the anti-Yo-associated syndrome. Spontaneous improvement has been seen in 15 percent of cases. In one case, effective treatment of HD resulted in remission of the lymphoma and significant neurologic improvement. As the patient responded to treatment, the anti-Tr antibody declined 10-fold in serum and disappeared from the CSF.[36]

Antibody-negative PCD may occur in conjunction with LES. Approximately 30 patients have been reported; in some no tumor has been identified.[45] The most common associated tumor is SCLC. The myasthenic syndrome has the typical features of LES, and antibodies directed against the voltage-gated calcium channel are usually present. The myasthenic component usually responds to plasmapheresis or ivIgG, whereas PCD frequently does not.

Approximately 15 percent of patients with anti-Hu antibodies present with PCD as the first manifestation of disease. In these patients, signs suggesting multisystem involvement are often present. Identification of the anti-Hu antibody directs the search for SCLC.

Progressive cerebellar degeneration has been associated with a variety of other solid tumors and with myelogenous leukemia and monoclonal gammopathy.[2] No conclusions can be reached about the causal relationship or the prognosis for these rare patients.

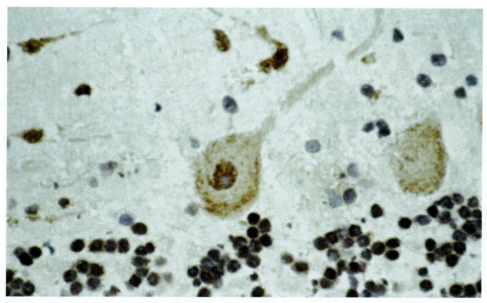

Figure 22–4. Immunocytochemical staining of human Purkinje cells with anti-Yo antiserum (H & E stain; ×250 original magnification). (Photo courtesy of Dr. Jerome B. Posner.)

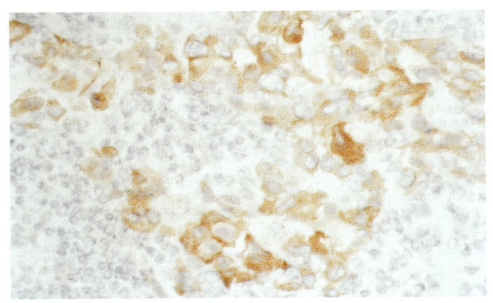

Figure 22–5. Anti-Yo antibodies react with antigen expressed by human breast adenocarcinoma (H & E stain; ×100 original magnification). (Photo courtesy of Dr. Jerome B. Posner.)

The pathophysiologic relevance of anti-Yo and anti-Tr antibodies is unclear. Attempts to passively transfer the disorder in animals[46] or to produce the syndrome by active immunization with Yo antigen have been unsuccessful.[47] Recently, major histocompatability complex (MHC) class 1 restricted cytotoxic T cells were found in all of three patients with paraneoplastic cerebellar degeneration and anti-cdr2 antibodies.[48] The cytotoxic T cells specifically recognized epitopes derived from cdr-2. This observation suggests that cellular immunity is important in at least some forms of PCD.

PARANEOPLASTIC VISUAL SYNDROMES

Paraneoplastic syndromes are a rare cause of visual loss in cancer patients. Paraneoplastic visual syndromes may be identified by the clinical history, ophthalmologic examination, retinal electrophysiologic studies, and the presence or absence of autoantibodies.[49] Retinal disorders are the most common disorders, with photoreceptor degeneration being the best characterized.[50]

Patients with photoreceptor degeneration commonly note night blindness, photopsias, and blurred vision. If cones are involved, loss of color perception may occur. Electroretinography demonstrates diminution and then loss of "a" waves. Cortical evoked potentials are usually preserved. Ophthalmoscopic examination may show retinal arteriolar attenuation.[50]

A number of different autoantibodies have been described in association with photoreceptor degeneration, but the most common is the anti-CAR (carcinoma-associated-retinal antigen). The target antigen is recoverin, a calcium-binding molecule involved in the transduction of light signaling in vertebrate photoreceptors.[51,52] The majority of patients with anti-CAR have cancer, usually SCLC,[52] but a similar syndrome has been reported in patients with no detectable cancer.[53] Usually the visual loss is relentlessly progressive and blindness is the ultimate result, but occasional patients have responded to high-dose corticosteroids, plasmapheresis, or intravenous γ-globulin.[53] At present, there are no clinical or immunologic features that identify patients likely to respond to therapy.

Antibodies directed against a variety of retinal antigens, including neurofilaments,[54,55] have been reported in patients with photoreceptor degeneration in addition to CAR. Most patients suffered from SCLC, non–small cell lung cancer, or breast cancer. Some patients with anti-Hu syndrome develop retinal photoreceptor degeneration; in these patients, other neurologic signs are frequently present. Again, the visual loss usually is relentlessly progressive. Treatment of the underlying tumor usually does not modify the course of the visual syndrome.

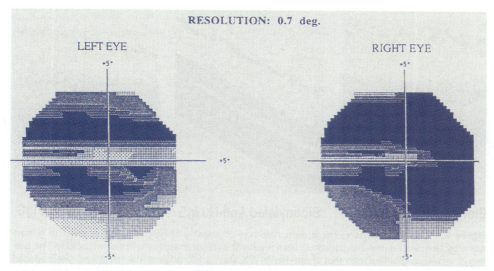

Figure 22–6. Computerized visual fields demonstrate bilateral pericentral scotomata in the patient with reversible paraneoplastic neuropathy. (Reproduced with permission from Lieberman FS, Odel J, Hirsh J, et al. Bilateral optic neuropathy with IgG multiple myeloma improved after myeloablative chemotherapy. Neurology 1999;57:414–7.)

Progressive visual loss with retinal pigmentary abnormalities has been separated into several syndromes. Most commonly associated with melanoma[55] or adenocarcinomas of the gut,[56] these disorders have distinctive ophthalmoscopic appearances.

Acquired night blindness has been reported in association with melanoma.[57,58] Isolated cone dystrophy also has been reported as a paraneoplastic syndrome.[59]

A small number of patients with paraneoplastic optic neuropathies have been reported.[60,61] Ophthalmoscopic examination may reveal optic disk pallor but not retinal pigmentary changes or vascular attenuation. Electroretinograms are normal, but visual evoked potentials are delayed. Patients do not complain of photopsia and develop progressive scotomata related to optic nerve dysfunction (Figure 22–6). The small number of patients and the heterogeneity of the immunologic findings preclude conclusions about the efficacy of treatment. The author has treated a patient with multiple myeloma and an antibody directed against an antigen in retinal ganglion cells in whom the visual loss completely resolved after high-dose chemotherapy and stem cell transplantation obliterated the autoantibody[62] (Figure 22–7).

The antibody-associated photoreceptor cell degenerations and optic neuropathies are examples of paraneoplastic syndromes in which localization of injury is incompletely explained by the distribution of the target antigen. Although recoverin is a photoreceptor molecule, immunoreactivity of CAR patient sera frequently reacts with optic nerve. Recently, a target antigen of 22 kD was identified as the target for antibodies in patients with autoimmune retinal degeneration and optic neuropathy.[53] One of these patients was diagnosed with melanoma-associated retinopathy.

OPSOCLONUS-MYOCLONUS

This disorder of ocular motility and multifocal myoclonus (OM) was first described in children with neuroblastoma. Probably 50 percent of pediatric cases are paraneoplastic.[2] Since OM antedates the discovery of neuroblastoma in many children, search for underlying neuroblastoma is necessary in any child who develops OM. The peak age of onset for the disorder is 18 months, and girls are preferentially afflicted.

Antineurofilament antibodies were implicated in one pediatric case[32] and anti-Hu antibodies in another.[63] A novel antibody, termed anti-Ri, has been reported in several adult patients with opsoclonus and truncal ataxia or other cerebellar signs and associated breast or gynecologic cancers.[64,65] Anti-Ri antibodies recognize 55-kD and 80-kD bands on denaturing Western blots of cortical neurons. The gene has been cloned and is not related to Hu or Yo.

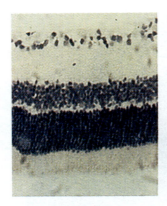 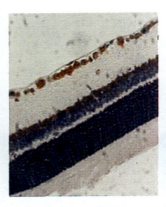 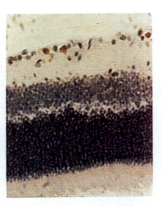

Figure 22–7. Immunocytochemical demonstration of staining of bipolar ganglion cells in human retina by biotinylated immunoglobulin G from a patient with paraneoplastic optic neuropathy. The pattern of localization differs from that of anti-Hu (H & E stain; ×100 original magnification). (Reproduced with permission from Lieberman FS, Odel J, Hirsh J, et al. Bilateral optic neuropathy with IgG multiple myeloma improved after myeloablative chemotherapy. Neurology 1999;57:414–7.)

It is unclear whether the neurologic prognosis is different for antibody-negative versus anti-Ri-associated OM. The role of antibody in producing disease is again unclear. The target antigen is an RNA-binding protein, and antibodies derived from patients recognize a region of the protein necessary for RNA interaction,[66] suggesting a mechanism for antibody-mediated toxicity.

Significant neurologic dysfunction frequently persists in children with OM and neuroblastoma.[67,68] Successful treatment of the neuroblastoma with chemotherapy may be associated with a good neurologic outcome.[39]

Opsoclonus-myoclonus also occurs in adults, usually in association with lung cancer.[40] These patients do not have anti-Ri antibodies. Some patients have improved after treatment with thiamine, suggesting the presence of a vitamin-deficiency disorder. Symptomatic treatment with benzodiazepines may suppress myoclonus.

PARANEOPLASTIC MOTOR NEURON DISORDERS

After a quarter century of controversy regarding the existence of paraneoplastic motor neuron disorders, (PMNDs) consensus is emerging. Most cases of PMND in patients with cancer represent the concomitant occurrence of two common disorders in the same patient. However, PMNDs do occur, and diagnosis is important because patients may improve after tumor removal or immunosuppression.[69] Experienced clinicians believe that PMNDs can be differentiated from amyotrophic lateral sclerosis (ALS) with the use of clinical and electrophysiologic criteria. Extensive search for occult malignancy in patients with typical ALS is probably unwarranted. However, PMNDs with a variable mixture of upper and lower motor neuron signs have been reported in association with both lymphoproliferative malignancies and solid tumors.[70–72]

A review of patients with PMNDs seen at Memorial Hospital identified three groups of patients.[71] One group was identified by the presence of anti-Hu antibodies in serum, corresponding with reports of similar cases elsewhere.[73] In these patients, progressive motor neuron dysfunction is part of a more complex syndrome incorporating features of the anti-Hu syndrome. In the second group, five women with primary lateral sclerosis and breast cancer were identified; none had anti-Hu antibodies or other autoantibodies. A third group of patients developed a syndrome resembling ALS and had a variety of underlying solid tumors.

Patients with HD or non-Hodgkin's lymphoma, paraproteinemia, and a mixed upper and lower motor neuron syndrome have been reported. Lower motor neuron syndromes, as well as a mixture of lower and upper motor neuron signs, have been reported in association with myeloproliferative disorders and paraproteinemias.[70,73,74] A rapidly progressive, painless, lower motor neuron syndrome has occurred in a patient with angiocentric lymphoma.[75]

Case reports suggest that patients may improve substantially after effective treatment of the underlying malignancy or, less often, with immunosuppression.[8,69] Remission of the motor neuron syndrome has been reported after nephrectomy in a patient with renal cell carcinoma and with successful treatment of lung cancer.[76]

Posner has suggested that the predominantly lower motor neuron disorder, termed subacute motor neuronopathy or spinal muscular atrophy, is an opportunistic viral syndrome.[2] This syndrome has been reported to occur with HD and non-Hodgkin's lymphoma.[77,78] Patients present with multifocal motor weakness. Sensory complaints may be present. The CSF is usually acellular with mildly elevated protein levels.

The author recently treated a patient who survived 15 years after diagnosis of metastatic adenocarcinoma of the colon and who developed a rapidly progressive motor neuron disorder and dementia. An antibody that was reactive with anterior horn cells in the spinal cord and pyramidal cells in the cortex was identified in the patient's serum. Treatment with ivIgG produced a transient improvement in leg strength and ambulation; however, the patient died of neurogenic respiratory failure despite continued ivIgG and a subsequent trial of high-dose methylprednisolone.

PARANEOPLASTIC PERIPHERAL NEUROPATHY

Progressive polyneuropathies are commonly the result of metabolic and nutritional disturbances, chemotherapeutic toxicity, and concurrent medical illness in cancer patients. The diagnosis of paraneoplastic peripheral neuropathy (PPN) is a diagnosis of exclusion. Cancer patients are frequently malnourished, and vitamin-deficiency disorders should be carefully considered.

When patients with peripheral neuropathy were evaluated at a neuromuscular disease center, PPN was an uncommon diagnosis.[79] In one series of 422 patients evaluated in a neuromuscular disorder referral center, 26 were considered possibly to have paraneoplastic neuropathies related to solid tumors.

SUBACUTE SENSORY-MOTOR NEUROPATHY

Subacute sensorimotor neuropathy (SSMN) usually presents with progressive, distal, symmetric sensory loss and weakness that is most severe in the legs.[80] Lung cancer is the most common associated malignancy. In approximately two of three patients, the neuropathy precedes the diagnosis of cancer or is noted at the time of diagnosis. Cerebrospinal fluid is usually acellular and protein levels may be mildly elevated. Neurophysiologic studies usually indicate an axonal process, but occasional patients show slowing consistent with demyelination.[81] Biopsy of nerve usually shows a mixture of axonal injury and demyelination. This disorder usually is relentlessly progressive, but some patients stabilize after tumor removal.[82] Posner indicates that some patients appear to benefit from corticosteroid therapy.[2]

Women with breast cancer may develop a slowly progressive sensorimotor neuropathy with proximal weakness and upper motor neuron signs.[83] Babinski's sign may be present. (Perhaps this disorder is a form of myeloneuropathy.) This disorder is frequently indolent, and patients remain functional and ambulatory.

ACUTE POLYRADICULONEUROPATHY

Acute polyradiculoneuropathy (APN) appears to occur in increased frequency in patients with HD. The clinical features of APN in HD are similar to those of idiopathic Guillain-Barré syndrome.[84] Treatment of HD does not clearly modify the course of the neuropathy. No specific autoantibodies have been identified in these patients. The APN associated with HD may respond to plasmapheresis or intravenous γ-globulin.[85] Acute polyradiculoneuropathy also has been reported to occur with leukemia, non-Hodgkin's lymphoma, and multiple myeloma.[86] Leukemic or lymphomatous infiltration of the peripheral nerves may be clinically indistinguishable from APN; biopsy may be required to confirm the diagnosis.[87] Relapsing and remitting forms of APN also have been reported to occur with a variety of solid tumors, leukemia, and lymphoma,[87] but it is possible that these cases represent the coincidental occurrence of idiopathic inflammatory polyneuropathy in a patient with cancer.

Several cases of chronic inflammatory demyelinating polyneuropathy (CIDP) have been associated with melanoma.[79,88] Concomitant vitiligo suggests the presence of an autoimmune disorder, perhaps directed against shared cell surface ganglioside antigens.

NEUROPATHIES ASSOCIATED WITH PLASMA CELL DYSCRASIAS

A number of different syndromes are associated with plasma cell dyscrasias.[89] Typical osteolytic multiple myeloma is only rarely associated with clinically significant peripheral neuropathy. Most commonly, the neuropathy is a sensorimotor neuropathy and is relatively mild. Pure sensory neuropathy also has been reported.[90] Patients with osteolytic myeloma also develop more severe neuropathies that clinically resemble Guillain-Barré syndrome or CIDP.[89] Secondary amyloidosis also may cause a relentless sensorimotor neuropathy (often painful) in these patients. Unfortunately, the progressive neuropathies rarely respond to immunosuppressive therapy of any form.[91]

Although osteosclerotic myeloma represents only 2 percent of cases of multiple myeloma, it is crucial that the association with progressive sensorimotor neuropathy is recognized since this neuropathy frequently improves after radiation therapy or chemotherapy.[89] Bone scanning is insensitive; a metastatic bone survey is necessary to identify the sclerotic bone lesion. Open biopsy or computed tomography (CT)-guided biopsy of bone lesions confirms the diagnosis. M protein (IgG or IgA) may be missed unless immunoelectrophoresis or immunofixation is performed on the serum specimen and urine. Osteosclerotic myeloma is a treatable cause of an otherwise relentless and disabling peripheral neuropathy.

Discussion of the nonmalignant plasma cell dyscrasias is beyond the focus of this chapter. When sensorimotor neuropathy complicates these disorders, the response to treatment is quite variable.[89] One study suggests that patients with IgA or IgG paraproteins respond more favorably to plasmapheresis than do the IgM-associated neuropathies.[91]

A distinctive syndrome combining polyneuropathy, organomegaly, endocrinopathy, M protein, and skin changes, known as the POEMS syndrome, is associated with osteosclerotic myeloma. The natural history and features of the neuropathy are the same as those for patients with osteosclerotic myeloma who do not have all the diagnostic criteria for POEMS syndrome.[89] When the syndrome is associated with solitary plasmacytoma, radiation therapy may produce slow resolution of the syndrome. Chemotherapy may be beneficial for patients with POEMS syndrome and disseminated plasmacytoma.

MONONEURITIS MULTIPLEX AND VASCULITIS

Painful mononeuritis multiplex due to small vessel vasculitis has been linked to underlying malignancy in a small number of patients. Prostate cancer, SCLC endometrial cancer, lymphoma, and renal cell carcinoma have been implicated.[92–95] In some patients, the mononeuritis multiplex is part of a more generalized vasculitis, with muscle involvement and an elevated sedimentation rate. In other patients, the vasculitis appears limited to the peripheral nerves. Nerve biopsy is necessary for diagnosis. Mononeuritis multiplex may be a presentation of the anti-Hu syndrome. Interestingly, the cases of prostate carcinoma associated with the vasculitic syndrome have been small cell, undifferentiated carcinomas.[13] In one case, the prostate cancer was associated with anti-Hu. Immunosuppression or plasmapheresis may be beneficial. Surgical removal of an associated cancer has been followed by improvement as well.

BRACHIAL NEURITIS

Inflammatory brachial neuritis is most commonly associated with HD.[2] Since metastatic plexopathy is more common than the paraneoplastic disorder, imaging studies should be performed to identify tumor infiltration of the plexus when paraneoplastic neuritis is considered. Unlike radiation-induced plexopathy, the inflammatory disorder is frequently painful at onset.

NEUROMUSCULAR JUNCTION DISORDERS

Typical myasthenia gravis is associated with thymoma in approximately 15 percent of cases, and the presence of autoantibodies against striated muscle contractile proteins is associated with increased probability of underlying thymoma.[6] All patients with myasthenia gravis should undergo CT scanning of the chest to identify thymic neoplasms. In patients with underlying thymoma, the myasthenia gravis may remit after thymectomy.[7] In most cases, the thymoma is not invasive and can be treated definitively by thymectomy. The paraneoplastic syndrome is similar to those cases that occur in the absence of thymoma.

LAMBERT-EATON SYNDROME

Lambert-Eaton syndrome is a paraneoplastic neurologic disorder for which the immunobiology is clinically relevant and the molecular understanding of the disease has direct clinical application[96] (Figure 22–8). In approximately 60 percent of patients with LES, the disorder is associated with an underlying cancer, usually SCLC.[97] Proximal weakness is a common presenting complaint, but bulbar symptoms are uncommon. In most patients, LES is not a pure motor syndrome. Paresthesias frequently are reported. The abnormality of autonomic function has been termed "cholinergic dysautonomia";[98] patients may report dry mouth or erectile dysfunction. Characteristic electrophysiologic abnormalities include augmentation of the compound motor action potential with repetitive stimulation.[96]

The autoimmune nature of LES is well established. Antibodies directed against protein epitopes in the voltage-gated calcium channel of presynaptic neurons are present in most patients with LES. Passive transfer of an antibody will reproduce the characteristic electrophysiologic abnormality in animal models of LES.[99] Immunization with a component of the P/Q-type calcium channel, synaptotagmin, will produce autoantibodies and clinical disease in an animal model of LES.

Most patients with LES benefit from plasmapheresis and immunosuppressive therapy.[96] Drugs that increase presynaptic acetylcholine release may also decrease symptoms; 3,4-diaminopyridine is one such agent that has relatively minimal side effects.[100]

Occasional patients with SCLC may develop more than one paraneoplastic syndrome. Patients with LES and PCD as well as those with LES and EMN have been reported. In such patients, anti-Hu or anti-Yo and antibodies directed against the voltage-gated calcium channel may be present independently. The LES may respond to immunosuppression independently of the other syndromes, and amelioration of weakness related to the LES may improve quality of life.

MOVEMENT DISORDERS

If one excludes cerebellar syndromes and paraneocoplastic opsoclonus-myoclonus (POM), paraneoplastic movement disorders are rare. Usually the movement disorder accompanies other signs of brainstem dysfunction. Disorders of excess movement predominate. Chorea has been reported in association with brainstem signs in patients with SCLC,[101–103] in a patient with acute lymphocytic leukemia,[104] and in patients with HD.[105] Rubral tremor in an extremity has been described as a paraneoplastic syndrome.[106]

Paraneoplastic parkinsonian syndromes appear to be extremely rare.[107] Rapidly progressive parkinsonism and autonomic failure have been reported in a man suffering from multiple myeloma. At necropsy, no inflammatory changes were detected in the basal ganglia or elsewhere in the brain.[108]

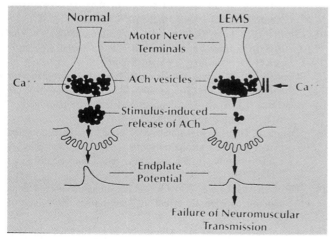

Figure 22–8. Pathophysiology of Lambert-Eaton syndrome. ACh = acetylcholine.

FUTURE DIRECTIONS

The past 7 years have seen significant advances in the clinical nosology and in our understanding of the immunobiology of paraneoplastic neurologic disorders.[109–113] New onconeural antigens are being identified.[24,114] This area of neurologic investigation is particularly exciting due to the collaboration of careful and inquisitive clinical neurologists, molecular biologists, and immunologists. Together, they have made significant advances; however, important questions remain.

For a number of paraneoplastic syndromes, treatment is currently unsatisfactory. When localized cancer is identified, surgical resection may remove an antigenic stimulus, but frequently the neurologic disorder does not improve with successful tumor ablation. Immunosuppression with corticosteroids, plasma exchange, ivIgG, or immunoadsorption is variably effective.[8] A small series of patients treated with extracorporeal immunoadsorption reported a 75 percent response rate;[115] this approach may warrant further clinical trials. For many paraneoplastic syndromes, we have no evidence-based rationale for choosing the type or sequence of immunotherapy. The ease and safety of ivIgG leads to its frequent use as first-line therapy in the antibody-mediated or antibody-associated disorders.[116]

We do not understand the variation in distribution of neural injury among patients with autoimmune processes directed against apparently identical antigens. We do not understand why tissue injury is localized to specific regions in disorders where the target antigen is ubiquitously distributed throughout the brain. We are just beginning to identify the cellular immune mechanisms in these disorders.[117]

Systematic study of a large serum bank has led to the characterization of a novel 62kd antigen, a member of the collapsin response mediator protein (CRMP) family, named CRMP-5.[118] Similar to the Hu antigen, this plays a crucial role in early nervous system development. The most common related tumors were lung cancer and thymoma. A spectrum of neurologic disorders is associated with anti-CRMP-5 antibody seropositivity, including paraneoplastic optic neuropathy, movement disorders, neuromuscular junction disorders, and OM. This antigen may be identical or closely related to that reported in previously reported cases of paraneoplastic optic neuropathy.[59,119] Development of consistently effective therapies awaits a more profound understanding of the mechanisms of disease. Hopefully, continued application of clinical and molecular expertise will lead to advances in therapy over the next few years.

REFERENCES

1. Clouston PD, De Angelis LM, Posner JB. The spectrum of neurologic disease in patients with systemic cancer. Ann Neurol 1992;31:268–73.
2. Paraneoplastic syndromes. In: Posner JB, editor. Neurologic complications of cancer. Philadelphia: FA Davis; 1995. p. 353–85.
3. Dalmau J, Posner JB. Neurologic paraneoplastic antibodies (anti-Yo, anti-Hu, anti-Ri): the case for a nomenclature based on antibody and antigen specificity. Neurology 1994;44:2241–6.
4. Posner JB, Furneaux HM. Paraneoplastic syndromes. In: Waksman BH, editor. Immunologic mechanisms in neurologic and psychiatric disease. New York: Raven Press; 1990. p. 187–219.
5. Leys K, Lang G, Johnston I, et al. Calcium channel autoantibodies in Lambert-Eaton myasthenic syndrome. Ann Neurol 1991;29:307–14.
6. Williams CL, Hay JE, Huiatt TW, et al. Paraneoplastic IgG striational autoantibodies produced by clonal thymic B cells in serum of patients with myasthenia gravis and thymoma react with titin. Lab Invest 1992;66:331–6.
7. Verma P, Oger J. Treatment of acquired autoimmune myasthenia gravis: a topic review. Can J Neurol Sci 1992;19:360–75.
8. Das A, Hochberg FH, McNelis S. A review of the therapy of paraneoplastic neurologic syndromes. J Neurooncol 1999;41:181–94.
9. Hormigo A, Lieberman F. Nuclear localization of anti-Hu antibody is not associated with in vitro cytotoxicity. J Neuroimmunol 1994;55:205–12.
10. Smitt PAE, Manley G, Posner JB. High titer antibodies but no disease in mice immunized with the paraneoplastic antigen HuD. Neurology 1994;44(Suppl 2):376.
11. Henson RA, Hoffman Hl, Urich H. Encephalomyelitis with carcinoma. Brain 1965;88:449–64.
12. Dorfman LJ, Forn LS. Paraneoplastic encephalomyelitis. Acta Neurol Scand 1972;48:556–74.
13. Dalmau J, Graus F, Rosenblum MK, et al. Anti-Hu associated paraneoplastic encephalomyelitis/sensory neuronopathy. A clinical study of 71 patients. Medicine (Baltimore) 1992;71:59–72.
14. Horwich MS, Cho L, Porro RS, et al. Subacute sensory neuropathy: a remote effect of carcinoma. Ann Neurol 1979;2:7–19.
15. Donofrio PD, Alessi AG, Alberts JW, et al. Electrodiagnostic evaluation of carcinomatous sensory neuronopathy. Muscle Nerve 1989;12:508–13.

16. Henson RA, Russell DS, Wilkinson M. Carcinomatous neuropathy and myopathy: a clinical and pathological study. Brain 1954;77:82–121.
17. Chalk CH, Windebank AJ, Kimmel DW, et al. The distinctive clinical features of paraneoplastic sensory neuronopathy. Can J Neurol Sci 1992;19:346–51.
18. Font J, Valls J, Cervera R, et al. Pure sensory neuropathy in patients with primary Sjögren's syndrome: clinical immunological and electromyographic findings. Ann Rheum Dis 1990;49:775–8.
19. Graus F, Vega F, Delattre J-Y, et al. Plasmapheresis and antineoplastic treatment in CNS paraneoplastic syndromes with antineuronal autoantibodies. Neurology 1992;42:536–40.
20. Sagar HJ, Read DJ. Subacute sensory neuropathy with remission: an association with lymphoma. J Neurol Neurosurg Psychiatry 1982;45:83–5.
22. Dirr LY, Elster AD, Donofrio PD, et al. Evolution of brain MRI abnormalities in limbic encephalitis. Neurology 1990;40:1304–6.
23. Dalmau J, Furneaux HM, Rosenblum MK, et al. Detection of the anti-Hu-antibody in specific regions of the nervous system and tumor from patients with paraneoplastic encephalomyelitis/sensory neuronopathy. Neurology 1991;41:1757–64.
24. Voltz R, Guletkin SH, Rosenfeld MR, et al. A serologic marker of paraneoplastic limbic and brain-stem encephalitis in patients with testicular cancer. N Engl J Med 1999;340:1788–95.
25. Dalmau J, Guletkin SH, Voltz R, et al. Ma1, a novel neuron and testis-specific protein is recognized by the serum of patients with paraneoplastic neurological disorders. Brain 1999;122:27–39.
26. Brennan LV, Craddock PR. Limbic encephalopathy as a nonmetastatic complication of oat cell lung cancer: its reversal after treatment of the primary lung lesion. Am J Med 1983;75:518–20.
27. Kaniecki R, Morris JC. Reversible paraneoplastic limbic encephalitis. Neurology 1993;43:2418–9.
28. Dietl HW, Pulst SM, Engelhardt P, et al. Paraneoplastic brain-stem encephalitis with acute dystonia and central hypoventilation. J Neurol 1982;227:229–38.
29. Veilleux M, Bernier JP, Lamarche JB. Paraneoplastic encephalomyelitis and subacute dysautonomia due to an occult atypical carcinoid tumour of the lung. Can J Neurol Sci 1990;17:324–8.
30. Babikian VL, Stefansson K, Dieperink MF, et al. Paraneoplastic myelopathy: antibodies against protein in normal spinal cord and underlying neoplasm. Lancet 1985;2:49–50.
31. Siemsen JK, Meister L. Bronchogenic carcinoma with severe orthostatic hypotension. Ann Intern Med 1963;58:669–76.
32. Lennon VA, Sas DF, Busk MF, et al. Enteric neuronal autoantibodies in pseudoobstruction with small-cell lung carcinoma. Gastroenterology 1991;100:137–42.
33. Szabo A, Dalmau J, Manley G, et al. HuD, a paraneoplastic encephalomyelitis antigen, contains RNA-binding domains and is homologous to Elav and Sex-lethal. Cell 1991;67:325–33.
34. Furneaux HM, Reich L, Posner JB. Autoantibody synthesis in the central nervous system of patients with paraneoplastic syndromes. Neurology 1990;40:1085–91.
35. Hammack J, Kotanides H, Rosenblum MK, et al. Paraneoplastic cerebellar degeneration II. Clinical and immunologic findings in 21 patients with Hodgkin's disease. Neurology 1990;42:1938–43.
36. Peltola J, Hietaharju A, Rantala I, et al. A reversible neuronal antibody (anti-Tr) associated paraneoplastic cerebellar degeneration in Hodgkin's disease. Acta Neurol Scand 1998;98:360–3.
37. Peterson K, Rosenblum MK, Kotanides H, et al. Paraneoplastic cerebellar degeneration. A clinical analysis of 55 anti-Yo positive patients. Neurology 1992;42:1931–7.
38. Posner JB. Paraneoplastic cerebellar degeneration. Prin Pract Oncol Updates 1991;5:1–13.
39. Brain WR, Daniel PM, Greenfield JG. Subacute cortical cerebellar degeneration and its relation to carcinoma. J Neurol Neurosurg Psychiatry 1954;14:59–75.
40. Greenberg HS. Paraneoplastic cerebellar degeneration: a clinical and CT study. J Neurooncol 1984;2:377–82.
41. Brain WR, Wilkinson M. Subacute cerebellar degeneration associated with neoplasms. Brain 1965;88:465–78.
42. Hammack JE, Kimmel DW, O'Neill BP, et al. Paraneoplastic cerebellar degeneration: a clinical comparison of patients with and without Purkinje cell cytoplasmic antibodies. Mayo Clin Proc 1990;65:1423–31.
43. Graus F, Dalmau J, Valldeoriola F, et al. Immunological characterization of a neuronal antibody (anti-Tr) associated with paraneoplastic cerebellar degeneration and Hodgkin's disease. J Neuroimmunol 1998;74:55–61.
44. Graus F, Guletkin SH, Ferrer I, et al. Localization of the neuronal antigen recognized by anti-Tr antibodies from patients with paraneoplastic cerebellar degeneration and Hodgkin's disease in the rat nervous system. Acta Neuropathol (Berl) 1998;96:1–7.
45. Clouston PD, Saper CB, Arbizu T, et al. Paraneoplastic cerebellar degeneration III: cerebellar degeneration, cancer and the Lambert-Eaton syndrome. Neurology 1992;42:1944–50.
46. Graus F, Illa I, Agusti M, et al. Effect of intraventricular injection of an anti-Purkinje cell antibody (anti-Yo) in a guinea pig model. J Neurol Sci 1991;106:82–7.
47. Sakai K, Gofuku M, Kitagawa Y, et al. Induction of anti-Purkinje cell antibodies in vivo by immunizing with a recombinant 52-kd paraneoplastic cerebellar degeneration-associated protein. J Neuroimmunol 1995;60:135–41.
48. Albert ML, Darnell JC, Bender A, et al. Tumor-specific killer cells in paraneoplastic cerebellar degeneration. Nat Med 1998;4:1321–24.
49. Tang RA, Kellaway J, Young SE. Ophthalmic complications of systemic cancer. Oncology 1991;5:59–71.
50. Thirkill CE, FitzGerald P, Sergott RC, et al. Cancer-associated retinopathy (CAR syndrome) with antibodies reactive with retinal, optic nerve, and cancer cells. N Engl J Med 1989;321:1589–94.
51. Thirkill CE, Tait RC, Tyler NK, et al. The cancer-associated retinopathy antigen is a recoverin-like protein. Invest Ophthalmol Vis Sci 1992;33:2768–72.
52. Keltner JL, Thirkill CE. The 22kDa antigen in optic nerve and retinal diseases. J Neuroophthalmol 1999;19:71–83.
53. Kornguth SE, Kalinke T, Grunwald GV, et al. Anti-neurofilament antibodies in the sera of patients with small cell carcinoma of the lung and with visual paraneoplastic syndrome. Cancer Res 1986;46:2588–95.

54. Gass JDM. Acute Vogt-Koyanagi-Harada-like syndrome occurring in a patient with metastatic cutaneous melanoma. In: Sari KH, editor. Uveitis update: proceeding of the international symposium on uveitis. Amsterdam: Elsevier Scientific Publishers; 1984. p. 407–8.
55. Gass JDM, Gieser RG, Wilkinson CP, et al. Bilateral diffuse uveal melanocytic proliferation in patients with occult carcinoma. Arch Ophthalmol 1990;108:527–33.
56. Berson EL, Lessell S. Paraneoplastic night blindness with malignant melanoma. Am J Ophthalmol 1988;106:307–11.
57. Alexander KR, Fishman GA, Reachey NS, et al. "On" response defect in paraneoplastic night blindness with cutaneous malignant melanoma. Invest Ophthalmol Vis Sci 1992;33:477–83.
58. McKay CJ, Gouras P, Roy LR, et al. Paraneoplastic cone dystrophy. Invest Ophthalmol Vis Sci 1994;35:3721.
59. Malik S, Furlan AJ, Sweeney PJ, et al. Optic neuropathy: a rare paraneoplastic syndrome. J Clin Ophthalmol 1992;12:137–41.
60. Hoogenraad TU, Sanders EACM, Tan KE. Paraneoplastic optic neuritis and encephalomyelitis, report of a case. Neuro-ophthalmology 1989;9:247–50.
61. Lieberman FS, Odel J, Hirsh J, et al. Bilateral optic neuropathy with IgG multiple myeloma improved after myeloablative chemotherapy. Neurology 1999;57:414–7.
62. Noetzel MJ, Cawley LP, Janes VL, et al. Antineurofilament protein antibodies in opsoclonus/myoclonus. J Neuroimmunol 1987;15:137–45.
63. Fisher PG, Wechsler SD, Singer HS. Anti-Hu antineuronal antibody in neuroblastoma-associated paraneoplastic syndrome. Pediatr Neurol 1994;10:309–12.
64. Budde-Steffen C, Anderson NE, Rosenblum MK, et al. An antineuronal autoantibody in paraneoplastic opsoclonus. Ann Neurol 1988;23:528–31.
65. Buckanovich RJ, Posner JB, Darnell RB. Nova, a paraneoplastic Ri antigen is homologous to an RNA-binding protein and is specifically expressed in the developing motor system. Neuron 1993;11:1–20.
66. Buckanovich RJ, Yang YY, Darnell RB. The onconeural antigen Nova-1 is a neuron-specific RNA-binding protein, the activity of which is inhibited by paraneoplastic antibodies. J Neurosci 1996;16:1114–22.
67. Russo C, Cohn SL, Petruzzi MJ, de Alarcon PA. Long-term neurologic outcome in children with opsoclonus-myoclonus associated with neuroblastoma: a report from the Pediatric Oncology Group. Pediatr Med Oncol 1997;28:284–8.
68. Kay CL, Davie-Jones GAB, Singal R, et al. Paraneoplastic opsoclonus-myoclonus in Hodgkin's disease. J Neurol Neurosurg Psychiatry 1993;56:831–2.
69. Evans BK, Fagan MD, Arnold T, et al. Paraneoplastic motor neuron disease and renal cell carcinoma: improvement after nephrectomy. Neurology 1990;40:960–2.
70. Rowland LP. Paraneoplastic primary lateral sclerosis and amoytrophic lateral sclerosis. Ann Neurol 1997;41:703–5.
71. Forsyth PA, Dalmau J, Graus F, et al. Motor neuron syndromes in cancer patients. Ann Neurol 1997;41:722–30.
72. Rowland LP, Schneck SA. Neuromuscular disorders associated with malignant neoplastic disorders. J Chron Dis 1963;16:777–95.
73. Verma A, Berger JR, Snodgrass S, Petito C. Motor neuron disease: a paraneoplastic process associated with anti-Hu antibody and small cell lung carcinoma. Ann Neurol 1996;40:112–6.
74. Rowland LP, Sherman WH, Latov N, et al. Amyotrophic lateral sclerosis and lymphoma: bone marrow examination and other diagnostic tests. Neurology 1992;42:1101–2.
75. Rubio A, Poole RM, Bara HS, et al. Motor neuron disease and angiotropic lymphoma. Arch Neurol 1997;54:92–5.
76. Mitchell DM, Olczak SA. Remission of a syndrome indistinguishable from motor neuron disease after resection of bronchial carcinoma. BMJ 1979;2:176.
77. Walton NJ, Tomlinson BE, Pearce GW. Subacute "poliomyelitis" and Hodgkin's disease. J Neurol Sci 1968;6:435–45.
78. Schold SC, Cho ES, Somasundaram M, et al. Subacute motor neuronopathy: a remote effect of lymphoma. Ann Neurol 1979;5:271–87.
79. Antoine JC, Mosnier J-F, Absi L, et al. Carcinoma associated paraneoplastic peripheral neuropathies in patients with and without anti-onconeural antibodies. J Neurol Neurosurg Psychiatry 1999;67:7–14.
80. Croft PB, Wilkinson M. The course and prognosis in some types of carcinomatous neuromyopathy. Brain 1969;92:1–8.
81. Campbell MJ, Paty DW. Carcinomatous neuromyopathy: electrophysiological studies. An electrophysiological and immunological study of patients with carcinoma of the lung. J Neurol Neurosurg Psychiatry 1974;37:131–41.
82. Croft PB, Urich H, Wilkinson M. Peripheral neuropathy of sensorimotor type associated with malignant disease. Brain 1967;90:31–66.
83. Peterson K, Forsyth PA, Posner JB. Paraneoplastic sensorimotor neuropathy associated with breast cancer. J Neurooncol 1994;21:159–70.
84. Lisak RP, Mitchell M, Zweiman B, et al. Gullain-Barré syndrome and Hodgkin's disease: three cases with immunological studies. Ann Neurol 1977;1:72–8.
85. Halls J, Bredkjaer C, Friss ML. Gullain-Barré syndrome: diagnostic criteria, epidemiology, clinical course and prognosis. Acta Neurol Scand 1998;78:118–22.
86. Baron KD, Rowland LP, Zimmerman HM. Neuropathy with malignant tumor metastases. Neur Ment Dis 1962;56:10–31.
87. Smitt PS, Posner JB. Paraneoplastic peripheral neuropathy. In: Latov N, Wokke JH, Kelly JJ Jr, editors. Immunological infectious disease of the peripheral nerves. Cambridge: Cambridge University Press; 1998. p. 208–24.
88. Bird SDI, Brown MD, Shy ME, et al. Chronic inflammatory demyelinating polyneuropathy associated with malignant melanoma. Neurology 1996;46:822–4.
89. Kelly JJ Jr. Polyneuropathies associated with myeloma, POEMS, and non-malignant IgG and IgA monoclonal gammopathies. In: Latov N, Wokke JH, Kelly JJ Jr, editors. Immunological infectious disease of the peripheral nerves. Cambridge: Cambridge University Press; 1998. p. 225–37.
90. Horwich MS, Sho L, Proor RS, Posner JB. Subacute sensory neuopathy: a remote effect of carcinoma. Ann Neurol 1977;2:7–19.
91. Kelly JJ Jr, Kyle RA, Latov N. Polyneuropathies associated with plasma cell dyscrasias. Boston: Martinus-Nijhoff; 1987.

92. Johnson PC, Rolak LA, Hamilton RH, et al. Paraneoplastic vasculitis of nerve: a remote effect of cancer. Ann Neurol 1979;5:437–44.
93. Torvik A, Berntzen AE. Necrotizing vasculitis without visceral involvement. Postmortem examination of three cases with affection of skeletal muscles and peripheral nerves. Acta Med Scand 1968;184:69–77.
94. Oh SH, Slaughter R, Harrell L. Paraneoplastic vasculitic neuropathy: a treatable neuropathy. Muscle Nerve 1991;14:152–6.
95. Vincent D, Dubas F, Hauw JJ, et al. Nerve and muscle microvasculitis in peripheral neuropathy: a remote effect of cancer? J Neurol Neurosurg Psychiatry 49:1007–10.
96. Tim RW, Massey JM, Sanders DB. Lambert-Eaton myasthenic syndrome (LEMS). Clinical and electrodiagnostic features and repsponse to therapy in 59 patients. Ann N Y Acad Sci 1998;841:823–6.
97. O'Neil JH, Murray NM, Newson-Davis J. The Lambert-Eaton myasthenic syndrome. A review of 50 cases. Brain 1988;111:577–96.
98. Khurana RK, Koski CL, Mayer RF. Autonomic dysfunction in Lambert-Eaton myasthenic syndrome. J Neurol Sci 1988;85:77–86.
99. Takamori M. An autoimmune channelopathy associated with cancer: Lambert-Eaton myasthenic syndrome. Intern Med 1999;38:86–96.
100. McEvoy KM, Windebank AJ, Daube JR, et al. 3,4-diaminopyridine in the treatment of the Lambert-Eaton myasthenic syndrome. N Engl J Med 1989;321:1567–71.
101. Albin RL, Bromberg MB, Penney JB, Knapp R. Chorea and dystonia: a remote effect of carcinoma. Mov Disord 1988;3:162–9.
102. Dietl HW, Pulst SM, Engelhardt P, Meharaien P. Paraneoplastic brainstem encephalitis with acute dystonia and central hypoventilation. J Neurol 1982;227:22–38.
103. Heckmann JG, Lang CJ, Druschky A, et al. Chorea resulting from paraneoplastic encephalitis. Mov Disord 1997;12:464–6.
104. Schiff DE, Ortega JA. Chorea, eosinophilia, and lupus anticoagulant associated with acute lymphoblastic leukemia. Pediatr Neurol 1992;8:466–8.
105. Batchelor TT, Platten M, Palmer-Toy DE, et al. Chorea as a paraneoplastic complication of Hodgkin's disease. J Neurooncol 1998;36:185–90.
106. Simonetti F, Peergami P, Aktipi KM, et al. Paraneoplastic "rubral" tremor—a case report. Mov Disord 1998;13:12–4.
107. Fahn S, Brin MF, Dwork AF, et al. Case 1: rapidly progressive parkinsonism, incontinence, impotency, and a levodopa-induced moaning in a patient with multiple myeloma. Mov Disord 1996;11:298–310.
108. Golbe LI, Miller DC, Duvoisin RC. Paraneoplastic degeneration of the substantia nigra with dystonia and parkinsonism. Mov Disord 1989;4:147–52.
109. Giometto B, Taraloto B, Graus F. Autoimmunity in paraneoplastic neurological syndromes. Brain Pathol 1999;9:261–73.
110. Scaravilli F, An SF, Groves M, Thom M. The neuropathology of paraneoplastic syndromes. Brain Pathol 1999;9:251–60.
111. Dalmau J, Guletkin SH, Posner JB. Paraneoplastic neurologic syndromes: pathogenesis and physiopathology. Brain Pathol 1999;9:275–84.
112. Lliblau R, Benyahia B, Delattre JY. The pathophysiology of paraneoplastic neurological syndromes. Ann Med Interne (Paris) 1998;149:512–20.
113. Schor NF. Nervous system dysfunction in children with paraneoplastic syndromes. J Child Neurol 1992;7:253–8.
114. Anntoine JC, Absi L, Honnaorat J, et al. Antiamphiphysin antibodies are associated with various paraneoplastic neurological syndromes and tumors. Arch Neurol 1999;56:172–7.
115. Batchelor TT, Platten M, Hochberg FH. Immunoadsorption therapy for paraneoplastic syndromes. J Neurooncol 1998;40:131–6.
116. Blaes F, Strittmatter M, Merkelbach S. Intravenous immunoglobulins in the therapy of paraneoplastic disorders. J Neurol 1999;246:299–303.
117. Darnell RB. The importance of defining the paraneoplastic disorders. N Engl J Med 1999;340:1831–2.
118. Yu Z, Kryzer TJ, Griesmann GE, et al. CRMP-5 neuronal autoantibody: marker or lung cancer and thymoma-related autoimmunity. Ann Neurol 2001;49:146–54.
119. Honnarat J, Byk T, Kusters I, et al. Antibodies to a subpopulation of glial cells and a 66Kda development protein in patients with paraneoplastic neurological syndromes. J Neurol Neurosurg Psychiatry 1996;61:270–78.

23

Future Directions

MICHAEL PRADOS, MD

For many of the diseases described in this monograph, standard approaches result in temporary control of disease, and, clearly, we now are able to identify patients who probably will live a normal life expectancy. For the majority of patients with brain cancer, however, we still need more effective strategies. Fortunately, the pace of research has increased, and we can "translate" these efforts more efficiently than in the past. Within the previous chapters, various research approaches have been described toward the further understanding of the biology, pathology, imaging, and treatment of these diseases. The goal of future research is to accommodate all of these new ideas into treatment plans that are specific for each patient.

One may start with molecular epidemiology to study larger patient groups, correlating observations in those populations with candidate genes and hoping to identify some factor(s) that may influence the development or maintenance of the various brain cancers. If specific factors are found to be common within certain patient subgroups, further research can look more carefully at genetic alterations that may cause biologic change in vitro. These hypotheses can be tested in animal models and, ultimately, in humans. Confirmation of population-based observations that are corroborated with laboratory and clinical research should serve as the basis for future interventions in the clinic. It should be apparent that each tumor type potentially will have many unique molecular events that may result in the initiation of the transformation of a normal cell into a cancer cell. Indeed, many interim steps likely are necessary prior to the development of the malignant phenotype. However complicated this line of investigation may be, this type of research needs to be performed.

Complementary to molecular epidemiology research are the investigations of basic cellular biologists, which help us further understand normal cell biology. Differences between normal and abnormal cellular functions will provide the tumor cell biologist with additional insight concerning dysregulation of cell growth typical of neoplastic cells. The data that will result from the work of the Human Genome Project will be critical in understanding those differences from "normal" gene function. Technology has improved our ability to quickly screen ribonucleic acid (RNA) from tumor and normal tissue to contrast patterns of gene expression. There shortly will come a time when the neuro-oncologist will have unique information about genetic properties of individual tumors. Hopefully, this information will help us to choose therapy specific for each patient.

As molecular and cellular biologists gain more information about cell growth and regulation, data from research into mechanisms important for tumor maintenance are emerging quickly. We now have a much better understanding of the processes involved in angiogenesis and tumor cell migration through the extracellular matrix. Cells need to grow, divide, and move to make space for new cells. This process is an active, dynamic process that requires energy to allow the tumor cell population to survive. Specific inhibitors of the proteins that regulate these events are an important area of research. We now have drugs that prevent invasion and angiogenesis in vitro and in laboratory animal models, and we have begun initial testing in the clinic. Although these drugs are not directly cytotoxic in the classic sense, in modulating these cellular events, they hopefully will effect a "stable" tumor or one that ultimately will die over time.

Laboratory investigations provide the basis for therapeutic interventions. As ideas are formulated in the laboratory, clinical researchers must consider how best to apply this knowledge in designing treatment strategies. Clinical research requires an understanding of both the molecular events that need to be investigated to prove or disprove the laboratory hypothesis and the environment in which that therapy will be carried out. It is not sufficient to know that introduction of wild-type p53 into a tumor cell with a mutated p53 will cause death by apoptosis. One also needs to know how to translate that observation to the treatment of the patient population. How can p53 be delivered to a patient with glioblastoma? How can one detect biologic activity that confirms that tumor cells are changed in situ? Are there nonspecific events that also may occur that either impede or enhance gene transfer? Is gene transfer safe and, if so, how frequently can it be done in a patient? Are there noninvasive ways of following a patient to assess both biologic and antitumor activity? Which patients are the best candidates for this therapy as opposed to the variety of other approaches that surely will be available at the same time?

We have found ourselves in a setting in which new treatment strategies are being developed at such a rapid pace that it is difficult to prioritize these ideas without compromising the research or putting patients at undue risk. Fortunately, there is such a wealth of investigators interested in the many aspects of clinical research that we now are better able to achieve rapid, quality clinical research.

CURRENT STRATEGIES

As mentioned, the pace of laboratory research for central nervous system (CNS) tumors has increased over the past 10 to 15 years, particularly in the area of molecular biology. A greater awareness of specific genetic abnormalities and their cellular consequences gives one hope that this research ultimately will translate into novel, more specific treatment strategies for patients with these disorders. Specific areas of ongoing clinical research include testing of new agents, modulation of resistance to standard chemotherapy agents, inhibitors of growth factors and their receptors, inhibition of angiogenesis and invasion, and gene transfer.

Some of the new drugs currently being tested in phase I or II trials have been described in Chapters 12, 13, and 15 and include O6-benzylguanine, CPT-11 (irinotecan) and other topoisomerase inhibitors, retinoids, new platinum agents, and temozolomide, to name a few. Temozolomide is an analogue of DTIC (dacarbazine) with good oral bioavailability and minimal systemic toxicity. This classic alkylating agent has shown significant activity in patients with recurrent malignant gliomas, particularly anaplastic astrocytomas, and it is undergoing testing in patients with newly diagnosed tumors as well. Future studies will include combinations of temozolomide with other chemotherapy drugs such as CPT-11, carboplatin, *cis*-retinoic acid, and the nitrosoureas. Cellular resistance to temozolomide and other alkylators may occur because of deoxyribonucleic acid (DNA) repair mechanisms, such as alkylquanine DNA-alkyltransferase (AGT). Inhibitors of AGT such as O6-benzylguanine are currently available, and future studies using temozolomide with O6-benzylguanine are being planned.

Drugs that may inhibit the ability of tumors to invade or produce new blood vessels also are being tested. Several inhibitors of angiogenesis have completed phase I and II trials or soon will be tested. Drugs in this category include TNP-470, SU-5416, and thalidomide. Monoclonal antibodies to the vascular endothelial growth factor (VEGF), a factor important in neoangiogenesis, now have become available and hopefully will soon begin phase I testing in brain cancer patients. Inhibitors of enzymes that alter the matrix surrounding tumor cells also are being tested. An oral metalloproteinase inhibitor currently is in clinical trials, both in phase II and III studies, with the goal of reducing the invasive nature of these tumors. Combination studies of angiogenesis inhibitors and anti-invasion drugs soon will begin as well. Inhibition of signal transduction via multiple pathways has become an area of intense research. Inhibition of protein kinase C is one such strategy, and the drugs bryostatin, UCN-01, and tamoxifen are being used in this regard. Testing of flavoperidol and other new drugs should begin this year in an attempt to inhibit cell-cycle progression by regulation of the cyclin-dependent kinase family of genes. Other trials targeting platelet-derived growth factor (PDGR) and fibroblast growth factor (FGF) as substrates for inhibitors of these growth factors also have begun phase I and II testing.

One of the more novel strategies in clinical trials is the use of vectors to help with gene transfer experiments. As molecular biologists identify genes and gene products important in tumor cell biology, virologists have created a number of viral vectors that can be used to deliver those genes to tumor cells. The herpes simplex virus thymidine kinase gene (HSV-TK) was the first gene therapy trials to be used in humans with recurrent malignant brain tumors.[1] In this trial, a retrovirus was used as the vector-producing cell. The goal was to transfer the HSV-TK gene into tumor cells and then treat patients with the antiviral drug ganciclovir. The HSV-TK encodes for the viral enzyme thymidine kinase that phosphorylates ganciclovir. The phosphorylated metabolite is then toxic to the tumor cell. Phase I and II testing has been completed and a phase III study recently closed. Introduction of the gene requires surgical placement of the vector directly into the tumor. Early results of phase I trials show that some patients had regression of tumor, suggesting that gene transfer occurred. However, it is still not clear whether the antitumor effect was specifically due to gene transfer or some other, yet unexplained, effect. A nonspecific inflammatory response is possible as well. A series of new gene therapy trials recently have opened using an adenovirus as the vector for the HSV-TK gene. Finally, a new study just opened with the goal of transferring the p53 gene into tumor cells, again using an adenoviral vector.

Intratumor injection of toxins is another line of research being developed. In this strategy, various toxins are infused into the tumor-bearing area of brain using catheters and pump systems that slowly cause diffusion of the agent over a period of time. To select for tumor cells, the toxin is conjugated to substrates that ideally will only be able to bind to tumor cells rather than to normal brain cells. Various strategies are being developed, including the use of *Pseudomonas* exotoxin conjugated to interleukin-4 (IL-4) or transforming growth factor (TGF)-α. Receptors to both of these factors are expressed highly on tumor cells but not in normal brain cells. Phase I studies are just beginning.

Trials using tumor-specific vaccines also are in progress. In general, tumor cells removed from patients are modified using gene transfer techniques ex vivo, irradiated, and, finally, injected subcutaneously back into the patient. Various cytokines are used to enhance the immune response to the vaccine, such as granulocyte-macrophage colony-stimulating factor (GM-CSF). One variation includes a further step of removing draining regional lymph nodes following subcutaneous vaccination, harvesting, and then ex vivo expansion of autologous "stimulated" lymphocytes, which are then infused back into the patient. Results of these studies are eagerly awaited.

It is beyond the scope of this chapter to discuss all of the many novel ideas being tested in the clinic. Clearly, patients with malignant CNS tumors have many more options for participation in clinical research than was possible several years ago. Referral to specialized centers to discuss these options is highly recommended.

FUTURE CLINICAL INVESTIGATIONS

The following hypothetical protocol is just one example of how clinical research can be conducted for patients with brain cancer. This trial takes into account the need for clinical-laboratory interactions, which are crucial for the understanding of the outcome of the clinical research.

Patient "A" presents with a history of new-onset seizures. He is 35 years old and is found on neuroimaging to have a nonenhancing lesion in the left frontal lobe. A detailed history reveals no obvious family or environmental risk factors, but after informed consent, blood and tumor tissue taken at the time of surgery will be sent to the molecular epidemiologist for current and future studies. One such study may be to investigate genetic instability by assessing for various DNA repair proteins specific for exposure to environmental toxins. The patient then is studied with standard magnetic resonance (MR) imaging that is correlated with MR spectroscopy. A spectral "map" of high-risk areas of brain that are likely to contain tumor is created. At the same time, functional imaging is done to determine the location of motor cortical fibers; these are added to the tumor map. The lesion also is assessed by imaging for blood flow and diffusion characteristics that are used to correlate with the specific histology of the tumor. These data also are used to assess the results of surgery and subsequent therapies. Finally, metabolic imaging using glucose and fluoromisonidazole positron emission tomography (PET) is done, evaluating glucose use and degree of hypoxia within the lesion. At the time of surgery, functional speech and motor mapping are done with the patient awake. Directed tumor biopsies will be taken to correlate with specific areas of abnormality noted on the neuroimaging done preoperatively, and an image-directed tumor resection then is done. Fresh tumor tissue accompanied by normal skin tissue are sent to a tumor bank for future analysis, while other parts of the tumor are sent for routine pathologic diagnosis and assessment of proliferation and apoptotic markers, p53 status, epidermal growth factor receptor (EGFR) expression, PDGF expression, and analysis of other investigational markers. The degree of neovascularity is quantified and correlated with the preoperative imaging data. A diagnosis of oligoastrocytoma is made based on histologic findings, and, because of this diagnosis, specific cytogenetic studies are done to look for chromosomal changes on chromosomes 1 and 19. This analysis suggests that the tumor will likely be responsive to chemotherapy, and the patient is entered into a phase II study using a novel oral chemotherapy drug. Fresh tumor tissue is assayed in vitro for chemosensitivity studies of this and other agents. Additional cytogenetic studies are done to evaluate any patterns that may suggest a specific response to radiation for possible future treatments. Baseline testing of neurocognitive functioning, fatigue, and quality of life is done, and the fatigue/quality-of-life studies are continued throughout treatment as part of the toxicity assessment. Assessment of response is determined by sequential MR imaging and MR spectroscopy. Disease-free survival is correlated with the initial metabolic imaging and tumor marker profile. Patterns of tumor failure also are correlated with these imaging parameters, particularly those of the MR spectroscopy. Neurocognitive changes over time, if any, are compared with those of other patients who enter the study and correlated with tumor location and volume. At the time of tumor progression, a second surgical resection is encouraged, if possible, to obtain tumor tissue for molecular comparision with tissue from the primary lesion. Any molecular genetic changes are correlated with response, progression-free survival, and overall survival for the patients in the protocol. These data are also used to compare results with those of similar studies done at other institutions or by other cooperative groups. Results are published electronically and are automatically distributed to interested investigators. Sequential studies are designed, in part, on the data that come from the phase II trial.

This process of translational research with clinical-laboratory correlation is necessary to understand results of various clinical therapies. It also provides vital human tumor tissue and clinical information for basic and tumor cell biologists to use as they continue their investigations.

CONCLUSION

Although it is clear that brain cancers are a biologically complex, heterogeneous group of highly malignant tumors, there is a great deal of research along many lines of investigation that gives one hope that future therapies will be more successful. Success requires a cooperative effort of many scientists and clinicians and participation by patients in clinical research studies. The reader is encouraged to support this effort.

REFERENCE

1. Ram Z, Culver KW, Oshiro EM, et al. Therapy of malignant brain tumors by intertumoral implantation of retroviral vector-producing cells. Nat Med 1997;3:1354–61.

Index

Page numbers followed by f indicate figure. Page numbers followed by t indicate table.

Abscess, MRI of, 106
Accelerator radiosurgery (SRS), for pituitary adenoma, 181
Acoustic neuromas, 176–179
Acquired immunodeficiency syndrome (AIDS), 121–122, 135
Acute polyradiculoneuropathy (APN), 415–416
Adenocarcinomas, mucin secretion in metastases, 376
Adenomas, pituitary, 134, 179–182
Adenoviruses in gene therapy, 230–231, 233
Adoptive immunotherapy, experimental, 217t
Adrenocorticotropic hormone secretion by pituitary adenoma, 180–181
Age-related factors, 2–4, 5f, 198, 327, 329
AIDS. See Acquired immunodeficiency syndrome
Alkylating agents, in chemotherapy, 196, 198, 200–202
9–Aminocamptothecin, effect on uptake of chemotherapy agents, 196
Amyotrophic lateral sclerosis (ALS) differentiated from PMND, 414
Anaplastic astrocytoma, 29, 108–109, 135–137, 146f, 149–150, 174f, 211–213, 321
Anaplastic ependymoma, 32, 326, 371
Anaplastic meningioma, 19–22, 340–341
Anaplastic oligodendrogliomas, 211, 276
Anaplastic tumors, mixed, 211–213
Anatomy of metastases, 375
Anesthesia, in pediatric surgery, 316
Angiogenesis, 102–103, 227–228
inhibitors of, 205, 275–276
Angiography, magnetic resonance (MRA) of meningiomas, 352–353
Angiomatous meningioma, 340
Anomia, in pediatric surgery, 309
Antacids, effect on uptake of chemotherapy agents, 196
Anthacyclines, in chemotherapy, 203
Antibiotics, in chemotherapy, 203
Antibodies, 205, 217t, 394, 407, 409, 411, 413–414
Anticonvulsants
in chemotherapy, 196–197, 212
for pediatric seizures/epilepsy, 307
Anti-Hu antibody, 407, 409
Anti-inflammatory drugs, 323, 326, 329
Anti-Ma 2 antibody, and limbic encephalitis, 409
Antimetabolites, in chemotherapy, 203
Antineurofilament antibodies, 413–414
Antisense approach in gene therapy, 228f, 229
Anti-YO PCD, 411
Aqueduct of Sylvius, surgical options for, 249–251
Arteriovenous malformations (AVM), post radiosurgery, 188

Astroblastoma, pediatric, 311
Astrocytic tumors, 25–32
glioblastoma multiforme, 39, 93–103, 109–110, 133t, 149–150, 198–199, 213, 219–234, 308f, 321–329
Astrocytoma. See Astrocytic tumors
Ataxia, as pediatric symptom, 321–322
Atypical meningioma, 340, 361t
Autoimmune disorders, noncancer, 407
Autologous stem cell or bone marrow rescue, post chemotherapy, 198
Autonomic neuropathy (AN), 409
Autosomal dominant cancer predisposition syndromes, 100–101
AVM. See Arteriovenous malformations

Bacterial meningitis, 400
Basal cell carcinoma (BCC), Gorlin's syndrome, 81–82
Basic fibroblast growth factor (bFGF), 229
BAT. See Brain adjacent to tumor
BAX gene, 277
BBB. See Blood-brain barrier
BCC. See Basal cell carcinoma
BCNU, 195, 292
interstitial/intratumoral chemotherapy, 199–200
intra-arterial chemotherapy, 198–199
BED. See Biologically effective dose
Behavioral and mental symptoms, 282
β2 receptors, interaction of Cereport with, 198
bFGF. See Basic fibroblast growth factor
Biochemical markers of neoplastic meningitis, 394
Biodegradable polymer wafers, BCNU-impregnated for chemotherapy, 199–200
Biologic agents, tumor management in infants, 322–323
Biologically effective dose (BED), radiosurgery, 169–170
Biology of meningiomas, molecular, 341–342
Biomodulation of specific receptors on BBB, 198
Biopsy, 238–242, 283, 381
pediatric, 311–312, 315–316, 322
Birthmark, See Skin lesions
Blindness, risk factor for, 199, 315–316
Blindness and chemotherapy, 412–413
Blood-brain barrier (BBB), disruption of, 196–198, 205, 378
Blood-CSF barrier, 194–195
Blood-tumor barrier or interface, 196–198
Bone lesions, spinal. See Spinal tumors
Bone marrow transplantation, post chemotherapy, 198
Bone metastases, neoplastic meningitis, 396
Bourneville's disease, 69–75
Brachial neuritis, 416
Brachytherapy, 157–164, 173–174, 272–273, 290–291, 358–359, 383
isotopes, 158

Bradykinin analogue, in chemotherapy, 198
Bragg peak phenomenon, in radiosurgery, 168
Brain adjacent to tumor (BAT), 196
Brain stem encephalitis (BSE), 409
Brain stem tumors, 151, 311–312, 322, 330–331, 409
Brain tumor-polyposis (BTP), 75–78
5–Bromodeoxyuridine (BUdR) labeling index, 280–281
Bronchogenic carcinoma, metastases from, 376
BTP. See Brain tumor-polyposis
BUdR, 280–281
"Bystander effect," 228–229

Calcification in spinal ependymomas, 371
Camptothecin analogues, in chemotherapy, 204
Cancer registries, 4, 13
Capillaries, 23–24, 107
Carbamazepine, in chemotherapy, 205
Carbon-11 methionine, used with PET FDG, 133
Carboplatin, in chemotherapy, 198–199
Carboplatin/thymidine combination for malignant gliomas, 374
Carcinoma-associated-retinal (CAR) antigen, 412–413
Carcinomatous meningitis, 393
Carmustine, in chemotherapy, 195, 198–200, 292
Carotid artery, intra-arterial chemotherapy, 198–199
Cavernous sinus adenoid cystic metastasis, 185f
CCNU. See 1–(2–Chloroethyl)-3–Cyclohexyl-1–Nitrosourea
CDK genes, 99–100, 277
Cell count, CSF studies of leukemic meningitis, 393
Cell cycle
chemotherapy agents specific to, 194
optimizing radiation effects, 169
regulatory pathways, 277
See also Genes and Genetics
Cell migration
discorded congenital, 369–370
kinetic studies showing, 193
leptomeningeal spread of PNETs, 324
and tumor recurrence, 193
See also Intracranial dissemination
Central nervous system (CNS) pharmacology, 193–195
Central neurocytoma, 39–40, 41f
Cephalosporins, for uptake of chemotherapy agents, 197
Cerebellar breast metastasis, radiosurgery, 188
Cerebellar dysfunction or degeneration, 321, 410–412
Cerebellar herniation, pediatric, 306

Cerebral symptoms/signs of leptomeningeal
    metastases, 392t, 393–395
Cerebrospinal fluid (CSF), 373, 410
    cytometric study of neoplastic meningitis,
        392–397
    drainage of, 249–251, 304–307, 312–314,
        316
    drug distribution in chemotherapy,
        194–195, 197, 199
    in limbic encephalitis, 408–409
    total lumbar CSF exams, 392–395
Cereport, in chemotherapy, 198
Cervical laminectomy, pediatric, 313
Cervicomedullary tumors, pediatric, 311–312
Chemical meningitis, postsurgical, pediatric,
    314
Chemicals
    modifiers of radiation, 147–148
    residual, cancer risk factor, 10–12
Chemosensitivity, 195, 276, 323
Chemotherapeutic agents, 194–205, 212–214,
        275–276, 323, 399–401
    cell-cycle-specific, 194
    developmental/experimental, 195–196
Chemotherapy, 323, 329, 373
    BCNU-impregnated biodegradable
        polymer wafers, 199–200
    blindness, risk of, 199
    clinical trials, 211–218, 373–374
    clinical trials and experiments, 199,
        211–218, 292, 323, 326, 329, 373–374
    high-dose, 198
    immunomodulatory strategies, 211
    interstitial/intratumoral drug delivery,
        199–200
    intra-arterial and intrathecal, 198–200
    pediatric options, 312, 322–327
    pre-irradiation for, 374
    with radiosurgery, 174
    with radiotherapy, 193
    toxicity, 194, 196–198, 327, 359–360, 415
Chiasmatic gliomas, optic, 315–316
Childhood. See Pediatric, 303–304
1–(2–Chloroethyl)-3–Cyclohexyl-
    1–Nitrosourea (CCNU), 194–195, 292
Choline, 137, 189
Choline/N-acetylaspartate (NAA), 189
Chondroid chordoma, 45
Chondrosarcoma
    low-grade myxoid, 45
    petrous, 186f
Chordoid meningioma, 340
Chordoma, 44–45, 185f
Chorea, and brain stem signs of SCLC, 417
Choriocarcinoma, 316, 376
Choroid plexus tumors, 116–117, 307
Chromosomes, 17
    in low-grade gliomas, 281
    in astrocytic tumors, 100–102
    in familial syndromes, 49t
    in gene therapy target, 234
    INK4α locus
        in glioblastoma multiforme, 98–99
        in oligodendroglioma, 102
    locus maps for 9p21, 98
    See also Familial syndromes; Gene
        therapy; Genes and Genetics
Chronic inflammatory demyelinating
    polyneuropathy (CIDP), 416
Circle of Willis, 315

Cisplatin, in experimental chemotherapy,
    199, 323, 326, 374
Classification of tumors, 61t, 262–265,
    279–280
Clear cell meningioma, 340
Clinical target volume (CTV) in
    radiotherapy, 144–145
Clonal heterogeneity of tumors, 195
    See also Heterogeneity
CNS. See Central Nervous System
Collapsin response mediator protein (CRMP),
    418
Colloid cyst, 44
Coma, 316
Computed tomography (CT), 104, 131, 133,
        137, 266, 282–284, 304, 349–351,
        366, 375–377, 394–397, 407
    CE-CT, 394–395
    combined CE-CT, 394–395
    combined CT/MR imaging, 283
    combined CT/MRI, 282–284
    CT myelography, 396–397
    vs. MRI of CNS tumors, 104
Concorde position, for pediatric surgery,
    304–305, 313
Congenital cell migration, discorded,
    369–370
Consciousness, altered, 316
Contrast enhanced computed tomography
    (CE-CT), for neoplastic meningitis, 394
Cortex, mapping for pediatric surgery, 304,
    308–311, 314
Corticosteroids
    in chemotherapy, 204–205, 212
    in enhanced MRI, 107
Corticotropin-releasing factor (CRF), 378
Costimulatory molecules, in gene
    immunotherapy, 232
Cowden syndrome (CS), LDD associated
    with, 84–85, 86f
Cranial nerves
    neoplastic meningitis, 396–403
    palsy, as pediatric symptom, 322
Cranial symptoms/signs of leptomeningeal
    metastases, 393t
Craniopharyngioma, 44, 126
    pediatric, 316
Craniotomy or craniectomy, pediatric, 305,
    312, 317
CRF. See Corticotropin-releasing factor
Crossed cerebellar diaschisis, 132
CS. See Cowden syndrome
CSF. See Cerebrospinal fluid
CSF shunting for pediatric surgery, 305, 314,
    316
CTC. See National Cancer Institute Common
    Toxicity Criteria
CTV. See Clinical target volume
Cyclins and cyclin-dependent kinases. See
    Cell cycle; CDK genes; Genes and
    Genetics
Cyclophosphamide
    in chemotherapy, 198
    in pediatric combined drug
        chemotherapy, 323
Cyclosporine, for uptake of chemotherapy
    agents, 197
Cystic tumors
    cavernous sinus adenoid cystic
        metastases, 185f

epidermoid and dermoid, spinal, 369–370
microcystic meningioma, 340
neuroimaging of cystic cerebellar
    astrocytomas, 304–305
pediatric
    brain stem tumors, 311–312, 322,
        329–330
    cerebellar astrocytomas, 302–305
    optic nerve tumors, 315, 328
    pineal, 317
vs. solid tumors, 304
Cystoperitoneal shunt, 305
Cytarabine, in chemotherapy, 203
Cytokine-expressing tumor cells, in gene
    immunotherapy, 232
Cytokines, in clinical trials of chemotherapy,
    216
Cytology of leptomeningeal metastases,
    392–397
Cytomegalovirus (CMV) associated with
    transverse myelitis, 366
Cytoreduction, surgery for, 252–254
Cytosine arabinoside, in pediatric combined
    drug chemotherapy, 323
Cytotoxic agents in systemic chemotherapy,
    194, 196–197
    See also Chemotherapeutic agents
Cytotoxic chemotherapy, 359–360
    See also Chemotherapy
Cytotoxicity. See Toxicity

Decarbazine, for CSF melanoma, 371
Dementia in PCD, 410
Demyelinating disease, MRI of, 106
Deoxyribonucleic acid. See DNA
Dermoid tumors, 123–125, 316, 369–370
Desmoplastic infantile astrocytoma (DIA),
    39
Desmoplastic infantile ganglioglioma (DIG),
    39, 119, 307, 311, 327
Developmental milestones, loss of, 321
Dexamethasone, 196, 304
DIA. See Desmoplastic infantile astrocytoma
Diagnosis, histopathologic review, 211–212
Dibromodulcitol, in pediatric combined drug
    chemotherapy, 329
Diencephalic gliomas, pediatric, 314–316
Diencephalic syndrome in infants, 321–322
Diet, risk factor, 10–12
Differential diagnosis of spinal tumors, 366
Differentiating agents, chemotherapy
    advances using, 205
Diffuse astrocytomas, 280t, 285t, 290
Diffuse gliomas, 311, 322, 330–331
Diffuse intrinsic tumor, pediatric, 311
DIG. See Desmoplastic Infantile
    ganglioglioma
Diplopia in PCD, 410
Disconnection deficit, 317
Discorded congenital cell migration, 369–370
DNA
    $P53$ genetic sequencing, 98f
    repair of
        by fractionation in radiosurgery, 169
        interference with chemotherapy
            agents, 196–197
        by p53 protein, 169
    See also Genes and Genetics
DOPA, fluorine-18–labeled, in PET imaging,
    129–130

Dose
　for brachytherapy, 157
　for chemotherapy, 195–197, 212–214, 323, 360
　NCCTG dose-response trials, 292
　pediatric radiation, 325
　for radiosurgery, 169–170
　for radiotherapy, 143f, 289–290
Dropsy. See Cerebrospinal fluid; Edema
Dura, anesthetizing in pediatric cases, 308
Dural metastases, 396
Dysarthria in PCD, 410
Dysembryoplastic neuroepithelial tumors (DNET), 40–41, 118
　pediatric, 307, 327
Dysnomia, in pediatric surgery, 309

Edema, 249–251, 304–307, 312–314, 316, 378
　See also Hydrocephalus
EDTA. See Ethylenediaminetetraacetic acid
Effective dose. See Biologically effective dose
Efflux systems, agents in PET imaging, 129–130
EGFR. See Epidermal growth factor receptor
Electrocortical mapping, for pediatric surgery, 304, 308–311, 314
Electromyography, for pediatric surgery, 309
Embryonal tumors, 36–39, 123–125, 316
Emesis in children, 321
Encephalopathy, for chemotherapy, 199
Endocrine development, pediatric, 323
Endothelial cells, 102–103, 195f, 196, 371
Enzymes, chemotherapy inhibition by, 197
　See also DNA; Genes and Genetics
EORTC. See European Organization for the Research and Treatment of Cancer
Ependymal tumors
　anaplastic ependymoma, 32–34
　ependymoma, 32–34, 115, 151–152, 307, 312–314, 321, 325–326, 371–372
　subependymoma, 32
Epidemiology, 1–13
　low-grade gliomas, 279
　malignant tumors, 262–265
　metastases, 375
Epidermal growth factor receptor (EGFR)
　amplified proto-oncogene, 101–102
　in antisense gene therapy, 229, 234
　in prognosis for astrocytic tumors, 212
Epidermoid tumors, 123–125, 316, 369–370
Epidural spinal cord compression, 396
Epilepsy, and pediatric tumors, 307–308, 310–311
Epstein-Barr virus (EBV) associated with transverse myelitis, 366
Ethnic variation in primary tumor incidence, 4
Ethylenediaminetetraacetic acid (EDTA), in PET imaging, 129–130
Etoposide in experimental chemotherapy, 203, 323, 374
European Organization for the Research and Treatment of Cancer (EORTC) study of low-grade glioma patients, 285, 287–288, 290–291
EVD. See External ventricular drainage
Exophytic tumors, pediatric, 311–312, 315–316, 322, 328
Expression or Overexpression. See Genes and Genetics

External ventricular drainage (EVD), 249–251, 303–307, 312–314, 316

Facial weakness and nerve function, 178
Failure to thrive, 321–322
Familial adenomatous polyposis (FAP), 77
Familial syndromes, 49t
　APC, hMSH1, and hMLH2 germline mutations, 77, 87
　Familial adenomatous polyposis (FAP), 77
　features common in, 49t
　Gorlin's syndrome, 81–82
　Lhermitte-Duclow disease (LDD), 82–85
　Li-Fraumeni syndrome (LFS), 85–87
　neurofibromatosis, 48–58
　Nevoid basal cell carcinoma syndrome (NBCCS), 81–82
　$PTCH$ in Gorlin's syndrome, 82
　retinoblastoma, 58–64
　risk factors, 6–7
　Sturge-Weber syndrome (SWS), 78–81
　Tuberous Sclerosis (TS) complex, 69–75
　Turcot's syndrome (or BTP), 75–78
　Von Hippel-Lindau (VHL) syndrome, 64–69
FAP. See Familial Adenomatous Polyposis
FDG. See 2–[F-18]fluoro-2–deoxy-D-glucose
Fibrillary astrocytomas, pediatric, 307
Fibrous meningioma, 339
Flow cytometry of metastases, 394–395
2–[F-18]fluoro-2–deoxy-D-glucose (FDG) in PET imaging, 129–140, 377
Foramen of Monro, obstruction of, 44, 249–251, 311
Foramina of Luschka, 313
Fractionated radiotherapy, 147, 169–170
Frameless navigation systems for pediatric brain tumors, 304, 314
Functional cortex, pediatric mapping, 304, 308–311, 314
Functional deficit. See Neurologic deficits

Gadolinium, MRI enhancement, 106–107, 394–395
　See also Magnetic resonance imaging
Gamma knife, in radiosurgery, 168, 170–173
Ganciclovir in gene therapy, 228–229
Gangliocytoma, 39–40f
Gangliogliomas, 39–40f, 117–118, 296, 307, 311, 327
Ganglioneuroma, MRI, 117–118
Gastric acid inhibitors, 196
Gender variables, 282
Gene delivery system, 222t
Gene immunotherapy, 232
Gene therapy, 219–222, 221t, 232–234
　angiogenesis: VEGF as target, 227–228
　antisense approach, 228f, 229
　clinical trial results, 232
　costimulatory molecules, 232
　cytokine-expressing tumor cells, 232
　delivery and vectors, 221–222
　gene transfer protocols, 234t
　immunotherapy, 232
　in infants, 322–323
　metalloproteases, 228
　p53 paradigm, 222–224
　promoters, specific and inducible, 233–234

　Rb pathway, 224–227
　targets in gliomas, 220–221, 222t, 234
　tumor-rejection antigens, 232
　See also Chromosomes; Familial syndromes; Genes and Genetics
Genes and Genetics
　adeno- + HSV-TK gene therapy, experimental, 217t
　angiogenesis in gliomas, 102–103
　APC, hMSH1, and hMLH2 germline mutations, 77, 87
　astrocytic tumors, 93–102
　CDK genes, 99–100, 277
　costimulatory molecules expressed on cell surface, 232
　in diagnosing malignant gliomas, 212
　$EGFR$, amplified, 101
　molecular, of low-grade gliomas, 281–282
　NF1 and NF2, 51–54, 57
　oligodendroglioma, 102
　oncogenes/proto-oncogenes, 93, 101–102
　pBDZR levels in vitro, 139
　prodrug activation, 228–229
　$PTEN$, germline mutation, 100–101
　suicide genes, 228–229
　transcripts encoding p16^{INK} and p19^{ARF}, 98
　tumor-suppressor genes, 93, 96–102, 277
　See also Chromosomes; Familial syndromes; Gene therapy
Germ cell tumors, 42–43
　germinoma, 122, 152–153, 316
　nongerminoma tumors, 153
　pediatric, 316
　teratoma, 123
Germinoma, 122, 152–153, 316
Germline mutation. See Genes and Genetics
GFAP. See Glial fibrillary acid protein
Giant cell astrocytomas, 41, 311
Giant cells in spinal ependymomas, 371
Glial cells ontogeny of, 282
Glial fibrillary acid protein (GFAP) in metastases, 376
Glial tumors, spinal, 371–372
Glioblastoma multiforme (GBM), 29–32, 39, 93–103, 109–110, 133t, 149–150, 198–199, 213, 219–234, 308f, 321, 329
Gliomas, 39–41, 40f, 50–51, 54, 93–103, 94f, 102–103, 131–133, 137, 139, 150–151, 173–175, 198–199, 211–234, 276–277, 279–280, 280t, 282–284, 286t, 291–292, 294–296, 316
　clinical presentation, 282–284
　glioneuronal tumors, mixed, 39–41
　low-grade, 279–299
　malignant, 211–217, 276–277
　management and screening, 279–299
　pediatric tumors, 303–317
　recurrent, 158–162t, 217, 274–275, 296–298
　"secondary GBM," 94–95
Gliomatosis cerebri, MRI, 111
Glioneuronal tumors, 39–41
Glucose metabolism, and PET imaging, 133–134, 139
Glucose transporter (GLUT1), in PET imaging, 129–130
Gorlin's syndrome, 81–82
Grading systems for tumors

EORTC, 285, 287–288, 290–291
Helsinki, 337t
Kernohan, 280t
Ringertz, 280t, 370t
St. Anne/Mayo, 280t, 370t
WHO, 16–17, 50, 93, 262–265, 279–280, 281t, 337t, 370t
Gross tumor volume (GTV) in radiotherapy (external beam), 144–145
Growth and development of children, 321, 323, 331
Growth factors in antisense gene therapy, 229
Growth hormone secretion by pituitary adenoma, 180–181
GTV. See Gross tumor volume
Guanine, DNA repair and chemotherapy, 197

hCHK2, germline mutation in, 87
Hearing loss
  high-frequency, in children, 323
  radiosurgery for acoustic neuroma, 178
"Hedgehog signaling pathway" in Gorlin's syndrome, 82
Hemangioblastomas, 120–121, 182–183, 184t, 372–373
Hemangiopericytoma, 22
Hemispheric tumors, pediatric, 307–311
  large, 324
Hemorrhage in metastases, 376
Hemostasis, postsurgical, pediatric, 314
Hereditary syndromes. See Familial syndromes
Herniation, pediatric, cerebellar, 306
Herpes simplex virus (HSV) in gene therapy, 228–229, 231
Heterogeneity in chemotherapy, 195
Heterozygotes, LOH in glioma, 96–102
Hh-N (sonic hedgehog) ligand, 82
High-frequency hearing loss in children, 323
Hodgkin's disease (HD), 408, 411, 414–417
Hormones
  hypersecretion by pituitary adenoma, 180–182t
  medications for pediatric optic nerve glioma, 316
  receptor antagonists of, in chemotherapy, 359
  risk factors for meningiomas, 335–337
HSV. See Herpes simplex virus
HSV-TK gene in gene therapy, 228–229
Human checkpoint kinase 2 (hCHK2), 87
Hydrocephalus
  pediatric, 304, 312, 314, 321
  surgery to relieve, 249–251
Hydroxyurea, in chemotherapy
  pediatric combined drug trials, 323
  spinal progressive recurrent meningiomas, 374
Hyperthermia, use with brachytherapy, 157–158
Hypertonic mannitol solutions, to open BBB, 197–198
Hyperventilation to relieve ICP, 378
Hypothalamic dysfunction, 316
  pediatric, 321
Hypothalamic gliomas, optic, 315–316
Hypothalamic-chiasmatic tumors, pediatric, 322
Hypothalamic-optic tumors, pediatric, 327

Hypothermia during pediatric surgery, 303
Hypoxia agents, in PET imaging, 129t, 132

ICP. See Increased intracranial pressure
  See also Symptoms
Ifosfamide, in chemotherapy for aggressive meningeal tumors, 374
IGF. See Insulin-like growth factor
Immobilization mask for CNS irradiation, 143–144f
Immunohistochemistry of low-grade gliomas, 282
Immunotherapy, genetic, 232
Implants, interstitial brachytherapy, 157–164, 291
IMRT. See Intensity-modulated radiotherapy
Increased intracranial pressure (ICP)
  in metastases, 378
  pediatric, 303
  See also Cerebrospinal fluid; External ventricular drainage; Symptoms
Infants, 307, 321–325
  See also Pediatric
Infarcts, focal hyperintensity on MRI, 105–106
Infection
  mimicking spinal cord tumor, 366–367
  as pediatric symptom, 322
  as risk factor, 12
Influx systems, agents in PET imaging, 129–130
Infratentorial ependymomas, pediatric, 313
Inherited syndromes. See Familial
INK4α locus
  in glioblastoma multiforme, 98–99
  in oligodendroglioma, 102
Insulin-like growth factor (IGF), 229
Intensity-modulated radiotherapy (IMRT), 167
Interferon, in clinical trials of chemotherapy, 216
Interferon β, chemotherapy advances using, 205
Interleukin-2, in clinical trials of chemotherapy, 216
Interstitial brachytherapy. See Brachytherapy
Interstitial drug delivery in chemotherapy, 199–200
Intra-arterial chemotherapy, 198–199
Intracavitary IL-2 and LAK cell therapy, 217t
Intracranial dissemination, 307, 314–316, 324, 326, 374
  See also Cell migration
Intracranial hypertension, 306
Intra-CSF chemotherapeutic administration, 399–401
Intradural extramedullary tumors, 368–371
Intralumbar intra-CSF chemotherapeutic administration, 399–401
Intramedullary astrocytomas, 371–372
Intrathecal chemotherapy, 200
Intratumoral drug delivery in chemotherapy, 199–200
Intraventricular lesions, 314
Intrinsic pontine gliomas, pediatric, 322
Invasion of gliomas by metalloproteases, 228
Ionizing radiation
  DNA damage due to, 169
  as risk factor for tumors, 7–9

Irinotecan, in chemotherapy, 204, 212, 373–374
Irritability as symptom in children, 321
Isotopes for interstitial brachytherapy, 158

Juvenile pilocytic astrocytoma (JPA), 321–322, 326–328

Karnofsky Performance Scale (KPS), 291–292, 378
72-kDa gelatinase-A (MMP-2), in gene therapy, 228
92-kDa gelatinase-A (MMP-9), in gene therapy, 228
Keratin squamous cell carcinoma, metastases, 376
Kernohan grading system for tumors, 280t, 370t
Kinases in gene therapy, 228–229
KPS. See Karnofsky Performance Status

Lambert-Eaton syndrome (LES), 406, 417
Laminectomy
  for medulloblastoma, pediatric, 306
  for spinal tumors, 373
Language deficits in pediatric cases. See Mutism
  See also Neurologic deficits
Lateral medullary velum, 313
LDD. See Lhermitte-Duclow disease
LE. See Limbic encephalitis
Leksell Gamma Knife systems for radiosurgery, 168, 170–173
Leptomeningeal disease
  nodular, 396
  pediatric
    relapse, 307
    spread of PNETs, 324
Leptomeningeal metastases
  diagnosis, laboratory tests for, 392–395
  incidence of, 391
  prognosis and survival, 402t
  symptoms of, 392–395
  treatment modalities, 397t
  See also Neuroplastic meningitis
Lesions
  in familial syndromes, 49t
  intraventricular, pediatric ependymoma, 314
  NF1, common for, 54t
  pediatric astrocytoma, 305
  pediatric pineal tumor, 317
  supratentorial, pediatric ependymoma, 312–313
Lethargy as symptom in children, 321
Leukemia associated with APN, 415–416
Leukemic meningitis, CSF studies of metastases, 393
LFS. See Li-Fraumeni syndrome
Lhermitte-Duclow disease (LDD), 82–85, 84t
Li-Fraumeni syndrome (LFS), 85–87
Limbic encephalitis (LE), 408–409
LINAC. See Linear accelerator
LINAC accelerator radiosurgery (SRS), for pituitary adenoma, 181
LINAC stereostatic radiotherapy (SRT), for pituitary adenoma, 181
Linear accelerator (LINAC)-based systems for radiosurgery, 167–168

Lipomas, 316, 370
Lipophilic alkylating agent, for chemotherapy, 197
Liposomes, as gene therapy vectors, 222
See also Gene therapy
Lobradamil, in chemotherapy, 198
Location of meningiomas, 334
LOH, See Loss of heterozygosity
Lomustine, for chemotherapy, 194–195, 292, 323, 329
Long tract signs, as pediatric symptom, 322
Loss of heterozygosity (LOH), 96–102
Lumboperitoneal shunt, 305
Lung cancer, 414–415
Lymphoma, 42–43f, 135
   AIDS-related, 135
   MRI of PLCNS, 121–122
   pediatric, 322
   PET imaging, 135
   systemic chemotherapy, 197
Lymphomatous meningitis, CSF studies of metastases, 393
Lymphoplasmacyte-rich meningioma, 340

Ma2 antigens and limbic encephalitis, 408–409
MAb. See Monoclonal antibodies
mAChR, See Muscarinic cholinergic receptor
Magnetic resonance angiography (MRA), 352–353
Magnetic resonance imaging (MRI), 104, 106–120, 123–126, 131, 133, 137, 213, 282–284, 351–352, 366, 375–377, 394–395, 408
   combined CT/MR imaging, 283
   pediatric, 304, 310f, 311, 313, 315, 317, 321–325, 327–328
   radiation necrosis, 107–108
   sensitivity and lesion localization, 104
   specificity, lack of, 105–106
Magnetic resonance spectroscopy (MRS), 108, 377
Magnetic resonance venography (MRV), 352–353
Malignant tumors, 211–213, 307, 321, 323, 340–341, 360–361
   alternative strategies, 216–217t
   cellular adoptive immunotherapy, 216
   chemotherapy, 215–216, 274–276
   classification and grading of, 61t, 93, 262–265
   clinical presentation of, 265–266
   diagnostic neuroimaging, 266–267
   epidemiology, 262–265
   etiology of, 279
   gene therapy strategies for, 216
   hisopathology, 211–213
   management and screening, 262–277
   molecular pathogenesis, 276–277
   newly diagnosed, research strategies, 215t, 217t
   pathogenesis, 276–277
   PNETs, 324
   radiation and surgical strategies, 214–215
   terminal care, 276
Mannitol, 197–198, 378
Mass effect, radiation-related increase, 164
Matrix metalloproteinases, chemotherapy advances using, 205, 275
Maximum tolerated dose (MTD)
   for chemotherapy, 196–197, 212–214
   for radiosurgery, 168
Mechlorethamine, in pediatric combined drug chemotherapy, 323
Medulloblastoma
   MRI, 119–120
   pediatric, 306–307, 323
   radiotherapy (external beam), 152
Melanocytic lesions, 24–25
Melanoma
   metastases from, 376
   primary spinal, 370–371
Memory loss, 316
Meningeal sarcomatosis, 24
Meningiomas, 16–25, 120–121, 154–155f, 175–176, 249, 316, 333–334, 341–342, 348–353, 360–361, 368
   clinical presentation, 342–348
   Grade I: nonrecurrent with aggressive growth, 338–340
   Grades II and III: having aggressive behavior, 340–341
   grading and macro- or microscopic features, 337–338
   management, PET role in, 133–134
   pathology, 337–341
   radiation-induced, 334–335
   recurrence, 337t
   treatment options, 353–360
Meningitis
   bacterial, 400
   neoplastic, 391–403
Meningothelial meningioma, 338
Mental symptoms of low-grade glioma, 282
Mesenchymal chondrosarcoma, 24
Mesenchymal nonmeningothelial tumors, 22
Metabolic agents. See Drugs
Metabolism
   radiopharmaceuticals, 129–132, 139
   sedation, 138–139
   and PPN, 415
Metalloproteases in gene therapy, 228
Metaplastic meningioma, 340
Metastases, 61, 126, 135, 154–155, 185f, 186–188, 307, 376–378, 387–388
   anatomy of, 375
   clinical presentation, 376
   diagnosis, 376–377
   edema and intracranial pressure, 378
   epidemiology of, 375
   pathology of, 375–376
   seizures, 378
   treatment
      chemotherapy, 387
      medical management, 378
      radiosurgery, 386–387, 388t
      radiotherapy, 378–383, 385–386
      surgery, 383–385
Methohexital, 308
Methotrexate, in chemotherapy, 203
Methylating agents, in chemotherapy, 196
Methylprednisone, in pediatric combined drug chemotherapy, 323
Microcystic meningioma, 340
Mitoses in spinal ependymomas, abnormal, 371
MM. See Malignant meningiomas
MMAC genes as gene therapy targets, 234
MMP-2. See 72-kDa gelatinase-A
MMP-9. See 92-kDa gelatinase-A
Molecular targets in gene therapy, 220–222t, 234
Monoclonal antibodies (MAb), in chemotherapy, 205, 217t
Mononeuritis multiplex and vasculitis, 416
MOP, See Nitrogen mustard/vincristine/procarbazine regimen
Morbidity, avoidance of, 179, 304–305, 311, 314, 316
Mortality rates, 2–5
   age-related, 5f, 198
   of chemotherapy patients, 193, 195, 198, 212
   metabolism-related, 132
   of radiosurgery patients, 174–175, 187t
Motor cortex, pediatric surgery issues, 308–309
See also Sensitivity mapping
Motor neuron dysfunction, 414–415, 417
MRI. See Magnetic resonance imaging
MRS. See Magnetic resonance spectrography
MTS-1, in mapping chromosome 9p21, 98
Mucin secretion in adenocarcinomas, metastatic, 376
Multicentric optic gliomas, 315
Multidrug resistance-associated protein (MRP), resistance to chemotherapy agents, 196–197
Multiple sclerosis, MRI of, 106
Muscarinic cholinergic receptor (mAChR), levels in gliomas, 139
Mutation. See Genes and Genetics
Mutism in pediatric cases, 305–307, 309
Myasthenia gravis, associated with thymoma, 417
Myelitis, in conjunction with brain stem encephalitis, 409
Myelography
   of neoplastic meningitis, 396–397
   of the spine, pediatric, 322
Myeloma, 197, 415–416
Myelosuppression, treatment of, 198
Myxoid chondrosarcoma, low-grade, 45
Myxoid degeneration in spinal ependymomas, 371

N-acetylaspartate (NAA), 137, 377
National Cancer Institute Common Toxicity Criteria, 212
NBCCS. See Nevoid Basal Cell Carcinoma syndrome
NCCTG. See North Central Cancer Treatment Group
NCI. See National Cancer Institute
Necrosis
   in brachytherapy, 164
   in metastases, 375–376
   MRI, effect on, 107–108
   polymers in chemotherapy causing, 164
   in spinal ependymomas, 371
Neoplastic meningitis (NM), 391–397
   autopsy studies of, 391, 396–397
   chemotherapy, 399–401
   radiotherapy, 397–399
   surgery, 399
   symptomatic therapy, 401
   symptoms and signs of, 392–395
Nerve root compression, spinal tumor causing, 365
Nerve sheath tumors, spinal, 368–369

Neurilemoma, 41–42, 43f
Neurocytoma, central, 39–40, 41f
Neuroectodermal tumors, primitive (PNET)
  MRI, 119–120
  pediatric, 311
  radiotherapy, 152
Neuroepithelial tumor, dysembryoplastic, 40–41
Neurofibromas, spinal, 369
Neurofibromatosis
  optic pathway tumors, 315–316
  type 1, 48–54, 322, 327–328
  type 2, 54–58, 180
Neuroimaging, 266–267
  of brain stem gliomas, 331
  of cystic cerebellar astrocytomas, 304–305
  diagnostic, 266–267
  low-grade gliomas, 304–305
Neurologic deficit/deterioration
  in brachytherapy, 164
  in chemotherapy, 200
  cognitive and developmental, 331
  disconnection deficit, 317
  fatal, in SSN-EMN, 407
  growth and development, 321–323
  hearing loss, high-frequency, 323
  low-grade glioma, 284
  mutism and pharyngeal dysfunction, 305–307, 309
  vision deficit, 315–316
  See also Morbidity; Necrosis
Neurologic morbidity, avoidance of, 304–305, 311, 314, 316
Neuromas, acoustic, 176–179
Neuromuscular junction disorders, 417
Neuronal primary tumors, 39–41
  central neurocytoma, 39–40, 41f
  DIA and DIG, 39, 41f
  dysembryoplastic neuroepithelial tumor, 40–41
  gangliocytoma and ganglioma, 39–40f
  giant cell astrocytoma, subependymal, 41
Neuro-oncology, 213–214, 331
Neuropathy of SSN-EMN, 407
Neurotoxicity. See Toxicity
Nevoid Basal Cell Carcinoma syndrome (NBCCS), 81–82
NF1 and NF2. See Neurofibromatosis
Nirtosoureas, in chemotherapy, 197, 199–201
Nitrogen mustards, in chemotherapy, 202
Nitrogen mustard/vincristine/procarbazine (MOP) regimen, 292
Nongerminoma germ cell tumors, 153
Non-Hodgkin's lymphoma, 414–416
Non-ionizing radiation, risk factor, 7–9
Nonpapillary anaplastic meningioma, 19–22
Nuclear polymorphism in spinal ependymomas, 371
Nutritional causes of PPN, 415

O^6Benzylguanine, effect on uptake of chemotherapy agents, 197
Observation, 284–286
Occlusion of artery, radiation-induced, 164
Occupational risk factors, 9–10
Ocular toxicity in chemotherapy, 199
OEF. See Oxygen extraction
OER. See Oxygen extraction
Oligoastrocytomas
  pediatric, 326–327
  survival rates, 285t
Oligodendrogliomas, 34–36, 211–213
  choroid plexus tumors, 35–36
  mixed gliomas, 35
  MRI, 114–115
  pathogenesis of, 102
  pediatric, 307, 326–327
  radiotherapy (external beam), 150–151
  survival rates (WHO rate II), 285t
Ommaya reservoirs, for intrathecal chemotherapy, 200
Oncogenes, 93
  chromosomal markers for, 102
  down regulation, in gene therapy, 228f, 229
  proto-oncogenes, 93, 101–102
Ontogeny of glial cells, 282
Ophthalmologic features of familial syndromes, 49t
Opsoclonus myoclonus (OM), 413–414
Optic gliomas, pediatric, 314–316
Optic pathway glioma (OPG), 49t, 50–51, 54
Optic tract tumors, pediatric, 322
  chiasmatic, 328
  hypothalamic, 327
Oral delivery of chemotherapeutic agents, 194
Osmotherapy to relieve ICP, 378
Osmotic diuretics, for pediatric surgery, 313
Oxygen extraction, in PET
  fraction (OEF), 131
  rate of (OER), 130–131
Oxygen metabolism agents, in PET imaging, 129t, 131–132
Oxygenation/reoxygenation, optimizing radiation effects, 169

$P53$ gene, 277
  advances in research, 423
  DNA sequencing, 98f
  gene therapy paradigm, 222–224
  in $P53/MDM2/ARF$ pathway, 96–99
  in prognosis for astrocytic tumors, 212
P glycoprotein (Pgp)
  inhibition of, 197
  resistance to chemotherapy agents, 195–197
Paclitaxel, in chemotherapy, 196–197, 204, 212
Papillary meningiomas, 340
  anaplastic, 19–22
Paraneoplastic motor neuron disorders (PMND), 414–415
Paraneoplastic peripheral neuropathy (PPN), 415
Paraneoplastic syndromes, 406–418
Paraneoplastic visual syndromes, 412–413
Parenchyma
  chemotherapeutic drug distribution, 194–195
  infiltration by low-grade tumors, 283–284
Parenchymal brain metastases, 396
Pareneocoplastic opsoclonus-myoclonus (POM), 417
Parental exposure, risk factor, 10–12
"Park bench position," for pediatric surgery, 317
Pathogenesis
  astrocytic tumors, 93–96
  low-grade gliomas, 279
  malignant, 276–277
  oligodendroglioma, 102
Pathology
  meningiomas, 337–341
  metastases, 375–376
  neoplastic meningitis, 395–396
Pathophysiology
  of angiogenesis in gliomas, 102–103
  of neoplastic meningitis, 395–396
pBDZR. See Peripheral benzodiazepine receptor
PCD. See Progressive cerebellar degeneration
PCV (Procarbazine/CCNU/Vincrisine) regimen, 292
PDGF and PDGFR. See Platelet-derived growth factor
Pediatric tumors, 212, 294–296, 303–331, 382, 413–414
  risk factors, 8t, 10–12
  surgical considerations, 303–317
  survival patterns and rates, 198, 282, 290–291, 294–296
Peptide risk factors for meningiomas, 335–337
Perfusion agents, in PET imaging, 130–131
Periosteal patch, 314
Peripheral benzodiazepine receptor (pBDZR), levels in gliomas in vitro, 139
Peripheral stem cell transplantation, post chemotherapy, 198
Perivascular rosettes, in spinal ependymomas, 371
Permeability, in chemotherapy drug delivery, 194–200
PET. See Positron emission tomography
Petrous chondrosarcoma, 186f
Pharmacology
  of chemotherapy agents, 200–205
  of the CNS, 193–195
  neuro-oncology, dynamic and kinetic studies, 213
  radiopharmaceuticals in PET imaging, 129–131
Pharyngeal dysfunction in pediatric cases, 305–307, 309
Phenytoin, in chemotherapy, 205
Photodynamic therapy using porfimer sodium, 217t
Photon irradiation for radiosurgery, 169
Pilocytic astrocytomas, 26–27, 111–112, 146f, 295–296
  alternate radiation options, 290–291
  pediatric, 307, 311–312
P-450–inducing anticonvulsants, effect on uptake of chemotherapy agents, 196–197
Pineal region tumors
  pediatric, 316–317, 324
  radiotherapy (external beam), 152–154
Pinealomas, 134–135, 316
Pineoblastomas, 119, 154, 316, 324
Pineocytomas, 119, 154, 249, 316
Pituitary adenomas, 125, 134, 179–182
Planning target volume (PTV) in radiotherapy (external beam), 144–145
Plasma cell dyscrasia, neuropathies associated with, 416
Plasma levels of drugs, anticonvulsant effect on, 205

Platelet-derived growth factor (PDGF), 101–102
  receptor (PDGFR), 229, 275
Platinum agents in chemotherapy, 201–202, 326
PLCNS. See Primary lymphoma of the central nervous system
Pleomorphic xanthoastrocytoma (PXA), 27–29, 112, 294, 296, 307, 311, 327
Ploidy studies of low-grade gliomas, 280–281
P53/MDM2/ARF pathway, 96–99
  See also Tumor suppressor genes
PNET. See Primitive neuroectodermal tumors
Polymer wafers, BCNU-impregnated for chemotherapy, 199–200
Polyneuropathy, organomegaly, endocrinopathy, M protein, and skin changes (POEMS), 416
POM. See Pareneoplastic opsoclonus-myoclonus
Pontine glioma, astrocytic, 25–26
Positron emission tomography (PET), 108, 129, 138–140, 189
  astrocytoma, low-grade, 297
  glioma, 131–133, 137, 213, 297–298
  meningioma, management of, 133–134
  metastases, 377
  miscellaneous cerebral tumors, 134–137
  oligdendroglioma, low-grade, 297
  oligoastrocytoma, mixed, 297
  pediatric imaging, 137–139, 322
Post radiosurgery imaging (PRI), 188
Posterior cerebral aqueduct, 313
Posterior fossa tumors, pediatric, 312
Postoperative cerebellar mutism syndrome, 305–307
Pregnancy risk factors for meningiomas, 335–337
Prenatal exposure to pesticide, 11
Pressure atrophy in spinal ependymomas, 371
Primary lymphoma of the central nervous system (PLCNS), MRI of, 121–122
Primary spinal melanoma, 370–371
Primitive neuroectodermal tumors (PNET), 322
  MRI of, 119–120
  pediatric, 311, 321, 324–325
  radiotherapy for, 152
Procarbazine, 323, 326, 329
  in chemotherapy, 198, 200–202
  oral delivery in chemotherapy, 194
Procarbazine/CCNU/Vincrisine (PCV) regimen, 292
Prodrug activation in gene therapy, 228–229
Prognosis factors for metastases, 377–378
  See also Survival patterns
Progression of metastases, randomized trial of WBRT, 381
Progressive cerebellar degeneration (PCD), 410–412
Prolactin secretion by pituitary adenoma, 181, 183f
Prolactinomas, PET imaging, 134
Proliferation index for meningiomas, 338
Proliferation studies, 280–281
Promoters, specific and inducible for gene therapy, 233–234
Proteases in gene therapy, 228–229

Proteins
  and chemotherapy drug resistance, 195–197
  in familial syndromes, 49t
  GFAP in metastases, 376
  growth factors in antisense gene therapy, 229
Proton beam stereotactic radiotherapy, for pituitary adenoma, 181
Proton irradiation
  in radiosurgery, 167–189
  treatment facilities in U.S., 169
  vs. photon irradiation, 169
Proto-oncogenes, 93, 101–102
Psammomatous meningioma, 340
PSC833 cyclosporine analogue, for uptake of chemotherapy agents, 197
Pseudomeningocele indicating CSF diversion, 305, 314
PTCH gene, inactivated, 82
PTEN tumor-suppressor gene, 100–101
  as gene therapy target, 234
  germline mutation, 100–101
Ptosis, 316
PTV. See Planning target volume
Purkinje cells, loss of, 410–411

Radiation
  DNA damage due to, 169
  photon vs. proton irradiation, 169
  as risk factor, 7–9
  risk factors for meningiomas, 334–335
Radiation necrosis, 107–108, 164, 175f, 182, 249f
Radiation-induced meningiomas, 334–335
Radiobiology of radiosurgery, 169–170
Radiographic features
  Lhermitte-Duclow disease, 84
  meningiomas, 348–349
  neurofibromatosis, type 1, 51
  retinoblastoma, 62
  Sturge-Weber syndrome, 79
  Tuberous Sclerosis complex, 71
Radiology of meningiomas, 348–353
Radionuclide in meningitis studies, 394–395
Radiopharmaceuticals in cerebral tumor imaging, 129–131
Radiopharmaceuticals in PET imaging, 129–131
Radiosensitivity of pediatric PNETs, 325
Radiosurgery, 173–186, 273–274
  Bragg peak phenomenon, 168
  complications, 188–189
  delivery systems, 168–169
  facilities in U.S., 168
  fractionated radiotherapy vs., 169–170
  gamma knife system (Leksell), 168, 170–173
  for low-grade gliomas, 290–291
  metastases, 186–188, 386–387
    with/without WBRT, 388t
  morbidities avoided with, 179
  MTD, 168
  pediatric options for, 329
  radiobiology of, 169–170
  repeat time for malignant vs. benign tumors, 173
  side effects, 173
  with whole-brain radiotherapy, 188
Radiotherapy, 142–155, 271–272

  after spinal tumor surgery, 373
  anaplastic astrocytoma and glioblastoma multiforme, 146f, 149–150
  brain stem glioma, 151
  CTV, GTV and PTV definition, 144–145
  dose distribution, 143f
  ependymoma, 151–152
  fractionated radiotherapy, 145, 147, 169t
  imaging and simulation, 144
  low-grade astrocytoma and oligodendroglioma, 150–151
  for low-grade gliomas, 287–289t
    dose and volume considerations, 289–290
  medulloblastoma and primitive neuroectodermal tumor, 152
  meningiomas, 154–155f, 334–335
  metastases, 154–155
  patient assessment and immobilization, 143–144
  pediatric options, 312, 322–324
    delay of radiotherapy, 323
    for ependymomas, 326
    for high-grade astrocytomas, 329
    for low-grade gliomas, 329
    for pineal tumors, 317
    for PNETs, 324–325
  pineal region
    germinoma, 152–153
    nongerminoma germ cell tumor, 153
    pineocytoma and pineoblastoma, 154
  primary CNS lymphoma, 154
  radiation, 147–148
  spinal canal, 154–155
  toxicity, 148–149
  treatment planning and delivery, 145–147
  vs. radiosurgery, 169t
Radiotherapy, whole-brain
  for metastases, 378–383
  postoperative, 385–386
RB. See Retinoblastoma
Rb function, loss of, 99–100, 277
Rb pathway, 277
  in gene therapy, 224–227
  Rb1/INK4α/CDK4/CDK6 pathway, 99–100
Receptors of PDGF, TGF-ß and VEGF, 102–103, 275–276
Recurrence of metastases, randomized trial of WBRT, 381
Recurrent tumors
  astrocytomas, pediatric, 307
  brachytherapy, 158–162t
  chemotherapy, 217, 274–275
  ependymomas, pediatric, 314
  low-grade, 296–298
  malignant, 158–162t, 217, 274–275
  PET imaging, 297–298
  PNET, pediatric, 325, 328–329
Recursive partitioning analysis (RPA) of metastases, 377–378
Reese-Ellsworth classification of retinoblastoma, 61t
Regional heterogeneity of tumors, 195
Registries, use of, 4, 13
Re-irradiation after WBRT, for recurrent metastases, 383
Renal cell carcinoma, metastases from, 376
Reovirus (human), in gene therapy, 232
Repair enzymes inhibited by chemotherapy, 197

Resection, surgery for, 242–245, 254–260
Retinoblastoma (RB), 58, 62–63
　clinical features, 58–61
　genetics, 63–64
　management and screening, 64
　metastatic, 61
　presenting signs of, 61t
　radiographic features, 62
　Reese-Ellsworth classification of, 61t
　trilateral, 61–62
　See also Familial syndromes
Retinoblastomas, 58–61
Rhabdoid meningioma, 340
Ribonucleic acid, advances in therapy, 422
Ringertz grading system for tumors, 280t, 370t
Risk factors
　for cancer, 5–13, 282, 325, 334–337
　for treatment and therapy, 7–9, 199, 290, 334–335
　for treatment and therapy, pediatric, 305–307, 309, 315–316, 321–323, 326, 331
　See also Familial syndromes; Survival patterns
RMP-7, in chemotherapy, 198
RNA, advances in therapy, 422
Rolandic cortex, identification of, 309
　See also Sensitivity mapping
RPA. See Recursive partitioning analysis
RTOG clinical trials for low-grade tumors
　chemotherapy, 292
　radiotherapy, 290

Sacral myxopapillary ependymoma, 371
Sacrococcygeal region teratomas, 370
Saint Anne-Mayo grading system for tumors, 280t, 370t
Schwannoma-derived growth factor (SDGF), 229
Schwannomas, 41–42, 43f, 55
　radiosurgery, 180f
　radiosurgery treatment, 176–179
　SDGF in antisense gene therapy, 229
SDGF. See Schwannoma-derived growth factor
"Secondary GBM," 94–95
Secretory meningioma, 340
Sedation and metabolism in PET imaging, 138–139
Seizures
　and metastases, 378
　as pediatric symptoms, 307–308, 310–311, 321
　as risk factors
　　for cancer, 12
　　in chemotherapy, 212
Sella
　expanded, with pediatric optic nerve glioma, 315
　sellar chordoma, 185f
Sensory loss, in SSN-EMN, 407
Sensory-motor neuropathy, subacute, 415
Sex hormones and meningiomas, 335–337
Side effects
　of anticonvulsants, 205
　of camptothecin analogues, 204
　of radiosurgery, 173, 188–189
　of steroids, 205
Signal-transduction inhibitors in chemotherapy, 205, 275–276

Simulation, radiotherapy (external beam), 144
Single photon emission computed tomography (SPECT), 189, 297
　of metastases, 377
Sjögren's disease, MRI, 121–122
Skin lesions in familial syndromes, 49t
Skull base neoplasm, malignant, radiosurgery treatment, 183–186
Small cell lung cancer (SCLC), 406–408
　and anti-Hu antibody, 409
　and LES, 417
Small-cell glioblastoma, 39
Somatosensory evoked potentials (SSEP), 309
"Sonic hedgehog" (Hh-N) ligand, 82
Sonogram and sononavigation, for pediatric cases, 304, 308, 310–312
SPECT. See Single photon emission computed tomography
Speech mapping. See Stimulation/sensitivity mapping
Spinal canal, radiotherapy of, 154–155
Spinal neurophysiologic monitoring of sensory and motor pathways, 312
Spinal symptoms/signs of leptomeningeal metastases, 393t
Spinal tumors, 365–373
　clinical presentation, 365–366
　conditions mimicking, 366–368
　differential diagnosis, 366–373
　imaging, 366
　neuroplastic meningitis, 391–403
　treatment, 373–374
Spirohydantoin mustard, for chemotherapy, 197
SSN-EMN. See Subacute sensory neuronopathy-encephalomyeloneuritis
Stem cell transplantation, post chemotherapy, 198
Stereostatic radiotherapy (SRT), for pituitary adenoma, 181
　See also Radiotherapy
Steroids
　effect on MRI contrast enhancement, 106–107
　effect on uptake of chemotherapy agents, 196
　preoperative use, pediatric, 306
　side effects of, 205
Stimulation/sensitivity mapping of pediatric tumors, 304, 308–311, 314
Stroke, risk in chemotherapy, 199
Sturge-Weber syndrome (SWS), 78–80
　clinical features, 78–79
　management, 80–81
　radiographic features, 79
Subacute sensory neuronopathy-encephalomyeloneuritis (SSN-EMN), 407–408
　relating to autonomic neuropathy, 409
　relating to Hodgkin's disease, 408
Subacute sensory-motor neuropathy (SSMN), 415
Subcortical pathways, mapping for pediatric surgery, 304, 308–311, 314
Subendymal giant cell astrocytomas
　pediatric, 307, 311
Subependymal giant cell astrocytoma, 41
Subependymal giant cell astrocytomas, 41, 112, 311

　pediatric, 311
Subependymomas, 115–116
Suicide genes, 228–229
Supportive care agents used for chemotherapy, 204–205
Supratentorial ependymomas, pediatric, 313–314
Supratentorial lesions, pediatric, 312–313
Supratentorial low-grade gliomas, 279–299
Supratentorial primitive neuroectodermal tumors, pediatric, 324
Surgery, 269–271
　biopsy, 238–242
　brachytherapy, 157–164
　for cytoreduction, 252–254
　delivery of adjuvant treatments, 251–252
　EVD, 249–251
　for intramedullary tumors, 272
　for low-grade gliomas, 286–287
　for metastases, 383–385
　　gross-total vs. subtotal, 385
　　randomized clinical trials, 386t
　　with/without WBRT, 385–386
　pediatric, 303–317, 322
　　complications of hypothermia, 303
　　craniotomy or craniectomy, 305
　　epilepsy/seizures, 307–308, 310–311
　　EVD, 303–307
　　for high-grade astrocytoma, combined therapy, 329
　　for low-grade glioma, 327
　　morbidity, avoidance of, 304–305, 311, 314, 316
　　mutism and pharyngeal dysfunction, 306–307
　　neuroimaging and neurosurgery, 303–304
　　optic and diencephalic gliomas, 314–316
　　for PNETs, 324–325
　　stimulation/sensitivity mapping, 304, 308–311, 314
　　with/without radiation, for ependymomas, 326
　to relieve symptoms, 245–249
　resection, 242–245
　　improving extent of, 254–260
　　in supratentorial low-grade gliomas, 286t
　of spinal tumors, 373–374
Survival patterns and rates
　age-related, 5f, 198
　of chemotherapy patients, 193, 195, 198, 212
　pediatric, 198
　in general, 4–5
　for low-grade gliomas, 282, 285t
　　favorable variants, 294–296
　　gender variables, 282
　　with observation only, 285t
　　pediatric pilocytic astrocytomas, 294
　　using surgery with/without radiotherapy, 288t
　　with surgical resection, 287t
　for low-grade oligodendrogliomas
　　using surgery with/without radiotherapy, 289t
　　with surgical resection, 286t
　metabolism-related, 132
　for metastases, 387–388

pediatric
   age-related, 327, 329
   high-grade astrocytoma, 329
   of radiosurgery patients
      median, 174–175
      for metastasis, 187t
   time trends, 2–4
   See also Familial syndromes; Risk factors
Swallowing dysfunction, pediatric, 305
SWS. *See* Sturge-Weber syndrome
Symptoms
   of low-grade gliomas, 282
   of meningiomas, 342–348
   of metastases, 376
   of neoplastic meningitis, 392–395
   of PCD, 410
   of pediatric tumors, 303
      cerebellar astrocytomas, 304, 307
      cranial nerve palsy, ataxia, long tract signs, 322
      diffusely infiltrating lesions, 322
      epilepsy/seizures, 307–308, 310–311
      relieved by surgery, 245–249
   of spinal tumors, 365–366
   of SSN-EMN, 407
   of toxicity in WBRT of metastases, 382–383
Syringomyelia mimicking spinal cord tumor, 367
Systemic chemotherapy of CNS tumors, 193–205
Systemic solid tumors, carcinomatous meningitis from, 393

Tamoxifen, in chemotherapy, 194, 204
Tectal tumors, pediatric, 312
Temozolomide
   in chemotherapy, 194–195, 197, 202
      clinical trials, 213
      oral delivery, 194
Temperature
   hyperthermia, use with brachytherapy, 157–158
   hypothermia during pediatric surgery, 303
Temporal field defect, optic chiasm, 316
   See also Neurologic deficit; Vision deficit
Temporal lobe tumors, 164
Teratomas
   MRI of, 123
   pediatric, 316
   spinal, 370
Terminal care, adult tumors, 276
Therapy. *See* Treatment and therapy
6-Thioguanine, 329
Thiotepa, in chemotherapy, 198
Thymidine kinase/ganciclovir approach in gene therapy, 228–229
Thymidine/carboplatin combination for malignant gliomas, 374
Thymoma and thymectomy, 417
Time trends for primary tumors, incidence and mortality, 2–4
Topoisomerase inhibitors, in chemotherapy, 203–204

Topotecan, in chemotherapy, 204
Total lumbar CSF exams for leptomeningeal metastases, 392–393t
Toxicity
   anticonvulsants, 205
   in chemotherapy
      agents, 194, 198, 327
      pediatric, 327
      PPN associated with, 415
   delayed reaction in radiotherapy, 148–149
   hypertonic mannitol solutions, 197–198
   National Cancer Institute criteria (CTC), 212
   neuro-oncology clinical trials, 213
   neurotoxicity
      in chemotherapy, 198–199
      in WBRT of metastases, 382–383
   ocular, in chemotherapy, 199
   radiation-induced, 291–292
   radiosurgery factors, 189
   radiotherapy factors, 148–149
   suicide genes, 228–229
   symptoms of, 205
   in WBRT of metastases, 382–383
Toxoplasmosis, as differential diagnosis of CNS metastatic disease, 135
Transcripts, encoding p16INK and p19ARF, 98
Transduction inhibitors in chemotherapy, 275–276
Transitional (mixed) meningioma, 339
Transverse myelitis mimicking spinal cord tumor, 366
Trauma, risk factor for meningiomas, 335
Trilateral retinoblastoma, 61–62
TS. *See* Tuberous Sclerosis
Tuberous Sclerosis (TS), 69–74
   clinical features, 70–71
   diagnostic criteria, 70t
   management, screening and surveillance, 74–75
   pediatric, 311
   radiographic features, 71
Tuberous Sclerosis complex, 70t
Tumors. *See* specific listings
Tumor-suppressor genes, 93, 100–102, 222t, 277
Turcot's syndrome, 75
   clinical features, 75–77
   genetics, 77
   management, 77
   type 1 *vs.* type 2, 75t

Ultrasound imaging, for pediatric cases, 304, 308, 310–312
Upper clival and sellar chordoma, 185f

Vaccination with cytokine-expressing tumor cells, 232
Valproic acid, in chemotherapy, 205
Vascular endothelial growth factor (VEGF), 102–103, 227–228, 228f, 229
Vascular malformations mimicking spinal cord tumor, 367–368
Vascular remodeling regulated by TGF-β, 103

Vascular tumors, 372–373
Vasogenic brain edema, ICP in metastases, 378
Vectors of gene therapy. *See* Gene therapy
VEGF or VEGFR. *See* Vascular endothelial growth factor
Venography, magnetic resonance (MRV) of meningiomas, 352–353
Ventricular system, 306–307, 311–312, 314, 316, 325, 394–396
Ventriculoperitoneal shunt, 314
Ventriculostomy, pediatric, 313–314
Verapamil, for uptake of chemotherapy agents, 197
VHL. *See* Von Hippel-Lindau syndrome, 64–69
Vincristine, in chemotherapy, 202, 323, 326, 329
Viruses
   Epstein-Barr associated with transverse myelitis, 366
   as gene therapy vectors
      adenoviruses, replication-competent, 230–231, 233
      delivery system approaches, 222t
      Herpes simplex virus, 228–229, 231
      reovirus (human), 232
   as risk factor, 12, 335
Vision deficit, 315–316, 412–413
Vitamins, risk factors, 10–12
Vomiting as symptom in children, 321
Von Hippel-Lindau syndrome, 66
Von Hippel-Lindau (VHL) syndrome, 64, 67–68
   clinical and molecular features, 60t, 64–65
   diagnostic criteria, 66
   genetics, 68
   lesions characteristic in, 65t
   management, screening and surveillance, 68–69
   radiosurgery plan, 183f
Von Recklinghausen's neurofibromatosis type 1, 48–54
   See also Neurofibromatosis

WBRT. *See* Whole brain radiotherapy
Weight loss as symptom in children, 321
WHO. *See* World Health Organization
Whole brain radiotherapy (WBRT)
   with/without radiosurgery, 188
Whole brain radiotherapy (WBRT) for metastases, 378–388
   postoperative, 385–386
   randomized trials, 380t
   recurrent metastases, 383–385
   symptomatic response, 379
Wiskott-Aldrich syndrome, MRI, 122
World Health Organization (WHO) grading, 16–17
   familial syndromes, 50
   low-grade gliomas, 279–280t
   malignant, 93, 262–265
   of the spine, 370t

Yolk sac tumor, 316